Hepatocellular CARCINOMA

WILEY SERIES ON DISEASES OF THE LIVER

Series Editor: Robert L. Peters, M.D.
University of Southern California School of Medicine
and the John Wesley Hospital
Los Angeles, California

Hepatocellular Carcinoma, edited by Kunio Okuda, M.D., and Robert L. Peters, M.D.

HEPATOCELLULAR CARCINOMA

Edited by

KUNIO OKUDA, M.D.

Professor of Medicine
Chiba University School of Medicine
Chiba, Japan

ROBERT L. PETERS, M.D.

Professor of Pathology
University of Southern California School of Medicine
and the John Wesley Hospital
Los Angeles, California

A WILEY MEDICAL PUBLICATION

JOHN WILEY & SONS, New York • London • Sydney • Toronto

Library of Congress Cataloging in Publication Data:
Hepatocellular carcinoma.

   (Wiley series on diseases of the liver) (A Wiley medical publication)
   Includes bibliographical references.
   1. Liver—Cancer.   I.   Okuda, Kunio, 1921-
II.   Peters, Robert Lee, 1927-
RC280.L5H45   616.9′94′36   76-6500
ISBN 0-471-65316-0

Printed in the United States of America

10 9 8 7 6 5 4 3 2 1

CONTRIBUTORS

ELLIOT ALPERT, M.D.
  Assistant in Medicine
  Massachusetts General Hospital
  Boston, Massachusetts
  Assistant Professor of Medicine
  Harvard Medical School
  Cambridge, Massachusetts

EIJI ARAKI, M.D.
  Associate Chairman of Clinical Biochemis-
  try
  National Cancer Institute
  Tsukiji, Cho-o-ku
  Tokyo, Japan

HECTOR A. BATTIFORA, M.D.
  Associate Professor of Pathology
  Northwestern University School of
  Medicine
  Chicago, Illinois

MALCOLM COCHRANE, M.D., M.B.,
M.R.C.P.
Senior registrar
Liver Unit
King College Hospital Medical School
Denmark Hill
London, England

HUGH A. EDMONDSON, M.D.
  Professor of Pathology
  University of Southern California
  Los Angeles, California

EMMANUEL FARBER, M.D., PH.D.
  Professor and Chairman, Department of
  Pathology
  University of Toronto
  Toronto, Ontario, Canada

KAMAL ISHAK, M.D., PH.D.
  Hepatic and Pediatric Branch
  Armed Forces Institute of Pathology
  Washington, D.C.

F. LEONARD JOHNSON, M.D., M.B.B.S.
  Assistant Professor of Pediatrics
  Department of Hematology and Oncology
  Childrens Hospital
  and University of Washington
  Seattle, Washington

YASUHIKO KUBO, M.D.
  Assistant Professor of Medicine
  Second Department of Medicine
  Kurume University School of Medicine
  Kurume, Japan

BENJAMIN LANDING, M.D.
  Chief Pathologist
  Childrens Hospital of Los Angeles and
  Professor of Pathology, University of
  Southern California
  Los Angeles, California

TIEN-YU LIN, M.D.
  Professor of Surgery
  National Taiwan University Hospital
  Taipei, Taiwan
  Republic of China

WATARU MORI, M.D.
  Professor of Pathology
  Tokyo University School of Medicine
  Bunkyo-ku
  Tokyo, Japan

KOU NAGASAKO, M.D.
  Department of Pathology
  Tokyo University School of Medicine
  Bunkyo-ku
  Tokyo, Japan

TOSHIRO NAKASHIMA, M.D.
  Professor of Pathology
  Kurume University School of Medicine
  Kurume, Japan

AKIRA OHBAYASHI, M.D.
  Associate Professor of Internal Medicine
  First Department of Medicine
  Osaka Medical College
  Daigaku-cho
  Takatsuki City, Osaka, Japan

NOBUO OKAZAKI, M.D.
  Department of Internal Medicine
  National Cancer Institute
  Tsukiji, Chu-o-ku
  Tokyo, Japan

YASUYUKI OHTA, M.D.
  Associate Professor of Medicine
  First Department of Medicine
  Okayam University School of Medicine
  Bunkyo-ku
  Tokyo, Japan

KUNIO OKUDA, M.D.
  Professor of Medicine
  First Department of Medicine
  Chiba University School of Medicine
  Chiba, Japan

ROBERT L. PETERS, M.D.
  Professor of Pathology
  University of Southern California and
  Chief of Pathology Services
  John Wesley Hospital
  Los Angeles, California

TELFER REYNOLDS, M.D.
  Professor of Medicine
  University of Southern California
  Los Angeles, California

TOSHIO SHIKATA, M.D.
  Associate Professor of Pathology
  Tokyo University School of Medicine
  Okayama, Japan

YUTAKA SHIMOKAWA, M.D.
  Associate Professor of Medicine
  Second Department of Medicine
  Kurume University School of Medicine
  Kurume, Japan

ROGER WILLIAMS, M.D., F.R.C.P.
  Consultant Physician and Director
  Liver Unit
  King College Hospital Medical School
  Denmark Hill
  London, England

G. N. WOGAN, Ph.D.
  Professor of Toxicology
  Department of Nutrition and Food Science
  Massachusetts Institute of Technology
  Cambridge, Massachusetts

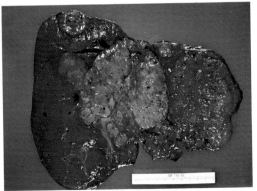

FIGURE 1 Gross photographs of megalonodular carcinoma arising in noncirrhotic liver.

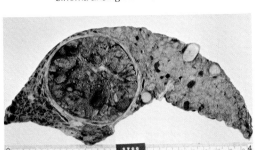

FIGURE 2 Encapsulated expanding hepatocellular carcinoma arising in cirrhotic liver. Note the multinodulated cirrhotomimetic character of the tumor.

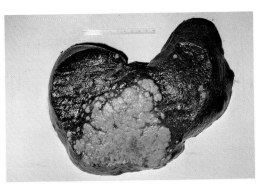

FIGURE 3 Hepatocellular carcinoma arising in deeply pigmented liver of child with familial cholestatic disease.

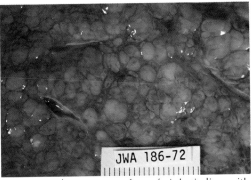

FIGURE 4 Close up cut surface of cirrhotic liver with multiple white foci of carcinoma arising within the cirrhotic nodules.

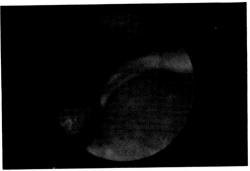

FIGURE 5 Peritoneoscopic view of bulging carcinoma arising in noncirrhotic liver near the falciform ligament before chemotherapy.

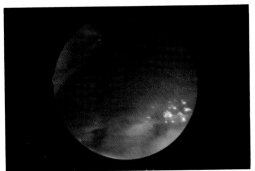

FIGURE 6 Liver from same patient as in Fig. 5 showing depressed area near the falciform ligament after chemotherapy.

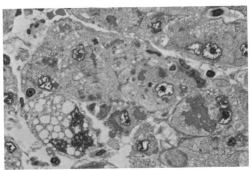

FIGURE 7 Well-differentiated liver cell carcinoma with alcoholic hyalin. The tumor arose in an alcoholic cirrhotic liver.

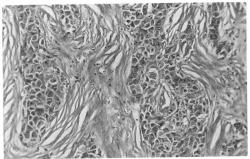

FIGURE 8 Eosinophilic hepatocellular carcinoma with lamellar fibrosis, an unusual histologic variant.

PREFACE

Liver cell carcinoma has long intrigued the pathologist and the epidemiologist alike in its relation to hepatic cirrhosis. The baffling question of the immensely differing racial and geographic incidence is beginning to unravel, thanks to the disclosure of the possible underlying factors such as mycotoxins and hepatitis B antigen. With sensitive methods now available for detecting alpha fetoprotein, a specific carcino-fetal antigen, the clinical study of primary hepatocellular carcinoma has entered a new era. Aided by the more sophisticated radiological techniques such as hepatic angiography and scanning, detection of minute, if not early, carcinoma is no longer an incidental discovery of laparoscopy. Reports on successful resection of small liver cell carcinomas are rapidly increasing.

The expression of "hepatoma" and "cholangioma," the preferred terms for years, was coined by Yamagiwa of Japan in 1911, who pioneered in the experimental production of carcinoma with coal tar seven years later. It was no surprise that announcement of the first experimental hepatic cancer came from Japan (Yoshida, 1932). The incidence of hepatocellular carcinoma in the United States has in the past been much lower compared with Southeast Asia. However, recent evidence has suggested strongly that it may be steadily and rapidly increasing among Caucasians. Many things that have become part of the modern life of Americans, such as more widespread ethanol consumption, blood transfusions, use of many drugs, poorly biodegradable pollutants of air, ground, and foods, could be linked to the rising incidence of hepatocellular carcinoma. The possible long latent period is brought out by the recognition that some of the Chinese immigrants to the United States who develop hepatocellular carcinoma as much as 30 years later, carry a subtype of the hepatitis B antigen seen almost exclusively in the Orient. Many important questions urgently need to be solved.

KUNIO OKUDA, M.D.
ROBERT L. PETERS, M.D.

January 1976
Chiba, Japan
Los Angeles, California

CONTENTS

Hepatocellular CARCINOMA

Part One PATHOGENESIS

CHAPTER 1 ON THE PATHOGENESIS OF EXPERIMENTAL HEPATOCELLULAR CARCINOMA

EMMANUEL FARBER, M.D., Ph.D.

The study of chronic diseases such as cancer and atherosclerosis, in the human, is subject to all the major difficulties, including false leads, irrelevant coincidences, and complex interactions associated with dynamic man living in a complicated environment and society. Although some clues to the etiology and pathogenesis of cancer have been obtained from the study of man, as evident from the discussion of hepatocellular caccinoma in this book, recourse to the experimental animal is increasing as we appreciate more and more the need for scientific analysis of disease processes. The experimental animal offers opportunities to manipulate and dissect the process in a fashion not possible in man, in order to formulate working hypotheses as well as to discover possible etiologic agents.

The author's research work included in this review was supported in part by research grants from the American Cancer Society and from the National Institutes of Health (CA-12218, CA-12227, and AM/14882) and by a contract with the National Cancer Institute (NO1-CP-33262).

Progress in our understanding of carcinogenesis has been considerable since the discovery of a model for liver cancer by Sasaki and Yoshida in 1935 (1). Among the areas of greatest development are the identification of an increasing number of hepatocarcinogens (a few of which may have importance in cancer in man), the establishment of carcinogen metabolic activation as an obligatory step in carcinogenesis, and the realization that the development of liver cancer, like that of cancer in many other organs or tissues, is not a single step but a multistep phenomenom in which we probably are seeing an example of cellular evolution from initiated preneoplastic hepatocytes to highly malignant hepatocellular carcinoma (HCC) (2). The major emphasis in this presentation is on the attempt to synthesize some ideas concerning the pathogenesis of HCC in the experimental animal. However, included also is a brief discussion of possible etiologic agents with emphasis on chemicals. The presentation is limited to hepatocellular carcinoma.

POSSIBLE HEPATOCARCINOGENS

There is general agreement today that no discussion of cancer is meaningful except in the context of an individual with a certain genetic background being influenced in a major way by the environment. In view of the extreme heterogeneity of the genetic potential of each human and the difficulty today in making any kind of systematic genetic analysis at the cellular level, it is natural that the major focus in looking for leads to the etiology of liver cancer should be the environment (3–9). Given the observations that (a) known carcinogens for man, with one possible exception—arsenic, are also carcinogenic for experimental animals (10), (b) HCC in animals resembles human HCC in its morphologic and biological characteristics, including such valuable and reasonably selective properties as the production of alpha fetoprotein (AFP) (11), and (c) the geographic distribution pattern of HCC in man shows as much dependence on the environment as does any cancer, it is only natural that the study of etiology and pathogenesis of HCC in animals should assume major importance in the concerted study of human HCC.

The liver in experimental animals is susceptible to the carcinogenic effects of a wide variety of chemicals, both man-made and naturally occurring (e.g., 12) of ionizing radiation (13) and at least one virus (14, 15). A list of some representative hepatic chemical carcinogens is given in Table 1. The number of man-made chemicals increases progressively with time, as dramatically witnessed by the very recent discovery of vinyl chloride as an hepatocarcinogen that induces angiosarcoma of the liver in man. In this category are the nitrosamines and nitrosamides, which are receiving increasing attention as potential carcinogens for man (10, 16–18). These are among the most versatile carcinogens for a wide variety of neoplasms in many different experimental animals. As a general group they are widespread by virtue of their ability to be easily

generated from nitrite and secondary amines. These compounds are quite easily formed not only in the environment but also in the gastrointestinal tract (17, 19). Nitrites (and nitrates) are common food additives, especially for packaged meat and meat products (20). Also, they occur in significant amount in saliva. Secondary amines are ubiquitous in nature, occurring in plants, animals, and microorganisms. The simultaneous addition of nitrite and any one of many different secondary amines, including some that are used as drugs, can lead to acute liver cell damage and liver cancer in experimental animals. Although no clear-cut evidence has been presented for any nitrosamine or nitrosamide being carcinogenic in man, the observation that the human liver can readily metabolize dimethylnitrosamine to active derivatives that can interact with cellular macromolecules including nucleic acids (21) offers presumptive support. The correlation between metabolism of nitrosamines and carcinogenicity is impressive (16).

The compounds currently considered to be the most important in relation to human liver cancer are the mycotoxins, especially the aflatoxins. These are considered in detail in Chapter 2.

Metabolic Activation of Carcinogens

Most hepatocarcinogens (e.g., almost all listed in Table 1) do not appear to be carcinogens per se, but are metabolically converted to highly reactive derivatives ("ultimate carcinogens") (22). So far, all such reactive compounds have been found to be positively charged "electrophilic reactants" or free radicals that can react with the many nucleophilic groups found in the macromolecules (DNA, RNA, protein) and small molecular weight compounds in many different cell organelles of the target cells.

Although it is becoming increasingly evident that many different cell types and perhaps all cells possess activating enzymes

Table 1   Representative Hepatocarcinogens in Experimental Animals

Naturally Occurring	*Aromatic Amines*
Aflatoxins[a]	p-Dimethylaminoazobenzene
Sterigmatocystin[a]	(butter yellow) and derivatives
Pyrrolizidine alkaloids	o-Aminoazotoluene
Cycasin and its aglycone,[a]	2-Acetylaminofluorene
methylazoxymethanol[a]	and derivatives
Safrole, isosafrole, dehydrosafrole[a]	m-Toluenediamine
Griseofulvin	2-Anthramine
Luteoskyrin	
Tannic acids	*Chlorinated Hydrocarbons*[a]
Thiourea	Carbon tetrachloride
	Chloroform
Nitrosamines and Nitrosamides[a]	*Miscellaneous*
Dimethylnitrosamine	Ethionine
Diethylnitrosamine	Aramite
N-Nitrosomorpholine	Thiocetamide
N-Nitrosopiperidine	Acetamide
N-Nitrosodihydrohydrouracil	Hycanthone
	Urethan
	7, 12-Dimethylbenzanthracene
	3-Hydroxyxanthine
	Dieldrin, aldrein
	Polychlorophenols

[a] Possibly of importance in human cancer.

for some carcinogens, the liver is particularly active in this respect (23). The liver appears to have the greatest concentrations and the widest versatility in its content of such enzymes. The detailed enzymologic analysis of the carcinogen-activating systems is only now beginning to be explored. To date, the majority have been located in the "microsomal fraction" of the liver, a fraction that consists predominantly of endoplasmic reticulum (ER) (smooth and rough), ribosomes, and probably other cell membranes. Where studied, they have been found to fall into the general group of enzymes called "mixed function oxidases" in which TPNH (NADPH) and TPNH reductase, cytochrome P450, and oxygen are three of the known reactants. The elucidation of the components, mechanisms of action, and controls are of great importance to our understanding of HCC, since modulations of the system can lead to inhibition or acceleration of the carcinogenic process (24, 25) Variations in dietary composition, drugs, and toxic agents including other carcinogens and hormones among other things can induce wide modulations in the activation process. Some of these modulations can prevent completely cancer induction by some potent hepatocarcinogens by interfering with the activation process (see 24, 26).

The procarcinogen *activation* process is closely connected functionally with the *inactivation* process that leads to the production of more soluble, less active derivatives. The latter, frequently hydroxyl derivatives in the case of aromatic compounds, are often excreted in the urine as conjugates with glucuronic acid, sulfate, or others. Even though the whole area of enzyme activation is still poorly understood mechanistically, it is already evident that at least two overall metabolic patterns can be discerned.

Pattern A, as exemplified by 2-acetylaminofluorene and other aromatic amines, consists of alternate pathways —one leading to activation and one to inactivation; for example,

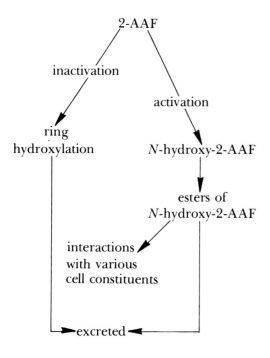

With carcinogens that are metabolized by this pattern, each of the pathways, the activation and the inactivation, may be modulated to different degrees. Presumably the inhibition of liver carcinogenesis by 3-methylcholanthrene or phenobarbitol operates through such a more or less selective effect. It is emphasized that where studied, the level of activation is only a very small fraction of that of inactivation. Perhaps, no more than 0.5 or 1% of the metabolized carcinogen follows the activation pathway.

In *Pattern B,* as exemplified by at least some polycyclic aromatic hydrocarbons (PHA) and possibly some nitrosamines such as dimethylnitrosamine, the activation and inactivation pathways are sequential, the inactivation process being reactions that follow the activation; for example,

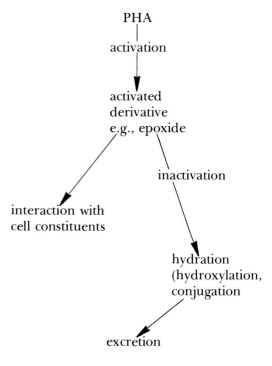

With Pattern B, the selective inhibition of activation is probably more difficult except by preventing any metabolism of the parent compound. The inhibition of the activation reaction(s) may be associated with a similar effect on the inactivation. The latter naturally might lead to an increase in the effective concentration of the activated derivative and thus could enhance carcinogenesis.

It is obvious that the activation and inactivation process for many carcinogens must be clarified to a considerable degree before any rational and highly predictable preventive measures can be entertained. Nevertheless, the possibility of eventually developing effective preventive therapy based on these principles is an exciting prospect for the future.

INTERACTIONS WITH TARGET CELLS

As anticipated from the chemical nature of the ultimate carcinogens, where known, carcinogens as activated electrophiles undergo a variety of reactions with components in nucleic acids, proteins, and probably many other cellular constituents (22). With proteins, they react with methionine, tyrosine, tryphtophan, and SH groups. With nucleic acids (both DNA and RNA), a variety of products are produced depending on the carcinogen. These include substitutions at N-7, C-8, O-6, and N-3 of guanine, N-1 and N-3 of adenine, and N-1 of cytosine (27–29).

The liver reacts rapidly to chemical carcinogens by the development of damage to DNA, as measured by a decrease in the size distribution of DNA on sedimentation in alkaline ("single strand breaks") and sometimes in neutral ("double strand breaks") sucrose gradients (30). This response is probably due to the chemical interaction between the ultimate form of the carcinogen and liver DNA. The damage-repair systems *in vivo* with many hepatic carcinogens seem to follow one of at least two patterns—single strand damage only with slow repair or double strand damage with rapid or slow repair (2,30). The majority of hepatocarinogens tested, as exemplefied by DMN, DEN (diethylnitrosamine), or 2-AAF, induce single strand breaks in DNA within 4 to 24 hours, followed by slow repair over the next 2 weeks or longer. This is in contrast to several other nonhepatic carcinogens that induce single strand damage with rapid repair (30). A few very active hepatocarcinogens, such as nitrosomorpholine (31). N-hydroxy-2-AAF or N-acetoxy-2-AAF (32), nitrosodihydrouracil (33), or 3-hydroxy xanthine (34), induce double strand breaks in DNA with repair within a few hours or a few days.

The mechanisms of repair of damaged DNA in liver *in vivo* remain unknown, although intensive research is going on in our laboratory (30, 35) and in a few other laboratories interested in chemical carcinogenesis. The possible importance of damage to other molecules, such as protein or RNA in facilitating or exaggerating the damage by, for example, inhibiting repair enzymes must be seriously entertained.

Carcinogens also induce a variety of functional and structural disturbances in virtually every cell organelle in the liver. Mitochondria, ER, ribosomes, nuclei, and nucleoli show reproducible ultrastructural changes as well as associated changes in RNA and DNA synthesis and metabolism, in protein synthesis, and in the oxidative generation of energy (see 23, 36–39). These various toxic effects are probably reflections of the interaction of the ultimate carcinogen with the proteins, RNA, and DNA characteristic of the various cell organelles.

Included among these effects are an interference with cell proliferation or mitosis and/or DNA synthesis in response to partial hepatectomy (see 40,41). A similar inhibition of regenerative response was found recently in our laboratory in animals pretreated with carcinogenic regimens such as feeding diets containing 2-AAF and then observing the response to a single necrogenic dose of CCl_4 or of dimethylnitrosamine. A regenerative response under such conditions is singularly lacking as the hepatocytes remain unresponsive. In contrast to the original hepatocytes, which we call en masse hepatocyte population I (hep. pop. I), ductular epithelial cells show proliferation in response to virtually every carcinogen (see 40, 42). This morphologic and functional response resembles that seen in cholangitis, cholestasis, and biliary obstruction. The functional stimulus for this ductular reaction and its physiologic or pathologic significance is still obscure. Conceivably, an appropriate stimulus could be generated by some metabolic disturbance in bile acid metabolism, since lithocholic acid is very active in inducing ductular cell proliferation in several animal species when incorporated in the diet (43, 44).

OTHER POSSIBLE ETIOLOGIC AGENTS

A variety of etiologic agents for human HCC, other than chemicals, have been suggested at various times during the course of research (see 3, 4, 6–10). These include poor nutrition (e.g., protein deficiency), parasitic infections, viruses and viral hepatitis, and irradiation. The evidence for disturbances in nutrition playing a major role in either experimental or human cancer has not been convincing (see 6–10, 22), although it was in vogue for several years in the 1940s and 1950s. However, one clear-cut effect of feeding protein-deficient diets has been reported (44)—the decrease in incidence of HCC with DMN with the concomitant increase in kidney cancer. This finding has been related to the dietary effect on the liver in decreasing metabolism of DMN and thereby making more DMN available for action in the kidney. Also, with butter yellow (4-dimethylaminoazobenzene) and some of its derivatives, the riboflavin concentration in the diet as well as other dietary components can have major effects on the induction of liver cancer. The site of action seems to be predominately, if not exclusively destruction of the carcinogen. One of the key enzymes that can destroy such azodyes contains riboflavin as an essential component of its coenzyme or prosthetic group (see 22).

With regard to parasites, no definite effects have been observed on the induction of hepatocellular carcinoma, but only on cholangiocellular carcinoma (46). The relationship of hepatitis and hepatitis B virus (HBV) is discussed in Chapter. Various forms of ionizing radiation can induce liver cancer in animals, especially when followed by treatment with CCl_4 (47, 48). Hepatocellular carcinoma as well as liver adenocarcinoma and sarcoma were found in hamsters inoculated intraperitoneally, subcutaneously, or intracerebrally as newborns with an avian adenovirus, chicken-embryo-lethal-orphan (CELO) virus, which is a DNA-containing virus (14, 15).

SOME OTHER VARIABLES IN THE INDUCTION OF HCC

The standard regimen for the induction of HCC in animals is to feed the carcinogen in stock or appropriate semipurified diets for periods of from 8 to 10 weeks. With many of the most active carcinogens this is sufficient to insure incidences of HCC from 80 to 100%. With shorter periods of feeding the incidence becomes correspondingly less.

A single exposure to a carcinogen in the intact adult animal is associated only rarely with the induction of liver cancer. However, with some carcinogens such as dimethylnitrosamine, diethylnitrosamine, urethan, or 7, 12-dimethylbenzanthracene, one dose induces a significant incidence of HCC if given during liver regeneration after partial hepatectomy (49–55). With urethan or 7,12-dimethylbenzanthracene, little or no incidence of HCC is seen in adult intact control rats, even with prolonged exposure. In addition, a weak or noncarcinogenic 2-methyl-4-dimenthylaminoazobenzene has been reported to be carcinogenic if the exposed animals are subjected to partial hepatectomy during the feeding regimen (56). Single exposure of pregnant rats to one of several carcinogens may result in development of HCC in the offspring (57,58). In addition, HCC can be induced with several compounds with a single exposure in newborn rats (59–61).

Thus, even a single administration to the partially hepatectomized adult, to the neonate, or transplacentally to the fetus, can set in motion a process that can eventuate in liver cancer. This occurs not only with water insoluble long-acting carcinogens such as the polycyclic aromatic hydrocarbons or some aromatic amines but also with short-acting water soluble compounds such as nitrosamines or urethan. These data indicate an essential similarity in at least some respects between carcinogenesis in liver and in skin and other organs.

It is evident that the hormonal status of the animal can play a critical role as a major variable in liver carcinogenesis (23, 62, 63). Hormones from the anterior pituitary, adrenal cortex, and thyroid as well as both male and female sex hormones influence to a striking degree the carcinogenic process in the liver. These have been reviewed recently (23).

Properties of the Neoplastic Hepatocyte

Many morphologic, biological, and biochemical differences between normal and neoplastic liver have been described (see 64–66). Many of the differences are not general but rather characteristic of one or a few neoplasms. However, in addition to invasion, metastasis, and cytologic (especially nuclear) aberrations, three general properties stand out as being the most reproducible in principle, and perhaps the most significant from a pathogenetic point of view. These all relate to alterations in gene expression and include *(a)* altered patterns of isozymes, *(b)* unusual production of hormones, and *(c)* excess production of fetal proteins (11, 67). All appear to fall under the general heading of *apparently inappropriate expression of genetic information.* This field has been reviewed extensively (see 2, 68–70) and therefore needs only passing reference. Isozymes of several glygolytic and other enzymes often appear

in neoplastic liver, especially in the more undifferentiated varieties. Insulinlike and erythopoitinlike substances have been found to be produced by some patients with hepatocellular carcinoma (see 25). Among the fetal proteins, alpha fetoprotein (AFP) stands out because of its obvious and great value as a diagnostic aid in liver cancer. This is covered in detail in Chapter 15. From the pathogenetic viewpoint, the most interesting aspect of AFP is its production by the liver *very early during liver carcinogenesis* and *long before there is any indication of HCC* (71–77). With one carcinogen, 2-AAF, the earliest new cell population, the hyperplastic nodule, stains positively for AFP by immunofluorescence at a time when the surrounding liver is essentially negative (78). The possible significance of this in the pathogenesis of HCC is discussed later.

ON THE PATHOGENESIS OF HEPATOCELLULAR CARCINOMA

The Initiation Process

Biologically, the process of initiation appears to consist of the induction of a population of new hepatocytes, population II,

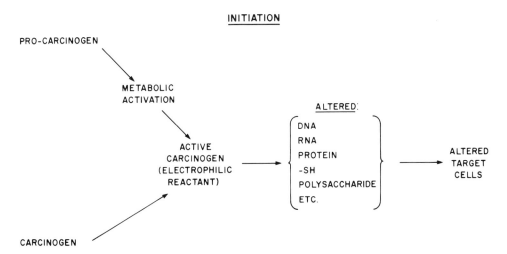

Figure 1 Diagrammatic representation of some of the steps thought to be active in the initiation of carcinogenesis by chemical carcinogens.

which differ in several respects from the original hepatocyte population (population I). First, it is more resistant to the cytotoxic environment created by the carcinogenic process. This allows it to respond to the carcinogen-induced liver damage by proliferation. Second, it contains an antigen (PN antigen) so far not found in normal liver (79, 80, 81, 82). Third, it proliferates in patterns resembling more fetal and neonatal liver than mature adult liver.

Biochemically, the process of initiation is most easily viewed as a more or less permanent change in its information content or its information retrieval system (Fig. 1-1). Today, the only clear-cut cellular information reservoir is DNA and perhaps some RNA in association with reverse transcriptase. Since DNA is a common target macromolecule for most carcinogens, it is natural that this should be the macromolecule most favored as being involved in initiation. The relatively long eclipse period between the termination of the life of many carcinogen molecules and the appearance of suspected preneoplastic or premalignant lesions strengthens the basis for the selection of DNA (2, 79).

The damage to DNA may be subject to repair (30, 35). However, if cell proliferation takes place near the time of damage, transitory or reparable damage of DNA may be converted to permanent damage by virtue of the replication of the DNA before adequate repair of the damage has occurred (35). Thus, the roles of partial hepatectomy and liver regeneration, fetal liver, or neonatal liver in allowing complete carcinogenesis with a single dose of one of several carcinogens are most easily interpreted as primarily due to their effects on DNA. However, it should be pointed out that fetal and neonatal liver have at least one other characteristic that may favor carcinogenesis—a primitive architectural pattern of liver cells (see below).

It must be emphasized that the focus on DNA is simply the most plausible hypothesis as of today. If and when other macromolecules, e.g., RNA, protein, surface membrane components, etc., are implicated in information receipt, storage, and/or retrieval, new rational and testable hypotheses should become available for analysis. Also, even if DNA is proven to be a major target, it is very probable that damage to other macromolecules such as proteins or RNAs may play important roles in facilitating or exaggerating the damage to DNA (e.g., by interfering with repair enzymes, etc.).

Although the biochemical and biological damage induced by carcinogens appears to involve the whole liver, only relatively few initiated cells seem to take part in the carcinogenic process. This is most easily explained in the following terms. Only very few combinations of sites of molecular and/or organelle damage allow the expression of the various properties involved in the beginning of the cellular evolution to neoplasia. In the case of DNA, since so much of the DNA at any moment in time and especially in the developed organism is not actively used, there must exist large "silent" regions. Since the induction of the "right" combination is probably a highly improbable event, large numbers of cells undergoing DNA replication must be the targets to allow an adequate number of initiated cells to occur. The replication of total DNA in the majority of cells remaining during liver regeneration following two-thirds hepatectomy or in the many cells undergoing cell proliferation during fetal and neonatal life would allow such an improbable event to occur over a short period of exposure to the carcinogen.

Neoplastic Development

Given the induction of the "right kind" of new altered or mutantlike cells, how can this population be selectively encouraged to proliferate? As already pointed out, carcinogens including hepatocarcinogens have long been known to be cytotoxic to normal cells (83, 84) and to inhibit cell proliferation and DNA synthesis in regenerating liver (85–87). The cytotoxicity stimulates a demand for regenerative cell proliferation. However, the original hepatocyte population (I), by virtue of the inhibitory effects of the carcinogen, cannot respond. In contrast, hepatocyte population II, the population of initiated cells, having acquired properties that now enable them to escape the susceptibility to the cytotoxicity, can respond to the proliferative stimulus. Thus the general toxic effect of the carcinogen creates an environment favoring the selective growth of the new focal population already induced by the carcinogen.

The nature of this resistance to the cytotoxic action of a carcinogen is unknown. The simplest hypothesis would state that, given the need for metabolic activation of most hepatocarcinogens prior to their becoming reactive chemically, the new cell population could acquire the resistance by failing to activate the procarcinogen. Thus, one of the properties that might go to make up the "right kind" of new cells could be such a loss. Since neoplastic cells in general and many hepatomas have low or no capacity for carcinogen activation, this suggestion seems reasonable. However, there has not yet been an adequate testing of this idea in the appropriate preneoplastic or premalignant cell population.

One of the striking characteristics of the presumptive preneoplastic or premalignant cell population, II, is that it remains focal and does not appear to integrate rapidly with the surrounding liver. This is in contrast to many examples of cell proliferation following acute toxic or viral hepatocyte damage where the regenerating cells become an integral part of the normal structure of the liver. Another striking feature is the apparent regression of nodules when the carcinogen is removed. If the initial proliferative response early in carcinogenesis is similar to that seen following partial hepatectomy or liver cell necrosis, why would the regenerating hepatocytes in population II disappear while "normal" regenerating liver obviously persist?

Considerable clarification of this puzzling phenomenon has come recently from careful studies of the early nodules in our laboratory. The nodules (population II, "hyperplastic liver nodules") do not regress, as we and others previously believed (42, 88, 89). They undergo remodeling or differentiation to mature liver. Unlike the original liver cell population in the adult, the first nodule population has its hepatocytes organized in two- or often more than two-cell-thick plates and in various other patterns such as tubules. This has, of course, been described before in so-called hyperplastic nodules in human cirrhosis (e.g., 90). This architectural pattern, which resembles the liver during embryologic development, persists for as long as the carcinogen is administered. On discontinuing the exposure to the carcinogen, the early nodule population (II) does not regress but undergoes remodeling and further differentiation to one-cell thick plates and to an architecture closely resembling normal adult liver (90). Grossly, the nodule is first grayish white in color and remains so as long as the carcinogen is fed. On removing the carcinogen, the nodules grossly acquire the color of normal adult liver. During this transition, as expected, nodules with a mottled grayish-white and brown appearance become common. When fully remodeled ("regressed") the nodule integrates almost imperceptibly into the structure of the surrounding liver. No evidence of cell necrosis, inflammation, or a rejection phenomenon is seen during this remodeling process. Careful histologic study shows many sites where the two-cell or more thick plates merge without transition with virtually normal-looking one-cell-thick plates. Also, the cells in the nodule, while unremodeled, are considerably larger than normal hepatocytes and many have a ground glass appearance or show abundant pale-staining cytoplasm often full of glycogen. The nuclei are almost uniformly

CARCINOGENESIS (PROMOTION)

DEVELOPMENT OR EVOLUTION

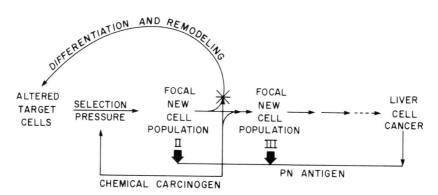

FIGURE 2 Diagrammatic representation of a working hypothesis of some steps in the development or evolution of liver cells from altered cells initiated by chemical carcinogenesis.

enlarged to about 1.5 to 2 times the diameter of liver nuclei, have a much looser open chromatin staining pattern than normal nuclei, and have one or two large nucleoli. During remodeling and differentiation, the nuclei and the cytoplasm assume an appearance essentially the same as normal adult hepatocytes, with one possible exception—the nucleoli often remain large.

Thus the carcinogen early during the development of liver cancer has at least three effects—the induction of a new cell population, which appears as multiple scattered foci, the creation of an appropriate selection pressure, and the interruption of differentiation or remodeling (see Fig. 2).

If the exposure to the carcinogen continues for a sufficiently long period of time (6 to 10 weeks) to assure a high incidence of cancer or if the exposure to some carcinogens occurs as a single pulse during liver regeneration after partial hepatectomy, a new hepatocyte population (III) appears which no longer becomes remodeled or does so only very slowly. Morphologically, this nodule population resembles closely the early nodule population (II) in that the hepatocytes are also ar-

ranged in two- or more cell-thick plates and show tubularization (see 90). In addition, they show many of the same biochemical properties as do the hepatocytes in population II, such as interference with glycogen breakdown, loss of iron accumulation, and low glucose-6-phosphatase and ATPase activities (see 40, 92 for references). Thus, a new population with a more permanent interruption in differentiation develops and remains as a presumptive precursor for the subsequent steps leading to liver cancer (40, 79, 80). This population seems to have acquired on a more permanent basis many of the same properties seen in the earlier focal population and thus is more independent of the environment. Exposure to carcinogen is no longer necessary. With the single exposure to carcinogen during liver regeneration, it seems as if the more adaptable differentiatable early population (II) is eliminated and only the more independent less differentiatable focal population III is seen. Judging by the differences between the findings on prolonged versus single exposure, it looks almost as if the relatively prolonged exposure to the carcinogen under the usual feeding regimen must either induce a more plastic population as a possible precursor for population III or induces both II and III independently.

As one examines livers at times after the appearance of population III, one can observe nodules with features not seen earlier. For example, not infrequently, discrete nodules often within nodules of population III are made up of much smaller cells with greater nuclear/cytoplasmic ratios and basophilic, not eonsinophilic, cytoplasm. Some of these may have quite pleomorphic nuclei and have some of the morphologic earmarks of malignancy (40, 92). The number of different populations occurring between population III and cancer is unknown. This remains a very important but difficult area for study. Preliminary comparisons between hepatocellular carcinomas and the early and later nodules point to simlarities in the architectural arrangements of the hepatocytes. Although the organization of malignant neoplastic liver cells shows quite a variability from section to section and from tumor to tumor, there is little doubt that these hepatocytes as a rule are arranged in two- or more cell-thick plates. They clearly resemble the patterns seen in fetal and nodule cell populations. Thus, even early in carcinogenesis, the putative precursor hepatocyte for the ultimate malignant liver cell is already arranged in a pattern that mimics, at least superficially, the fetal and neonatal liver.

It is noteworthy that Smetana (93) in careful studies of cirrhosis induced by dietary means in the primate suggested that some nodules may show a disturbance in complete maturation of the liver cell architecture, similar to that seen in the rat during carcinogenesis and in human cirrhosis (90). He also found that some nodules underwent maturation.

Some Important and Critical Considerations

No doubt, the most important single question concerns the relationship between these different cell populations and liver cancer. Perhaps they are not really related at all and have no pathogenetic significance in the development of liver cancer. Although the hyperplastic nodule has long been considered to be preneoplastic or premalignant in human and experimental cirrhosis (see 40), the basis for this judgment has been largely intuitive. To date the evidence in support of the hypothesis that hyperplastic nodules (population II, III, etc.) are components in a linear sequence of cellular evolution is as follows. (a) Virtually every hepatic carcinogen induces many changes in common including focal and nodular hyperplastic lesions and perhaps even earlier precursors, islands of altered enzyme histochemistry (see 40, 94). (b) Other compounds, often just as toxic, such as alpha-naphthylisothiocyanate, even though they induce many functional and structural changes in the liver cells and ductular cells, do not give rise to hyperplastic nodules in the rat and do not induce liver cancer in this species. (c) There is a large body of observational experience in human disease, correlating nodular hyperplasia and liver cancer (5–8, 95). (d) With one carcinogen, 2-acetylaminofluorene (2-AAF), a bound form of the carcinogen is found in the glycogen in hyperplastic nodules and in liver cancer but is apparently not present in liver surrounding nodules or cancer (96). (e) Areas of hyperbasophilia, along with histological and cytological atypia, indistinguishable from unequivocal hepatocellular carcinoma, can be seen arising in the interior of nodules, in the absence of any identifiable cancer elsewhere in the liver (40, 42, 92).

Although interesting and provocative, such evidence is largely probabilistic. Missing in our armamentarium for the study of histogenesis and pathogenesis of liver cancer are *positive markers* that tie various suggested precursors and product together mechanically. Naturally, until absolute markers (if such exist) for different types of cancer are discovered and until the essential relationship of such markers to the biological behavior of any one type of neop-

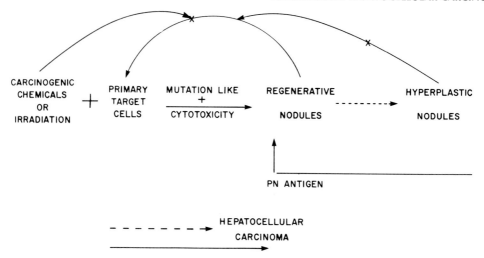

FIGURE 3   Some probable steps involved in the development of HCC induced by chemical carcinogens.

lasm is clarified, we must of necessity continue to explore on a less than firm foundation.

Alpha fetoprotein was thought to be one such marker. Recent studies on AFP during carcinogenesis have shown that this positive marker for hepatocellular carcinoma often appears very early during carcinogenesis (71–78). We have found it to be localized by immunofluoresence in hyperplastic nodules (population II and III) during carcinogenesis (78). Unfortunately, this marker is a product of normal adult liver as well as fetal liver and is increased in many situations associated with liver cell proliferation (11, 97). (See Chapter 15.) Also, it is not reliable as even a quantitative marker, since it is variable from nodule to nodule, from cancer to cancer, and from animal to animal (e.g., 78, 98).

A new positive marker for hepatocytes in preneoplastic or premalignant and primary liver cell cancer has recently been discovered (81, 82). This antigen, called PN (preneoplastic) antigen, is present in every hyperplastic nodule from the very earliest seen and in every primary hepatocellular carcinoma induced in one of three different strains of rats by one of five different carcinogens [2-AAF, ethionine, DMN,

DEN, 3'-methyl-4-dimethylaminoazobenzene (3'-MeDAB)]. It has not been found so far in any normal tissue or fluid, including adult liver, intact or regenerating, serum, fetal liver or amniotic fluid or in carcinomas of the kidney or earduct or in leukemia (81). It has been localized by immunofluorescence to every hepatocyte in nodules and liver cancer.

Most interestingly, the PN antigen seems to be closely tied to the state of differentiation or remodeling of population II. When unremodeled or with apparent arrest in differentiation, as seen during carcinogen administration, the nodules are positive for PN antigen. However, as they become remodeled, the more mature liver cells are negative. When fully remodeled, the original nodule becomes negative. Later nodules (population III) and HCC remain positive for PN antigen after removal of the carcinogen (Fig. 3).

Transplanted hepatomas are variable in their content of PN antigen. Some are highly positive, even after many transplants (up to 150). Others are negative. Thus it does not appear to be a marker for neoplastic liver cells per se (81).

The nature of the marker is now being studied but its essential meaning is not clear yet. The possibility of it being a viral antigen is very attractive but as yet unproven. Equally attractive is the hypothesis that it may be an antigen turned on as a response to interruption in differentiation. Conceivably, it might be an isozyme of a liver enzyme that appears early during liver carcinogenesis (see 99).

Regardless of its essential nature, if further work proves that the PN antigen is not present in normal cells but only in altered cells, one now has the possibility of the first selective marker for preneoplastic or premalignant liver cells. The potential use not only as a marker for different cell populations in cirrhosis but also for quantitative assay for discrete cell populations is interesting.

Arrested Differentiation and Development of Hepatocellular Carcinoma

If the hypothesis as here presented has an essential validity, then the phenomenon of arrested differentiation or aborted development might be an important principle in the pathogenesis of hepatocellular carcinoma. This is an old idea that has been suggested periodically for perhaps 50 or 75 years. This thought has been proposed on occasion in recent years, especially as a result of the biohhemical findings relating to fetal isozymes and other fetal proteins in a variety of hepatomas (100,101). It has received a variety of designations including "blocked ontogeny" "retrogenetic expression" (102), "disdifferentiation" (103), "retrodifferentiation" (104), "depression of fetal enzymes" (105), and "anomalous gene expression" (68). Also, very recently Bruni (37), on the basis of a careful ultrastructural study of liver carcinogenesis induced in the rat by DEN and in referring to malignant neoplastic liver cells ("former cells"), suggested that "the total fine structure of the former cells expresses permanently arrested differentiation more than dedifferentiation." In concluding his paper, Bruni again suggested that "studies should

aim to elucidate how DENA (diethylnitrosamine) blocks permanently the differentiation of the neoplastic hepatocytes, if we are to understand how this carcinogen induces permanent abnormal cell proliferation."

Of course, these considerations raise an issue of the greatest importance in our understanding of the pathogenesis of HCC. What is the ultimate cell of origin of the cancer—a fully mature hepatocyte, such as is obviously the precursor for almost all the hepatocytes during regeneration of the adult liver following partial removal of the liver or an undifferentiated stem cell? We have been carefully examining the liver of the rat daily for up to two weeks following partial hepatectomy and have failed to find any sign of an architectural pattern other than that of the mature liver. From our observations, the liver cells during regeneration divide in such a manner as to maintain a single cell plate organizational pattern. What then is the origin of the two-or more cell-thick plates seen in the experimental animal in the new cell hepatocyte populations during carcinogenesis and in some nodules in human cirrhosis (90)? Does "dedifferentiation" and "redifferentiation" really take place? A simpler hypothesis would suggest that under some pathologic conditions, such cirrhosis and liver cell carcinogenesis, perhaps a as-yet-to-be-identified stem cell, is altered and is stimulated to proliferate. Conceivably, this cell could more easily recapitulate the fetal liver developmental pattern and thus would be subject to interrupted differentiation by carcinogen. An origin of population II and III from a stem cell could more easily explain the selective effect of liver damage by carcinogens. Since fetal liver is often deficient in at least some activating enzymes, the hypothetical stem cell might be equally deficient. This would give it a tremendous advantage over the mature hepatocytes in carcinogenesis, since it might have a built-in resistance to the cytotoxic effects of the carcinogens. On this

16

basis, one could easily conceive of a dual origin for liver regeneration in cirrhosis. Man in high liver cancer areas might be exposed to an etiologic agent for cirrhosis which favors a selective proliferation of stem cells while in other areas, the cause of the cirrhosis might favor the simpler regeneration from mature liver cells.

The thesis for a stem cell origin for cancer is by no means original, although little has been said concerning liver and liver cancer in this context. Pierce (106) has been emphasizing the logical nature of the stem cell hypothesis of carcinogenesis. Unfortunately, the possible identification of such cells continues to remain a challenge.

These considerations naturally lead to the question of whether a stem cell or a mature liver cell might be the only precursor cells for liver cell cancer. With butter yellow (4-dimethylaminoazobenzene) and its active derivatives (e.g., 3'-Me-DAB), one observes an unusual enlargement of ductular cells and an apparent conversion of these cells to hepatocytes (42, 107, 108). As mentioned earlier, virtually every hepatocarcinogen induces ductular prolif-

eration in the liver early in carcinogenesis. With most carcinogens, this response either regresses or sometimes develops into areas of cholangiofibrosis. Also, with many carcinogens, cholangiofibrosis appears to be a nonneoplastic lesion which rarely if ever evolves into cholangiocarcinoma. However, with the carcinogenic azo dyes, an origin of liver cancer, not only cholangiocarcinoma but also HCC from ductular cells must be seriously entertained (107, 108). Such a histogenesis of HCC could account for the reported presence of AFP in ductular cells in rats on an azo dye carcinogenic regimen (71–73, 109) (Fig. 4).

General Considerations

These newer developments in the study of liver carcinogenesis in the experimental animal offer new insights into several aspects of the development of liver cancer. They emphasize that both *somatic mutation* and *altered differentiation* may each play an important role at different stages of the process.

The analysis of preneoplastic and pre-

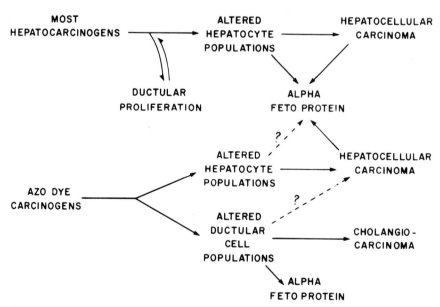

Figure 4 The suggested relationship of different cells in the liver in relation to $\alpha_1 F$ and HCC induced by most chemical hepatocarcinogens and azo dye carcinogens.

malignant cell populations for new antigens has been neglected generally, probably because of the general unavailability of sufficient amounts of uniform tissue. Two systems, skin papillomas and hyperplastic nodules in breast, have been studied from this point of view in Prehn's laboratory (111–113). In both instances, with chemical carcinogens, new antigens have been identified that have persisted through transplantation and were still present in the malignant neoplasms that developed. However, these antigens, unlike the PN antigen, were unique for each lesion and were not common to all of the similar lesions in each organ.

In regard to liver neoplasms, there are several reports of a marked decrease or loss of liver antigens in hepatomas (103–118). Also, Weiler reported (119) the loss of some liver antigens in focal islands of liver cells, considered to be a presumptive preneoplastic population.

In addition, new antigens have also been found in a variety of hepatomas (see Baldwin (67) for review). Some of these seem to be unique for each hepatoma or for each group of hepatomas induced by a single carcinogen while others are probably fetal in type.

In regard to immunological aspects of liver carcinogenesis, no mention has been made of the possible role of immunological surveillance during carcinogenesis. Friedrich-Freska and Hoffmann (120) reported that unlike normal rabbit serum the administration of rabbit anti-rat lymphocyte serum daily during exposure of animals to diethylnitrosamine resulted in many more islands and larger islands of liver cells showing one of the characteristics of nodular hyperplasia, low or absent glucose-6-phosphatase histochemically. Obviously, much more research into this general area is needed before immunologic surveillance can be implicated in liver carcinogenesis. It is noteworthy that the concept in general has been receiving some setbacks very recently (e.g., 121, 122).

Since the PN antigen appears to be a common link between all the putative preneoplastic or premalignant hepatocyte populations and liver cancer, its possible significance in the pathogenesis of liver cancer rests on its fundamental nature. Any definitive answer must obviously await purification and localization in the cell, etc. Such studies are in progress.

The relationship of the PN antigen to a carcinogen-protein product with new antigenic properties can be easily ruled out, since it is seen with five chemically quite different chemical carcinogens and is found in some hepatomas that have been transplanted more than 150 times over a period of almost 20 years.

The two most plausible hypotheses are that the PN antigen is (a) a viral component or (b) a protein, conceivably even an isozyme, that is turned on when normal differentiation or remodeling of the hepatocytes is interrupted.

In respect to a virus, there is of course considerable evidence for a viral component in many carcinogenic processes. The possible role of a virus in liver cancer, although often proposed over the years, has not received strong scientific support. Conceivably, the new finding in regard to PN antigen could allow a new approach.

In respect to the second hypothesis, since the presence or absence of the PN antigen seems to be linked to only certain types of hepatocytes, a response to disturbed differentiation is an attractive possibility, especially since different enzymes and isozyme patterns are intimately linked to differentiation.

Regardless of its fundamental nature, the observations with PN antigen, although still essentially preliminary, already indicate that the induction of certain type or types of altered hepatocytes by a chemical may play a crucial role in carcinogenesis. Thus, even if a virus is implicated, it remains clear that the future course of the process is determined in a major way by whether the "right kind" of hepatocyte population is induced for a sufficiently long time to allow the further evolution to malignancy.

The essential nature of the progressive cellular alterations leading ultimately to liver cancer remains a challenge. Although we can now begin to focus on certain key steps, much more progress will be needed before we can begin to devise rational ways to control and interrupt the process.

In my view, an important concept to stress in this context is probability. It appears increasingly evident from studies on carcinogenesis in different tissues, that, in many of the steps in carcinogenesis, we are dealing with a probability function, not a certainty. The whole liver is subjected to a carcinogen, yet only a few cells develop as nodules; many early nodules develop, yet only a few persist as such on removal of the carcinogen; the later nodules have many hepatocytes, yet only very few appear to develop into a population of malignant hepatocytes. Thus there appears to be a continual selection of smaller and smaller number of cells, each with an increasingly greater probability of development of cancer. If this ooncept of cellular evolution (2) or progression (123) is basically a valid one, then the challenges become the identification of the essential nature of each of the selected populations that are relevant to the u!umate liver cancer and of the selection pressure, exogenous or endogenous, that are operating at each stage. Although this is a tall order for any carcinogenic system, the possibility of approaching this in the liver seems less remote than in times past.

ACKNOWLEDGMENT

I thank D. S. R. Sarma, S. Rajalakshmi, H. Shinozuka, K. Okita, Gary Williams, and all my other colleagues and co-workers for their great assistance in our studies on liver cancer. I also thank my secretary, Mrs. Barbara Dole, for her diligence, devotion, and competence in the preparation of this chapter.

REFERENCES

1. Sasaki T, Yoshuda T: Experimentelle Erzeugung des Lebercarcinoms durch Fütterung mit o-amidoazotoluol. *Virchows Arch Pathol Anat Physiol* **295**:175–200, 1935.

2. Farber E: Carcinogenesis—Cellular evolution as a unifying thread: Presidential address. *Cancer Res* **33**:2537–2550, 1973.

3. Magee PN: Liver carcinogens in the human environment. *Liver Cancer—International Agency for Research on Cancer Scientific Publications No. 1*, 1971, pp 110–120.

4. Hutt MSR: Epidemilogy of human primary liver cancer. *Liver Cancer—International Agency for Research on Cancer Scientific Publications No. 1*, 1971, pp 21–29.

5. Steiner PE: Carcinoma of the liver in the United States. *Acta Unio Int Contra Cancrum* **13**:628–645, 1957.

6. Higginson J: The geographic pathology of primary liver cancer. *Cancer Res* **23**:1624–1633, 1963.

7. Higginson J, Svoboda D: Primary carcinoma of the liver as a pathologist's problem. *Pathol Ann* **5**:61–89, 1970.

8. Higginson J: Geographic considerations in liver disease. In *Progress in Liver Diseases*, Vol 2. Popper H, Schaffner F (Eds). Grune & Stratton, New York, 1965, pp 211–227.

9. Farber E: Environmental factors in the development of liver cancer. In *The Liver and Its Diseases*. Schaffner F, Sherlock S, Leevy C (Eds). Intercontinental Medical Book Corp., New York, 1974, pp 337–341.

10. Evaluation of carcinogenic risk of chemicals to man. *International Agency for Research on Cancer Monographs*, Vol 1, 1972.

11. Abelev GI: Alpha-fetoprotein in ontogenesis and its association with malignant tumors. *Adv Cancer Res* **14**:295–358, 1971.

12. Tomatis L, Partensky C, Montesano R: The predictive value of mouse liver tumour induction in carcinogenic testing—a literature survey. *Int J Cancer* **12**:1–20, 1973.

13. Cole LJ, Nowell PC: Radiation carcinogenesis: the sequence of events. *Science* **150**:1782–1786, 1965.

14. Anderson JP, McCormick KJ, Stenback WA, et al: Induction of hepatomas in hamsters by an avian adenovirus (CELO). *Proc SocExp Soc Med* **137**:421–423, 1971.

15. Stenback WA, Anderson JP, McCormick, et al: Induction of tumors in the liver of hamsters by an avian adenovirus (CELO). *J Natl Cancer Inst* **50**:963–970, 1973.

16. Magee PN, Barnes JM: Carcinogenic nitroso compounds. *Adv Cancer Res* **10**:163–256, 1967.

17. Lijinsky W, Epstein SS: Nitrosamines as environmental carcinogens. *Nature* **225**:21–23, 1970.

18. Druckery H, Preussmann R, Ivankovic S: *N*-Nitroso compounds in organotropic and transplacental carcinogenesis. *Ann N Y Acad Sci* **163**:676–695, 1969.

19. *N*-Nitroso Compounds: Analysis and formation. *International Agency for Research on Cancer Scientific Publications No. 3*, 1972.

20. Wolff IA, Wasserman AE: Nitrates, nitrites and nitrosamines. *Science* **177**:15–19, 1972.

21. Montesano R, Magee PN: Metabolism of dimethylnitrosamine by human liver slices *in vitro*. *Nature* **228**:173–174, 1970.

22. Miller JA: Carcinogenesis by chemicals: an overview. GHA Clowes Memorial Lecture. *Cancer Res* **30**:559–576, 1970.

23. Warwick GP: Metabolism of liver carcinogens and other factors influencing liver cancer induction. *Liver Cancer—International Agency for Research on Cancer Scientific Publications No. 1*, 1971, pp 121–157.

24. Miller JA, Miller EC: Chemical carcinogenesis: mechanisms and approaches to its control. *J Natl Cancer Inst* **47**:V–XIV, 1971.

25. Wattenberg LW: Enzymatic reactions and carcinogenesis. In *Environment and Cancer*. Twenty-fourth annual symposium on fundamental research at the University of Texas and MD Anderson Hospital and Tumor Institute. Williams & Wilkins, Baltimore, 1971, pp 241–255.

26. Farber E: Hepatic carcinogenesis. In *Progress in Liver Diseases*, Vol 4. Popper H, Schaffner F (Eds). Grune & Stratton, New York 1972, pp 173–182.

27. Sarma DSR, Rajalakshmi S, Farber E: Chemical carcinogenesis—carcinogens: Interactions with nucleic acids. In *Cancer: A Comprehensive Treatise*, Becker FF (Ed). Plenum Press, New York, in press.

28. Lawley PD: Some aspects of the cellular response to chemical modifications of nucleic acid purines. In *Purines, Theory and Experiment*. The Jerusalem Symposium on Quantum Chemistry and Biochemistry, Vol 4. Bergmann ED, Pullman P (Eds). Israel Academy of Sciences & Humanities, Jerusalem, 1972, pp 579–591.

29. Irving CC: Interaction of chemical carcinogens with DNA. In *Methods in Cancer Research*, Vol

7. Busch H (Ed). Academic Press, New York, 1973, pp 189–244.

30. Farber E, Sarma DSR: DNA damage and repair during carcinogenesis. In *Control Processes in Neoplasia*, Mehlman M, Hanson R (Eds). Academic Press, New York, 1974, pp 173–185.

31. Stewart BW, Farber E: Strand breakage in rat liver DNA and its repair following administration of cyclic nitrosamines. *Cancer Res* **33**:3209–3215, 1973.

32. Sarma DSR, Michael RO, Stewart BW, et al: Pattern of damage and repair of rat liver DNA induced by chemical carcinogens *in vivo*. *Fed Proc* **32**:833, 1973.

33. Stewart BW, Farber E, Mirvisch SS: Induction by an hepatic carcinogen, 1-nitroso-5,6-dihydrouracil, of single and double strand breaks of liver DNA with repid repair. *Biochem Biophys Res Commun* **53**:773–779, 1973.

34. Michael RO, Parodi S, Sarma DSR: *In vivo* repair of rat liver DNA damaged by 3-hydroxyxanthine. *Chem Biol Interactions*, in press.

35. Sarma DSR, Rajalakshmi S, Farber E: DNA repair and chemical carcinogenesis, *Biochim Biophys Acta*, in press.

36. Svoboda D, Higginson J: A comparison of ultrastructural changes in rat liver due to chemical carcinogens. *Cancer Res* **28**:1703–1733, 1968.

37. Bruni C: Distinctive cells similar to fetal hepatocytes associated with liver carcinogenesis by diethylnitrosamine. Electron microscopic study. *J Natl Cancer Inst* **50**:1513–1528, 1973.

38. Smuckler EA, Arcosay M: Structural and functional changes of the endoplasmic reticulum of hepatic parenchymal cells. *Int Rev Exp Pathol* **7**:305–418, 1969.

39. Bannasch P: The cytoplasm of hepatocytes during carcinogenesis; electron and light microscopical investigations of the nitrosomorpholine-intoxicated rat liver. In *Recent Results in Cancer Research*, Vol 19. Springer-Verlag, Berlin, New York, 1968.

40. Farber E: Hyperplastic liver nodules. In *Methods in Cancer Research*, Vol. 7. Busch H (Ed). Academic Press, New York, 1973, pp 345–375.

41. Farber E, Sarma DSR, Rajalakshmi S, et al: Liver Carcinogenesis; a unifying hypothesis. In *Principles of Liver Disease*, Becker FF (Ed). Marcel Dekker, New York, in press.

42. Farber E: Ethionine carcinogenesis. *Adv Cancer Res* **7**:383–474, 1963.

43. Hunt RD, Leveille GA, Sauberlich HE: Dietary bile acids and lipid metabolism. II. The ductul-

107. Price JM, Harman JW, Miller EC, et al: Pro-
     gressive microscopic alterations in the livers of
     rats fed the hepatic carcinogens 3'-methyl-4-
     dimethylaminoazobenzene and 4'-fluoro-4-
     dimethylaminoazobenzene. *Cancer Res* **12**:192–
     200, 1952.

108. Farber E: Similarities in the sequence of early
     histological changes induced in the liver of the
     rat by ethionine, 2-acetylaminofluorene and 3'-
     methyl-4-dimethylaminoazobenzene. *Cancer Res*
     16:142–148, 1956.

109. Onoe T, Dempo K, Kaneko A, et al: Signifi-
     cance of α-fetoprotein appearance in early stage
     of azo-dye carcinogenesis. *Gann Monogr Cancer
     Res* **14**:233–247, 1973.

110. Uriel J, Aussel C, Bouillon D, et al: Localization
     of rat liver α-fetoprotein by cell affinity labell-
     ing with tritiated oestrogens. *Nature* **244**:190–
     192, 1973.

111. Lappé MA: Evidence for the antigenicity of pa-
     pillomas induced by 3-methylcholanthrene. *J
     Natl Cancer Inst* **40**:823–846, 1968.

112. Lappe MA: Tumor specific transplantation an-
     tigens: Possible origin in premalignant lesions.
     Nature **223**:82–84, 1969.

113. Slemmer G: Host response to premalignant
     mammary tissues. *Natl Cancer Inst Monogr*
     35:57–71, 1972.

114. Abelev GI: Antigenic structure of chemically in-
     duced hepatomas. *Prog Exp Tumor Res* **7**:104–
     157, 1965.

115. Fisher E, Weiler E: Die histologishe Darstellung
     der leberspecifishen Antigens und diesen
     Schwund in Hepatoma mit Hilfe fluorescein-
     markierten Anticomplements. *Z Krebsforsch*
     64:441–447, 1962.

116. Hiramoto R, Gurand J, Bernecky J, et al: Im-
     munochemical differences among *N*-2-
     fluorenylacetamide-induced rat hepatomas.
     Cancer Res **23**:109–111, 1963.

117. Nairn RC, Richmond HG, Fothagill JE: Im-
     munological differences between normal and
     malignant cells. *Brit Med J* **2**:1335–1340, 1960.

118. Weiler E: Loss of specific cell antigen in rela-
     tion to cancer. In *Carcinogenesis—Mechanisms of
     Action*. Ciba Foundation Symposium, 1958, pp
     165–175.

119. Weiler E: Die Änderung der serologischen Spe-
     zificität von Leberzellen der Ratte während der
     Carcinogenese durch   dimethylaminobenzol.
     Z Naturforsch **116**:31–38, 1956.

120. Friedrich-Freksa H, Hoffmann M: Immunolo-
     gical defense against preneoplastic stages of
     diethylnitrosamine-induced carcinoma in rat
     liver. *Nature* **223**:1162–1163, 1969.

121. Stutman O: Tumor development after methyl-
     cholanthrene in immunologically deficient
     athymic-nude mice. *Science* **183**:534–536, 1974.

122. Prehn RT: Immuno-modulation of tumor
     growth. *Am J Pathol*, in press.

123. Foulds L: *Neoplastic Development*, Vol 1. Aca-
     demic Press, London, 1969.

Part Two *ETIOLOGY*

CHAPTER 2 AFLATOXINS AND THEIR RELATIONSHIP TO HEPATOCELLULAR CARCINOMA

GERALD N. WOGAN

INTRODUCTION

Knowledge about aflatoxins has developed during an era of increasing awareness of the importance of natural as well as man-made chemicals as environmental contaminants. The intensity with which this problem has been investigated is reflected in the large number of publications about it which have appeared since its emergence in 1960. Most of this literature is beyond the scope of this chapter which emphasizes recent developments, mainly in the areas of carcinogenicity of aflatoxins and their implications for man. This field has been the subject of previous specialized reviews (e.g., 1–3), and the entire subject has been comprehensively surveyed in a monograph (4) and in summary form (5). These sources give detailed references to the original literature on which the following general summary is based.

Several features of the aflatoxins problem have provided continuing stimuli for its further exploration. The fact that some food-spoilage fungi are capable of producing mycotoxins has been recognized for a long time. However, the importance of toxic mold metabolites as food contaminants used to be evident principally to veterinarians who frequently encounter outbreaks of poisoning of farm animals. The existence of aflatoxins was discovered as a consequence of mass outbreaks of poisoning of poultry, and it is possible that this episode might have been relegated to the miscellaneous problems of agriculture except for several features of the problem whose importance became increasingly obvious as early developments unfolded.

Important among these was the early recognition that the toxic agents were produced by *Aspergillus flavus,* a common and widely distributed food spoilage fungus. The problem assumed global dimensions when aflatoxins were identified in agricultural products, especially peanut meals, originating in many different parts of the world. Coupled with this information was the eventual discovery that toxin-producing fungal strains could produce aflatoxins whenever conditions permitted their growth on practically any natural substrate, thereby providing for a high probability of appearance of the toxins as contaminants of human foods. Perhaps the strongest impetus to investigation was provided by the poisonous properties of aflatoxins and especially their extraordinary potency as hepatocarcinogens in animals. The obvious implications of these various facets of the problem to public health stimulated research into occurrence of the toxins, means for prevention and control of contamination of human foods, and their toxicology and pharmacology.

In addition to their importance as public health hazards, the aflatoxins have become useful model compounds for investigations in experimental chemical carcinogenesis. In this group of substances, nature has provided compounds of closely related chemical structure but widely differing potency and tissue specificity. Although various members of the series are effective in inducing toxic or other manifestations of biological activity in many kinds of test systems, there are great variations in carcinogenic response among animal species. The underlying mechanisms responsible for these structure-activity relationships and species differences in responses are unidentified. Their elucidation can reasonably be expected to improve our understanding of some of the mechanisms involved in carcinogenesis and fully warrant continued investigation. This is particularly important in view of increasing evidence that human populations in some parts of the world are being exposed to aflatoxins and that such populations are at higher risk of developing liver cancer than unexposed groups.

tuted coumarins and contain a fused dihydrofurofuran configuration peculiar to a limited number of compounds of natural origin. The compounds occur in two series, aflatoxin B_1 and derivatives and aflatoxin G_1 and derivatives. Structures of presently known aflatoxins from biological sources are shown in Figs. 1 and 2.

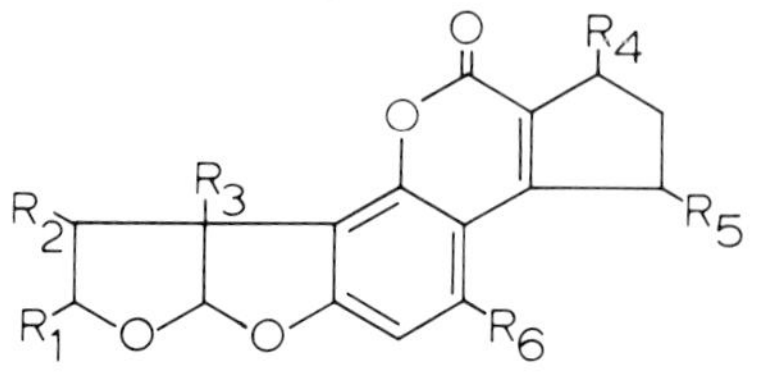

Aflatoxin	R_1	R_2	R_3	R_4	R_5	R_6
B_1	H	H	H	=O	H	OCH_3
B_2	H_2	H_2	H	=O	H	OCH_3
B_{2a}	HOH	H_2	H	=O	H	OCH_3
M_1	H	H	OH	=O	H	OCH_3
M_2	H_2	H_2	OH	=O	H	OCH_3
P_1	H	H	H	=O	H	OH
Q_1	H	H	H	=O	OH	OCH_3
R_0	H	H	H	OH	H	OCH_3

Figure 1   Aflatoxin B_1 and derivatives.

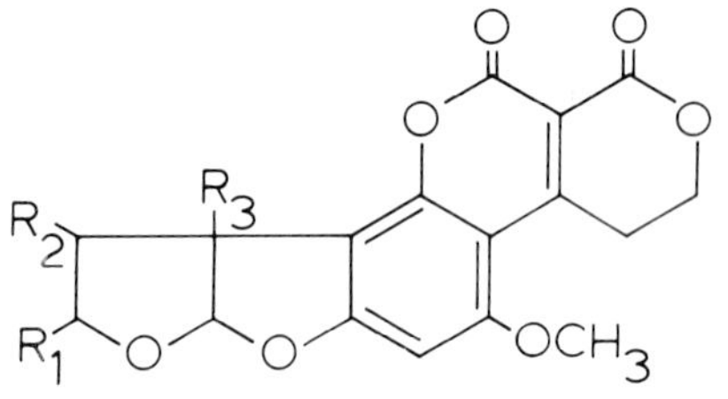

Aflatoxin	R_1	R_2	R_3
G_1	H	H	H
G_2	H_2	H_2	H
G_{2a}	OH	H_2	H
GM_1	H	H	OH

Figure 2   Aflatoxin G_1 and derivatives.

CHEMISTRY

Chemically, the aflatoxins are highly substi-

Aflatoxins B_1, B_2, B_{2a}, M_1, G_1, G_2, and G_{2a} have been isolated from mold cultures and/or from contaminated foods. Certain of these, as well as the remaining derivatives whose structures are shown in Figs. 1 and 2 are metabolites produced from the parent toxins by animals or animal tissues as discussed subsequently.

The aflatoxins are produced by only a few strains of *Aspergillus flavus* and *A. parasiticus,* fungi whose spores are widely distributed, especially in soil. Those organisms that are capable of toxin production generally synthesize only two or three aflatoxins under a given set of conditions. When they occur as food contaminants, aflatoxin B_1 is always present. Although aflatoxins B_2, G_1, and G_2 have sometimes been found in contaminated products, they generally occur less frequently than B_1 and have never been reported in the absence of B_1. This is an important point, since B_1 has the highest potency of the group as a toxin and as a carcinogen.

With respect to substrate, requirements for toxin production are relatively nonspecific, and the mold can produce the compounds on virtually any food (or indeed on simple synthetic media) that will support growth. Thus any food material can be subject to aflatoxin contamination if it becomes moldy. However, experience has shown that the frequency and levels of aflatoxins found vary greatly among foods collected within a given region and among different regions, which we discuss subsequently.

CARCINOGENICITY AND OTHER BIOLOGICAL EFFECTS

The carcinogenicity, toxicity, and biochemical effects induced in biological systems by aflatoxins have been reviewed in detail recently (1, 5), and only a brief summary is necessary here to indicate the present status of these facets of the field. Acute or subacute poisoning can be produced in animals by feeding aflatoxin-contaminated diets or by dosing with purified compounds. Although there are wide species differences in responsiveness to acute toxicity, no completely refractory species is known. Symptoms of poisoning are produced in most domestic animals by aflatoxin levels of 10 to 100 mg/kg (ppm) or less in the feed. As regards lethal potency to experimental animals, the oral or parenteral LD_{50} values are generally in the range of 5 to 15 mg/kg body weight for aflatoxin B_1. The value for trout, the most sensitive species, is < 0.5 mg/kg, whereas the value for the mouse, the least sensitive, is 60 mg/kg. In both acute and subacute poisoning the liver is the main target organ for aflatoxin B_1. The chief pathologic lesions in liver associated with acute or chronic toxicity are periportal or centrilobular necrosis, bile duct proliferation, and in some species, cirrhosis.

Many of the biochemical changes induced in various biological systems by aflatoxin B_1 follow a consistent pattern. Administration of the toxin to rats is quickly followed by pronounced inhibition of DNA and RNA polymerases in liver, and similar responses have been observed in human and animal cell cultures. Protein synthesis is also impaired, particularly under conditions where synthesis is strongly influenced by alterations in messenger RNA synthesis. Available evidence indicates that polymerase inhibition is an indirect consequence of impaired template activity of chromatin subsequent to toxin-chromatin interaction. Consequently, interaction between aflatoxin or some derivative of it with DNA or other component of chromatin is viewed as the initiating event in the observed series of reactions. Much of the current literature deals with one or another facet of this sequence of biochemical events. Another line of evidence that may be related to the mode of action of the toxins deals with their ability to interact with membranes of the endoplasmic reticulum and thereby alter polysomal binding to those membranes. However, the available evidence is as yet inadequate to explain in detail the biochemical basis of the

Table 1   Dose-Response Characteristics of Aflatoxin B$_1$ Carcinogenesis in Male Fischer Rats

Dietary Aflatoxin Level (ppb)	Duration of Feeding (weeks)	Liver Carcinoma Incidence	Preneoplastic Liver Lesions
0	74–109	0/18	0/18
1	78–105	2/22	7/22
5	65–93	1/22	5/22
15	69–96	4/22	13/22
50	71–97	20/25 [a]	5/25
100	54–88	28/28 [b]	—

[a] Two animals had pulmonary metastases.
[b] Four animals had pulmonary metastases.

cytotoxicity and carcinogenic effects of these toxins.

Aflatoxins have been shown to have carcinogenic activity in many species of animals including rodents, nonhuman primates, birds, and fish. The liver is the organ principally affected, in which the toxins induce hepatocellular carcinomas and other tumor types. However, under some circumstances, significant incidences of tumors at sites other than liver have been recorded, their distribution depending on the specific aflatoxin used, species, strain, and dose level administered.

Various aflatoxin preparations have been used in carcinogenesis experiments. Much of the literature, particularly that appearing in the earlier stages of the problem before purified aflatoxins became available, deals with carcinogenic properties of dietary ingredients such as peanut meal contaminated through mold spoilage of the raw material by aflatoxin-producing fungi. Availability of mixed aflatoxin concentrates and eventually of highly purified individual compounds facilitated experimental manipulation of parameters such as dose, route, etc., and also has permitted evaluation of structure-activity relationships between aflatoxins and structural analogs.

The majority of published information on aflatoxin carcinogenicity deals with ex-

periments in rats in which the toxins have a high order of potency. In addition to experiments dealing with dose-response characteristics, influences of such factors as route, dosing regimen, strain, sex, and age have been investigated. Also, effects of various other modifying factors on carcinogenic responses have been evaluated, including diet, hormonal status, liver injury, microsomal enzyme activity, and concurrent exposure to other carcinogenic agents.

Many early experiments involved the feeding of diets containing aflatoxin-contaminated ingredients. Levels of the toxin were determined by chemical assays and manipulated by dilution with uncontaminated material. As a group, these experiments established the fact that aflatoxin levels of 0.1 ppm (mg/kg diet) and higher consistently induced liver carcinomas in rats. This conclusion has been confirmed and extended in later experiments in which purified aflatoxin B$_1$ was added to diets at various levels. The results of a recent dose-response study (6) in a particularly susceptible rat strain (Fischer) fed a semipurified diet to which aflatoxin B$_1$ was added are summarized in Table 1. It is evident from these observations that the compound has demonstrable carcinogenic properties at a level of 1 ppb (μg/kg diet), and the response is dose-related up to 100

Table 2 Hepatocarcinogenicity of Aflatoxin B_1 in Rodents

Species	Dosing Regimen	Duration of Treatment	Period of Observation	Liver Tumor Incidence	Reference
Rat, Fischer	1.0 ppm in diet	33 weeks	52 weeks	3/6	(48)
Rat, Fischer	1.0 ppm in diet	41–64 weeks	Same	18/21	(12)
Rat, Porton	1.0 ppm in diet	20 weeks	90 weeks	19/30	(9)
Rat, Wistar	1.0 ppm in diet	21 weeks	87 weeks	12/14	(4)
Mouse, C57Bl/6NB	150 ppm in diet [a]	20 months	Same	0/60	(1)
	1.0 ppm in diet	20 months	Same	0/30	
Mouse, C3HfB/HEN	1.0 ppm in diet	20 months	Same	0/30	
	6.0 μg/g body wt.	3 doses i.p.	80 weeks	16/16	(50)
Mouse, hybrid F_1, 4 days old					

[a] A mixture of aflatoxins B_1 and G_1 was used in this experiment.

ppb at which level liver carcinoma developed in all animals surviving for approximately 18 months. The sensitivity of this rat strain is further demonstrated by results of another experiment in which a level of 20 ppb induced liver tumors in 11 of 41 animals (7).

Considerable variation exists among rat strains with respect to sensitivity to carcinogenic effects of low levels of aflatoxins. However, a dietary level of 1.0 ppm consistently induces liver carcinoma at high incidence in several rat strains even when feeding is not continued throughout the entire period of observation as shown by representative data in Table 2. In contrast, inbred mice showed no evidence of carcinogenic response at this level. In fact, a dietary level of 150 ppm was ineffective in inducing liver tumors in a random-bred mouse strain fed that level for their entire lifespan. On the other hand, infant mice of an F_1 hybrid strain (C57Bl × C3H) developed a high incidence of hepatocellular carcinomas when given repeated injections of aflatoxin B_1 during the perinatal period.

The primary target organ for aflatoxin B_1 in most rat strains is the liver in which it induces hepatocellular carcinomas and cholangiocarcinomas among other lesions (8–10). Tumors of other tissues that have been observed in aflatoxin B_1-treated rats include carcinomas of the glandular stomach (11) and mucinous adenocarcinomas of the colon (12). Both are infrequently observed in rats trated with carcinogens, and although only a relatively small number have been observed in aflatoxin-treated animals, a causative association has been suggested. More recent experiments suggest that the incidence of the colon tumor is enhanced by vitamin A deficiency (13).

Published evidence of carcinogenicity of aflatoxin B_1 in nonrodent species is summarized in Table 3. Liver carcinomas have been induced in subhuman primates in three separate experiments. Although the total number of positive responses is very small, it seems clear that aflatoxin B_1 is an effective carcinogen for the liver of these species.

Among the remaining animals that have been studied, the rainbow trout and duck appear to be of comparable sensitivity, responding to levels of 4 to 30 ppb in the diet. Effective levels in the guppy and ferret were in the ppm range, and the salmon

Table 3 Hepatocarcinogenicity of Aflatoxin B₁ in Nonrodent Species

Species	Dosing Regimen	Duration of Treatment	Period of Observation	Liver Tumor Incidence	Reference
Monkey, rhesus (M)	1.655 g total [a]	5.5 years	8.0 years	1/1	Gopalan (51)
Monkey, rhesus (F)	0.504 g total	6.0 years	Same	1/1	Adamson (52)
Marmoset	3.0 mg total	50–55 weeks	Same	1/3	Lin (53)
	5.04–5.84 mg total [b]	87–94 weeks	Same	2/3	
Ferret	0.3–2.0 ppm in diet	28–37 months	Same	7/9	Butler (9)
Duck	30 ppb in diet	14 months	Same	8/11	Carnaghan (54)
Rainbow trout	4 ppb in diet	12 months	Same	15%	Sinnhuber (55)
	8 ppb in diet	12 months	Same	40%	
	20 ppb in diet	12 months	Same	65%	
Rainbow trout embryos	0.5 ppm in water	1 hour	296–321 days	38%	Sinnhuber and Wales (56)
Salmon	12 ppb in diet [c]	20 months	Same	50%	Wales and Sinnhuber (57)
Guppy	6 ppm in diet	11 months	Same	7/113	Sato (58)

[a] A mixture of aflatoxins B₁ and G₁ was used in this experiment.
[b] These animals were simultaneously infected with hepatitis virus.
[c] This diet also contained 50 ppm cyclopropenoid fatty acids.

responded only when exposed concurrently to aflatoxin B_1 and fatty acids that have a cocarcinogenic property in fish.

Numerous reports have dealt with a variety of factors that modify the carcinogenic response of rats to aflatoxin B_1, including experimental alteration of nutritional and endocrine status, various types of liver insults, and simultaneous exposure to aflatoxins and other pharmacologically active compounds.

Because of the possibility that exposure to aflatoxins could occur in human populations suffering from malnutrition, the influence of nutritional status on aflatoxin carcinogenesis in rats has received attention by a number of investigators. The effect of dietary protein has been evaluated with somewhat contradictory results. Madhaven and Gopalan (14) found that rats fed a low-protein (5%) diet were sensitized to the toxic effects of aflatoxin, but developed liver tumors at a lower incidence than controls fed a 20% protein ration. On the other hand, Newberne et al. (15) and Newberne and Wogan (8) found that diets containing 9% protein resulted in a higher incidence of liver tumors in a shorter period of time than a diet containing 22% protein when both groups of rats were intubated with 375 μg aflatoxin B_1 per animal. The reasons for these disparate results are unclear, and this important problem requires further investigation.

Rogers and Newberne (16, 17) have focused attention on the possible importance of simultaneous occurrence of marginal insufficiency of dietary lipotropic agents such as methionine and vitamin B_{12} and aflatoxin exposure and have studied these conditions in rats. Marginal lipotrope deficiency protected rats against doses of aflatoxin B_1 that were letal to 60 to 100% of rats on an adequate diet. However, when treated with a carcinogenic regimen, animals with a lipotrope deficiency developed liver tumors much earlier and at higher frequency than did control animals. The

mechanisms responsible for these interactions have not been identified.

Several investigations have been concerned with the influence of endocrine status on responses of rats to aflatoxin carcinogenesis. Goodall and Butler (18) studied the effects of hypophysectomy on rats fed a diet containing 4 ppm aflatoxin B_1. Whereas control animals developed liver tumors in 49 weeks, hypophysectomized rats failed to develop tumors in the same period despite the fact that they received aflatoxins at a higher rate than the controls. Newberne and Williams (19) reported that rats fed diets containing 0.2 ppm aflatoxin B_1 and 4 ppm diethylstilbestrol developed fewer liver tumors than those fed aflatoxin alone. Appropriate controls indicated that the decreased tumor incidence associated with diethylstilbestrol was not the result of decreased food intake. A more direct association is implied, but the specific mechanisms responsible for protection are not known.

Experimentally induced liver insults of a variety of types have also been studied with respect to their interactions with the carcinogenic effects of aflatoxins (15). Concurrent cirrhosis and exposure to low dietary levels of aflatoxin B_1 (0.07 ppm) appeared to increase tumor incidence, while animals returned to a normal diet after cirrhosis and then exposed to aflatoxins at a level of 1 ppm developed a much higher tumor incidence. Repeated biopsy was without effect and partial hepatectomy performed before or after administration of aflatoxin B_1 had no effect on development of hepatocarcinoma, compared to either sham operation or no operation (20).

Simultaneous administration of aflatoxin B_1 with other pharmacologically active compounds including other carcinogens has been investigated. Newberne et al. (15) found ethionine fed at a level of 0.2% of the diet to act syncarcinogenically with aflatoxin B_2 at 0.4 ppm. In contrast, aflatoxin B_1 alone at dietary levels of 0.4 or

1.5 ppm was more effective in inducing liver tumors when fed alone than in combination with urethan at 0.1 to 0.6% of the diet (21). Simultaneous treatment of rats with maximal tolerated doses of rubratoxin B (a toxic but not carcinogenic mycotoxin) and aflatoxin B_1 resulted in potentiation of the toxicity of rubratoxin, but no evidence of sensitization to aflatoxin carcinogenesis (22).

Reddy and Svoboda (23) studied the effects on rats of lasiocarpine, a pyrrolizidine alkaloid that is strongly hepatotoxic, on carcinogenesis by feeding aflatoxin B_1 at 2 ppm. They found that the alkaloid did not prevent initiation of liver tumors by aflatoxin but did alter the pathogenic pattern in which the tumors developed.

McLean and Marshall (24) demonstrated a protective action of phenobarbitone against the carcinogenicity of aflatoxin B_1. Continuous administration of phenobarbitone in drinking water during a nine-week period in which aflatoxin B_1 was fed at 5 ppm in the diet resulted in a smaller incidence and delayed appearance of liver tumors than in rats fed aflatoxin alone. These investigators suggested that phenobarbitone induces liver microsomal enzymes to metabolize aflatoxin to noncarcinogenic products.

AFLATOXIN METABOLISM

Considerable research on the metabolic fate of aflatoxin B_1 is intended mainly to produce data bearing on mechanisms that might explain mode of action and differences in susceptibility to the toxin among various animal species. Information generated to date is inadequate to provide complete explanations, but some general outlines of metabolic patterns are beginning to emerge (25, 26).

Patterns of tissue distribution and excretion of aflatoxin B_2 following oral or parenteral dosing have been studied in several species. Experiments with ^{14}C-labeled toxin indicated that more than 90% of a single dose is excreted within 24 hours by rats (25). Feces represents the principal excretory route, accounting for up to 75% of the dose, with urine containing an addition 15 to 20%. Retained radioactivity is present mainly in liver. This pattern of tissue distribution and excretion is generally similar in mice (25), in rhesus monkeys given a single dose intraperitoneally (27) or orally (28), and in chickens dosed repeatedly by intubation (29, 30). In all of these experiments, the identity of the radioactive material retained or excreted is largely unknown, except that unmetabolized aflatoxin B_1 does not account for more than 5% of the total in any instance. In a few cases, major metabolites have been isolated and identified chemically.

All of the metabolic transformations of aflatoxins B_1 and G_1 known to take place in animals are indicated by the structural derivatives in Figs. 1 and 2. The identity of some metabolites has been established from compounds isolated from *in vivo* sources, others have been produced *in vitro*. Most of the work has been done on aflatoxin B_1, but in a few cases parallel pathways have been shown for G_1 as indicated in Fig. 2.

Hydroxylated derivatives of aflatoxin B_1 are formed through several routes. Ring hydroxylation at the 4 position, producing M_1, appears to be a common pathway. This derivative has been found in milk, tissues, and urine of animals and people ingesting B_1, and is also produced *in vitro* by liver microsomes of birds, rodents, and primates including man (26). Ring hydroxylation of the carbon atom to the carbonyl function of the cyclopentenone ring to form aflatoxin Q_1 was recently discovered in monkey liver preparations (31), and represents the major *in vitro* conversion by human liver microsomes (32). This pathway seems to be of only minor importance in rodent and bird liver (26), and free aflatoxin Q_1 has not yet been found in tissues or excreta of any animal exosed to B_1 *in vivo*.

Aflatoxin P_1, a phenolic derivative, is produced by 0-demethylation of B_1. Although this metabolite is a major excretory product in monkeys (27), the free phenol is only a minor *in vitro* metabolite of liver microsomes of monkeys, mice, and rabbits and is apparently not formed by other species *in vitro*.

A further pathway leading to a hydroxylated derivative is the hydration of the 2,3 vinyl ether double bond producing the hemiacetal called B_{2a}. This transformation is accomplished readily by liver microsomes of the rabbit, guinea pig, mouse, chick, and duck, but much less efficiently by the rat (26). Nonenzymatic addition of water also occurs readily under strongly acidic conditions.

All of the preceding metabolic transformations have been demonstrated with crude and purified microsomal preparations. An additional conversion leading to a hydroxylated derivative involving an $NADPH_2$-dependent soluble enzyme is the reduction of the cyclopentenone function of aflatoxin B_1 to produce the cyclopentenol called R_0 (or aflatoxicol). This pathway is especially prominent in the livers of rabbits and several avian species, and the reaction is blocked by 17-ketosteroid sex hormones, suggesting that a soluble $NADPH_2$-linked 17-hydroxysteroid dehydrogenase may be involved (26).

It must be emphasized that current knowledge about aflatoxin metabolism is very incomplete. All of the available information on the relative importance of known pathways is at best semiquantitative in character. This is true because only unconjugated metabolites extractable from excreta or incubation media by organic solvents have thus far been identified. Whenever quantitative experiments using radioactive toxin have been done, thus permitting accurate monitoring of all substrate and product fractions, it has been found that significant portions, often a majority, of metabolites are not recovered by solvent extraction and thus remain unidentified. These undoubtedly include, among other possible derivatives, conjugates of known metabolites; all such components will remain unidentified until methods are developed for their isolation.

Recent evidence for an additional pathway seems particularly important to the question of metabolic activation of aflatoxin B_1. Rodent liver microsomes convert the toxin to its reactive 2,3 oxide, which has been trapped as an RNA-adduct (33, 34). This system generates a product lethal and mutagenic to bacteria (35) through the production of an electrophilic derivative that reacts with cellular nucleophiles. Production of a derivative lethal to bacteria, presumably through a similar pathway, has also been observed in trout liver (36). Although the epoxide itself has not yet been isolated owing to its great reactivity, a more stable model compound, aflatoxin B_1-2,3 dichloride has been synthesized (37). This electrophilic analog of the epoxide is more potent than the parent toxin in several biological and chemical assay systems. Thus it seems likely that the epoxidation pathway may represent an important activation step in aflatoxin metabolism.

STRUCTURE-ACTIVITY RELATIONSHIPS

The aflatoxins provide an interesting set of structural homologs for investigations of relationships between chemical structure and biological activity (1). These relationships have not been systematically examined with respect to all biological and biochemical effects of the compounds, but enough work has been done to permit some general statements about this point.

Relatively few comparative carcinogenesis experiments have been done with aflatoxin other than B_1; those that have can be summarized as follows (Figs. 1 and 2). In rats, aflatoxin G_1 induces liver tumors similar to those induced by B_1, but with considerably reduced potency, and the same pattern of responses is observed in rainbow trout. In addition to liver tumors, kidney tumors are also induced in rats by G_1. Aflatoxin G_2 is inactive in trout, and has not been tested in other species.

Aflatoxin B_2 induces liver tumors in trout with the same potency as G_1, but in rats the dose level required to induce liver tumors is about 150 times the effective dose of B_1.

Aflatoxin M_1 is hepatocarcinogenic to rainbow trout with about 30% of the potency of B_1. It is also carcinogenic to rats (38), but has a greatly reduced potency compared to B_1 in that species.

Data regarding various toxic and biochemical actions of aflatoxins consistently indicate a structure-activity series with decreasing potency in the order $B_1 > G_1 > B_2 > G_2$. This generalization holds for toxicity to ducklings, rainbow trout, zebra fish larvae, chick embryos, and cultures of various mammalian cells. A similar order of potency has also been described for their ability to bind to DNA, alter biochemical processes *in vitro,* and induce functional changes in rat liver.

Collectively, this information indicates that two functionalities of the aflatoxin molecule are important determinants of its biological activities. Substituents fused to the coumarin nucleus determine activity to the extent that the G configuration is less potent than the B configuration (Figs. 1 and 2). Further indication of the importance of this part of the molecule is the fact that R_0 is less potent than B_1. Even stronger evidence exists for the importance of the dihydrofurofuran segment of aflatoxin B_1. Compounds lacking this portion of the molecule are inactive in every system tested. Moreover, reduction of the double bond of the terminal furan ring (B_1 vs. B_2; B_{2a}) brings about significant reduction of potency in most systems. These findings are consistent with the postulated importance of epoxidation as an activation mechanism. On the other hand, hydroxylation in the 4 position (B_1 vs. M_1) appears not to affect acute toxicity, but significantly reduces carcinogenic potency for rats.

For the most part, structure-activity relationships established *in vitro* agree well with those obtained *in vivo.* Continued investigations of both types should ultimately reveal the cellular and molecular bases of action of those toxins.

AFLATOXINS AND HUMAN LIVER CANCER

Direct information on the responsiveness of humans to chemicals known to be carcinogenic to animals is lacking except in a very few instances. Evaluation of the importance of chemical agents in the induction of human cancers therefore currently depends on assessment of exposure to specific carcinogens in populations with different disease incidence. Existing information of this kind has come mainly from exposures in industrial or occupational settings.

Aflatoxins are among the few chemically identified and widely disseminated environmental carcinogens for which quantitative estimates of human exposure have been systematically sought. Despite the fact that significant differences in responsiveness are known to exist among animal species, it is reasonable to assume that man might respond to either acute or chronic effects of the toxins in the event that exposure takes place through contamination of dietary components. It also seems reasonable to assume that the character and intensity of the human response might vary depending on factors such as age, sex, nutritional status, concurrent exposure to other agents (e.g., herbal medicines), genetic factors, concurrent illness (e.g., viral hepatitis or parasitic infestation) as well as level and duration of exposure to aflatoxins.

As information has accumulated on various aspects of the aflatoxin problem (4), it has become evident that the risk of exposure to aflatoxins is much less in technologically developed countries than in developing areas. The lower risk is attributable to the combined effects of several factors contributing to prevention of contamination of

Table 4   Geographical Distribution of Malignant Hepatoma in Swaziland 1964 to 1968

	Highveld	Middleveld	Lowveld
Number of cases	11	34	44
Crude rate/10^5/year	2.2	4.0	9.7
Population ratios	1.0	1.7	0.9
Relative risk	1.0	1.8	4.5
Corresponding aflatoxin assays in groundnuts			
Positive samples (%)	20	57	60

Source.   Keen and Martin (41).

foods or food raw materials. The use of such agricultural practices as rapid post-harvest drying of crops and controlled storage conditions tend to reduce mold damage in general and thereby also reduce the likelihood of aflatoxin contamination.

In societies not equipped technologically to apply such practices, the risk of aflatoxin exposure is clearly much greater. Since their discovery, reports have occasionally been made of the identification of aflatoxins in many kinds of human foods collected in various parts of the world (39, 40). Although these findings indicate the widespread geographic nature of the problem, they provide little useful information on human exposure, since samples were randomly collected and it was unknown whether they would actually have been eaten.

Information has recently become available from studies carried out by several groups of investigators in different countries of Africa and Asia. All of these investigations were designed to obtain estimates of aflatoxin intake by populations in which primary carcinoma of the liver occurs at different incidences. The pertinent findings of these investigations can be briefly summarized in the following way.

Keen and Martin (41) analyzed for aflatoxins market samples of peanuts collected in various localities within Swaziland and attempted to estimate aflatoxin intake by interviews concerning habitual patterns of peanut ingestion. Data obtained are summarized in Table 4. In the highveld

region, 20% of the peanut samples contained detectable levels of aflatoxins, whereas those from the middleveld and lowveld regions were contaminated at rates of 57% and 60%, respectively. The geographical distribution of liver cancer in Swaziland, derived from cancer registry data, are also summarized in Table 4, and the authors suggest a higher disease risk in those areas with highest frequency of aflatoxin contamination. These data provide only a general impression of a pattern of potential exposure, since measurements were made on only one dietary component and intake was not measured. The data are, however, suggestive enough to warrant further investigation.

The results of a study of somewhat similar design conducted in Uganda (42) are summarized in Table 5. In this instance, an attempt was made to collect samples of all major diet ingredients from home granaries. In all, a total of 480 food samples were analyzed during one year (1966 to 1967). Among these samples, 29.6% contained detectable amounts of aflatoxins and 3.7% contained more than 1 ppm. Most frequently contaminated diet ingredients were beans, maize, and sorghum, although most staples were contaminated to some extent. The data in Table 5 are arranged in order of decreasing frequency of aflatoxin contamination and include tribal distribution of hepatoma incidence as determined by identification of new cases. Highest incidence of the disease was recorded in tribal regions in which frequency

Table 5   Aflatoxin Contamination of Foods Versus Hepatoma Incidence in Ugandan Tribes

	Hepatoma Incidence (Cases/10^5/year)	Aflatoxin-containing Foods (%)	Number of Samples
Bwamba	No data	79	29
Karamojong	15.0	44	105
Baganda	2.0	29	149
West Nile	2.7	23	26
Acholi	2.7	15	26
Soga	2.4	10	39
Nakole	1.4	11	37

Source.   Alpert et al *(42).*

of aflatoxins contamination was also high (44% of samples). Although these data provide a somewhat clearer indication of patterns of aflatoxin intake among the tribal groups involved, accurate values for actual intakes cannot be calculated since food intake measurements were not made, nor were cooked foods analyzed.

Results of a study by Peers and Linsell (43) who investigated aflatoxin ingestion and hepatoma incidence in Kenya are summarized in Table 6. Aliquots of total diet (as eaten) and of beers (as consumed) were systematically collected and analysed for aflatoxins. In three subareas circumscribed on the basis of altitude, the frequency of contamination of diet samples varied from 4.8 to 9.5%, and of beer samples from 3 to 9%. Average aflatoxin intakes were calculated on the basis of assumed daily intakes of food and beverages. As in previous studies, the groups with higher average aflatoxin intakes also had elevated incidence of hepatoma.

A study with similar general objectives was previously completed in Thailand (44-46). The investigation was conducted in three phases, the first being a survey of market samples of foods. Over a 23-month period, 2180 samples of more than 170 varieties of foods and foodstuffs were collected from markets, mills, warehouses, distributors, farms, and homes throughout Thailand. A total of 204 (9%) of these sam-

ples were contaminated with aflatoxin (Table 7). Peanuts and corn were the most frequently contaminated foodstuffs (49% and 35% of the samples contaminated, respectively) while 11% of millet and dried chili pepper samples contained aflatoxins. Total aflatoxin concentrations in what superficially seemed to be wholesome foods or foodstuffs destined for human consumption were as high as 772 ppb in dried fish, 966 ppb in dried chili peppers, 2.7 ppm in corn, and more than 12 ppm in peanuts.

Such extensive contamination of market foods and foodstuffs was used to design a dietary survey to measure more accurately the amounts of aflatoxins actually consumed. Based on results from the market study, three areas in Thailand representing suspected high, intermediate, and low levels of contamination were chosen for such a dietary survey. Three representative villages were selected in each area and 16 families randomly chosen in each village constituted the survey population (Table 8). A portion of the diet of each family was collected and assayed for aflatoxins for three separate two-day intervals over a period of one year. Samples of as many prepared foods as were feasible were collected, and a sample of cooked rice was obtained from almost every meal of each family. In most cases, 30 to 50% of the prepared foods in the diet were analyzed.

Table 6   Daily Aflatoxin Intake and Liver Cancer Incidence in Kenya (Data for Males ≥ 16 Years Old)

	Altitude Subarea		
	High	Middle	Low
Frequency of diet contamination	39/808	54/808	78/816
Mean aflatoxin level (ppb)	0.121	0.205	0.351
Frequency of beer contamination	3/101	4/101	9/102
Mean aflatoxin level (ppb)	0.050	0.069	0.167
Mean aflatoxin ingested [a]			
ng/kg b.w./day	4.88	7.84	14.81
Liver cancer incidence	3.11	10.80	12.12

Source.   Peers and Linsel (43).
[a.] *Assuming intake of 2 kg food and 2 liters beer/day/70 kg.*

Table 7   Aflatoxin Contamination of Selected Thai Foods (Market Samples 1967 to 1969)

Foodstuff	Contamination (%)	Aflatoxin (mean)	Content (ppb) (maximum)
Peanuts	49	1530	12,256
Corn	35	400	2,730
Chili peppers	11	125	966
Millet	11	67	248
Dried fish	5	166	772
Mung beans	5	16	112
Rice	2	20	98

Source.   Shank et al (46).

As shown in Table 8, the proportion of contaminated samples was lowest in Songkhla (1%) and highest in Ratburi (16%). Similarly, levels of contamination were lowest in Songkhla (only one sample containing more than 50 ppb) and higher in the other regions.

Based on weights of cooked foods eaten at each meal, aflatoxin intake was calculated, on a family basis, for each region (Table 8). In the Singburi area, an average of 73 to 81 ng total aflatoxins per kilogram of body weight on a family basis were consumed each day. In the second area, Ratburi, the average was 45 to 77 ng/kg body wt/day; in Songkhla (the area of lowest contamination) the average was 5 to 8 ng/kg body wt/day. In a few instances, it was possible to measure the amount of aflatoxins

consumed in one day by individual members of survey families. The highest single day's consumption measured was for a 75-year-old woman who ingested aflatoxins totaling 1072 ng/kg body wt; the contaminated food in this case was cooked rice, probably leftover and resteamed several times.

The most heavily contaminated foods were a dish containing cabbage fried with pork and garlic (1.3 ppm total aflatoxins), sun dried fish (0.8 ppm total aflatoxins), and a dish containing fresh shrimp fried with pork, garlic, and chili peppers (0.4 ppm total aflatoxins). While it would not be anticipated that these foods (none of which contained peanuts) would be among the most heavily contaminated dishes, the data are consistent with the results from the

Table 8   Aflatoxin Contamination of Thai Foods (Cooked Samples in Three Regions)

	Number of Foods or Samples		
	Singburi District	Ratburi District	Songkhla District
Foods eaten	2640	2943	2008
Samples assayed	1021	1005	922
Samples contaminated	45	159	11
Aflatoxin content (ppb)			
Trace	22	129	10
< 50	4	19	0
50–100	10	7	1
100–200	3	3	0
> 200	6	1	0

Source.   Shank et al *(45).*

Table 9   Daily Aflatoxin Intake and Liver Cancer Incidence in Thailand (Data for Both Sexes ≥ 16 Years Old)

Region	Mean Aflatoxin Intake (ng/kg body wt/family)	Liver Cancer Incidence (new cases/10^5/Year)
Songkhla	5–8	2
Ratburi	45–77	6
Singburi	73–81	

Source.   Shank et al *(44).*

market study indicating significant contamination in garlic, dried chili peppers, and dried fish, all common ingredients in Thai foods.

Peanuts were found not to be common to many prepared foods in Thailand. Indeed, peanuts and peanut products were usually eaten as snacks away from home; thus it was not possible to determine aflatoxin intakes from peanut sources for this reason. However, several observations were made that are of interest to this discussion. It was noted, for example, that children consumed peanuts more frequently and in larger quantity on a body weight basis than adults. Children aged about 3 years and weighing 10 to 12 kg were observed to eat up to 250 g of shelled boiled peanuts in one day during harvest season. The aflatoxin B_1 content of boiled peanuts has been as high as 6.5 ppm; thus a 10 kg child could con-

sume as much as 163 μg aflatoxin B_1 per kilogram body weight in one day by eating 250g of such highly contaminated peanuts.

Although the absolute values of aflatoxin ingestion appear to be quantitatively small, the potency of these compounds as carcinogens in animals must be kept in mind in order to put these data into perspective. The highest values, in Singburi, based on the yearly average total aflatoxin consumption amount to 20 to 30% of comparable intakes that induce nearly 100% tumor incidence in rats following continuous exposure. Also, because these are family averages, exposures to individual family members are undoubtedly higher.

Included in Table 9 are incidence values for liver cancer in the lowest and intermediate aflatoxin intake regions. These values, calculated from new cases identified during the third phase of the study, showed a three-fold difference between the low and intermediate intake regions, being higher in Ratburi than in Songkhla. Unfortunately, incidence in the third district was not determined.

The relationship between aflatoxin intake and liver cancer incidence has recently been examined in the highest known incidence area of the world, namely the Inhambane district of Mozambique (47). Based on a hospital registration program and health record of gold miners originating from the study area, the incidence of liver carcinoma for the period 1969 to 1971 was calculated as 25.4 per 100,000 annually.

The extent of aflatoxin contamination of prepared foods consumed by the study population was determined by chemical assay of 880 meals collected at random. Aflatoxin was found in 9.3% of all samples, with a mean concentration of 7.8 g/kg food (ppb). The mean daily per capita ingestion of aflatoxins was calculated to be 222.4 ng/kg body wt (15 μg/adult/day).

Pooling of these observations with the data from similar studies in other regions reveals a significant correlation between the level of aflatoxin consumption and liver cancer incidence (Table 10). This evidence cannot be regarded as constituting unequivocal proof that aflatoxins are the single cause of liver cell carcinoma in man. However, the data are sufficient to suggest that exposure to these carcinogens substantially elevates risk of this disease and therefore warrant continued investigations into effective means for monitoring and control of their appearance as food contaminants.

REFERENCES

1. Wogan GN: Aflatoxin carcinogenesis. In *Methods in Cancer Research*, Vol 7. Busch H (Ed). Academic Press, New York, 1973, pp. 309–344.

2. Rodricks JV: Fungal metabolites which contain substituted 7,8-dihydrofuro (2,3-b) furans (DHFF) and 2,3,7,8-tetrahydrofuro (2,3-b) furans (THFF). *J Agric Food Chem* **17**:457–461, 1969.

3. Wogan GN: Biochemical responses to aflatoxins. *Cancer Res* **28**:2282–2287, 1968.

4. Goldblatt LA: *Aflatoxin: Scientific Background, Control, and Implications*. Academic Press, New York, 1969, 472 pp.

5. Detroy RW, Lillehoj EB, Ciegler A: Aflatoxin and related compounds. In *Microbial Toxins*, Vol 6. Ciegler A, Kadis S, Ajl SJ (Eds). Academic Press, New York, 1971, pp. 4–178.

6. Wogan GN, Paglialunga S, Newberne PM: Carcinogenic effects of low dietary levels of aflatoxin B1 in rats. *Food Cosmet Toxicol* **12**:681–685, 1974.

7. Nixon JE, Sinnhuber RO, Lee DJ, et al: Effect of cyclopropenoid compounds on the carcinogenic activity of diethylnitrosamine and aflatoxin B1 in rats. *J Natl Cancer Inst* **53**:453–458, 1974.

8. Newberne PM, Wogan GN: Potentiating effects of low-protein diets on effect of aflatoxin in rats. *Toxicol Appl Pharmacol* **11**:51A, 1969.

9. Butler WH: Aflatoxicosis in laboratory animals. In *Aflatoxin: Scientific Background, Control and Implications*. Goldblatt LA (Ed). Academic Press, New York, 1969, pp 223–236.

10. Newberne PM, Butler WH: Acute and chronic effects of aflatoxin on the liver of domestic and laboratory animals: A review. *Cancer Res* **29**:236–250, 1969.

Table 10 Summary of Current Evidence on Aflatoxin Intake and Liver Cancer Incidence

Population	Aflatoxin Intake (ng/kg body wt/day)	Liver Cancer Incidence (cases/10⁵/year)
Kenya—high altitude	4.88	3.11
Thailand—Songkhla	5.00	2.00
Kenya—middle altitude	7.84	10.80
Kenya—low altitude	14.81	12.12
Thailand—Ratburi	45.00	6.0
Mozambique—Inhambane	222.40	25.4

11. Butler WH, Barnes JM: Carcinoma of the glandular stomach in rats given diets containing aflatoxin. *Nature (Lond)* **209**:90, 1966.

12. Wogan GN, Newberne PM: Dose-response characteristics of aflatoxin B_1 carcinogenesis in the rat. *Cancer Res* **27**:2370–2376, 1967.

13. Newberne PM, Rogers AE: Rat colon carcinomas associated with aflatoxin and marginal vitamin A. *J Natl Cancer Inst* **50**:439–448, 1973.

14. Madhavan TV, Gopalan C: The effect of dietary protein on carcinogenesis of aflatoxin. *Arch Pathol* **85**:133–137, 1968.

15. Newberne PM, Harrington DH, Wogan GN: Effects of cirrhosis and other liver insults on induction of liver tumors by aflatoxin in rats. *Lab Invest* **15**:962–969, 1966.

16. Rogers AE, Newberne PM: Aflatoxin B_1 carcinogenesis in lipo trope-deficient rats. *Cancer Res* **29**: 1965–1972, 1969.

17. Rogers AE, Newberne PM: Nutrition and aflatoxin carcinogenesis. *Nature (Lond)* **229**:62–63, 1971.

18. Goodall CM, Butler WH: Aflatoxin carcinogenesis: Inhibition of liver cancer induction in hypophysectomized rats. *Int J Cancer* **4**:422–429, 1969.

19. Newberne PM, Williams G: Inhibition of aflatoxin carcinogenesis by diethylstilbestrol in male rats. *Arch Environ Health* **19**:489–498, 1969.

20. Rogers AE, Kula NS, Newberne PM: Absence of an effect of partial hepatectomy on aflatoxin B_1 carcinogenesis. *Cancer Res* **31**:491–495, 1971.

21. Newberne PM, Hunt CE, Wogan GN: Neoplasms in the rat associated with administration of urethan and aflatoxin. *Exp Mol Pathol* **6**:285–299, 1967.

22. Wogan GN, Edwards GS, Newberne PM: Structure activity relationships in toxicity and carcinogenicity of aflatoxins and analogs. *Cancer Res* **31**:1936–1942, 1971.

23. Reddy JK, Svoboda D: Effect of lasiocarpine on aflatoxin B_1 carcinogenicity in rat liver. *Arch Pathol* **93**:55–60, 1972.

24. McLean AEM, Marshall A: Reduced carcinogenic effects of aflatoxin in rats given phenobarbitone. *Brit J Exp Pathol* **52**:322–329, 1971.

25. Wogan GN: Metabolism and biochemical effects of aflatoxins. In *Aflatoxin: Scientific Background, Control and Implications*. Goldblatt LA (Ed). Academic Press, New York, 1969, pp. 151–186.

26. Patterson DSP: Metabolism as a factor in determining the toxic action of the aflatoxins in different animal species. *Food Cosmet Toxicol* **11**:287–294, 1973.

27. Dalezios JI, Wogan GN, Weinreb S: Aflatoxin P_1: A new aflatoxin metabolite in monkeys. *Science* **171**:584–585, 1971.

28. Dalezios JI, Hsieh DPH, Wogan GN: Excretion and metabolism of orally administered aflatoxin B_1 by rhesus monkeys. *Food Cosmet Toxicol* **11**:605–616, 1973.

29. Mabee MS, Chipley JR: Tissue distribution and metabolism of aflatoxin B_1-^{14}C in broiler chickens. *Appl Microbiol* **25**:763–769, 1973.

30. Mabee MS, Chipley JR: Tissue distribution and metabolism of aflatoxin B_1-^{14}C in layer chickens. *J Food Sci* **38**:566–570, 1973.

31. Masri MS, Haddon WF, Lundin RE, et al: Aflatoxin Q_1: A newly identified major metabolite of aflatoxin B_1 in monkey liver. *J Agric Food Chem* **22**:512–515, 1974.

32. Büchi GH, Muller PM, Roebuck BD, et al: Aflatoxin Q_1: A major metabolite of aflatoxin B_1 produced by human liver. *Res Commun Chem Pathol Pharmacol* **8**:585–592, 1974.

33. Garner RC: Microsome-dependent binding of aflatoxin B_1 to DNA, RNA, polyribonucleotides and protein *in vitro*. *Chem Biol Interactions* **6**:125–129, 1973.

34. Garner RC: Chemical evidence for the formation of a reactive aflatoxin B_1 metabolite, by hamster liver microsomes. *FEBS Lett* **36**:261–264, 1973.

35. Garner RC, Miller EC, Miller JA: Liver microsomal metabolism of aflatoxin B_1 to a reactive derivative of *Salmonella typhimurium* TA 1530. *Cancer Res* **32**:2058–2066, 1972.

36. Schoenhard GL, Lee DJ, Sinnhuber RO: Aflatoxin B_1 activation and aflatoxicol toxicity in rainbow trout *(Salmo gairdneri)*. *Fed Proc* **33**:247, 1974.

37. Swenson DH, Miller EC, Miller JA: Aflatoxin B_1-2,3-oxide: Evidence for its formation in rat liver *in vivo* and by human liver microsomes *in vitro*. *Biochem Biophys Res Commun* **60**:1036–1043, 1974.

38. Wogan GN, Paglialunga S: Carcinogenicity of synthetic aflatoxin M_1 in rats. *Food Cosmet Toxicol* **12**:381–384, 1974.

39. Wogan GN: Aflatoxin risks and control measures. *Fed Proc* **27**:932–937, 1968.

40. Barnes JM: Aflatoxin as a health hazard. *J Appl Bacteriol* **33**:285–298, 1970.

41. Keen P, Martin P: Is aflatoxin carcinogenic in man? The evidence in Swaziland. *Trop Geog Med* **23**:44–53, 1971.

42. Alpert ME, Hutt MSR, Wogan GN, et al: Association between aflatoxin content of food and hepatoma frequency in Uganda. *Cancer* **28**:253–260, 1971.

43. Peers FG, Linsell CA: Dietary aflatoxin and liver cancer: A population based study in Kenya. *Brit J Cancer* **27**:473–484, 1973.

44. Shank RC, Bhamarapravati N, Gordon JE, et al: Dietary aflatoxins and human liver cancer. IV. Incidence of primary liver cancer in two municipal populations of Thailand. *Food Cosmet Toxicol* **10**:171–179, 1972.

45. Shank RC, Gordon JE, Wogan GN, et al: Dietary aflatoxins and human liver cancer. III. Field survey of rural Thai families for ingested aflatoxins. *Food Cosmet Toxicol* **10**:71–84, 1972.

46. Shank RC, Wogan GN, Gibson JB, et al: Dietary aflatoxins and human liver cancer. II. Aflatoxins in market foods and foodstuffs of Thailand and Hong Kong. *Food Cosmet Toxicol* **10**:61–69, 1972.

47. van Rensburg SJ, van der Watt JJ, Purchase IFH, et al: Primary liver cancer rate and aflatoxin intake in a high cancer area. *S Afr Med J* **48**:2508a–d, 1974.

48. Svoboda D, Grady H, Higginson J: Aflatoxin B_1 injury in rat and monkey liver. *Am J Pathol* **49**:1023–1051, 1966.

49. Epstein SM, Bartus B, Farber E: Renal epithelial neoplasms induced in male Wistar rats by oral aflatoxin B_1. *Cancer Res* **29**:1045–1050, 1969.

50. Vesselinovich SD, Mihailovich N, Wogan GN et al: Aflatoxin B_1, a hepatocarcinogen in the infant mouse. *Cancer Res* **32**:2289–2291, 1972.

51. Gopalan C, Tulpule PG, Krishnamurthi D: Induction of hepatic carcinoma with aflatoxin in the rhesus monkey. *Food Cosmet Toxicol* **10**:519–521, 1972.

52. Adamson RH, Correa P, Dalgard DW: Occurrence of a primary liver carcinoma in a rhesus monkey fed aflatoxin B_1. *J Natl Cancer Inst* **50**:549–553, 1973.

53. Lin JJ, Liu C, Svoboda DJ: Long term effects of aflatoxin B_1 and viral hepatitis on marmoset liver. A preliminary report. *Lab Invest* **30**:267–278, 1974.

54. Carnaghan RBA: Hepatic tumours in ducks fed a low level of toxic groundnut meal. *Nature (Lond)* **208**:308, 1965.

55. Sinnhuber RO, Lee DJ, Wales JH, et al: Dietary factors and hepatoma in rainbow trout *(Salmo gairdnerii)*. II. Cocarcinogenesis by cyclopropenoid fatty acids and the effect of gossypol and altered lipids on aflatoxin-induced liver cancer. *J Natl Cancer Inst* **41**:1293–1299, 1968.

56. Sinnhuber RO, Wales JH: Aflatoxin B_1 hepatocarcinogenicity in rainbow trout embryos. *Fed Proc* **33**:247, 1974.

57. Wales JH, Sinnhuber RO: Hepatomas induced by aflatoxin in the sockeye salmon *(Oncorhynchus nerka)*. *J Natl Cancer Inst* **48**:1529–1530, 1972.

58. Sato S, Matsushima T, Tanaka N, et al: Hepatic tumors in the guppy *(Lebistes reticulatus)* induced by aflatoxin B_1, dimethylnitrosamine and 2-acetylaminofluorene. *J Natl Cancer Inst* **50**:765–778, 1973.

CHAPTER 3

GENETIC AND FAMILIAL ASPECTS OF LIVER CIRRHOSIS AND HEPATOCELLULAR CARCINOMA

AKIRA OHBAYASHI, M.D.

Except for the rare inherited diseases in which cirrhosis develops, the etiologic factors for the more common types of cirrhosis as well as hepatocellular carcinoma (HCC) in man have long been considered to be environmental rather than genetic. In experimental animals, however, genetic susceptibilities to cirrhosis (1, 2, 3) and also to hepatoma (4, 5) are already recognized. Recently, a trend of these diseases to appear in families is being realised in humans. Therefore, our study on familial clustering of cirrhosis and hepatoma is presented here with a discussion of the possible involvement of genetics as a predisposing factor or factors.

FAMILIAL CIRRHOSIS WITH OR WITHOUT HEPATOMA

Familial occurrence of cryptogenic cirrhosis in adults has only rarely been reported in the literature of Europe and the United States, except for the observations by Iber and Maddrey (6). In Japan, however, there have been reports on 10 families with clustering of chronic liver disease during the past decade from 1963 to 1972 (7–14). In these families, chronic hepatitis, cirrhosis of the liver, and HCC occurred frequently among adult members (Table 1). Of the 39 affected members of the 10 families, 11 died of cirrhosis and 9 died of cirrhosis with HCC. The other 5 died with a diagnosis of liver cancer, although it could not be confirmed by autopsy.

In these reported cases, the onset of the disease was usually insidious, and symptoms such as jaundice or ascites appeared either at the advanced stage of cirrhosis or at the time of well-developed liver cancer. The clinical features were of the usual cryptogenic cirrhosis.

It is noteworthy that a successive occurrence of the disease for two generations was recognized in 7 of the 10 families, and

Table 1 Familial Occurrence of Cirrhosis and Liver Cancer in Adults Reported in Japan from 1963–1972.

Reporter	Patient	Sex	Age of Diagnosis or Death	Diagnosis
Tokuda (7)	Mother[a]		69	Cirrhosis
	*2nd sib	M	40	Cirrhosis
	3rd sib[a]	M	38	Cirrhosis
Ueda et al (8)	Mother[a]	M	48	Cirrhosis
	1st sib[a]	F	44	Liver cancer
	*2nd sib	M	41	Cirrhosis[c]
	3rd sib[a]	F	34	Cirrhosis with liver cancer[c]
	4th sib[a]		28	Liver cancer
	5th sib			Chronic hepatitis
	Father[a]		37	Liver cancer
	Mother[a]	F	48	Cirrhosis
	1st sib[a]	M	44	Cirrhosis
	*2nd sib[a]	M	47	Cirrhosis with liver cancer[c]
	5th sib		42	Chronic hepatitis[c]
Morimoto et al (9)	Maternal aunt[a]	F	50	Cirrhosis with liver cancer[c]
	1st sib[a]	M	48	Cirrhosis with liver cancer
	*3rd sib[a]	M	41	Cirrhosis with liver cancer[c]
	5th sib[a]	M	38	Cirrhosis with liver cancer[c]
	6th sib	F		Chronic hepatitis
Yuta et al (10)	*1st half sib[a,d]	M	36	Cirrhosis with liver cancer[c]
	2nd half sib[a,d]	M	46	Cirrhosis with liver cancer[c]

Reference	Relationship	Sex	Age	Diagnosis
Fukuhara et al (11)	*Mother[a]		54	Postnecrotic cirrhosis[c]
	3rd sib[a]	M	19	Postnecrotic cirrhosis[c]
	4th sib	M		Jaundice and hepatic dysfunction
Wada et al (12)	*1st sib[a]	M	42	Postnecrotic cirrhosis[c]
	2nd sib[a]	M	38	Postnecrotic cirrhosis[c]
Ohbayashi et al (13, 14)	Mother[a]	F	54	Cirrhosis
	1st sib[a]	F	36	Liver cancer
	*2nd sib	M	41	Chronic aggressive hepatitis[c]
	4th sib	M	35	Chronic aggressive hepatitis[c]
	5th sib	F	28	Postnecrotic cirrhosis[c]
	*2nd sib	F	58	Cirrhosis
	5th sib[a]	M	47	Liver cancer
	9th sib	M	41	Postnecrotic cirrhosis[c]
	Mother[a]		49	Liver cancer
	Maternal uncle[a]		56	Liver cancer
	Maternal uncle[a]		61	Liver cancer
	*3rd sib[a]	M	38	Cirrhosis with liver cancer[c]

[a] Dead.
[b] Proband indicated by asterisk (*).
[c] Morphologically confirmed by autopsy or biopsy.
[d] Brothers from same mother but different fathers.

the mother and/or her siblings were inevitably affected in all of these 7 families.

Ohbayashi et al (14) in testing for hepatitis B antigen (HBAg) by means of the immune adherence hemagglutination method (15), found that in such families many carriers of HBAg, either symptom-free or with obvious chronic liver disease, cluster principally on the maternal lines of their pedigrees (Fig. 1).

Since this discovery, such families have been successively identified in Japan. Therefore, it is likely in retrospect that nearly all the patients in these families studied in the past, as shown in Table 1, were associated with HBAg also. Similar families were also reported in Chile (16) and the United States (17).

A summary of the results of HBAg tests on the five families observed up to 1973 by Ohbayashi et al are given in Table 2. Out of 26 siblings, 25 (96%) were positive for HBAg, and 26 of the 33 offspring of

Table 2 Prevalence of HBAg in Five Families with Multiple Occurrence of Cirrhosis and Hepatoma

Relation to Probands	Cumulative Number (Positive/Total)
Father	0/1
[a] Mother	0/1
Paternal uncle	0/1
Maternal uncles	2/2
Siblings	25/26(96%)
Male siblings	8/8
Female siblings	17/18
Spouses	0/10
Children of male siblings	4/12(34%)
Children of female siblings	26/33(79%)
Spouses	0/2
Children of HBAg-positive daughters	0/3

[a] Only a few were alive.

the female siblings (79%) were also positive. In contrast, positive tests were obtained in 4 (34%) of the 12 offspring of the male siblings, and in none of the 10 spouses of the siblings so far tested (18). Thus the majorities of the HBAg-positive individuals in the five kindreds were on the maternal lines of their pedigrees as well as the patients themselves as shown in Table 1.

These observations suggest that, in such families, infections with hepatitis B (HB) virus occurred frequently among family members, principally from mother to child, and that many of the infected persons became carriers of HBAg—some of them developed chronic hepatitis, cirrhosis of the liver, and eventual HCC in their adult ages.

Ohbayashi and Mayumi (19) have lately determined HBAg subtypes of the familial carriers with respect to adr, adw, ayr, and ayw (20, 21). In four families so far studied, the subtypes were always identical within each family: adr in 7, 8, and 11 carriers from three families, and adw in 5 carriers from the other family. These results are highly suggestive that infections with HB virus were intrafamilial.

The hypothesis of maternal transmission of HB virus has already gained support from many publications demonstrating that infants who were born of HBAg-positive mothers, whether with acute hepatitis or symptom-free, developed acute type B hepatitis or became persistent carriers of HBAg (22–29). According to the observations in Japan (25) and Taiwan (26), about 40% of infants born of asymptomatic, HBAg-positive mothers became positive for HBAg within their several months of life, and the majority subsequently developed a chronic carrier state of HBAg. Schweitzer et al (27–29) have also reported that mother-to-infant transmission of HB virus was recognized with an extremely high rate (76%) in the subjects whose mothers had acute type B hepatitis during the third trimester of pregnancy or within

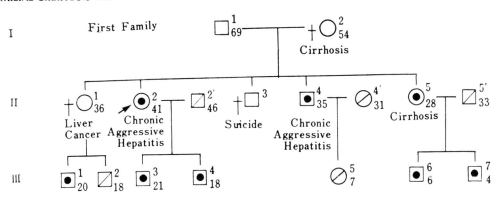

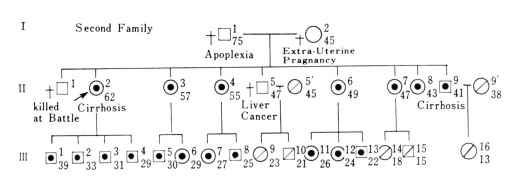

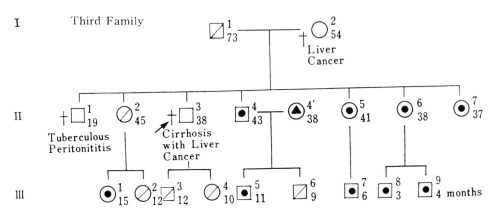

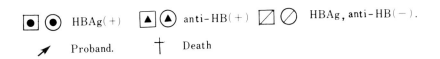

FIGURE 1 Detection of HBAg in three families with clustering of chronic liver disease.

two months after delivery, and that once the infants became positive for HBAg, it persisted in all except two babies who had overt, acute hepatitis. These bits of evidence suggest that primary infection with HB virus in the neonatal period leads the host to a chronic carrier-state of the virus or, if rephrased, that newborns are in a state prone to develop immunological tolerance to HB virus.

As for the mode of maternal transmission of HB virus, three routes are now considered (30): transplacental transmission, oral contamination from the mother's blood during delivery, and postpartum oral transmission as a result of close contact. These three possibilities are supported by the fact that HBAg was detected in some cord sera from HBAg-positive mothers, and that even newborns with a HBAg-negative test in the cord serum frequently became positive for HBAg later (25–29).

Thus, it seems that familial clustering of HB antigenemia develops principally as a result of maternal transmission of HB virus. However, infection to infant by a close contact with the father or the other family members and close relatives harboring HBAg can by no means be ignored since the offspring of the fathers with HBAg were found positive for HBAg with a relatively high rate as mentioned above.

However, even though chronic carriage of HBAg is relatively easily established by infection in early life, it may be difficult to explain by this reason alone the extremely high, familial clustering of chronic HB antigenemia. Since 1967 Blumberg and his co-workers (31) have asserted that susceptibility to persistence of HBAg is controlled by a genetic trait. They have also found lately in a study of 109 families collected from five different locations that there was a higher frequency of HBAg in offspring of families with positive mothers and negative fathers than in offspring of positive fathers and negative mothers. However, if only families with HBAg-negative parents were considered, the data

were consistent with the hypothesis of autosomal recessive inheritance. From these observations, Sutnick (32), one of Blumberg's co-workers, has recently reasoned that the mechanism for the development of HBAg persistence is by autosomal recessive inheritance with a superimposed factor of maternal transmission. As additional evidence against the hypothesis of intrafamilial infection alone, he cited that, of 32 families with the clustering of HB antigenemia in Bougainville, 11 families had different subtypes of HBAg among the family members. However, to give a satisfactory explanation for this problem further studies are definitely needed.

Incidentally, our recent observations have shown that, among families with clustering of HB antigenemia, there are large differences in the frequency of chronic liver disease. Some families have multiple occurrence of cirrhosis and HCC as described here, and others have only a few or no obvious chronic liver disease. Moreover, among the families with high incidences of both HB antigenemia and liver disease, the occurrence rates of hepatoma are different. Such familial differences in the incidence of chronic liver disease and hepatoma suggest that some genetic predispositions to cirrhosis and to hepatoma do exist.

Iber and Maddrey (6) asserted for the first time in the United States that familial cryptogenic cirrhosis is not so rare, and they even stated that alcoholic cirrhosis would occur familially. It was concluded on these observations that the heredity in their family cases was compatible with an autosomal recessive mode of transmission.

Familial autoimmune hepatitis reported by Australian investigators in recent years is also of interest. Whittingham et al (33) described a family that had two cases of autoimmune-type chronic hepatitis, one case of chronic persistent hepatitis, and one case of myasthenia gravis. Joske and Laurence (34) reported a kindred in which five members had chronic liver disease with abnormal immunological findings and eight others had abnormal immunological findings without liver disease—one of the five affected members subsequently died of HCC arising in a cirrhotic liver (35). There was a sibship aggregation of typical lupoid hepatitis reported by Hilberg et al (36) in the United States, in which two white sisters had active chronic hepatitis and positive lupus erythematosus preparations at ages of 18 and 15 years, respectively.

Regarding the cause of familial occurrence of autoimmune hepatitis, Whittingham et al (33) have suggested that a combination of three processes is required to account for the disease in a family: a genetic predisposition to chronic liver disease in particular, a genetic predisposition to autoimmune reaction in general, and "triggering" effect of infection with hepatitis virus. Dudley et al (37) have explained the pathogenesis of liver damage associated with HBAg as follows: the development of viral hepatitis must depend on a complex interaction between HB virus and the immune response of the host, particularly cell-mediated immunity. Chronic hepatitis is associated with persistence of HB virus and inadequate T-cell function. If this hypothesis is correct, there may exist a genetic factor such as one which is associated with an inadequate immunological response to HB virus, allowing it to persist in the host. The hypothetical genetic susceptibility may be accentuated in certain individuals and also in certain families.

There have recently been a few papers that attempted to study familial or racial differences in the occurrence of serologic abnormalities usually associated with autoimmune chronic liver diseases. Feizi et al (38) reported that mitochondrial antibodies were found in 7% of 126 close relatives of 27 patients with primary biliary cirrhosis, while none of healthy controls paired with them for sex and age comparisons were positive for this antibody. Whittingham et al (39) have also recognized higher prevalence of autoantibodies (antinuclear antibody, smooth muscle antibody, and mi-

tochondrial antibody) among patients with "idiopathic" chronic liver disease from Australia than among the patients from other parts of Asia, and they have inferred that the variations in chronic liver disease associated with autoimmune markers between races are related to genetic differences that have evolved between peoples of European and Asian descent. Mackay and Morris (40) have also found that among Australian Caucasian patients with active chronic hepatitis, there was a high frequency of two histocompatibility antigens, HL-A1 and HL-A8 (60% and 68%, respectively). Based on these observations, Whittingham et al (39) have discussed that genetic differences expressed through histocompatibility antigens could account for differences in racial prevalence of disease in general, and for the autoimmune type of active chronic hepatitis in particular. Further surveys on families of patients with chronic liver disease and HCC are needed for understanding of the interplay of immunity with neoplasia.

FAMILIAL HEPATOCELLULAR CARCINOMA WITHOUT CIRRHOSIS

Hepatocellular carcinoma without cirrhosis per se is relatively rare in humans. Edmondson and Steiner (41) reported that 89.2% of HCC in the United States were complicated by cirrhosis of the liver. Nevertheless, a few instances of familial occurrence of hepatomas without cirrhosis have been reported.

Kaplan and Cole (42) described three Jewish male siblings who had HCC at the ages of 64, 59, and 64 years. Hagstrom and Barker (43) reported another case of familial occurrence of HCC in which three Caucasian male siblings were affected at the ages of 11, 22, and 31 years. In these cases, there had been no cirrhosis or other conditions known to be related to this neoplasm, such as hepatitis, hemochromatosis, and parasitic or syphilitic liver disease, nor was there a clue to the pathogenesis in personal, family, and environmental studies. Since no clear hint was obtained in these cases regarding the etiology, genetic susceptibility, or common exposures to hepatocarcinogens, as yet unknown, both hereditary and environmental factors would have to be considered.

No familial clustering of HCC without cirrhosis or other preexisting hepatic changes has as yet been reported in Japan, and the relationship between HBAg and HCC without cirrhosis or fibrosis is still largely unknown.

Also of interest is a sibship aggregation of hepatoblastoma reported by Fraumeni et al (44), in which two Caucasian infant sisters out of four siblings were affected in a family. In this case, however, there was no evidence to clarify an etiological relationship.

REFERENCES

1. Gillespie RJG, Lucas CG: Different response to the production of dietary and alcoholic cirrhosis in "Webster" rats from two sources. *Can J Biochem* **39**:249–255, 1961.

2. Kalow W: Genetic differences in drug metabolism. *Ann N Y Acad Sci* **104**:894–904, 1963.

3. Patek AJ, DeFritsch NM: Evidence for genetic factors in the resistence of the rate to dietary cirrhosis. *Pro Soc Exp Biol (N Y)* **113**:820–824, 1963.

4. Heston WE, Vlahakis G: Influence of the A^y—A high hepagene on mammary-gland tumors, hepatoma, and normal growth in mice. *J. Natl Cancer Inst* **26**:969–982, 1961.

5. Heston WE, Vlahakis G: C3H-A^{vy}— A high hepatoma and high mammary tumor strain of mice. *J Natl Cancer Inst* **40**:1161–1166, 1968.

6. Iber FL, Maddrey WC: Familial hepatic diseases with portal hypertension with or without cirrhosis. In *Progress in Liver Diseases,* Vol 2. Popper H, Schaffner F (Eds). Grune & Stratton, New York, 1965, p. 290–302.

7. Tokuda M: Multiple occurrence of cirrhosis in a family (in Japanese) *J Ehime Prefect Hosp* **1**:68–72, 1963.

8. Ueda H, Kameda H, Harada S, et al: Familial chronic liver disease (in Japanese). *J Jap Soc Intern Med* **54**:675, 1965.

9. Morimoto Y, Okochi J, Higashino K, et al: Familial cirrhosis with hepatoma (in Japanese). *J Jap Soc Intern Med* **58**:89, 1969.

10. Yuta K, Yasui S, Katoh J, et al: Cirrhosis with hepatoma in two uterine brothers (in Japanese). *Acta Hepatol Jap* **10**:592, 1969.

11. Fukuhara G, Ohi M, Ishihara H, et al: Two cases of cirrhosis of the liver in a family (in Japanese). *J Jap Soc Intern Med* **59**:366, 1970.

12. Wada M, Nakai Y, Hananouchi M, et al: Cirrhosis of the liver occurring in siblings (in Japanese). *Jap J Gastroenterol* **67**:280, 1970.

13. Ohbayashi A, Yoshinaka M, Gotoh N, et al: Active chronic hepatitis and post-necrotic cirrhosis occurring in three siblings—Some notes on familial cryptogenic cirrhosis (in Japanese). *Jap J Clin Med* **27**:2592–2601, 1969. *Advance Abstracts of Fourth Congress of Gastroenterology, 1970, p. 179.*

14. Ohbayashi A, Okochi K, Mayumi M: Familial clustering of asymptomatic carriers of Australia antigen and patients with chronic liver disease or primary liver cancer. *Gastroenterology* **62**:618–623, 1971.

15. Mayumi M, Okochi K, Nishioka K: Detection of Australia antigen by means of immune adherence hemagglutination test. *Vox Sang* **20**:178–181, 1972.

16. Velasco M, Sorenson R, Carmona A, et al: Australia antigen and primary carcinoma of the liver. *Gastroenterology* **60**:729, 1971.

17. Denison EK, Peters RL, Reynold TB: Familial hepatoma with hepatitis-associated antigen. *Ann Intern Med* **74**:391–394, 1971.

18. Ohbayashi A, Nakamura Y, Kakehi K: Familial clustering of HB antigenemia and of chronic liver disease and hepatoma. *Abstracts of International Symposium on Hepatitis in Taipei, 1974, p. 2.*

19. Ohbayashi A, Mayumi M: HBAg subtypes in familial carriers. *Lancet* **1**:507, 1974.

20. Le Bouvier G: The heterogeneity of Australia antigen. *J Infect Dis* **123**:671–675, 1971.

21. Bancroft WH, Mundon FK, Russel PK: Determination of additional antigenic determinants of hepatitis B antigen. *J Immunol* **109**:842–848, 1972.

22. Schweitzer IL, Spears RL: Hepatitis-associated antigen in mother and infant. *New Engl J Med* **283**:570–572, 1970.

23. Wright R, Perkins JR, Bower BD, et al: Cirrhosis associated with the Australia antigen in an infant who acquired hepatitis from her mother. *Brit Med J* **2**:719–721, 1970.

24. Gillespie A, Dorman D, Walker-Smith JA, et al: Neonatal hepatitis and Australia antigen. *Lancet* **2**:1081, 1971.

25. Okuda K: Maternal transmission of Australia an-

tigen. *Regional Meeting on Australia Antigen and Hepatocellular Carcinoma.* National Cancer Center Research Institute, Tokyo, December 7, 1971.

26. Stevens CE, Tu'si J, Beasley RP: Vertical transmission of hepatitis B antigen in Taiwan. *Abstracts of International Symposium on Hepatitis in Taipei,* 1974, p. 1–2.

27. Schweitzer IL, Wing A, MacPeck C, et al: Hepatitis and hepatitis-associated antigen in 56 mother-infant pairs. *JAMA* **220**:1092–1095, 1972.

28. Schweitzer IL, Mosley JW, Ashcarai M, et al: Factors influencing neonatal infection by hepatitis B virus. *Gastroenterology* **65**:277–283, 1973.

29. Schweitzer IL, Dunn AEG, Peters RL, et al: Viral hepatitis B in neonates and infants. *Am J Med* **55**:762–771, 1973.

30. Zuckerman AJ: *Hepatitis-associated Antigen and Viruses.* North-Holland Publishing Co., Amsterdam, London, p. 618.

31. Blumberg B, Friedlander J, Woodside A, et al: Hepatitis and Australia antigen: Autosomal recessive inheritance of susceptibility to infection in humans. *Proc Natl Acad Sci USA* **102**:1108–1115, 1969.

32. Sutnick AI: Australia antigen and the immune response in human diseases. *J Allergy Clin Immunol* **55**:42–51, 1974.

33. Whittingham S, Mackay IR, Kiss ZS: An interplay of genetic and environmental factors in familial hepatitis and myastenia gravis. *Gut* **11**:811–816, 1970.

34. Joske RA, Laurence BH: Familial cirrhosis with autoimmune features and raised immunoglobulin levels. *Gastroenterology* **59**:546–552, 1970.

35. Joske RA, Laurence BH, Matz LR: Familial active chronic hepatitis with hepatocellular carcinoma. *Gastroenterology* **62**:441–444, 1972.

36. Hilberg RW, Mulhern LM, Kenny JJ, et al: Chronic active hepatitis. Report of two sisters with erythematose preparations. *Ann Intern Med* **74**:937–941, 1971.

37. Dudley BS, Fox RA, Sherlock S: Cellular immunity and hepatitis-associated antigen-liver disease. *Lancet* **1**:723–726, 1972.

38. Feizi T, Naccarato R, Sherlock S, et al: Mitochondrial and other tissue antibodies in relatives of patients with primary biliary cirrhosis. *Clin Exp Immunol* **10**:609–622, 1972.

39. Whittingham S, Mackay IR, Thanabalasundrum RS, et al: Chronic liver disease: Differences in autoimmune serological reactions between Australians and Asians. *Brit Med J* **4**:517–519, 1973.

40. Mackay IR, Morris PJ: Association of autoimmune active chronic hepatitis with HL-A1, 8. *Lancet* **2**:793–795, 1972.

41. Edmondson HA, Steiner PE: Primary carcinoma of the liver. A study of 100 cases among 48,900 necropsies. *Cancer* **7**:462–503, 1954.

42. Kaplan L, Cole SL: Fraternal primary hepatocellular carcinoma in three male, adult siblings. *Am J Med* **39**:305–311, 1965.

43. Hagstrom RM, Barker TD: Primary hepatocellular carcinomas in three male siblings. *Cancer* **22**:142–150, 1968.

44. Fraumeni JF, Rosen PJ, Hull EW, et al: Hepatoblastoma in infant sisters. *Cancer* **24**:1086–1090, 1969.

CHAPTER 4

PRIMARY LIVER CARCINOMA AND LIVER CIRRHOSIS

TOSHIO SHIKATA, M.D.

INTRODUCTION

It has long been accepted that cirrhosis of the liver has an intimate causal relationship with hepatocellular carcinoma (HCC) since they are frequently associated with each other. However, the relationship of cirrhosis to HCC must be studied with other variables in mind.

1. *Morphologic type of liver carcinoma.* Most investigators undertaking epidemiologic studies of liver cancer have grouped all primary hepatic malignancies together. Although HCC and cholangiocarcinoma constitute the primary epithelial malignancies of the liver, they are quite different, not only in geographic distribution but in clinical and pathologic features as well. They probably differ in etiology and should be considered separately in their relationship to cirrhosis which is present in more than 80% of patients with HCC. In contrast, cirrhosis is found in only 10 to 20% of patients with cholangiocarcinoma. Hepatocellular carcinoma is usually related to coarsely nodular types of cirrhosis, whereas cholangiocarcinoma may be associated with chronic cholangitis, biliary cirrhosis, or bile duct parasitosis.

Chemical carcinogens have been reported to induce cholangiocarcinoma and HCC under similar experimental conditions, even in the same animal (1). However, the experimental adenomatous neoplasm, designated as cholangiocarcinoma, may be thought of as a variant of hepatocellular carcinoma derived from parenchymal cells. The true cholangiocarcinoma is less common in experimental hepatocarcinogenesis (2, 3).

In humans, combination of both types of carcinoma as well as adenomatous variants of hepatocellular carcinoma that resemble cholangiocarcinoma are rather rare. Very few cases of primary liver carcinomas are microtubular and because they are believed to arise from cholangioles (rather than ductal epithelium or hepatocytes), they are designated cholangiolocellular carcinomas. However, most of the human cholangiocarcinomas are ductal or cystopapillary adenocarcinoma and histologically resemble extrahepatic bile duct carcinoma, gallbladder carcinoma, and pancreatic carcinoma. They are less frequently associated with cirrhosis, except for biliary cirrhosis. Thus it may be inferred that hepatocellular carcinoma and cholangiocarcinoma have different causal factors in man and warrant separate considerations.

2. *Geographic features.* Association of HCC and cirrhosis varies geographically. For instance, 40 to 50% of livers with cirrhosis give rise to HCC in Africa and Southeast Asia which is in sharp contrast to Europe and the United States where the corresponding figure is only 5 to 10%. The difference is accounted for in part by the predominant type of cirrhosis which varies from country to country. Therefore, one has to analyse the associated cirrhosis very carefully.

3. *Hepatocellular carcinoma and precirrhotic changes.* In the study of the relation between HCC and cirrhosis, one has to give special attention to liver fibrosis. HCC is not only closely associated with fully developed cirrhosis, but also with incomplete cirrhosis in which fibrous tissue is increased in the portal area, connecting with each other in places but not completely forming pseudolobules as yet. Furthermore, HCC even develops in livers with slight fibrosis. Such incomplete cirrhosis and hepatic fibrosis are probably an abortive form of cirrhosis, sharing some etiologic features with fully developed cirrhosis. Therefore, it is more appropriate to divide HCC into those with cirrhosis or fibrosis and those without cirrhosis or fibrosis, instead of into HCC with or without cirrhosis. At least, some of the HCC without cirrhosis or fibrosis may have a different etiology.

GEOGRAPHICAL CONSIDERATIONS OF LIVER CIRRHOSIS AND FREQUENCY OF ITS ASSOCIATION WITH HEPATOCELLULAR CARCINOMA

Incidence of hepatocellular carcinoma in cirrhotic livers

The incidence of liver cirrhosis varies considerably from country to country, as evidenced by the mortality rates ranging from 3 to 35 per 100,000 population (4). The incidences are highest in the south European countries, especially France, Portugal, Austria, Italy, and West Germany. This is in sharp contrast to the low mortality rate in the United Kingdom. A high incidence of cirrhosis is also observed in Mexico and Chile. The United States and Japan have an incidence intermediate between southern Europe and Great Britain, similar to those of Belgium and Denmark. In Africa and South Asia, the incidence of cirrhosis as a cause of death may be artificially lower because of the prevalence of infectious diseases with their effect on mortality figures. Such geographic distribution of cirrhosis suggests variation of the etiologic relationship between cirrhosis and HCC, since the latter is uncommon in Europe and the United States (5). The epidemiology of HCC, which has been studied by a number of investigators has clearly shown that HCC is prevalent in Africa and Southeast Asia (6-8), and that the degree of association between cirrhosis and hepatocellular carcinoma varies from area to area. In fact, the frequency of association varies markedly between these two representative locations, namely Africa and South Asia versus Europe and the United States.

In calculating statistics on the frequency of this association, some investigators based their data on cases with cirrhosis and "liver carcinoma" without subdividing liver carcinoma into cholangiocarcinoma and hepatocellular carcinoma. As already discussed, HCC and cholangiocarcinoma are quite different. Among various types of cirrhosis the former is seldom associated with cardiac fibrosis, biliary cirrhosis, or Wilson's disease although it is with hemochromatosis. The more common types of cirrhosis such as so-called "posthepatic," "postnecrotic," and alcoholic are of importance as predisposing conditions.

Studies on the association of cirrhosis and hepatocellular carcinoma have mostly been undertaken on postmortem material, and thus clinical data are often inadequate.

Table 1 Types of Liver Cirrhosis with and Without HCC at Tokyo University

	Number of subjects	Number of subjects with HCC	Percentage of cirrhosis with HCC	Percentage among total HCC
A. Common types of liver cirrhosis				
Not remarkable liver	13			6.2
Fibrosis	17			8.0
Precirrhotic liver	43	10	23.3	
Posthepatitic cirrhosis	337 } 378	166 } 169	49.3 } 44.7	85.8
Postnecrotic cirrhosis	41	3	7.3	
Nutritional cirrhosis	17	2	11.8	
Toxic cirrhosis	5	0	0.0	
Total	443	211	40.9	100.0
B. Other types of liver cirrhosis				
Schistosomiasis	17	1		
Cardiac cirrhosis	35	0		
Budd-Chiari disease	7	1		
Hemochromatosis	14	3		
Wilson's disease	13	1		
Biliary cirrhosis	68	1		
Thorotrast	5 [a]	1		
Syphilitic cirrhosis	1	1		

[a] Cholangiocarcinoma, 2; hemangioendothelioma, 1.

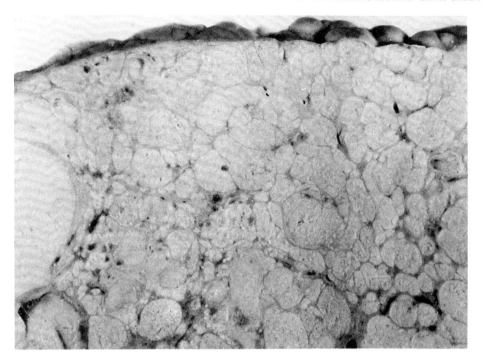

FIGURE 1   Hepatocellular carcinoma associated with macronodular thin-septal cirrhosis.

In Africa and Southeast Asia HCC is well known to occur in high incidence as the carcinoma is seen in 40 to 50% of the patients with cirrhosis; Stewart gave a figure as high as 40% (9), Davis and Steiner found 17% of cirrhotic livers to have HCC in Uganda (10), and Backer and Chatigidakis found a rate of 44% among South African Bantus (11). In Japan, Miyaji calculated this rate of incidence of liver carcinoma occurring in cirrhotic livers to be 26.3%, but this figure was based on all cases of primary liver carcinoma including HCC and cholangiocarcinoma (12). In our study, the frequency of development of HCC in livers of patients with the common types of nodular cirrhoses excluding cardiac, biliary, and other less common varieties, was 40.9% (Table 1). In our previous report in 1959 the rate was 49% (13).

The percentage of cirrhotic patients who develop HCC is low in the United States and Europe. According to Stewart, only 5% of patients with cirrhosis developed hepatocellular carcinoma in Chicago (9), and a similar figure has recently been given by Purtilo and Gottlieb (14). Pequignot et al indicated a rate of 2 to 4% in 1959–1960 and a sharp increase to 14 to 17% in 1965–1966 in Europe (15).

In South Africa, ethnic differences are evident from the report of Backer and Chatgidakis who indicated that 44% of African Negroes with cirrhosis had HCC whereas only 6% of cirrhotic Caucasians had HCC (11). Similar findings have been shown by Rose (16). The varying statistics may be principally due to the differences in the predominant type of cirrhosis among countries.

The morphologic type of cirrhosis that is followed most frequently by HCC is essentially similar in geographic areas that have a high incidence of HCC and those with a low incidence. Although a classification of cirrhosis has never been agreed upon, HCC is most frequently associated with macronodular cirrhosis, (including types commonly referred to as posthepatic and as postnecrotic cirrhosis) (Fig. 1), but less commonly with micronodular (alcoholic, nutritional) cirrhosis (17, 18). Miyai and Ruebner found hepatocellular carcinoma in 15% of cases of "postnecrotic" cirrhosis and in only 4% of those with "portal" cirrhosis (19). Purtilo et al studied the combination of the two diseases, demonstrating association in 3.2% in "nutritional" (presumably alcoholic) cirrhosis, 24% in "postnecrotic" cirrhosis, and 0.4 in a type undetermined (13). In other words, even in Europe and the United States where the incidence of hepatocellular carcinoma is low, if one limits the type of cirrhosis to macronodular cirrhosis, the percentage of such patients with HCC is high. Our study demonstrated an association rate of HCC in 44.7% of patients with macronodular cirrhosis and 11.8% in micronodular cirrhosis.

Backer and Chatgidakis pointed out in their report on the differences between Africans and Europeans that the predominant type of cirrhosis in the former is macronodular, whereas that in the latter is micronodular (11). In fact, in Africa the majority of cirrhosis is macronodular (20). In Japan over 90% of the cirrhosis is macronodular and only less than 5% micronodular. In Europe and in the United States micronodular type constitutes 40 to 60% of all cirrhosis (21), and the close relationship between alcohol consumption and incidence of cirrhosis is obvious (22). A comparison of the types of cirrhosis between Japan and the United States is given in Table 2. It may be concluded, therefore,

that one of the main reasons for the differing rates of association among countries is the difference in the predominant type of cirrhosis. Thus, hepatocellular carcinoma develops in 40 to 50% of the livers that have a background of macronodular cirrhosis. In contrast, this carcinoma is associated in less than 10% in micronodular cirrhosis regardless of its incidence in the particular country.

Among other types of cirrhosis, hemochromatosis is known for its frequent association with HCC, the figure being put at about 19% (23). Other types of cirrhosis, such as cardiac, biliary, Wilson's, and metabolic disease-associated cirrhosis, are seldom accompanied by HCC (Table 1).

Incidence of cirrhosis found in livers with hepatocellular carcinoma

In contrast to the percentage of cirrhotic patients who develop HCC, if one carefully studies various reports, it appears that the frequency of associated cirrhosis in patients with HCC is rather consistent among those countries in the two representative areas with differing incidences of HCC. Reported low figures of incidences of cirrhosis in patients with HCC may again be due in part at least to inclusion of cholangiocarcinoma in the statistics. The percentage of HCC arising in cirrhotic livers given by Berman, who extensively reviewed the literature, was 67.2%. However his report encompassed all cases of primary liver carcinoma that included cholangiolar and HCC (6). Other reports dealing with the percentage of HCC that arise in cirrhotic livers include figures of 86% by Hutt and Anthony in Uganda (24), 80% among the

Table 2 Types of Liver Cirrhosis in Japan and the United States

	Postnecrotic (%)	Posthepatitic (%)	Nutritional (%)
Tokyo University	41 (10.4)	337 (85.3)	17 (4.3)
Gall (21)	61 (11.0)	262 (47.3)	231 (41.7)

Table 3   Age distribution of HCC

Age (years)	HCC with Cirrhosis or Fibrosis	HCC Without Cirrhosis or Fibrosis
−10	1	0
11–20	0	4
21–30	4	4
31–40	21	1
41–50	49	1
51–60	69	3
61–70	39	3
71–	13	0

Bantu race (type of liver cancer not specified), 100% in whites, and 45% in Cape colored by Rose (16). In Japan, the figure stands at 85.8% in the present review. Even in low incidence areas, the frequency of association is similar or at least as high. Edmondson and Steiner found cirrhosis in 89.2% in the livers with hepatocellular carcinoma in the United States (25).

Thus, there may be two reasons for inconsistency of the reported figures that range from 60 to 90%. One is the inclusion of cholangiocarcinoma, which is associated with cirrhosis much less frequently, and another, the criteria for the diagnosis of cirrhosis. Distinction between hepatic fibrosis and cirrhosis is rather arbitrary and subject to the diagnostic criteria which vary among pathologists. Nonetheless, it may be concluded from the aforegoing discussion that the frequency with which livers involved by HCC are also cirrhotic is perhaps closer than previously thought among those countries with differing incidences of HCC.

LIVER CHANGES ASSOCIATED WITH HEPATOCELLULAR CARCINOMA

Changes, especially cirrhotic changes, in the liver involved by HCC have characteristic features as already mentioned. Careful review and analyses of liver pathology were

made of 220 necropsies of patients with HCC performed at the Department of Pathology, University of Tokyo, in the period of 1940 to 1972, excluding hepatoblastoma of infants. Nine of the cases of HCC were associated with special less common types of liver cirrhosis, such as parasitic, biliary cirrhosis, Wilson's disease, and so on. Among 211 cases, excluding those 9, 181, (85.8%) were associated with the common types of cirrhosis, and 17 (8.0%) were associated with hepatic fibrosis. There were only 13 cases (6.2%) that were seen with unremarkable liver pathology in the areas not involved by neoplasm (Table 1).

Age distribution was quite different between the cases with and those without cirrhosis or fibrosis (Table 3). Some patients without liver pathology were rather young, and the histology of the neoplasm somewhat resembled hepatoblastoma of infants. Such tumors may be related to hepatoblastoma and hence have a different etiology.

In patients with HCC associated with hepatic fibrosis rather than cirrhosis, fibrosis was seen in areas of the liver that were remote from the carcinoma, and the possibility of secondary fibrosis due to neoplastic expansion may be excluded (Figs. 2 and 3). The degree of fibrosis varied from case to case, and scanty infiltration by small round cells was seen in the stroma in some cases (Fig. 4). In 10 of the 17 cases in this category, examination for hepatitis B sur-

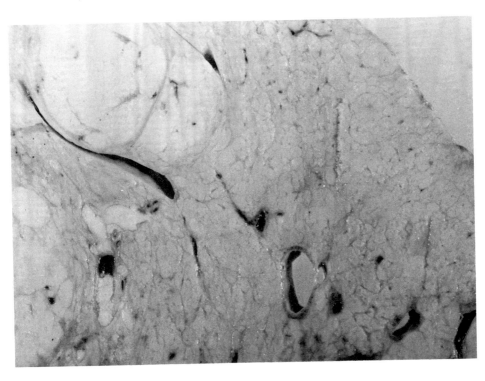

FIGURE 2 Hepatocellular carcinoma with portal fibrosis.

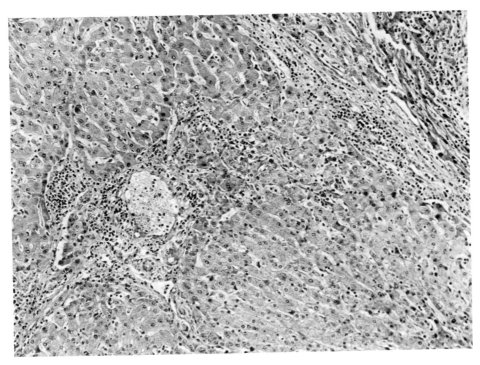

FIGURE 3 Liver fibrosis seen in a case of HCC. Fibrosis is mild and there is some distortion of the lobular architecture. A small carcinoma nodule is seen in the upper right portion (hemotoxylin and eosin stain).

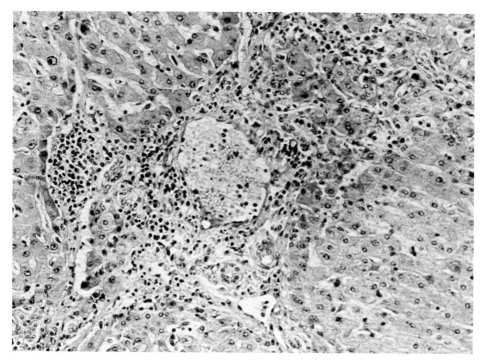

FIGURE 4   Liver changes in a case of HCC. Very mild portal fibrosis and few round cells are in the portal area (hematoxylin and eosin stain).

face antigen (HBsAg) was made on the paraffin sections using a new stain method for demonstrating what appears to be disulfide bonds. Both orcein and aldehyde fuchsin have been shown to stain the same cells that demonstrate HBsAg by immunofluorescent techniques (26). HBsAg was found in hepatocytes in the noncancerous areas in 4 out of the 10 livers with fibrosis only and HCC. Thus it may be presumed that some of the fibrosis associated with HCC was related to hepatitis B and may have represented an abortive form or precursor to cirrhosis.

Previously, it was thought by most pathologists that the relationship between HCC and hepatitis B only occurred in fully developed macronodular cirrhosis. However, this carcinoma may develop not only in livers with cirrhosis but also on the basis of mild chronic hepatitis and, rather, it re-

sembled chronic persistent hepatitis by the European criteria (27) [persistent viral hepatitis (28, 29)]. The age distribution of patients with fibrosis was about the same as that for those with cirrhosis.

Detailed histologic analysis was made of the liver with cirrhosis and hepatocellular carcinoma with respect to the histologic type of cirrhosis. There were some livers with incomplete cirrhosis, namely, fibrous tissue was increased in the portal and central vein areas, connecting each other in places, but not having quite surrounded pseudolobules as yet. HBsAg was detected in some of these livers with incomplete cirrhosis and coexisting hepatocellular carcinoma. Thus, complete cirrhosis is not a prerequisite for the development of this type of carcinoma. Although destruction and regeneration occurring in fully developed cirrhosis may promote hepatocarcin-

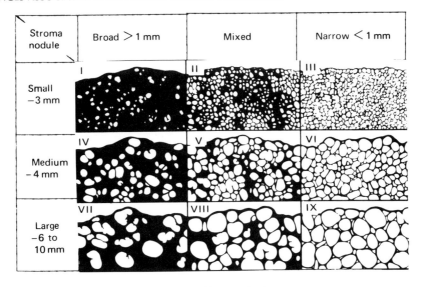

FIGURE 5   Macroscopic classification of liver cirrhosis.

Stroma nodule	Broad > 1 mm	Mixed	Narrow < 1 mm
Small −3 mm	I o o o o o	II o o o o o o	III o o o o o o o o o o • • • • •
Medium −4 mm	IV o o o o o	V o o o o o o o o o o • • •	VI o o o o o o o o o o o o o o o o o o o o o • • • • • • •
Large −6 to 10 mm	VII o o o o o	VIII o o o o o o o o o o • • • • • • • • •	IX o o o o o o o o o o o o • • • • • • • • • • •

o Cirrhosis without HCC
• Cirrhosis with HCC

FIGURE 6   Number of cases in various types of liver cirrhosis with or without HCC.

ogenesis, carcinoma can develop even on the ground of chronic hepatitis in livers without lobular distortion or with only a minimal lobular distortion.

One of the classifications of cirrhosis relies on the gross balance between fibrous stroma and parenchyma at the postmortem examination. Pseudolobules are classified by their sizes into three groups of "micronodular," "mesonodular," and "macronodular," and the stroma into "thin stromal," "broad stromal," and "mixed." Combination of these produces nine groups in this classification, for example, "micronodular thin septal," "macronodular mixed stromal," etc. Using this method, livers with and without hepatocellular carcinoma were classified into nine categories as illustrated in Figs. 5 and 6. It is apparent from these figures that hepatocellular carcinoma is most frequently associated with the macronodular group. Of course, the broad-septal group represents what Gall called "postnecrotic" cirrhosis (21). Macronodular thin-septal cirrhosis is the type Gall referred to as "posthepatitic" cirrhosis.

ETIOLOGY OF LIVER CIRRHOSIS ASSOCIATED WITH HEPATOCELLULAR CHANGES

Determination of the exact etiology of liver cirrhosis in each case is difficult, especially after it has fully developed. Popper insisted that the same factor would lead to different morphological patterns and contrariwise, that various etiologic factors might all result in a morphologically indistinguishable type of cirrhosis (30). It has been shown that alcoholic liver disease may progress not only to a fine granular, monolobular type to the so-called Laennec or portal cirrhosis, but also may develop into an irregular, coarsely nodular multilobular form, or even to the macronodular ("postnecrotic"). Rubin et al found such postnecrotic type in chronic alcoholics (31). Recent studies have demonstrated a higher incidence of HBsAg in alcoholics compared with nonalcoholics (32), but no convincing studies have indicated that viral hepatitis plays a role in the etiology of alcoholic cirrhosis.

The type of cirrhosis that is related to chronic active hepatitis and develops within two or three years is characterized by rather small monolobular pseudolobules. On the other hand, posthepatitic cirrhosis of long duration which may develop in 10 years or more, has relatively large multilobular pseudolobules. Generally speaking, however, fine granular monolobular cirrhosis is somewhat more characteristic of chronic alcoholism, and coarsely nodular multilobular cirrhosis is more often the pattern following chronic active hepatitis caused by hepatitis virus.

In Japan, HBsAg has been detected in the serum in about 30% of the patients with postnecrotic or posthepatitic cirrhosis and in 40% of those with hepatocellular carcinoma (33). Namely, HBsAg is found more frequently in sera of patients with hepatocellular carcinoma than in those with cirrhosis alone. This phenomenon suggests that most of the macronodular cirrhotic livers in which HCC develop are of hepatitis B origin.

The type of cirrhosis associated with HCC is often designated as "posthepatitic" cirrhosis, but HBsAg is still detected in the serum, and noncancerous hepatocytes contain relatively large amounts of antigen in some cases. Furthermore, inflammatory cell infiltration, which does not correlate with the existence of HBsAg, is prominent in some. Therefore, it may be more desirable to designate it as "hepatitic" cirrhosis in certain instances instead of posthepatitic. The seropositivity rate for HBsAg of patients with HCC varies among the reports, but it is generally high compared to the control groups. It is about 40% in Japan, and as high a figure of 80% has been reported from Taiwan (34) and Uganda (35). The concentration of the antigen in serum is usually low, and unless sensitive methods are employed, the positivity rate will turn out to be low (36).

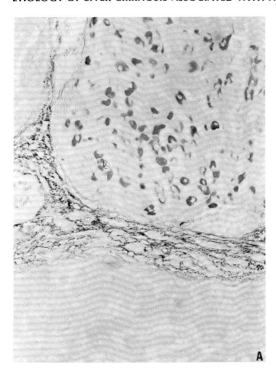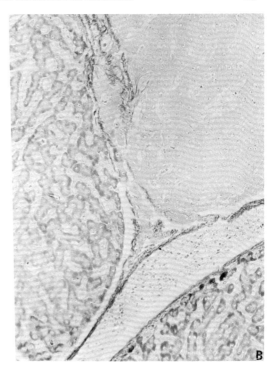

FIGURE 7 Distribution pattern of HBsAg in a noncancerous area of liver bearing HCC. Showing scattered strongly positive cells in one nodule with none in adjacent *(a)*, and membranous distribution in two nodules also adjacent to a nodule that has no demonstrable antigen *(b)* (orcein stain).

In spite of the low titers of HBsAg in serum, it is demonstrable abundantly in liver tissue as demonstrated by the immunofluorescent technique or orcein staining method (26), compared with acute or active stages of chronic active hepatitis. In the latter types of hepatitis, HBsAg concentrations in serum may be relatively high, while in liver tissue the antigen is scanty. In fulminant hepatitis tissue antigen is particularly sparse. An explanation is not readily available at the moment, and it may be that for the release of HBsAg, necrosis of HBsAg-containing hepatocytes is also important. During the long period of quiescent cirrhosis, those HBsAg-containing cells do not display any destructive changes despite the fact that they do contain the antigen.

It has been postulated that hepatitis virus or HBsAg alone produces a very mild cytopathic effect, and that cell destruction is caused by an immunological reaction either humoral or cellular (37, 38). In the case of cirrhosis and hepatocellular carcinoma, an immunodeficient state develops with minimal destruction of HBsAg containing cells. Orcein or aldehyde fuchsin methods (26) can be applied to conventional paraffin sections. With this stain technique, the details of HBsAg in its relation to the hepatocytes are more clearly demonstrated.

Distribution of HBsAg in the noncancerous tissue in hepatocellular carcinoma is very irregular, and the amount of antigen varies from case to case. Two major patterns of antigen distribution are recog-

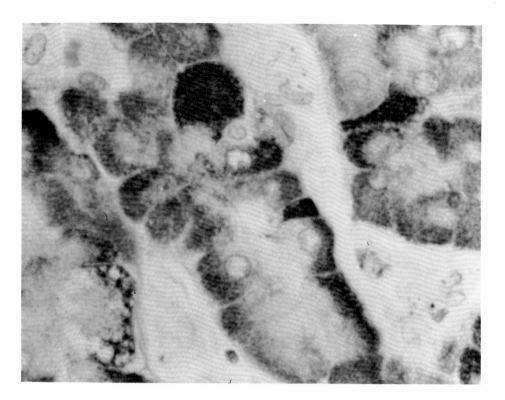

FIGURE 8 Diffuse distribution of HBAg in the hepatocytes. Almost all hepatocytes in this area contain HBAg, especially in the perisinusoidal areas (orcein stain).

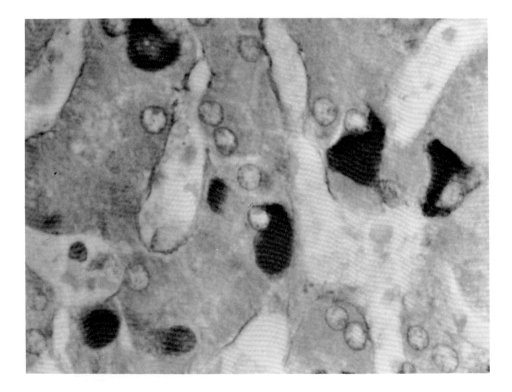

FIGURE 9 Cytoplasmic inclusion bodies of HBAg. Some of them contain neutral fat in its center (orcein stain).

nized in such cases—lobular, in which almost all hepatocytes appear in some areas of the lobule or pseudolobule, or focal, in which single cells are scattered in the liver tissue (Fig. 7). In the former pattern, HBsAg is distributed diffusely in the cytoplasm, particularly in areas of the hepatocytes adjacent to the sinusoids, showing a fine granular structure (Fig. 8). In the latter pattern, round, oval or irregularly shaped aggregates of HBsAg nearly replace the cytoplasm and, at the same time, some of the antigen is diffusely distributed in the cytoplasm (Fig. 9). The electron microscopic findings corresponding to diffuse distribution of HBsAg have not been elucidated. Early cytoplasmic inclusions correspond to the localized proliferation of smooth endoplasmic reticulum, and occasional filamentous structures are seen in the cisterna of the smooth endoplasmic reticulum (Fig. 10) (37, 38). In a late stage, filamentous structures are not restricted to the smooth endoplasmic reticulum and they exist diffusely in the matrix (Figs. 11 and 12). It is supposed that HBsAg, as an abnormal lipoprotein, might form a filamentous structure in some physiochemical conditions. In a more advanced stage, those structures are destroyed to be replaced by an amorphous structure. Those inclusion bodies are stainable with the peroxidase antibody technique, and particles with unstained center are sometimes found in them (39). The complete hepatitis virus has a duality of antigenic components, the core material (HBcAg) localized in hepatocyte nuclei and the surface antigen (HBsAg) localized in cytoplasm (40). Although both HBsAg and HBcAg can be demonstrated by immunofluorescence, only the former is demonstrated by the orcein and aldehyde fuchsin stains referred to by Shikata et al (26). Distribution of core antigen (HBcAg) in the liver tissue of HCC is still obscure.

The author's hypothesis on hepatocar-

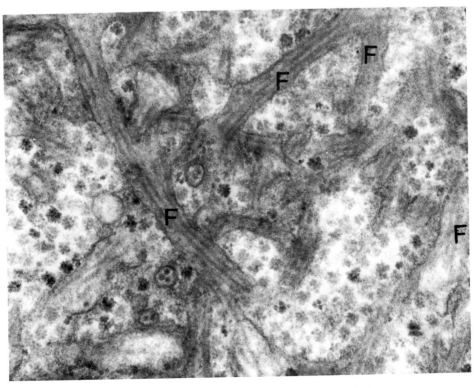

FIGURE 10 Filamentous structures *(f)* in the cisternae of proliferated endoplasmic reticulum.

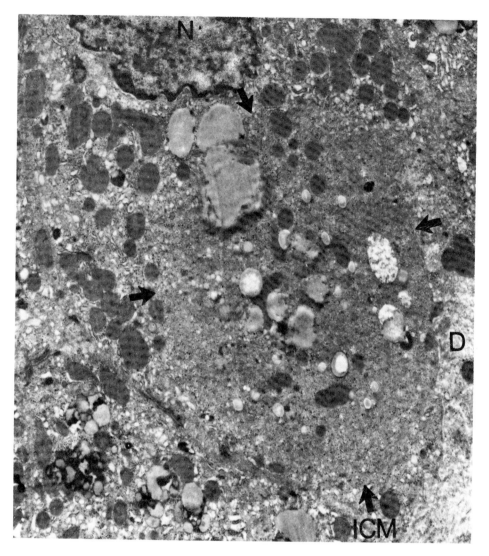

FIGURE 11 Electron micrograph of the cytoplasmic inclusion body (indicated by arrows).
D: space of Disse; ICM: intercellular membrane; N: nucleus.

cinogenesis associated with hepatitis virus is as follows: in acute and in active stages of chronic active hepatitis, HB antigen-containing hepatocytes and perhaps hepatitis virus are removed by immunological processes. Persistent, long-term infection of hepatitis virus is associated with an immunodeficient state against HBsAg or other hepatitis B virus-associated antigens. Therefore, hepatitis virus or HBsAg-containing cells cannot be removed by the usual mechanisms of cellular immunity. In

fact, HBsAg-containing cells are seen most numerously in noncancerous portions of the liver with hepatocellular carcinoma. On the other hand, frequency of antibody to HBsAg is very low in cases with HCC who do not have HBsAg. Obviously free anti-HBs cannot be demonstrated in the presence of HBsAg. Immunoblasts producing anti-HBs can be demonstrated in spleen and lymph nodes by the immunofluorescent antigen method. Such immunoblasts are seen most numerously in patients with fulminant hepatitis, sparsely in patients with HCC, and not at all in healthy cariers.

Persistence of hepatitis virus of HBsAg in hepatocytes may lead to malignant change of the hepatocyte, but only in rare instances is HBsAg found in the cytoplasm of the HCC cells (Figs. 13 and 14).

OTHER TYPES OF LIVER CIRRHOSIS AND HEPATOCELLULAR CARCINOMA

Although hepatocellular carcinoma occurs in highest incidence in HBsAg positive macronodular cirrhosis, it sometimes develops in other types of cirrhosis.

Alcoholic Liver Disease

Nutritional cirrhosis can become the basis for HCC, but the frequency of association is relatively lower. Purtilo et al found hepatocellular carcinoma in 3.2% of the cases of "nutritional" cirrhosis in comparison with 24.2% in "postnecrotic" cirrhosis (14). The chapter by Peters dealing with morphology of HCC also discusses alcoholic cirrhosis and HCC in the United States. Hemochromatosis is known to be associated with hepatocellular carcinoma (23), the frequency being put at 22.3% by Purtilo et al (14). In contrast, in Wilson's disease, which is associated with the deposit of a heavy metal, HCC is rare. We have so far seen only one patient with Wilson's disease complicated by HCC, and such reports are scanty throughout the world.

Thorotrast

Thorotrast, a well-known cause of cholangiocarcinoma and hemangioendothelioma,

FIGURE 12   High power view of inclusion area of Fig. 11. Filamentous structures are not restricted in the cisternae of endoplasmic reticulum. They exist diffusely in the matrix.

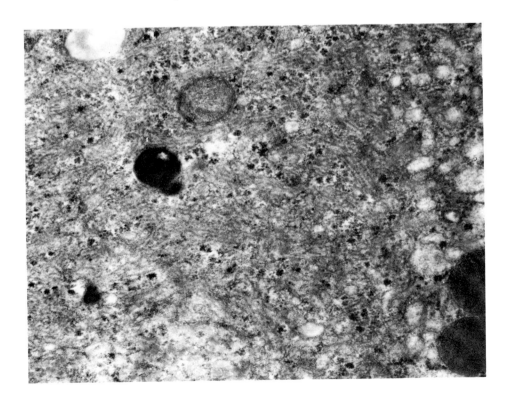

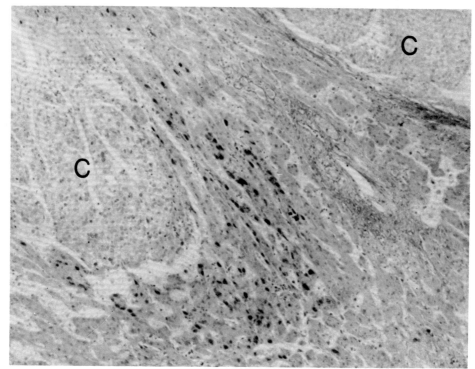

FIGURE 13 HBs Ag usually existed in the noncancerous areas (center) and not in carcinoma tissue *(c)* (orcein stain).

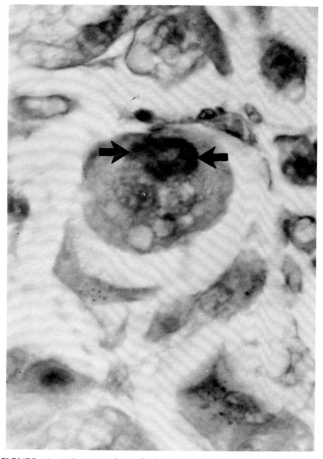

FIGURE 14 HBs Ag in the cell of HCC (aldehyde-fuchsin stain).

sometimes produces hepatocellular carcinoma and is covered elsewhere in this book.

Budd-Chiari's Disease

In parts of the world where it is more common, Budd-Chiari's disease is often associated with hepatocellular carcinoma for unknown reasons (42). However, the possible relationship of Budd-Chiari's disease to plant toxins make it unclear whether the HCC is related to Budd-Chiari's disease in reported cases, or whether it results from the same plant alkaloids that cause the hepatic vein disease (43, 44). Production of the Budd-Chiari's syndrome secondary to a mass lesion impinging on the hepatic venous outflow is more common (45).

Alpha 1 Antitrypsin

Reports of isolated patients with HCC who also have aberrant pi genotypes (alpha-1-antitrypsin) have appeared (46, 47, 48). The data are yet too scanty for analysis and may reflect anomalies more common in one geographic or population group than another. Peters mentions the experience with aberrant pi types and HCC in Los Angeles in his chapter.

Diseases of Abnormal Carbohydrate Metabolism

A case of glycogen-storage disease has been reported to terminate in HCC. Similarly, an example of galactosemia with development of cirrhosis and HCC has been recorded.

CHOLANGIOCARCINOMA AND LIVER CIRRHOSIS

Cholangiocarcinoma is quite different from hepatocellular carcinoma in its pathogenesis and association with cirrhosis. The proportion of cirrhotic livers in which this type of carcinoma develops is very small, and the type of cirrhosis that is associated with cholangiocarcinoma is almost restricted to biliary cirrhosis. Gibson found 2 cases (12%) associated with cirrhosis among 17 cases of cholangiocarcinoma (42). In the present series this rate was 16.3%. Cholangiocarcinoma is often associated with chronic cholangitis with fibrosis, and it is very difficult to determine whether biliary tract pathology preceded carcinogenesis.

Cholangiocarcinoma develops in some of the livers with thorotrast deposit. We have seen one case of cholangiocarcinoma that developed in a liver with congenital intrahepatic bile duct dilation. Hepatic distomiasis has long been thought to predispose the liver to cholangiocarcinoma, although biliary cirrhosis is produced by liver flukes infrequently. *Clonorchis sinensis* in South China and *Opisthorchis viverrine* in Thailand are the common species. Gibson reported that 65% of the patients with cholangiocarcinoma had been infected by *Clonorchis sinensis,* whereas the corresponding figure for hepatocellular carcinoma and the control group was 29% and 23%, respectively, in series of consecutive autopsies in Hong Kong.

Areas of cholangiocarcinoma may be found in areas of the so-called combined form of hepatocellular and cholangiolar carcinomas. Such tumors are often associated with the usual type of hepatitic cirrhosis. The latter may be regarded as variants of hepatocellular carcinoma.

REFERENCES

1. Sasaki T, Yoshida T: Experimentelle Erzeugung des Lebercarcinoms durch Fütterung mit *o-amidoazotoluol. Virchows Arch Pathol Anat Physiol* **295**:175–200, 1935.
2. Stewart HL, Snell KC: The histopathology of experimental tumors of the liver of the rat. *Acta Unio Int Contra Cancrum* **13**:770–803, 1957.
3. Butler WH: Pathology of liver cancer in experiment animals. *Liver Cancer—International Agency for Research on Cancer Scientific Publication No. 1.* London, 1971, pp. 30–41.
4. World Health Statistics Report. **26**(4), 1973.
5. Higginson J: The geographic pathology of primary liver cancer. *Cancer Res* **23**:1624–1633, 1963.

6. Berman C: *Primary Carcinoma of the Liver*. Lewis, London, 1951.

7. Doll R, Payne PM, Waterhouse JAH: *Cancer Incidence in Five Continents*. Springer Verlag, Berlin (UICE publication), 1966.

8. Hutt MSR: Epidemiology of human primary liver cancer. In *Liver Cancer—International Agency for Research on Cancer Scientific Publication No. 1*. London, 1971, pp. 21–29.

9. Stewart HL: Geographic distribution of hepatic cancer. In *Primary Hepatoma*. Burdette WJ (Ed). University of Utah Press, Salt Lake City, 1965, pp. 31–36.

10. Davis JNP, Steiner PE: Cirrhosis and primary liver carcinoma in Uganda Africans. *Brit J Cancer* 11:523–534, 1957.

11. Backer BJP and Chatgidakis CB: Primary carcinoma of the liver in Johannesburg. *Acta Unio Int Contra Cancrum* 17:650–653, 1961.

12. Miyaji T: Primary liver carcinoma in Japan—especially its relationship with liver cirrhosis (in Japanese). *Tr Soc Pathol Jap* 54:23–38, 1965.

13. Shikata T: Studies on the relationship between hepatic cancer and liver cirrhosis. *Acta Pathol Jap* 9:267–311, 1959.

14. Purtilo DT, Gottlieb LS: Cirrhosis and hepatoma occurring at Boston City Hospital (1917–1968). *Cancer* 32:458–462, 1973.

15. Pequignot H, Etienne JP, Delavierre P, et al: Cancers primitifs du foie sur cirrhose. *Presse Med* 75:2595–2600, 1967.

16. Rose AG: Primary carcinoma of the liver in Cape Town. In *Liver* Saunders SJ, Terblanche J (Eds). Pitman Medical, London, 1973, pp. 310–311.

17. Sherlock S: *Diseases of the Liver and Biliary System*, 4th ed. Blackwell, Oxford.

18. Sheuer PJ: Pathogenesis and morid anatomy of human primary liver cancer. In *Liver Cancer—International Agency for Research on Cancer Scientific Publication No. 1*, 1971, pp. 13–20.

19. Miyai K, Ruebner BH: Acute yellow atrophy, cirrhosis, and hepatoma. *Arch Pathol* 75:609–617, 1963.

20. Anthony PP: Primary carcinoma of the liver: A study of 282 cases in Ugandan Africans. *J Pathol* 110:37–48, 1973.

21. Gall EA: Posthepatitic, postnecrotic and nutritional cirrhosis. *Am J Pathol* 36:241–271, 1960.

22. Martini GA, Bode C: Zur Epidemiologie der Leberzirrhose. *Internist (Berl)* 11:84–93, 1970.

23. Warren S, Drake EL: Primary carcinoma of the liver in hemochromatosis. *Am J Pathol* 27:573–609, 1951.

24. Hutt MSR, Anthony PP: Tumours of liver, biliary system and pancreas in tumours in a tropical country. Templeton AC (Ed). Springer-Verlag Berlin, 1973, pp. 57–78.

25. Edmondson HA, Steiner PE: Primary carcinoma of the liver: An autopsy study of 100 cases among 48,900 necropsies. *Cancer (Phila)* 7:462–502, 1954.

26. Shikata T, Uzawa T, Yoshiwara N, et al. Staining methods of Australia antigen in paraffin section. *Jap J Exp Med* 44:25–36, 1974.

27. DeGroote J, Desmet VJ, Gedigk P, et al: A classification of chronic hepatitis. *Lancet* 2:626–628, 1968.

28. Ishak KG: Viral hepatitis, the morphologic spectrum. *The Liver, International Academy of Pathology Monograph*. Gall EA, Mostofi FK (Eds). Williams & Wilkins, Baltimore, 1973.

29. Peters RL: Viral hepatitis, a pathologic spectrum. *Am J Med Sci*, in press.

30. Popper H: *Cirrhosis in Liver*. Saunders ST, Terblanche J (Eds). Pitman Medical, London, 1973, pp. 204–251.

31. Rubin E, Krus S, Popper H: Pathogenesis of postnecrotic cirrhosis in alcoholic. *Arch Pathol* 73:288–299, 1962.

32. Traswell HF, Shorter R, Poncelet TK, et al: Hepatitis-associated antigen in blood donor populations. Relationship to posttransfusion hepatitis. *JAMA* 214:142–144, 1970.

33. Nishioka K: *Report of WHO Associated Workshop of Hepatitis B Antigen*. 1973.

34. Tong MJ, Sun SC, Schaeffer BT, et al: Hepatitis-associated antigen and hepatocellular carcinoma in Taiwan. *Ann Int Med* 75:687–691, 1971.

35. Vogel CL, Anthony PP, Sadikall F, et al: Hepatitis-associated antigen and antibody in hepatocellular carcinoma. *J Natl Cancer Inst* 48:1583–1588, 1972.

36. Almeda JD, Waterson AP: Immune complexes in hepatitis. *Lancet* 11:893–986, 1969.

37. Dudley FJ, Fox RA, Sherlock S: Cellular immunity and hepatitis-associated, Australia antigen liver disease. *Lancet* 1:723–726, 1972.

38. Huang, SN, Groh V, Beausoin JG, et al. A study of the relationship of virus-like particles and Australia antigen in liver. *Hum Pathol* 5:209–222, 1974.

39. Gerber MA, Hadziyannis S, Vissoulis C, et al: Electron microscopy and immunoelectron microscopy of cytoplasmic hepatitis B antigen in hepatocytes. *Am J Pathol* 75:489–502, 1974.

40. Shikata T: Australia antigen in liver tissue—and immunofluorescent and immunoelectron microscopic study. *Jap J Exp Med* 43:231–243, 1973.

41. Brzosko WJ, Madalinski K, Krawczynski K, et al: Duality of hepatitis B antigen and its antibody. I. immunofluorescent studies. *J Infect Dis* 127:424–428, 1973.

42. Simpson IW, Middlecote BD: The Budd-Chiari syndrome in the Bantu. In *Liver*. Saunders SJ, Terblanche J (Eds). Pitman Medical, London, 1973, p. 257.

43. Schoental R: Pyrolizidine alkaloids. *Cancer Res* **28**:2237–2246, 1968.

44. Cook JW, Duffy E, Schoental R: Primary liver tumors in rats following feeding with alkaloids of senecio jacobaea. *Brit J Cancer* **4**:405–410, 1950.

45. Reynolds TB, Peters RL: Budd-Chiari syndrome. In *Diseases of the Liver*, 4th ed. Schiff L (Ed). Lippincott, Philadelphia, 1975.

46. Ganrot PO, Laurell CB, Eriksson S: Obstructive lung disease and trypsin inhibitors in alpha-1-antitrypsin deficiency. *Scand J Clin Lab Invest* **19**:205–208, 1967.

47. Berg NO, Eriksson S: Liver disease in adults with alpha-1-antitrypsin deficiency. *NEJM* **287**:1264–1267, 1972.

48. Rawlings W, Moss J, Coper HS, et al: Hepatocellular carcinoma and partial deficiency of alpha-1-antitrypsin. *Ann Intern Med* **81**:771–773, 1974.

49. Gibson JB: Parasites, liver disease and liver cancer. In *Liver Cancer—International Agency for Research on Cancer Scientific Publication No. 1*, Lyon, 1971, pp. 42–50.

CHAPTER 5 VIRAL HEPATITIS AND HEPATOCELLULAR CARCINOMA

YASUYUKI OHTA, M.D.

INTRODUCTION

The geographic incidence of hepatocellular carcinoma (HCC) varies considerably (1–4). Areas of high incidence are also noted for the frequency of liver cirrhosis (LC), notably of the posthepatitic variety which is *a sequela* to viral hepatitis, but not of the nutritional type (fatty cirrhosis) seen among alcoholics (5). Kalk presented evidence for a direct relationship between viral hepatitis and LC in a serial study of viral hepatitis by peritoneoscopy (6). The recent discovery of hepatitis B antigen (HBAg) and its etiological implications in viral hepatitis B lend further support to this relationship (7, 8).

Before the discovery of HBAg, viral hepatitis was not seriously considered as the cause of HCC, although several investigators suggested this possibility. Sheldon and James (9) described five patients with LC following infectious hepatitis. Two of their patients, both males, developed HCC. One patient, who had a history of chronic alcoholism and malnutrition, developed HCC 10 years after infectious hepatitis.

The postmortem study demonstrated HCC arising on the seat of regenerative LC nodules of varying sizes, 1 to 20 mm in diameter. These investigators emphasized postnecrotic cirrhosis rather than Laennec's cirrhosis as the matrix of HCC. Walshe and Wolff (10) reported on two male patients who had developed hepatitis followed by LC and finally HCC. In both cases the interval between viral hepatitis and HCC was seven years: neither patient had a history of alcoholism. In one, the postmortem examination revealed HCC on the grounds of coarsely granular cirrhosis which consisted of nodules of 5 to 20 mm in diameter. In the other, HCC arose on an atrophic postnecrotic scar (toxic cirrhosis of Marchand). Recently, Sherlock and her associates (7) described 17 patients from three countries with chronic liver disease and with serum positive for HBsAg; of the 5 patients with HCC, 4 had cirrhosis. They suggested that B virus hepatitis could proceed to cirrhosis and HCC. In this chapter, I summarize my own findings in addition to other data on the relationship between viral hepatitis and HCC.

Table 1   Clinical course of patients with HCC with antecedent acute viral hepatitis [a]

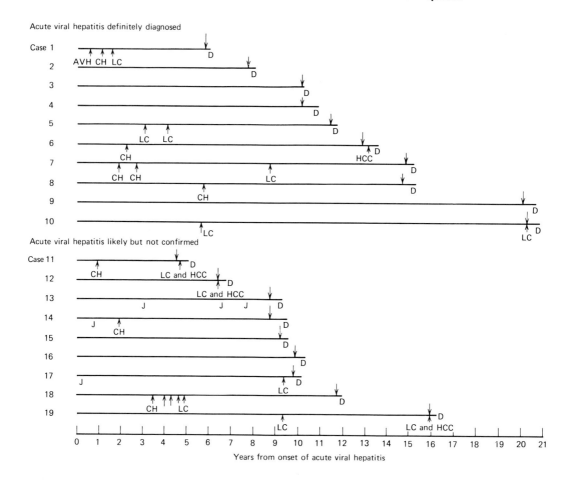

[a] AVH, acute viral hepatitis; CH, chronic hepatitis; LC, liver cirrhosis, HCC, hepatocellular carcinoma; D, death; J, jundice; ↓, time of HCC diagnosis; ↑, time of liver biopsy and diagnosis.

CLINICAL OBSERVATIONS

During the period from 1958 to 1974, 83 patients (68 males, 15 females) with HCC were hospitalized at the Okayama University Hospital (OUH). Most male patients were between the fifth and the seventh decade, but the age of female patients varied widely. Diagnosis was established by autopsy in 46, by peritoneoscopy and liver biopsy in 16, by surgical biopsy in 5, and clinically with the aid of liver scans and serum alpha fetoprotein (AFP) in 16. Thus in 80.7% of the cases (67 patients) some histological evidence was available. Of these histologically verified cases, 52 (77.6%) developed HCC superimposed on cirrhosis. Livers with fibrosis but not cirrhosis underlay the HCC of three of them. In one case, HCC was followed by Budd-

Chiari syndrome. In 11 cases HCC developed without any morphologic evidence of previous or underlying liver disease.

A history of viral hepatitis was elicited from 19 patients (Table 1). They were all males, and 5 were in their fifties, 9 in their sixties, and 5 in their seventies. Family clustering of chronic liver diseases was a feature of 6 patients; 4 had sibs with a liver disease, 1 a parent, and 1 a cousin. One patient developed acute viral hepatitis during a local 1958 epidemic in his work environment. Two others lived within the area of the same outbreak.

The interval from confirmed acute viral hepatitis to the diagnosis of HCC was from 6 to 20 years with a mean of 12.8 years; in patients with unconfirmed acute viral hepatitis it ranged from 4.5 to 16 years with a mean of 9.5 years (Table 1). The time interval from the clinical diagnosis of LC to HCC ranged from 5 to 15 years with a mean of 8 years. Three patients with a history of earlier hepatitis developed HCC without LC. One of these patients, however, developed HCC superimposed on what might be considered to be posthepatic fibrosis 13 years after viral hepatitis. This patient was free of symptoms for about 10 years; he then developed general malaise and dull pain in the upper abdomen which were signs of HCC. In this case both HBsAg and anti-HBs were negative in the serum but the antigen was detected in the liver. In the other two without LC, minimum fibrosis of the portal areas was the underlying histologic change.

Serum HBsAg was detected with the immune adherence hemagglutination technique (IAHA), anti-HBs by the passive hemagglutination method (PHA). Liver HBsAg was studied by immunofluorescent technique. In our experience the immuno:uorescent method was more sensitive than IAHA for detecting antigen in HCC. By IAHA, the rate of positive HBsAg was 60% in patients developing HCC with a previous history of viral hepatitis, whereas it was 61.5% in patients with HCC who had no history of viral hepatitis (control group). The rate of positive anti-HBs was 40% in patients with a history of viral hepatitis, but the anti-HBs incidence was 27.3% in the control group. Therefore, on purely statistical basis these data indicate little difference between the two groups. The clinical and histological data of individual patients were more suggestive of a relationship between clinically acute viral hepatitis type B and HCC, however. In the following two cases, acute viral hepatitis was diagnosed from family occurrence and histology (Case 1) and from laboratory tests (Case 7).

ILLUSTRATIVE CASES

CASE 1. Male, age 43. In June 1967 the patient underwent examinations at another hospital because his younger brother had a liver tumor. Although he had no complaints, he was told he had a liver disease. In October 1967 he was admitted to a hospital for a duodenal ulcer. Marked impairment of liver function was noted in December 1967. He began to complain of nausea, anorexia, and epigastric pain, and was referred to us in January 1968. There was a history of moderate drinking. On admission, a soft liver was palpable 2.5 fingerbreadths below the costal margin in the midline. Laboratory findings included a total serum bilirubin level of 1.2 mg/100 ml, SGOT activity of 105 u, SGPT activity of 89 u, alkaline phosphatase activity 3.0 Bessey-Lowry (BLU), albumin 3.7g –-globulin 1.3 g/100 ml, and BSP test within normal limits. Peritoneoscopy disclosed a firm, reddish, smooth-surfaced liver. Histologically, the liver showed changes of a convalescent stage of acute viral hepatitis.

The patient was discharged on May 2, 1968 and remained without symptoms until mid-June 1968, when he again complained of nausea and anorexia. SGOT activity was 24u, SGOTu, ALP 1.9 BLU. Liver biopsy in September 1968 demonstrated chronic aggressive hepatitis of moderate activity. A third biopsy performed on March 7, 1969 revealed extensive fibrosis linking the central veins with the portal triads. Activation of Kupffer cells and proliferation of the ductules were conspicuous. Toward the end of September 1974, he complained of malaise and developed jaundice. At the time of admission to Kawasaki Hospital, neither the liver nor spleen was palpable below the costal margin. His abdomen was markedly distended with ascites. HBsAg was positive, anti-HBs negative, and serum AFP 1.3 10⁴ ng/ml (normal 2–9 ng/ml). The patient died in hepatic coma on October 30, 1974.

At the time of autopsy, the liver weighed 2130 g and the surface was distorted by coarse 0.1 to 1.0 cm nodules. About two-thirds of the right lobe was occupied by a grayish yellow tumor. Lymph node metastases were found around the porta hepatis, pancreas, peritoneum, paraaortic region of the abdomen, and in Virchow's nodes. Histological examination revealed HCC of Edmondson's grade II developing in a cirrhotic liver characterized by multilobular regenerative nodules and thin stroma infiltrated by a moderate number of round cells.

CASE 7.   Male, age 66. The patient had a history of alcohol abuse in his younger years. In May 1959 he was admitted to the hospital for investigation of jaundice. Before clarification of the cause of jaundice or complete recovery, gastrectomy was carried out for duodenal ulcer. During the operation, it was observed that his liver had a smooth surface and appeared normal; there were no gall stones. He received 4 u of blood. Jaundice continued after the operation and a diagnosis of acute hepatitis was made on July 19 based on the liver function data which, by that time, included total bilirubin 4.5 mg/100 ml, SCOT 148 u, SGPT 106 u, serum albumin 3.8 g%, serum globulin 3.4 g% with 2.0 gamma fraction, and BSP 12.5% retention at 45 minutes. He was treated with prednisolone for one month and except for BSP which remained at 10% retention at 45 minutes, liver tests were normal by August 27. It is unclear whether it was considered that acute hepatitis resulted from blood transfusion or was the cause of his initial jaundice episode.

In February 1960, slight jaundice developed again and the patient was admitted to another hospital. In October 1960, he developed malaise and right upper quadrant pain and was readmitted to OUH. The first biopsy on January 10, 1961 showed enlarged portal areas with moderately heavy lymphocyte infiltrations. The lobular structure was slightly distorted, suggesting a severe chronic aggressive hepatitis. After three months of prednisolone therapy, a marked reduction in cell infiltration was observed. Glycosuria was noted at that time, and the patient stopped alcohol intake. However, he resumed alcoholic intake in 1964, gradually increasing consumption up to 200 g of ethanol per day. On December 28, 1967, after drinking heavily, he developed fever, dyspnea, diarrhea, and then jaundice. Ascites developed for the first time and he was readmitted on January 22, 1968. Palmar erythema and vascular spiders on the forechest were noted. Peritoneoscopy revealed a nodule in the left lobe of the liver, and the right lobe was not visible due to adhesions. A blind liver biopsy done in April revealed established cirrhosis. He was discharged on August 3, 1968 and placed on insulin, and he remained without symptoms.

When he was admitted on February 1, 1974 for dark urine, he was emaciated and icteric. The liver was palpable three fingerbreadths below the xiphoid process and HCC was indicated by serum AFP (62,000 ng/ml). HBsAg was negative by IAHA, and anti-HBs positive (32 to 64x by PHA). He died on April 25, 1974. At the time of autopsy, the liver weighed 900 g. Remarkably coarse nodules of ping pong ball size projected from the surface of the right lobe. The centers of some nodules were softened. On the cut surface, the tumor appeared dark brown with greenish spots. Histological examination revealed HCC of Edmondson's grade II in a multilobular thin stromal cirrhotic liver.

HBAg, LIVER CIRRHOSIS, AND HCC

LC and HCC have often been found in the same patient, the LC appearing about 7 to 10 years prior to the development of HCC. It is tempting, therefore, to speculate that the etiological agents for both diseases are the same or at least closely related. In the cases in which hepatitis B preceded HCC, hepatitis B virus (HBV) appeared to be a possible etiological agent as there is a high incidence of HBsAg in HCC, although a number of unknown variables still remain to be elucidated.

The incidence of serum HBsAg in patients with HCC is remarkably high in comparison with that for chronic hepatitis and for liver cirrhosis. The geographical and family studies on high HBsAg incidence in HCC also suggest an etiological relationship between HBV and HCC. Table 2 summarizes the available data on HBsAg from various regions. Incidences vary by the method used for HBsAg detection, but the data indicate high figures in those areas where HCC is frequent. In areas of high HCC incidence, such as South Africa, Southeast Asia, and the Far East, hepatitis B incidence is higher than in populations of less affected areas. In the

Table 2 Hepatitis B Antigen and Hepatocellular Carcinoma

Author	Country	Method[a]	Hepatoma Patients			Comparison Groups		
			Number	HBsAg	%	Number	HBsAg	%
Smith et al (20)	USA	MO	12	0	0	2412	2	0.1
Prince et al (11)	USA	IEOP	55	2	3.6	55,956	58	0.1
Alpert et al (12)	USA	IEOP	51	3	5.8	–	–	–
Smith et al (20)	East Africa	MO	11	0	0	511	8	1.5
Vogel et al (14)	Uganda	CF	45	18	40.0	122	4	3.3
Prince et al (11)	Senegal	IEOP	210	88	42.0	1160	140	9.0
Hadziyannis et al (21)	Greece	MO	13	4	30.8	–	–	–
Reed et al (22)	Great Britain	RIA	38	9	24.0	–	–	–
Teres et al (23)	Spain	MO	26	9	34.0	900	3	0.3
Anand (24)	India	IEOP	11	7	63.6	–	–	0.1
Simons et al (25)	Singapore	IAHA	156	55	35.3	1516	114	7.5
Smith et al (20)	Hong Kong	MO	42	2	4.7	50	2	4.7
Welsh et al (26)	South Vietnam	IEOP	26	0	0	–	–	–
Tong et al (27)	Taiwan	MO	55	44	80.0	943	138	14.6
Nishioka et al (28)	Japan	IAHA	260	93	37.3	4387	113	2.9
Masuda et al (13)	Japan	IEOP	216	34	15.7	–	–	–

[a] CF, complement fixation; IAHA, immune adherence hemagglutination; IEOP, immunoelectroosmophoresis; MO, micro-Ouchterlony; RIA, radioimmunoassay.

United States the incidence of HBsAg in HCC patients is low; the patients diagnosed as having HCC with positive HBsAg were found to be from Africa and not natives of the States in one study (12). The positive rate of HBsAg in HCC appears to be generally low among Caucasians, but reports from Spain and Greece indicate fairly high incidence (21, 23). The genetic-racial susceptibility to HCC, therefore, is not altogether clear and other factors may also be involved, such as sanitation, nutrition, and toxic chemicals.

The geographic distribution is reported to be closely related to the type of LC. In areas of low HCC incidence the prevailing types of cirrhosis are the alcoholic and the micronodular Laennec type of cirrhosis (15). In areas of intermediate HCC incidence, such as Japan, the so-called posthepatitic or mixed macro- and micronodular nonalcoholic type cirrhosis is common. Higginson et al (5) felt that the histological picture of LC in South Africa was suggestive of a cirrhosis following "infectious" hepatitis, and this idea that the etiology was in truth viral although of type B was further substantiated by the relatively high incidence of HBsAg.

The matrix of the HCC liver is coarsely nodular macroscopically, and histologically multilobular with thin stromas (16, 17). In the areas of high incidence such as Mozambique and Senegal, HCC develops in noncirrhotic livers of young subjects (18, 19). In these areas, HCC and LC may appear at closer time proximity compared to the areas of intermediate incidence. At present, the reason for these latency differences are not clear. It is also uncertain whether carcinoma arises with consistent frequency in each morphological pathogenetic or etiologic type of cirrhosis.

Family studies provide some support to the relationship between HBV and HCC. Denison et al (29) described two adult male siblings who died of HCC; the one with available serum had HBsAg. The father of

these two was said to have died of liver cancer, and later another sibling was found to have HBsAg positive HCC (30). Ohbayashi et al (31) reported HCC with positive serum HBsAg along with the adult type of LC in three Japanese families. According to the latter investigators, chronic liver diseases and asymptomatic HBsAg carriers were found on the maternal side; they concluded that transmission occurred from the mother probably during delivery or the postpartum period. In this model, the infected offspring may then be a latent carrier, later manifesting hepatitis, to proceed to chronic hepatitis, LC, and finally to HCC.

IMMUNOLOGICAL INVOLVEMENT OF HBAg IN HCC

Immunotolerance can be conceived as a strong possibility in cases of newborn infants infected by hepatitis virus from the mother. Nishioka and his associates (28) obtained evidence of possible immunological involvement in a survey of HBsAg in three population groups. Using a haemagglutination technique with sheep red cells tagged with purified HBsAg, specific antibody to HBsAg was detected in the sera of normal healthy subjects in 69 out of 367 cases (18.4%), in patients with malignant diseases other than HCC in 33 out of 229 cases (14.4%), and in HCC patients in 6 out of 80 cases (7.5%). In HCC patients positive for HBsAg, anti-HBs was rarely detected by techniques for demonstration of free anti-HBs. These investigators interpreted the low antibody-forming response against HBsAg in HCC as possibly indicating a specific immunotolerance against HBsAg. Our preliminary observations indicate that the lymphocytes of patients with HCC and LC show a low percentage of blastic transformation to nonspecific mitogens, such as phytohemagglutinin, and that lymphocyte response was also low in contact dermatitis following application of dinitrochlorobenzene (DNCB). However, other investigators report that anti-HBs did not differ between HCC and various control cases (14).

A small amount of ribonucleic acid was first reported in HBsAg by a group of Polish investigators (32), but its presence was not confirmed by later investigators. A collaborative study in the United States gathered evidence that Dane particles contain nucleic acid as well as DNA polymerase which serves as the genetic material for many viruses (33). Their experiments revealed that the core of the Dane particle most likely contains a template that directs the synthesis of DNA, and that the hepatitis virus is a DNA virus. Both DNA polymerase and the postulated DNA template are within the core of the Dane particle found in sera, and it is quite possible that the Dane particle is the human hepatitis B virion and that the core structure is the virion nucleocapsid. From these observations and inferences, a theoretical model may be possible of human HCC carcinogenesis based on animal carcinoma induced by either ONCORNA or ONCODNA. Blumberg (34) has proposed the idea that HBsAg is a new biological unit particle and coined the name ICRON. The physiocochemical and biological properties of ICRON are more similar to ONCORNA than ONCODNA. In animals, if the primary infection of either ONCORNA or ONCODNA occurs at the newborn stage, carcinoma first develops in adulthood. By analogy a newborn infant infected by HBV from his mother may obtain immunological tolerance to HBsAg as a result of constant exposure to HBV. Thus, specific antibody formation to HBsAg may not appear. The present findings on HCC patients appear to support this hypothesis but further investigations are necessary for complete understanding of the disease processes.

LIMITATIONS OF THE PRESENT DATA

The involvement of HBV as the cause of HCC can be established if the three so-called Koch's principles are satisfied. First, the causal relationship of HBV in HCC must be clear. Second, HBsAg should be specific to HCC, or at least specific in cases with a previous history of viral hepatitis B. Third, HBV should be isolated in culture studies, and inoculation of the cultured HBV into susceptible animals should induce hepatitis and later HCC. Serum HBsAg is often found in asymptomatic carriers and in other diseases, such as leukemia, Hodgkin's disease, Down syndrome, tuberous leprosy, and periarteritis nodosa. Several investigators have reported success in isolating and culturing HBV with human fetal lymph node cells or hepatic cells. The reported success by Purcell (35) in production of hepatitis by inoculation of HBsAg positive material into the chimpanzee and rhesus monkey is promising. However, further confirmation and extension of all these studies are essential for definitive conclusions.

CONCLUSIONS

The positive rate of HBsAg in serum is significantly high in patients with HCC. The geographical frequency of HCC patients parallels the frequency of viral hepatitis B. Furthermore, long-term follow-up studies of hepatitis patients reveal a close relation between viral hepatitis and HCC in some patients, but it is incontrovertible that most patients with HCC and with HBsAg in serum give no history of prior jaundice episodes. The subclinical character of the initial disease may relate to the subdued immunity that such patients appear to have HBsAg. Clustering of HCC and LC in families does not contradict but supports a hypothesis of viral hepatitis forming an important basis for development of HCC. In such families, HBsAg infection at the newborn stage may be a critical event for a later disease development.

References

1. Higginson J: The geographic pathology of primary liver cancer. *Cancer Res* **23**:1624–1633, 1963.

2. Higginson J: The epidemiology of primary carcinoma of the liver. in *Tumors of the Liver.* Pack GT, Islami AH (Eds). Springer-Verlag, Berlin, 1970, pp. 39–52.

3. Steiner PE, Davies JNP: Cirrhosis and primary liver carcinoma in Uganda Africans. *Br J Cancer* **11**:523–534, 1957.

4. Isaacson C: The aetiology of cirrhosis and hepatoma in the Bantu—an appraisal. *S Afr Med J* **40**:11–13, 1966.

5. Higginson J, Grobbelaar MB, Walker ARP: Hepatic fibrosis and cirrhosis in man in relation to malnutrition. *Am J Pathol* **23**:29–53, 1957.

6. Kalk H: *Cirrhose und Narbenleber.* Ferdinand Enke, Stuttgart, 1957.

7. Sherlock S, Fox RA, Niazi SP, et al: Chronic liver diseases and primary liver-cell cancer with hepatitis-associated (Australia) antigen in serum. *Lancet* **1**:1243–1247, 1970.

8. Sutnick AI, Millman I, London WT, et al: The role of Australia antigen in viral hepatitis and other diseases. *Ann Rev Med* **23**:161–176, 1972.

9. Sheldon WH, James DF: Cirrhosis following infectious hepatitis—A report of five cases, in two of which there was superimposed primary liver cell carcinoma. *Arch Int Med* **81**:666–689, 1948.

10. Walshe JM, Wolff HH: Primary carcinoma of the liver following viral hepatitis; report of two cases. *Lancet* **2**:1007–1010, 1952.

11. Prince AM, Leblanc L, Krohn K, et al: SH antigen and chronic liver diseases. *Lancet* **2**:717–718, 1970.

12. Alpert E, Isselbacher KJ: Hepatitis-associated antigen and hepatoma in the U.S. *Lancet* **2**:1087, 1971.

13. Masuda M, Takino T, Toyoda E, et al: Hepatitis B antigen in primary liver cancer (in Japanese). *Gendai no Rinsho* **7**:301–307, 1973.

14. Vogel CL, Anthony PP, Sadikali F, et al: Hepatitis-associated antigen and antibody in hepatocellular carcinoma: results of a continuing study. *J Natl Cancer Inst* **48**:1583–1588, 1972.

15. Lopez-Corella AE, Ridula-Sanz C, Albores-Saavedra J: Primary carcinoma of the liver in Mexican adults. *Cancer* **22**:678–685, 1968.

16. Shikata T: Studies on relationship between hepatic cancer and liver cirrhosis. *Acta Pathol Jap* **9**:267–311, 1959.

17. Mori W: Cirrhosis and primary cancer of the liver, comparative study in Tokyo and Cincinnati. *Cancer* **20**:627–631, 1967.

18. Prates MD, Torres FA: A cancer survey in Lourenco Marques, Portuguese East Africa. *J Natl Cancer Inst* **35**:729–757, 1965.

19. Payet M: Etiology and pathogenesis of primary liver cancer in Black Africa. *Acta Unio Int Contra Cancrum* **20**:565–566, 1964.

20. Smith BM, Blumberg BS: Viral hepatitis, postnecrotic cirrhosis and hepatocellular carcinoma. *Lancet* **2**: 953, 1969.

21. Hadziyannis SJ, Merikas GE, Afroudakis AP: Hepatitis-associated antigen in chronic liver disease. *Lancet* **2**:100, 1970.

22. Reed WD, Eddleston ALWF, Stern RB, et al: Detection of hepatitis B antigen by radioimmunoassay in chronic liver disease and hepatocellular carcinoma in Great Britain. *Lancet* **2**:690–694, 1973.

23. Terés J, Guardia J, Brugera M, et al: Hepatitis-associated antigen and hepatocellular carcinoma. *Lancet* **2**:215, 1971.

24. Anand S: Hepatitis-associated antigen in primary liver cell carcinoma. *Lancet* **2**:1032, 1971.

25. Simons MJ, Yap EH, Yu M, et al: Australia antigen in Singapore Chinese patients with hepatocellular carcinoma and comparison groups: Influence of technique sensitivity on differential frequencies, *Int J Cancer* **10**:320–325, 1972.

26. Welsh JD, Brown JD, Arnold K, et al: Hepatitis-associated antigen and hepatoma in South Vietnam. *Lancet* **1**:592, 1972.

27. Tong MJ, Sun Shih-Chien, Schaffner BT, et al: Hepatitis-associated antigen and hepatocellular carcinoma in Taiwan. *Ann Intern Med* **75**:687–691, 1971.

28. Nishioka K, Hirayama T, Sekine T, et al: On

CONCLUSIONS **81**

the relationship between primary carcinoma of the liver and Australia antigen (in Japanese). *Nihon Rinsho* **30**:1154–1158, 1972.

29. Denison EK, Peters RL, Reynolds TB: Familial hepatoma with hepatitis-associated antigen. *Ann Intern Med* **74**:391–394, 1971.

30. Tepfer BD: Hepatoma and HAA *Ann Int Med* **76**:145–146, 1972.

31. Ohbayashi A, Okochi K, Mayumi M: Familial clustering of asymptomatic carriers of Australia antigen and patients with chronic liver disease or primary liver cancer. *Gastroenterology* **62**:618–625, 1972.

32. Jozwiak W, Koscielak J, Madalinski K, et al: RNA of Australia antigen. *Nature* **229**:92, 1971.

33. Kaplan PM, Greenman RL, Gerin JL, et al: DNA polymerase associated with human hepatitis B antigen. *J Virol* **12**:995–1005, 1973.

34. Blumberg BS, Millman I, Sutnick AI, et al: The nature of Australia antigen and its relation to antigen-antibody complex formation. *J Exp Med* **134**:320–329, 1971.

35. Purcell R: *Viral Hepatitis Symposium*, Melbourne, 1974.

CHAPTER 6 THOROTRAST AND TUMORS OF THE LIVER

HECTOR A. BATTIFORA, M.D.

Malignant liver tumors have developed in patients many years after the administration of thorium dioxide (ThO₂) suspensions as a radiological contrast media. To date approximately 120 cases are documented in the world literature (1–59). It is estimated that there are between 50,000 and 100,000 carriers of this substance, and in view of a long latent period of approximately 20 years many additional liver tumors are likely to occur.

HISTORIC BACKGROUND

Thorium dioxide was initially used for lacrimography as early as 1915 (60). In 1928 a ThO₂ solution known as Umbrathor was developed. It was used mostly for bronchography because of its tendency to flocculate when given intravascularly (61). Discovery of the concentration of this product in the liver and spleen led to the development of another technique known as hepatolienography (62).

In 1930 the Hyden Company of Germany developed a new suspension called thorotrast. Because of the fine particle dispersion and apparent absence of deleterious effects, it quickly found extensive use in many countries as a multipurpose contrast medium, particularly for arteriography. However, because of its radioactivity, early questions about safety were raised in several quarters. In 1932 and again in 1937 the Council on Pharmacy and Chemistry of the American Medical Association warned against the possible hazards, restricting its use to patients with malignant tumors, advanced age, or otherwise shortened life expectancy (63, 64). Despite similar warnings in several other countries, the use of thorotrast was continued until the late fifties when it was discontinued because of increasing documentation of its carcinogenicity and other late deleterious effects.

GENERAL DATA ON THOROTRAST

Nature of the Compound

Thorotrast is an aqueous, colloidal solution containing approximately 25% ThO₂. The size of the particles varies from 3 to 10 mμ. The solution also contains 25% dextran and 0.15% methyl p-hydroxybenzoate, the latter as a preservative. Thorium is a radioactive element emitting about 90%

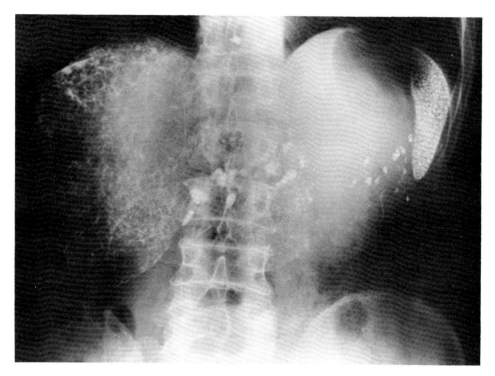

Figure 1 Typical thorotrast deposits in a plain abdominal film, visualizing the liver, spleen, and peripancreatic lymph nodes. This 57-year-old man had a leg fracture 35 years ago, at which time thorotrast angiography was performed. The density in the liver slowly changes with time from the original uniform distribution to an uneven nubecula or arborization pattern. Courtesy of Professor K. Okuda.

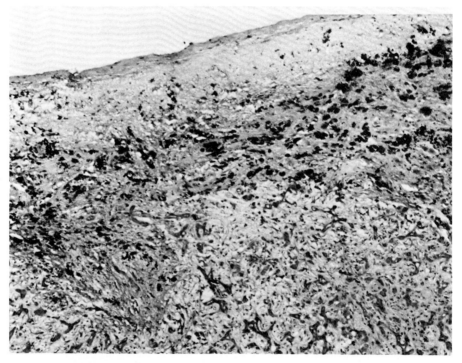

Figure 2 Section of liver including Glisson's capsule. Note marked fibrous thickening of the capsule and abundance of deposits immediately beneath. There is reactive fibrosis and ductular proliferation in the underlying parenchyma (hemotoxylin and eosin X50).

alpha, 9% beta, and 1% gamma particles. During its decay, radium daughter products and thoron are formed. The daughter products are deposited within the bones while thoron is largely exhaled by the lungs (65).

Excretion and Distribution

Thorotrast is excreted so slowly that from a practical standpoint it is thought to remain in the body indefinitely. Its biological half life has been estimated to be 400 years (66). The bulk of the administered ThO_2 is deposited in the liver ($\pm$ 70%), while the spleen and bone receive about 15% and 8%, respectively. The remainder is distributed in lymph nodes, adrenal glands, and lungs. The cells of the reticuloendothelial system absorb most of the ThO_2 where its progressive concentration leads to formation of increasingly larger aggregates. With time destruction of the phagocytic cell releases the product into the stroma where it causes a reactive fibrosis. After several years, large extracellular deposits are common, which, in the liver, are irregularly distributed, being more abundant near Glisson's capsule (Figs. 1 and 2).

Dose and Mode of Administration

The amount of thorotrast administered depended on the type of study carried out. A fraction of a milliliter was used for lacrimography and from 60 to 80 ml were given for hepatolienography. For the latter, 20 to 25 ml of the contrast medium was often given intravenously every other day for three days. Radiographs of the abdomen were usually started the day after the last injection. Intermediate amounts were used for arteriography.

Dosimetry

It has been estimated that the radioactive effect of 75 ml of thorotrast (the amount used for hepatolienography) is comparable to 1.5 to 3.0 μg of radium. The average dose in rads per week has been estimated to be 1.5 for the liver, 2.5 for the spleen, and 0.3 for the bone marrow (65, 66). It is difficult to accurately determine the extent of radiation dose to tissues. Given the short penetrability of alpha particles (1.2 mm) the degree of self-absorption by the ThO_2 aggregates also cannot be estimated accurately. Another important factor in estimating radiation dose is the state of equilibrium at any given time between thorium and its daughter products. The most important problem is produced by the irregular distribution of the radioactive deposits. Because of this, it is estimated that after 50 years, a patient's liver may receive 700 rads in some areas, but as much as 15,000 rads at sites of concentrated particle deposition (67).

Functional and Morphologic Impairment of the Liver

Early studies failed to reveal any functional or morphologic impairment of the liver (11). Later studies disclosed interference with the Bromsulphalein retention test and an elevation in serum alkaline phosphatase (68). These features occurred in patients many years after administration of thorotrast. Some authors have attributed the development of cirrhosis to the presence of thorotrast deposits in the liver, although in most reports, only periportal fibrosis and increased lobulation are described. Fibrosis has been described in other sites of deposition of thorotrast, but most notably the spleen which most authors describe as shriveled, atrophic, and fibrotic. The tendency for the deposits to induce fibrosis has led to serious complications at some sites, for example, around the cauda equina after myelography (69).

CARCINOGENICITY OF THOROTRAST

Experimental Data

In 1936 Selbie produced sarcomas in 58%

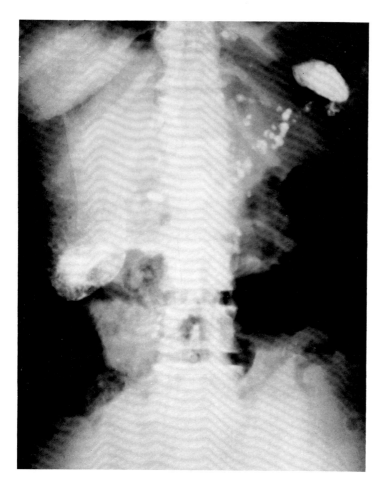

Figure 3 AP X-rays of the abdomen 28 years after administration of thorotrast for hepatolienography. Thorotrast deposits in liver, spleen, and abdominal lymph node are demonstrated.

of rats injected with 0.6 ml of thorotrast and observed for up to 73 weeks (70). Long periods of latency preceded the neoplasms. Later in mice inoculated subcutaneously with 0.2 ml, tumors developed in 43% of those surviving over 62 weeks. Most of the tumors were spindle-cell sarcomas occurring at the site of injection, but an ostiosarcoma, histiocytoma, and angiosarcoma were also reported (71).

Foulds obtained three sarcomas and one carcinoma from 20 guinea pigs three years after 0.3 ml of thorotrast was injected into the mammary region (72). Oberling and Guérin observed subcutaneous and peritoneal sarcomas in rats after the in-

traperitoneal injection of thorotrast (73).

Human Extrahepatic Tumors Induced by Thorotrast

Tumors have been described following extravasation of thorotrast, as well as near deposits caused by the injection of the contrast medium into hollow organs or fistulous tracts. Many were exuberant fibrous reactive processes ("thorotrastomas") rather than true neoplasms. There have been rare sarcomas and various types of epithelial neoplasms in the maxillary sinuses, the renal pelvis, the lung, and so on. The evidence for a etiologic role of thorotrast in these cases is largely circums-

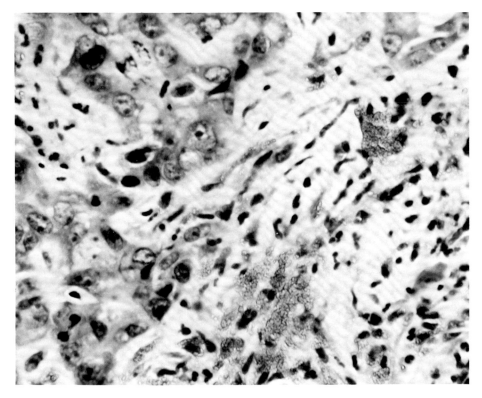

Figure 4 Liber biopsy showing presence of refractile thorotrast deposits within macrophages (although some may be extracellular). To the left of the deposits, atypical hepatocytes are seen (hemotoxylin and eosin, X600).

tantial. Experimental data, however, tend to substantiate a direct cause-effect relationship.

Tumors of the Liver Induced by Thorotrast

To date approximately 120 liver tumors have been attributed to the use of thorotrast. In many cases these followed large doses used for hepatolienography, but in others the patients received smaller doses for arteriography.

Essential criteria for a case to be classified as thorotrast-induced is the presence of the tumor in the immediate vicinity of the deposits and a prolonged period of latency that averages at least 20 years. The deposits of thorotrast are recognized by a characteristic light microscopic appearance and radioactivity, which is easily demonstrated by autoradiographs of tissue sections (Figs. 3 and 4).

The tumors have the usual histologic spectrum of spontaneous liver neoplasms, but with a disproportionally high number of angiosarcomas. Approximately 20% are classified as hepatocellular carcinoma, 32% as cholangiocarcinoma, and 15% as bile duct carcinoma, or histologic combinations of these types. The remaining 33% are predominantly hemangiosarcomas (Kupffer cell sarcoma, angiosarcoma).

Initially, because of the low incidence of hepatic tumors in patients receiving thorotrast, it was difficult to demonstrate a significant statistical relationship between it and the inducement of liver tumors. Indeed, in many of the earlier series (with short follow-up periods) no statistically significant increase could be demonstrated.

However, in later studies, clear-cut increases over the control groups were found (5, 6, 8, 20, 36, 43).

The rather large number of hemangiosarcomas developing in patients receiving thorotrast suggest that this otherwise exceedingly rare neoplasm is a characteristic thorotrast-induced tumor. On the other hand, it may be a peculiar response of the liver to various carcinogens, as suggested by reports of angiosarcoma found in chronic arsenic (73–75) and vinyl chloride poisoning, the latter only recently (76).

The mechanism by which thorotrast induces cancer remains open to question. Although the induction of malignant tumors by ionizing radiation has long been established, the occurrence of liver cancer in response to nonradioactive, chemical poisoning (arsenic, vinyl chloride, iron) raises serious doubts concerning the cancer-inducing mechanism.

Rapidly dividing cells are known to be more sensitive to irradiation, and those in a regenerating liver may be more susceptible to malignant changes through constant bombardment by radioactive particles; thus chemical and radiation damage may combine in the production of tumors by thorotrast.

ILLUSTRATIVE CASE REPORT

CASE 1. R. V., a 60-year-old Caucasian woman, was admitted to Chicago Wesley Memorial Hospital Hospital on October 1, 1971 with complaints of intermittent spasms of the left facial muscles, occasional fever, chills, and mild upper abdominal distress. She denied alcoholism.

Past history revealed hospitalizations for cholecystectomy in 1943, subtotal thyroidectomy for hyperthyroidism in 1949 (hepatomegaly was noted at this time), and medical evaluation of hypothyroidism at another hospital two months prior to admission. Again, hepatomegaly was noted, but no other abnormality was reported.

Physical examination was unremarkable except for evident hepatomegaly, the liver edge being palpated 7 cm below the right costal margin.

X-ray studies revealed large opaque densities in the liver, spleen, and upper abdominal lymph nodes (Fig. 1). At this time it was suspected that the patient might have been given thorotrast in 1943 at the time of her cholecystectomy, and this was subsequently substantiated. A liver scan reported a mass defect in the right lobe corresponding to the opacity on x-ray with markedly distorted and decreased activity in the left lobe. Tumor was suspected. A percutaneous liver biopsy done on October 12, 1971 revealed portal fibrosis and pigmentation in the Kupffer cells. An alpha fetoglobulin test was negative. On October 17, 1971 an open liver biopsy was performed. Sections revealed a mixed hepatocellular carcinoma (Fig. 2). The patient had a difficult postoperative course, but was finally discharged on November 18, 1971. A course of chemotherapy was considered but was not given.

R. V. was readmitted on January 5, 1972 in poor general condition. She complained of weakness and abdominal pain. On physical examination, the patient was jaundiced, ascites was present, and she was diagnosed as being in liver failure.

Abnormal laboratory findings were as follows: hemoglobin, 9.0 g/100 ml; hematocrit, 27%; WBC, 13,500; LDH, mu/ml; SGOT, 422 mu/ml; total bilirubin, 13 mg/100 ml; blood urea nitrogen, 45 mg/100 ml.

Morphological Findings

Light Microscopy

The hepatic architecture was severely distorted. Portal areas were widened by broad adjoining bands of connective tissue containing numerous chronic inflammatory cells and histiocytes. The latter, which often appeared in clusters, contained a variable amoung of an amorphous crystalline material which was not birefringent or stainable (Fig. 4). The hepatic lobules were markedly distorted, and nodules of regenerating liver cells of variable size were conspicuous. Around these regenerating nodules, there were numerous proliferatting ductules. Occasional atypia of hepatocytes and ductule cells were seen.

One of the biopsies was almost entirely composed of neoplastic tissue. The tumor cells were grouped in anastomosing cords and were slightly larger than normal hepatocytes. They had abundant, eosinophilic cytoplasm, round or oval nuclei with one or more eosionphilic nucleoi. Mitoses, often atypical, were numerous.

Electron Microscopy of the Tumor

Abundant collagenous stroma containing macrophages and fibroblasts surrounded the nests of tumor cells (Fig. 5). Electrondense material, presumably thorotrast, was seen within some of the macrophages. The tumor cells were characterized by irregular outlines and abundant endoplasmic reticulum

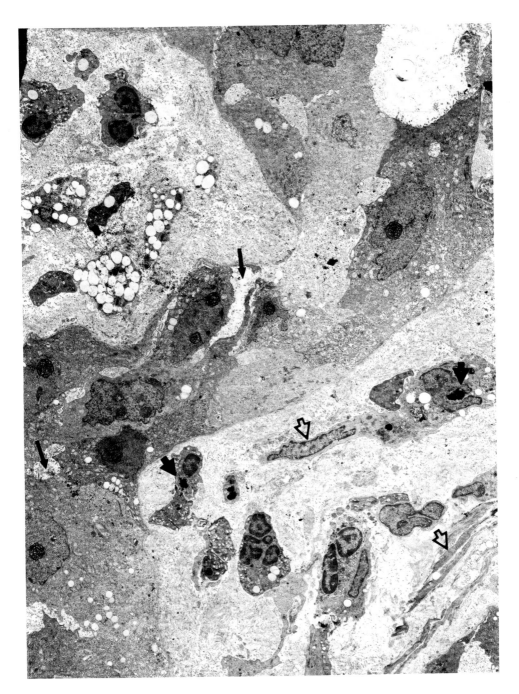

Figure 5 Low-power electron micrograph showing HCC cells. Note presence of biliary canaliculi (arrows) between the tumor cells. The macrophages contain clear vacuoles, presumably lipid and electron dense thorium deposits (thick solid arrows), and are associated with collagen and fibroblasts (hollow arrows).

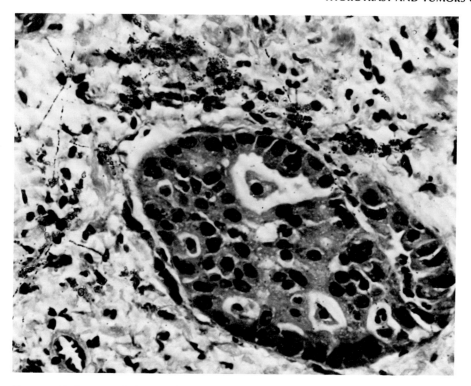

Figure 6 Radioautograph showing characteristic alpha tracks radiating from the thorotrast deposits. A large nest of HCC is seen about the deposits (hemotoxylin and eosin counterstained, X600).

and mitochondria. Their nuclei had variable amounts of chromatin and often multiple, sharply outlined nucleoli. The most distinctive feature was the presence of biliary canaliculi between tumor cells. Microvilli and tight junctions, structures normally present in biliary canaliculi, were conspicuous in the tumor cells.

Autoradiography

Autoradiography disclosed numerous short, straight tracks emanating in spokelike fashion from the intracellular crystalline material (Fig. 6). The number of tracks was proportional to the amount of foreign material present, the tracks being typical of those produced by alpha particles.

REFERENCES

1. Abo M, Sugiwara T, Shinao K: Case of liver cancer caused by Thorotrast. *Jap J Cancer Clin* **15**:822–826, 1969.

2. Akagi G, Hizawa K, Kitamura T, et al: Primary hepatoma 31 years after injection of thorium dioxide sol (abstract). *Tokushima J Exp Med* **13**:111–119, 1966.

3. Baserga R, Yokoo H, Henegar G: Thorotrast-induced cancer in man. *Cancer* **13**:1021–1031, 1960.

4. Batzenschlager A, Dorner A, Weil-Bousson M: La pathologie tumorale du Thorotrast chez l'homme. Revue de la littérature—données statistiques personnelles. *Oncologia* **16**:28–63, 1963.

5. Batzenschlager A, Wilhelm E: Hepatoma in Thorotrast cirrhosis. *Ann Anat Pathol (Paris)* **2**:39–50, 1957; (abstract, *Exc Med*, Section 5, Vol 11, 1958, p 185.

6. Batzenschlager A, et al: Hepatic and biliary carcinoma due to thorotrastosis of the hepatic lymph nodes (abstract). *Arch Anat Pathol (Paris)* **15**:295–300, 1967.

7. Bauer KH: Thorotrast and Krebsgefahr. *Chirurg* **15**:204, 1943.

8. Blomberg RL, Larsson E, Lindell B, Lindgren E: Late effects of Thorotrast in cerebral angiography. *Acta Radiol* **1**:995–1006, 1963.

9. Caroli J, Eteve J, Platteborse R: Thorotrast et

hemangioreticulome malin du foie. *Rev Med Chir Mal Foie* **31**:53–65, 1956.

10. Dahlgren S: Thorotrast tumors: a review of the literature and report of two cases. *Acta Pathol Microbiol Scand* **53**:147–161, 1961.

11. da Silva Horta J: Lebersarkom einer Frau, 3 Jahre und 2 Monate nach Thorotrastinjektion. *Chirurg* **24**:218–223, 1953.

12. da Silva Horta J: Late lesions in man caused by thorium dioxide. (Thorotrast). A new case of sarcoma of the liver 22 years after the injection. *Arch Pathol* **62**:403–418, 1956.

13. da Silva Horta J: Late effect of Thorotrast on the liver and spleen, and the efferent lymph nodes. *N Y Acad Sci* **145**:676–699, 1967.

14. Ellis PA: A case of thorium-induced cholangioma. *Br J Surg* **51**:74–76, 1964.

15. Faber M: Thorium dioxide patients in Denmark. *Ann N Y Acad Sci* **145**:843–848, 1967.

16. Fallot P: Commentaire à propos d'une observation de cancer du foie consecutif a'l'administration de Thorotrast. *Rev Med Chir Mal Foie* **31**:60–68, 1956   cited by Caroli (9)

17. Federlin K, Scior H: Late damages and tumors after injection of Thorotrast (abstract). *Frankfurt Z Pathol* **68**:225–253, 1957.

18. Forbes IJ, Geddes RA, Wood NM: Thorotrast-induced hepatoma with dysimmunoglobulinaemia. *Med J Aust* **55**:18:762–765, 1968.

19. Freese P, Kemnitz P: The development of malignant tumors after Thorotrast (abstract). *Zentralbl Allg Pathol* **105**:161–169, 1964.

20. Fruhling L, Gros CM, Batzenschlager A: Sarcome endothelial angioplastique generalisé chez un malade ayant subi 12 ans auparavant une injection intraartérielle et para-arteriélle de Thorotrast. *Bull Cancer* **42**:559–563, 1955.

21. Gardner DL, Ogilvie RF: The late results of injection of Thorotrast: Two cases of neoplastic disease following contrast angiography. *J Pathol Bacteriol* **78**:133–144, 1959.

22. Grampa G, Tommasini Degna A: Hemangioendothelioma of the liver following intravenous injection of Thorotrast. *Acta Genet Stat Med* **8**:65–78, 1958.

23. Grases PJ: Delayed hepatic and splenic damage from Thorotrast. A case report and review of the literature (abstract). *GEN (Caracas)* **20**:755–788, 1966.

24. Grossiord A, et al: Adenocarcinoma of the liver with cirrhosis, 21 years after an arteriography with Thorotrast (abstract). *Sem Hop Paris* **32**:184–193, 1956.

25. Hassler O, Bostroem K, Dahlback LO: Thorotrast tumors. Report of 3 cases and microradiolog-

ical study of the deposits of Thorotrast in man. *Acta Pathol Microbiol Scand* **61**:13–20, 1964.

26. Heger N, Bayindir MD: Thorotrast: primary liver sarcoma 22 years after the administration. *Minn Med* **53**:1137–1139, 1970.

27. Heitmann W: Carcinoma of the biliary tract and the liver following injection of Thorotrast (abstract). *Chirurg.* **25**:223–225, 1954.

28. Hieronymi G: Kritische Untersuchung sogenannter Thorotrasttumoren nebst Mitteilung zweier Falle. *Zentralbl Allg Pathol* **97**:513–523, 1958.

29. Howard RJ, Todd EP, Dietzman RH, Filleher RC: Thorotrast-induced endothelial cell sarcoma of liver. *Minn Med* **54**:685–688, 1971.

30. Kahn HL: Two cases of carcinoma after Thorotrast administration. *Ann NY Acad Sci* **145**:700–717, 1967.

31. Kemnitz P: Multicentric angioplastic reticuloendotheliomatosis of the liver after Thorotrast arteriography (abstract). *Zentralbl Allg Pathol Anat* **106**:189–197, 1964.

32. Kiely JM, Titus JL, Orvis AL: Thorotrast-induced hepatoma presenting as hyperparathyroidism. *Cancer* **31**:1312, 1973.

33. Kido C, Kaneko M: Radiological study on Thorotrast liver with an additional report of 2 cases of liver cancer caused by Thorotrast (abstract). *Jap J Clin Radiol* **14**:673–680, 1969.

34. Kohoutek J, Novak D: Cholangiogenni Karcinom jater po Thorotrastu. *Cesk Renitgenol* **14**:110–116, 1960 (cited by Dahlgren).

35. Larson B: A case of postangiographic Thorotrast deposition and primary squamous cell carcinoma of the liver. *Acta Pathol Microbiol Scand* **58**:389, 1963.

36. Looney WB, Hursch JB, Colodzin M, Stedman LT: Tumor induction in man following Thorotrast (thorium dioxide) adminstration *Acta Unio Int Cancer* **16**:435–447, 1960.

37. Ludin M: Hemangioendotheliomatosis of liver and spleen after administration of thorium dioxide sol (Thorotrast) (abstract). *Schweiz Z Allg Pathol* **16**:987–994, 1953.

38. MacKay JS, Ross RC: Hepatoma induced by thorium dioxide (Thorotrast). *Can Med Assoc J* **94**:1298–1303, 1966.

39. MacMahon E, Murphy AS, Bates MI: Endothelial cell sarcoma of the liver following Thorotrast injections. *Am J Pathol* **23**:585–613, 1947.

40. Matthes TH: Damage due to thorium dioxide ("Thorotrast") and cancer risks (abstract). *Arch Geschwulstforsch* **6**:162–182, 1954.

41. Mobius G, Lembke K: Thorotrast tumors of the liver (abstract). *Zentralbl Allg Pathol* **105**–41–56, 1963.

42. Morgan A, Jayne W, Marrack D: Primary liver cell carcinoma 24 years after intravenous injection of Thorotrast. *J Clin Pathol* **11**:7–18, 1958.

43. Mori T, Sakai T, Nozue Y, et al: Malignancy and other injuries following Thorotrast administration: Follow-up study of 147 cases in Japan. *Strahlentherapie* **134**:229–254, 1967.

44. Nettleship A, Fink WJ: Neoplasms of the liver following injection of Thorotrast. *Am J Clin Pathol* **35**:422–426, 1961.

45. Ogawara S: Case report of liver cancer induced by Thorotrast and a study of the metabolism of daughter nuclides (abstract). *Nippon Ika Daigaku Zasshi* **40**:169–175, 1965.

46. Okinaka S, Nakao K, Ibayashi H, et al: A case report on the development of biliary tract cancer 11 years after the injection of thorotrast. *Am J Roentgenol* **78**:812–818, 1957.

47. Person DA, Isaac E: Thorotrast induced carcinoma of the liver. *Arch Surg* **88**:503–510, 1964.

48. Rakov HL, Smalldon TR, Derman H: Hepatic hemangioendotheliosarcoma. Report of a case due to thorium. *Arch Intern Med* **112**:173–178, 1963.

49. Roberts JC, Carlson K: Hepatic duct carcinoma seventeen years after injection of thorium dioxide. *AMA Arch Pathol* **62**:1–7, 1956.

50. Rosenbaum FJ: Hepatic sarcoma after Thorotrast. *Dtsch Med Wochenschr* **84**:428–433, 1959.

51. Smoron J, Battifora H: Thoratrast induced hepatoma. *Cancer* **30**:1252–1259, 1972.

52. Stemmermann G: Adenocarcinoma of the intrahepatic biliary tree following Thorotrast. *Am J Clin Pathol* **32**:446–454, 1960.

53. Suchow E, Henegar GC, Baserga R: Tumors of the liver following administration of Thorotrast. *Am J Pathol* **38**:663–677, 1961.

54. Tesluk H, Nordin WA: Hemangioendothelioma of liver following thorium dioxide administration. *AMA Arch Pathol* **60**:493–501, 1955.

55. Vallenga LR: A case of hemangiosarcoma of the liver 25 years after Thorotrast injection for cerebral angiography. *J Belg Radiol* **45**:682–688, 1962.

56. Verhaak R: A case of carcinoma in a Thorotrast liver (abstract). *Fortschr Geb Roentgenstr Nuklearmed* **101**:539–543, 1964.

57. Wenz W, Ott G: Actual Thorotrast problems: Hepatic sarcoma with intraperitoneal hemorrhage (abstract). *Strahlentherapie* **127**:463–469, 1965.

58. Yanagi T, Suga S, Mekata H, et al: Case of Thorotrast and cancer of the liver with epidural metastasis to the spinal cord. *Saishin Igaku* **24**:2149–2159, 1969.

59. Yamada K, Autopsy case of Thorotrast-induced liver cancer complicated by thyroid cancer. *Rinsho Haska* **13**:751–759, 1968.

60. Rudolphi H: Spatentwieklung eines Unterlidkarzinoms nach Thoriumoxydinjektion. *Beitr Pathol Anat* **111**:158–164, 1950.

61. Blubaum T, Frick K, Kalkbrenne H: Eine neue Anwendungasast der Kolloide in der Rontgendiagnostik. *Fortschr Geb Roentgenstr Nuklearmed* **37**:18–29, 1928.

62. Oka M: Eine neue Methode zur rontgenologischen Dorstellung der Milz (Lienographie). *Fortschr Geb Roentgenstr Nuklearmed* **40**:497–501, 1929.

63. Editorial: Council on pharmacy and chemistry: Thorotrast. *JAMA* **99**:2183–2185, 1932.

64. Editorial: Potential hazards of the diagnostic use of thorium dioxide. *JAMA* **108**:1656–1657, 1937.

65. Looney WB: An investigation of the late clinical findings following Thorotrast (thorium dioxide) administration. *Am J Roentgenol* **83**:163–185, 1960.

66. Hursh JB, Stedman LT, Looney WB, Colodzin M: Excretion of thorium and thorium daughters after Thorotrast administration to human subjects. *Acta Radiol* **47**:481–498, 1957.

67. Rundo J: Thesis, University of London, 1958.

68. Janower ML, Miettinen OS, Flynn MJ: Effects of long-term Thorotrast exposure. *Radiology* **103**:13, 1972.

69. Boyd JT, Langlands AO, Maccabe JJ: Long-term hazards of Thorotrast. *Br Med J* **2**:517–521, 1968.

70. Selbie FR: Experimental production of sarcoma with Thorotrast. *Lancet* **2**:847, 1936.

71. Selbie FR: Tumours in rats and mice following the injection of Thorotrast. *Brit J Exp Pathol* **29**:100, 1938.

72. Foulds L: Production of transplantable carcinoma and sarcoma in guinea pigs by injections of Thorotrast. *Am J Cancer* **35**:363, 1939.

73. Oberling C, Guérin M: Action du Thorotrast sur le sarcome de Jensen du rat blanc. *Bull Assoc Fr Cancer* **22**:469–489, 1933.

74. Roth F: Chronic arsenic poisoning in vineyard workers of the Moselle with special reference to arsenic cancer (abstract). *Z Krebforsch* **61**:287–319, 1956.

75. Roth F: Arsen-Leber-Tumoreum (Hemangioendotheliom). *Z Kresforsch* **61**:468–503, 1957.

76. Block JB: Angiosarcoma of the liver following vinyl chloride exposure. *JAMA* **229**:53–54, 1974.

CHAPTER 7 ANDROGENIC-ANABOLIC STEROIDS AND HEPATOCELLULAR CARCINOMA

F. LEONARD JOHNSON, M.D., M.B.B.S.

The hepatic toxicity of oral androgenic-anabolic steroids has frequently been documented (1, 2). Ranging from a symptomless elevation in liver function tests such as BSP excretion (3) to a clinical and histologic picture of cholestatic jaundice (4), such toxicity has appeared benign and reversible on withdrawal of the steroid (2). More recently, however, there has been an increasing number of reports of more serious side effects seemingly attributable to these agents, including hepatocellular carcinoma (HCC) and peliosis hepatis (5–9). This chapter is a review of the evidence available that suggests these hormones have a role in hepatoma pathogenesis—evidence which, although presently circumstantial in humans, becomes more significant with each case report.

The evidence centers around two major observations: (1) epidemiological and rodent studies indicating that a predominantly "androgenic environment" in the absence of primary hepatic disease favors hepatoma formation in certain mouse strains; and (2) the increasingly frequent reports since 1971 of hepatomas arising in patients with aplastic anemia or impotence treated with long term oral C-17 alkylated androgenic-anabolic steroids (Table 1).

EPIDEMIOLOGICAL AND ANIMAL DATA

In humans there is an increased incidence of HCC in males beyond puberty (4, 10) which suggests the possibility of a relationship between androgens and HCC formation. In rodent strains with a high incidence of spontaneous HCC, for example, C3H and CBA mice, the neoplasm is three to six times more common in males (11). The most direct experimental data, however, come from rodent strains where a direct effect of hormonal manipulation on HCC development has been demonstrated. Such studies have shown the following:

95

Table 1   Summary of Reported Cases of Oral Adrenogenic-Anabolic Steroid-Associated with HCC

Patient	Age	Fanconi's Anemia	Transfusions Before Liver Disease	Agent	Dose (mg/day)	Duration (months)	Ref.
1	6	−	+	Oxymetholone	30–100	46	(9)
2	20	−	+	Oxymetholone	150–250	28	(9)
3	27	+	+	Methyltestosterone	20	40	(9)
4	21	+	−	Methandrostenolone	10–50	89	(9)
5	20	+	−	Oxymetholone	100	10	(7)
6	16 [a]	−	+	Methyltestosterone	40–80	21	(16)
				Norethandrolone	10	3	
				Oxymetholone	100	35	
				Stanazalol	15	18	
7	68 [b]	−	−	Methyltestosterone	?	360	(17)
8	6	−	+	Oxymetholone	40–60	41	(18)
9	6	−	+	Methyltestosterone	60	> 24	(19)

[a] Not histologically proved, alpha fetoprotein positive.
[b] History of "infectious jaundice" 40 years previously.

1. Castration of male mice of the C3H and CBA strains reduces the incidence of spontaneous HCC from over 33% to less than 12% (11), with suggestive evidence that injection of the less hepatoma-prone female mice of these strains with testosterone increases their rate of spontaneous hepatoma formation (12).

2. In rats with chemically induced hyperplastic nodules that precede the formation of HCC, testosterone administration increases both HCC formation and the degree of nodular undifferentiation, whereas castration results in some protective benefit (13).

3. In C57BL x C3H F' mice castration of males decreases the frequency of HCC formation from 96 to 62% of animals, and ovariectomy of females increases the incidence from 20 to 67% of animals (14).

4. Diethylsilbestrol decreases the incidence of HCC in male C3H mice from 90.5% to 55% (15).

Until this decade these observations had appeared to have little relevance to the pathogenesis of human hepatomas. This has changed however with the documenta-

tion of HCC arising in nine patients receiving long-term therapy with oral androgenic-anabolic steroids (7–9, 16–19).

HUMAN EVIDENCE

Speculation that oxymetholone, a C_{17} alkylated testosterone derivative, might have been involved in the development of a hepatocellular carcinoma was first made in 1971 by Bernstein and his colleagues. They described development of this neoplasm in a 21-year-old male with Fanconi's anemia who was treated with oxymetholone for 10 months (7). Four similar cases were subsequently detailed in 1972 (9) followed by a series of individual case reports (16–19). The relevant details of these patients are given in Table 1. One further patient has been reported who developed HCC 24 years after receiving a short course of androgenic-anabolic steroids (20). A relationship between drug and tumor seems remote and this patient is not included in the present discussion.

The reason that one cannot state with absolute certainty that the androgenic-anabolic steroid given was directly implicated in the development of the HCC observed is that obviously other factors are present in every patient so far described which may also play a role in hepatoma development. In three of the nine patients the underlying disease was Fanconi's anemia, a syndrome complex known to be associated with a higher than normal incidence of acute leukemia and squamous cell carcinoma (21). There has also been reported a girl with Fanconi's anemia diagnosed at age 7 and treated with multiple transfusions, who 17 years later developed an alpha-fetroprotein (AFP) positive HCC in the apparent absence of androgen therapy (22). Macronodular cirrhosis and hemochromatosis were also present however, preventing a clear statement of association between Fanconi's anemia and HCC in this patient.

The multiple transfusions necessary to treat aplastic anemia also complicate the issue leading as they do to hepatic iron deposition and postnecrotic cirrhosis following serum hepatitis, known factors in HCC formation (4). All five patients whose indication for androgenic-anabolic steroids was idiopathic aplastic anemia had received prior transfusions. The two patients who had not received multiple transfusions prior to HCC development carried the diagnosis of Fanconi's anemia. Nevertheless, the absence of an increased incidence of HCC in patients with other conditions requiring multiple transfusions over a similar time period such as the congenital hemoglobinopathies, thalassemia, and sickle cell anemia, raise doubts that transfusions alone account for this high incidence of HCC in such a small selected group of patients.

UNIQUE BEHAVIOR OF ANDROGEN ASSOCIATED HEPATOMAS

Supporting the contention that these tumors are not basically transfusion-related or a malignancy arising in a patient predisposed by Fanconi's anemia, but rather directly related to the long-term exposure to androgenic steroids, is the unusual biological behavior of the tumors so far reported. No evidence of metastatic spread beyond the liver has yet been documented and particularly fascinating is the demonstrated hormone dependence of the neoplasm in one patient (9). A five-year-old girl with idiopathic aplastic anemia developed what appeared grossly at the time of laparotomy to be nodules of HCC scattered throughout the liver. She had previously been treated with oxymetholone for 46 months. Histopathological examination of a biopsy of one of these nodules revealed polyhedral cells of hepatic origin arranged in trabeculae 2 to 5 cells in width. Bile production was seen in occasional cells. Large groups of cells with decreased eosinophilic staining, increased nuclear to cytoplasmic ratio, and a compact growth pattern that represented dedifferentiation of the hepatocellular elements were seen in 40% of the biopsy specimen submitted. Pseudoglandular and psuedoalveolar arrangements of hepatocellular tumor cells were also noted in this area. Only one normal structure, a single portal area, was seen; nodular hypoplasia was not seen.

The morphologic features of this tumor satisfied the criteria of the Armed Forces Institute of Pathology for HCC.

Following laparotomy oxymetholone was stopped, and within 11 months complete clinical resolution of this hepatic neoplasm, usually associated in children with a prognosis of less than 6 months (23), had occurred (Figs. 1 and 2).

Exogenous androgen dependence has also been reported in a patient developing peliosis hepatis, a lesion whose pathogenesis is not only linked to long-term androgenic-anabolic steroid use, but one which has also been present concomitantly with HCC in reported cases (24).

MECHANISMS

How androgenic hormones could give rise

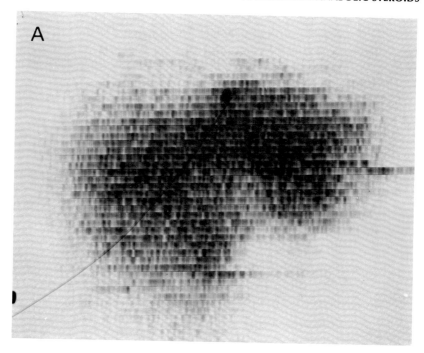

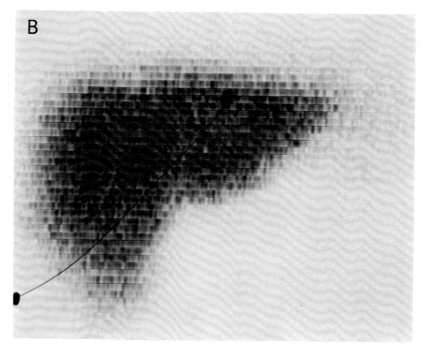

Figure 1   Regression of androgenic steroid associated with HCC following cessation of steroid. *(a)* Liver scan of July 1971 showing hepatomegaly, diffuse infiltrative process, and focal defects. *(b)* Liver scan of same patient made in July 1972 showing resolution of original lesion (markers show outlines of right rib cage).

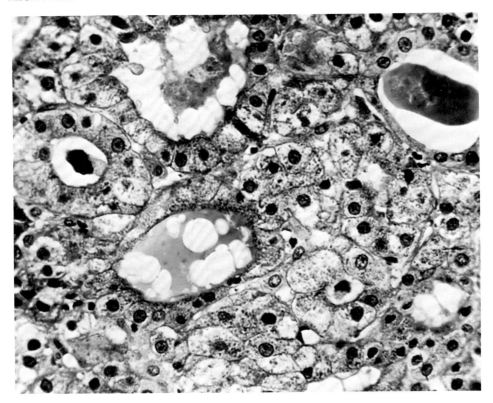

Figure 2 Histopathology of androgenic-anabolic steroid associated with HCC shown in liver scan of Fig. 1 (hemotoxylin and eosin, 142.50X).

to hepatic tumors remains an unanswered question. The simplest concept is that following androgen-induced injury compensatory liver cell hypertrophy occurs and if this becomes uncontrolled, a malignant HCC results (7). Experience in the mouse HCC model, however, suggests that many factors affect the influence of hormones on the formation of hepatomas. Lingeman best expressed it when he reported that "assessment of carcinogenicity of hormones will require attention to the many variables . . . including variation in inducibility of metabolizing enzymes and interference with or enhancement of their activity by endogenous hormones, other drugs, or chemical compounds in the environment" (25).

Along these lines may lie a clue to more complete understanding of the effect of androgens on the human liver in the seemingly paradoxical documentation since 1973 of hepatic adenomata in normal women taking the mixed contraceptive pill (26–33). Details of reported cases are summarized in Table 2.

Based on these observations it has been hypothesized that androgens predispose to HCC and estrogens to benign hepatic adenoma (26), but the situation may be far more interrelated than this.

For example, the role of the progesterone component in contraceptive agents has perhaps been overlooked. "Enovid" and "Ortho-Novum," two agents implicated in hepatic adenoma production, contain norethynodrel and norethindrone, respectively. Norethynodrel is a derivative of

Table 2 Summary of Reported Cases of Contraceptive Agent Associated Benign Hepatic Adenomas

Patient	Age	Agent[a]	Duration (years)	Massive Hemorrhage	Result	Survived	Reference
1	26	Enovid	2	Yes	Left hepatectomy	Yes	(26)
2	27	Ovin, Oracon	Several	Yes	Right hepatectomy	No	(26)
3	25		6	–	Left hepatectomy	Yes	(26)
4	25	Ovral	0.5	–	Right hepatectomy	Yes	(26)
5	29	Enovid	6	–	Quadrate lobectomy	Yes	(26)
6	30	Multiple	7	Yes	Right hepatectomy	Yes	(26)
7	39	Enovid	7	Yes	Right hepatectomy	Hepatic insufficiency	(26)
8	28	Enovid	7	–	Right partial hepatectomy	Yes	(27, 28)
9	37	Ovral	Several	Yes	Right hepatectomy	No	(29)
10	30	Ordol	3	–	Left lobectomy	Yes	(30)
11	33	Ortho-novum	Several	Yes	Right hepatectomy	No	(31)
12	36	Ovral	5–6	Yes	Right hepatectomy	No	(32)
13	26	?	Several	–	Biopsy right lobe	Yes	(27, 33)

[a] Enovid: norethynodrel + mestranol; Ovin, Oracon: dimethisterone + ethinyloestradiol; Ovral: norgestrol + ethinyloestradiol; Ortho-novum: norethindrone + mestranol.

the androgenic norethisterone (34) and norethindrone (17 α-ethyl-19-nortestosterone) has both anabolic and androgenic actions. As Groos and his colleagues have pointed out, the androgenic "17 -alkylated norandrostane derivatives and other gestagens present in these mixed contraceptive agents may indeed be implicated in the liver tumors seen" (24).

In the mouse model norethynodrel, norethisterone, and norethisterone plus mestranol were found to produce an increase over expected frequency of hepatoma in male mice (35). In female mice norethynodrel has not been reported to produce hepatomas but rather hepatic cellular swelling with sinusoidal aberrations (36). Thus the androgenic effects of norethynodrel may well be modified and the animal protected from malignant hepatoma formation by the estrogen environment of the female.

These observations then raise an alternative postulation to the simple androgen-carcinoma estrogen-adenoma hypothesis. What has been observed may well be a spectrum of basically androgenic-induced liver changes, with a hepatocellular carcinomalike lesion on one end of the spectrum, a lesion with as yet undefined malignant potential, and benign adenoma of the liver at the opposite end. The adenoma formation has been modified by the influence of estrogen either endogenously circulating or exogenously taken in the form of the mixed contraceptive pill.

Such a hypothesis helps explain the three interesting case reports in humans which previously have seemed only to confuse this issue of sex hormones and hepatic tumors. In the first report Nosonyi reported the case of a 61-year-old woman who was found to have three hepatic nonmalignant nodules in association with an androgen secreting ovarian adenoma (37).

This is further evidence of an androgenic sensitivity of liver cells, but the fascinating aspect of this report was the dis-covery in these nodules of "estrogenic material," material that may well have had protective benefit, preventing frank hepatocellular carcinoma formation.

In the second case Contostavlos reported the unsuspected finding of peliosis hepatis, the hitherto well-described androgen-induced change, in a 37-year-old woman with a norgestrel plus ethinyloestradiol-associated hepatoma. In such instances the androgenic effect of the progesterone component may account for peliosis hepatis (29).

In the third case Thalassinos and colleagues described a 30-year-old woman who following pregnancy induced by fertility agents developed a hepatocellular carcinoma thought secondary to "estrogen-like" drugs (38). She had, however, received long-term clomiphene therapy prior to receiving the estrogens. Clomiphene is a potent "anti-estrogen" (34) and may explain the development of a carcinoma rather than adenoma in this patient if indeed the neoplasm was hormone related.

IMPLICATIONS

Despite our ignorance as to the precise nature and pathophysiology of this correlation between hepatomas and sex hormones, several implications are apparent. Epidemiologically it may give a clue as to the pathogenesis of hepatomas in children and young adults who develop this lesion spontaneously without any known predisposing factor. If indeed an imbalance between the androgen-estrogen environment favors the development of HCC-adenoma, therapeutic advantage of this might also be taken.

Most important are the clinical implications of these lesions. Patients on androgenic-anabolic steroids need to be closely monitored. With the observed regression of both a hepatocellular carcinoma and peliosis hepatis following cessation of exogenous androgen, the best course of action in a patient with either lesion appears to simply be to stop the androgenic agent (9, 24) and not subject the patient to the risks of extensive surgery and hepatic lobectomy or chemotherapy of limited value. This is particularly relevant to the patient with aplastic anemia where granulocytopenia and thrombocytopenia mitigate against any surgical procedures aimed at diagnosis or therapy.

Conversely, although histologically "benign," the adenomas developing in women taking the contraceptive pills were responsible for the death from unremitting hemorrhage of 4 of the 13 illustrated cases (39).

Knowledge of these particular hepatic effects of hormonal agents dictates a course of therapy that in the usual circumstances appears to be completely inadequate in one instance and excessive in the other. It prevents inappropriate or overaggressive therapy in the patient on androgenic-anabolic steroids who develops a hepatocellular carcinomalike lesion, and stresses the need for prompt diagnosis and aggressive therapy in the woman on contraceptive pills who develops a benign adenoma.

Recently there has been extension of the use of androgenic-anabolic steroids in high dose for long periods of time beyond the patient with disease to the healthy athlete aiming to improve muscle strength (40). Unless there is more active discouragement of the use of these agents in normal individuals, it may not be very long before it actually takes the development of a significantly damaging side effect of androgenic steroids in a normal athlete to defer others.

Because these tumors are so rare, and a justifiable controversy exists over whether they are even malignant, the most rapid answer to this association of liver tumors and sex hormones will most likely come from basic research. Beaconsfield has stated that "to investigate the existence of an association like the one we are discussing

without waiting half a generation to collect enough cases, it is necessary to look for corroborative evidence, and this is to be found in the study of cell metabolism and cellular dynamics" (36). Notwithstanding this, it is important that these liver tumors are reported whenever they occur and particularly that more detail than has currently been evident is directed toward the clinical history and precise histopathological descriptions of such lesions to aid comparison between reports.

REFERENCES

1. Sanchez-Medal L, Gomez-Leal A, Duarte L, et al: Anabolic-androgenic steroids in the treatment of acquired aplastic anemia. *Blood* **34**:283–300, 1969.

2. Shahidi NT: Androgens and erythropoiesis. *N Engl J Med* **289**:72–79, 1973.

3. Silink SJ, Firkin BG: An analysis of hypoplastic anemia with special reference to the use of oxymetholone (Adroyd) in its therapy. *Australas Ann Med* **17**:224–235, 1968.

4. Sherlock S: *Diseases of the Liver and Biliary System*, 4th ed. Scientific Publications, F. A. Davis Co., Philadelphia, 1968, p. 371.

5. Kintzen W, Silny J: Peliosis hepatis after administration of Fluoxymesterone. *Can Med Assoc J* **83**:860–862, 1960.

6. Gordon BS, Wolf J, Krause T, et al: Peliosis hepatis and cholestasis following administration of norethandrolone. *Am J Clin Pathol* **33**:156–165, 1960.

7. Bernstein MS, Hunter RL, Yachnin S: Hepatoma and peliosis hepatis developing in a patient with Fanconi's anemia. *N Engl J Med* **284**:1135–1136, 1971.

8. Recant L, Lacy P (Eds). Fanconi's anemia and hepatic cirrhosis. Clinopathological conference. *Am J Med* **39**:464–475, 1965.

9. Johnson FL, Feagler JR, Lerner KW, et al: Association of androgenic-anabolic steroid therapy with development of hepatocellular carcinoma. *Lancet* **ii**: 1273–1276, 1972.

10. Fraumeni JF, Miller RW, Hill JA: Primary carcinoma of the liver in childhood: an epidemiologic study. *J Natl Cancer Inst* **40**:1087–1099, 1968.

11. Andervont HB: Studies on the occurrence of spontaneous hepatomas in mice of strains C3H and CBA. *J Natl Cancer Inst* **11**:581–591, 1952.

12. Agnew LRC, Gardner WU: The incidence of spontaneous hepatomas in C_3H, C_3H (low milk factor), and CBA mice and the effect of estrogen and androgen on the occurrence of these tumors in C_3H mice. *Cancer Res* **12**:757–761, 1952.

13. Reuber MD: Influence of hormones on N-2-fluorenyldiacetamid-induced hyperplastic hepatic nodules in rats. *J Natl Cancer Inst* **43**:445–451, 1969.

14. Vesselinovitch SD, Mihailovich N: The effect of gonadectomy on the development of hepatomas induced by urethan. *Cancer Res* **27**:1788–1791, 1967.

15. Deringer MK: Occurrence of tumors, particularly mammary tumors, in agent-free strain C_3HeB mice. *J Natl Cancer Inst* **22**:995–1002, 1959.

16. Henderson JT, Richmond J, Sumerling MD: Androgenic-anabolic steroid therapy and hepatocellular carcinoma (letter). *Lancet* **i**: 934, 1972.

17. Ziegenfuss J, Carabasi R: Androgens and hepatocellular carcinoma (letter). *Lancet* **i**:262, 1973.

18. Meadows AT, Naiman JL, Valdes-Dapena MV: Hepatoma associated with androgen therapy for aplastic anemia. *J Pediatr* **84**:109–110, 1974.

19. Johnson W: personal communication.

20. Guy JT, Auslander MO: Androgenic steroids and hepatocellular carcinoma (letter). *Lancet* **i**: 148, 1973.

21. Dosik H, Hsu LY, Todaro GJ, et al: Leukemia in Fanconi's anemia: Cytogenetic and tumor virus susceptibility studies. *Blood* **36**:341–352, 1970.

22. Cattan D, Vesin P, Wantier J: Liver tumours and steroid hormones (letter). *Lancet* **i**:878, 1974.

23. Ishak KG, Glunz PR: Hepatoblastoma and hepatocarcinoma in infancy and childhood. *Cancer* **20**:396–422, 1967.

24. Groos G, Arnold OH, Brittinger G: Peliosis hepatis after long term administration of oxymetholone (letter). *Lancet* **i**: 874, 1974.

25. Lingeman CH: Liver cell neoplasms and oral contraceptives (letter). *Lancet* **i**:64, 1974.

26. Baum J, Holtz F, Bookstein JJ, et al: Possible association between benign hepatomas and oral contraceptives. *Lancet* **ii**:926–931, 1973.

27. Horvath E, Kovacs K, Ross RC: Ultrastructural findings in a well differentiated hepatoma. *Digestion* **7**:74–82, 1972.

28. Horvath E, Kovacs K, Ross RC: Benign hepatoma in a young woman on contraceptive steroids (letter). *Lancet* **i**: 357–358, 1974.

29. Contostavlos DL: Benign hepatomas and oral contraceptives (letter). *Lancet* **ii**: 1200, 1973.

30. Tountas C, Paraskevas G, Deligeorgi H: Benign hepatoma and oral contraceptives (letter). *Lancet* **i**: 1351–1352, 1974.

31. Knapp WA, Ruebner BH: Hepatomas and oral contraceptives (letter). *Lancet* **i**: 270–271, 1974.

32. Kelso DR: Benign hepatomas and oral contraceptives (letter). *Lancet* **i**: 315–316, 1974.

33. Kay S, Schatzki PF: Ultrastructure of a benign liver cell adenoma. *Cancer* **28**:755–761, 1971.

34. Astwood EB: Estrogens and progestins. in *The Pharmacological Basis of Therapeutics,* 3rd ed. Goodman LA, Gilman A (Eds). The Macmillan Co., New York, 1965, pp. 1540–1565.

35. Carcinogenicity tests of oral contraceptives. A report by the committee on the ssafety of medicines. London, 1972.

36. Beaconsfield P: Liver tumors and steroid hormones (letter). *Lancet* **i**: 516–517, 1974.

37. Mosonyi L: Multiple benign hepatomas and virilization by ovarian tumor (letter). *Lancet* **ii**: 1263–1264, 1974.

38. Thalassinos HC, Lymberatos C, Hadjioannou J, et al: Liver-cell carcinoma after long-term estrogen-like drugs. *Lancet* **i**: 270, 1974.

39. Liver tumors and steroid hormones (editorial). *Lancet* **ii**: 1481, 1975.

40. Wade N: Anabolic steroids: doctors denounce them but athletes aren't listening. *Science* **176**:1399–1403, 1972.

Part Three PATHOLOGY

CHAPTER 8 PATHOLOGY OF HEPATOCELLULAR CARCINOMA

ROBERT L. PETERS, M.D.

INTRODUCTION

A classification of hepatocellular carcinoma (HCC) and description of the various morphologic forms that the tumor assumes was originally proposed in the latter part of the nineteenth century by Hanot and Gilbert (1) but was supplemented by a detailed and classic work of Eggel in 1901 (2). Prior to that time microscopic studies of tumors involving the liver were sparse. The best developed and most accepted characterization of HCC is probably that of Edmondson in *Tumors of the Liver and Intrahepatic Bile Ducts* published by the Armed Forces Institute of Pathology in 1958 as fascicle #25 (3). The statistical data presented in the fascicle were based in part on experiences of Edmondson and Steiner with 75 cases of HCC (including 5 mixed hepatocellular-ductal) and 18 peripheral choangiocarcinomas and 7 hilar bile duct carcinomas from among the 48,900 autopsies at Los Angeles County Hospital from 1918 through 1953 (4). The population used as the basis of the pathologic characterization of HCC in this chapter is similar

to that of Edmondson and Steiner in that it is drawn in large part from the autopsy material of Los Angeles County-USC Medical Center (LAC-USCMC) and USC-John Wesley County Hospital (USC-JWCH) but at a later time, from January 1954 through December 1973. Thus both studies represent the hepatocellular carcinomas found in the indigent population of Los Angeles County. With time there have undoubtedly been some population shifts and environmental changes. The principal effort in the following chapter is (1) to further characterize the gross appearances of HCC, (2) to describe the background hepatic histologic disorders on which HCC may become engrafted, (3) to describe the histologic patterns that HCC may assume, (4) to describe the biologic behavior of the neoplasm, and (5) to relate morphologic pattern to the background lesion and to biologic behavior if possible.

The incidence of HCC in the western hemisphere at the turn of the century ranged between 0.05% and 0.13% of autopsies (2, 5). At LAC-USCMC in the 35 years from 1918 to 1953, 48,915 autopsies

Table 1   Changing of HCC in indigent population of Los Angeles

	Guy's Hospital	LAC-USCMC	LAC-USCMC and JWCH	
Years	pre-1900	1918 to 1953	1954 to 1963	1964 to 1973
Number of autopsies	18,500	49,915	23,476	15,380
HCC	24	81	78	147
Autopsies (%)	0.13	0.17	0.33	0.96
HCC c̄ Cirrhosis (%)	25 to 50	85	90.8	81.8
Admitted alcoholism (%)	?	50±	48	48

yielded 81 cases of HCC (0.17%). From January 1954 to the end of 1963, half as many autopsies (23,476) yielded essentially the same number of cases of HCC (78 cases or 0.33%) whereas 1964 through 1973 showed a further drop in number of autopsies (15,380) with an increase in HCC to 147 (0.96%). (See Table 1.)

In the United States the incidence of HCC seems to vary from one type of environment to another. The variation may partly depend on the immigrant population but is also related to the number of indigent patients. Becker noted a fivefold difference in incidence of HCC between a charity and a university hospital only 1/5 mile apart (6). The principal difference in HCC incidence between the two kinds of hospital seems to rest with the larger number of patients with alcoholic cirrhosis in the charity hospital.

PRENEOPLASTIC CONDITIONS

CIRRHOSIS. The relationship of nonalcoholic kinds of cirrhosis to HCC is discussed in detail in a separate chapter (Chapter 4, Shikata). Hepatocellular carcinoma is usually associated with some variety of cirrhosis. As a general rule in parts of the world where HCC is a very common neoplasm, its association with cirrhosis is high, in the range of 90%, whereas in those geo-graphic areas with a low incidence of HCC the concurrence of cirrhosis is decreased to about 65%. Shikata has questioned the accuracy of this general observation and has proposed that cirrhosis in many instances may have been overlooked (7). He has correctly pointed out that many studies that have resulted in reports of an incidence of cirrhosis in patients with HCC of only 65 to 75% have not been based on material that convincingly excluded cholangiocarcinoma (8). Shikata's complaint is undoubtedly well founded. Certainly in regions with a low incidence of HCC, cholangiocarcinoma may make up a larger percentage of the cases of total primary liver cancer. Since cholangiocarcinoma is less frequently superimposed on a cirrhotic liver, grouping cholangiocarcinoma and hepatocellular carcinoma together would cause a significant error in the relationship to cirrhosis. However, MacSween in reviewing 64 cases of histologically established HCC in Scotland, a country with low HCC incidence, found only 49 patients (75%) to have cirrhosis (9). Conversely, certain African populations with high incidence of HCC have relatively lower percentage associated with cirrhosis. Geddes and Falkson, in a study of 189 Bantu patients with histologically established liver cancer, found in autopsies of 167 patients including 2 with cholangiocarcinomas that 40% had no evidence of cirrhosis (10).

Table 2   Sex Incidence of HCC

	Total	Male (%)	Female (%)
Autopsies	38,856	56.9	43.0
Cirrhosis	3,465	63.7	36.3
HCC	225	84.3	15.7
HCC in cirrhosis	190	90	10
HCC without cirrhosis	35	51.5	48.5

Apparently the relationship of HCC with cirrhosis has in the past been even less definite, at least in the western hemisphere. In 1888 Hanot and Gilbert indicated that about one-third of their patients who had HCC also had cirrhosis (1), whereas Rolleston reported in 1912 that of the 41 patients with liver cell carcinoma at Middlesex Hospital in London, 10 also had cirrhosis of the liver (11). On the other hand, Eggel, whose 1901 report originated the gross morphologic classification of HCC, found in reviewing gross descriptions that cirrhosis was positively identified in 57 of 99 patients with HCC (57.6%) but that only nine times was a statement made excluding cirrhosis (2). Thus one might conclude that cirrhosis was present in 86.4% of the 66 patients with HCC on which an adequate description of the liver was made, or in 57.6% of the total group—a considerable discrepancy which bears out Shikata's suspicion that quoted percentages of cirrhotic patients in many series may be inaccurate. In the United States, between 69% (12) and 89% (3, 4) of HCC patients have been reported to have cirrhosis. The percentage of patients with HCC studied at LAC-USCMC and USC-JWCH in the 20 years from 1954 through 1973 who had frank cirrhosis with developed nodules described grossly has been 67%. But when those with poorly defined nodules and "precirrhotic" fibrosis were included, the incidence was 85%. Almost invariably those livers with granular surfaces not called

clearly cirrhotic on gross description were cirrhotic microscopically at least in the region of the tumor. Even more striking than the relationship of HCC to cirrhosis is the sex difference in relationship of HCC to cirrhosis. HCC arising in the cirrhotic liver is predominantly a disease of men whereas the tumor developing in the noncirrhotic liver is of about equal sex incidence (Table 2).

Additional variations that affect the relationship between cirrhosis and HCC is related in some way to factors that are noticeable after a racial breakdown of patients studied. Edmondson noted variations related to racial factors (3). Table 3 shows that 2/3 of the autopsies at LAC-USCMC and USC-JWCH are performed on Caucasians and that a similar percentage of the cirrhotic patients are Caucasian. However only one-half of the HCC arising in cirrhotic or noncirrhotic livers are from Caucasians. Black patients, making up 20% of the autopsies, constitute only slightly over 10% of the cirrhotic patients but yield 20% of the HCC associated with cirrhotic livers and 30% arising in noncirrhotic livers. This suggests that the kind of cirrhosis occurring in black patients is less common or occurs later in life but more often results in development of HCC. Oriental patients, making up a small percentage of the total patients on which autopsies were obtained and a similar percentage of cases of cirrhosis, have a 10-fold increase in development of HCC on cirrhotic livers; the number of Oriental patients with HCC in noncirrhotic livers is too small to be significant.

Hepatocellular Carcinoma and Alcoholic Cirrhosis

Several attempts have been made over the years to classify cirrhosis in some orderly fashion. Unfortunately cirrhosis is a dynamic complex condition of varied etiologies in which cellular destruction, variably prominent inflammatory reaction, and fibro-

Table 3 Racial Distribution of Autopsies, Cirrhosis, and HCC

	Autopsies (%)	Cirrhosis (%)	Hepatocellular Carcinoma	
			With Cirrhosis (%)	Without Cirrhosis (%)
Number of cases	38,856	3456	190	35
Racial breakdown				
Caucasian	64.50	69.60	52.0	50.0
Negro	20.50	11.80	23.0	29.4
Spanish surname	13.80	17.30	14.0	17.6
Oriental	0.89	0.95	10.6	2.9
American Indian	0.25	0.51		

	Incidence of cirrhosis in autopsy series (%)	Incidence of HCC in cirrhotics patients (%)	Incidence of HCC in noncirrhotic patients (%)
Caucasian	9.6	4.1	0.08
Negro	5.1	10.7	0.14
Spanish surname	11.2	4.4	0.13
Oriental	9.5	61.2	0.32 [a]
American Indian	18.2		

[a] Numbers too small for accuracy.

genesis occur in "active" phases of disease, whereas nodular regeneration generally is maximal when destructive activity has subsided. Moreover, in more advanced cirrhosis, the independence of individual regenerative nodules becomes apparent wherein one nodule may be undergoing cellular destruction while a neighboring nodule has only exuberant hepatocellular regeneration and still another area has reactive hyperplasia of reticuloendothelial tissue. Thus, although a purely morphologic classification could be devised, that classification may not reflect etiologic or pathogenetic categories of liver disease, and the terminology used would require change with different stages and phases of the cirrhotic process.

The most commonly used classification of cirrhosis in recent years has been based on the work of Gall in 1960 (13) which was undertaken prior to the widespread use of the liver biopsy, peritoneoscopy, or serum transaminase determinations—data that were not available in the autopsy cases in Gall's study. The methods for detecting hepatitis B surface antigen (HBsAg) were not available to most facilities for another ten years. Thus the pathogenesis and etiology of end-stage cirrhosis found at autopsy were largely conjectural. The use of terminology that implied either pathogenesis (postnecrotic) or etiology (posthepatitic, nutritional) while defining those types of cirrhosis by purely morphologic means (13) should be discontinued. There is no good evidence for and ample evidence against the concept that nodular cirrhosis ever develops as a result of a single episode of submassive necrosis of either toxic or viral etiologies (14–16). Whereas cirrhosis does occasionally develop in association some forms of viral hepatitis, the initial episode is invariably mild, usually subclinical, and there is good evidence that the viral agent persists in an uncomfortable antagonistic relationship when chronic liver disease results from viral hepatitis. As pointed out by Shikata (8), there is no single morphologic pattern of cirrhosis that can be uniquely associated with the chronic liver disease of hepatitis B. Similarly, alcoholic liver disease includes morphologic patterns far beyond that of fatty cirrhosis, patterns that include some instances of coarsely nodular cirrhosis that may have been called "postnecrotic" or "posthepatitic" under the old classification (17). It should be recognized that many past surveys in the United States comparing incidence of HCC in "nutritional" versus "postnecrotic" and "posthepatitic" actually represented comparisons of the early stages of alcoholic liver disease with well-developed quiescent cirrhosis, both alcoholic and nonalcoholic (18).

Unfortunately, for epidemiologic purposes, 86% of the patients at LAC-USCMC who developed HCC in a background of cirrhosis had no prior clinical evidence of any earlier liver disease; no record was made of questioning regarding the alcohol consumption in 22.8%. In addition, the fact that a patient may have been alcoholic is not proof that his or her cirrhosis was of alcoholic type any more than absence of admission of history of alcoholism excludes alcoholic cirrhosis. This silent development of cirrhosis has hampered both a prospective and retrospective study of the liver disorders underlying HCC. It would appear that patients who have chronic liver disease of sufficient severity which prompts them to seek medical care of it do not live long enough to develop HCC, whether that underlying disorder is alcoholic, viral, or toxic. A more inclusive but still imperfect classification of cirrhosis has been proposed (19).

We propose that the complete terminology for cirrhosis include four categories: (1) a morphologic term that incorporates nodular size (granular, finely nodular, coarsely nodular, megalonodular with a modifying term to indicate extent of fibrosis (sclerosing, hard, firm, loose) and a term designating discreteness of regenerative units; (2) a term indicating the major established feature related to etiology or pathogenesis (i.e. alcoholic, B-viral, cryptogenic, hemochromatotic, etc.); (3) a term indicating true cirrhosis versus a nearly cirrhotic (i.e., paracirrhosis) condition; and (4) a term indicating function or activity (i.e., with chronic active hepatitis, quiescent, with extensive alcoholic hyaline necrosis, etc.). The terminology used within each category may best be fluid to suit local prejudices and needs. The terminology will allow the clinical term to be expressed without attempting to apply a morphologic term (e.g., alcoholic cirrhosis with hepatic failure).

Although the typical pattern of development of alcoholic liver disease in the United States is characterized by diffuse and progressive intrasinusoidal deposition of collagen fibers with early partial obliteration of the smallest hepatic venous structures (20, 21, 22), cessation or diminution of alcohol intake apparently reduces the stimulus for collagen production, regenerative activity becomes more pronounced, and the small poorly defined nodules of the sclerosing finely nodular alcoholic cirrhotic liver are transformed into larger, discrete nodules. These nodules often become macronodules that results in the quiescent sclerosing coarsely nodular alcoholic cirrhotic liver, (Fig. 1) or occasionally the loose coarsely nodular alcoholic cirrhotic liver. The patients who discontinued their alcohol consumption before developing a fatal complication of cirrhosis apparently constitute a significant number of those alcoholics who develop HCC. Of our HCC patients who admitted prior moderate to heavy alcoholism, 21% had a history of cessation of alcoholic intake from one to several years prior to development of signs of carcinoma of the liver. Admittedly such histories are notoriously unreliable; however, Lee (23) found that 16 of 29 alcoholic cirrhotic patients studied at au-

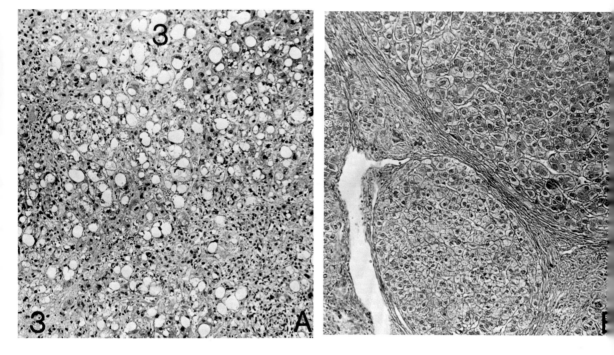

Figure 1   Acute alcoholic liver disease in liver of 55-year-old alcoholic patient in 1974. *(a)* Note the obliteration in zone 3 (3) with neutrophilic infiltrate and arachnoid intrasinusoidal collagenosis (hematoxylin and eosin, X65; JWS4005-74). *(b)* One year later after a period of medical management, there are well-formed, discrete regenerative nodules without fat or intrasinusoidal collagen (hematoxylin and eosin, X65; JWS1188-75).

topsy who had discontinued drinking after onset of cirrhosis had HCC (55%) whereas only 9 of 55 of those who had not given up alcohol had HCC (16.4%). Those who gave up alcohol had a higher incidence of coarsely nodular cirrhosis. Lee also pointed out that whether the HCC developed in a finely nodular alcoholic cirrhotic liver or in a coarsely nodular alcoholic cirrhotic liver, patients with HCC were about 10 years older than those alcoholic patients who died with similar patterns of cirrhosis but without HCC. The age difference suggests only that the HCC patients had less functional impairment and lived long enough to develop what may be considered a natural sequel to cirrhosis. The age distribution of our patients dying of cirrhosis is compared with the age distribution of those dying

with HCC who admitted chronic alcoholism in Table 4.

Not all HCC developing in the liver of the alcoholic cirrhotic patient arises in the setting of coarsely nodular cirrhosis. About half of such livers are either sclerogranular or scleromicronodular, the more typical alcoholic type but still lacking fat (24, 6). Figure 2 shows a typical scleromicronodular alcoholic cirrhosis with HCC, whereas Fig. 3 shows more macronodular alcoholic cirrhosis with HCC.

Hepatitis Antigen Positive Liver Cell Carcinoma

Shikata has dealt with the subject of liver cell carcinoma arising in various morphologic types of B-virus cirrhosis and paracirrhosis (Chapter 4). The status in the

Table 4 Age Distribution at Death of Patients with HCC and Alcoholic Cirrhosis, Alcoholic Cirrhosis Without HCC, and HCC in HBsAg Positive Cirrhosis

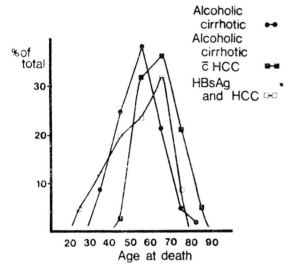

Alcoholic cirrhotic •—•
Alcoholic cirrhotic c̄ HCC ▪—◼
HBsAg and HCC □—□

United States is somewhat different as indicated in Table 5 which includes the 70 cases of HCC studied at USC-JWCH since HBsAg testing began on this material. Staining of the nontumor liver tissue of patients with HCC from 1953 to present by both the orcein method of Shikata (25) and the immunoperoxidase technique of Afroudakis (26) show that the relative incidence of HBsAg positive HCC may have changed (Table 6). The sharp rise in HCC incidence alone in the years 1963 to 1968 with subsequent drop in 1969 to 1973 (Table 7) might have caused conjecture as to whether a single early epidemic of widespread subclinical hepatitis B might not have been responsible. However, although a widespread single pulse exposure to the same carcinogen or agent could have occurred and might be the basis for the 1964 to 1968 peak, evidence is against HBV as

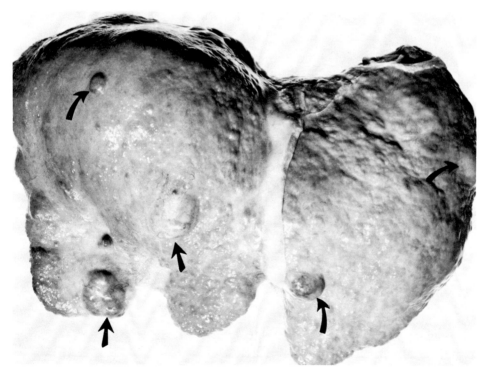

Figure 2 Typical finely granular alcohol cirrhosis with multiple foci of HCC (arrows) incidental in 63-year-old Caucasian man with portal vein involvement and pulmonary tumor emboli (JWA15-66).

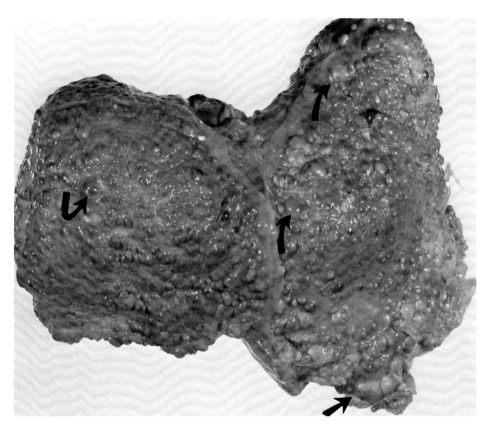

Figure 3 Alcoholic cirrhotic liver with somewhat more coarse nodules than the liver of Fig. 2. The left lobe and some of the right have multiple softened tumor nodules, some pale, some dark (arrow marks a few) (JWA160-72).

Table 5 Coincidence of HBsAg with HCC in Nonalcoholic but Cirrhotic Livers

Underlying Disease	Cases	+ HBsAg	+ AFP	M:F	Average Age	Caucasian (%)
Nonalcholic cirrhosis	28	71.4%	71.4%	14:1	53.3	30
Alcoholic liver disease	22	4.5	66.7	63:1	60.8	48
Nonalcoholic, noncirrhotic	15	6.6	46.7	7:8	40	33
Cholangio, mixed, sclerosing, other	5	0	0	3:2	54	100

Table 6   Changing Incidence of HCC at LAC-USCMC and JWCH with Incidence of Demonstrability of HBsAg in Livers Bearing HCC

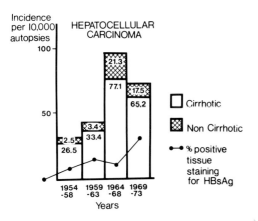

the cause. Some other anomaly related to national shifts in attitude toward socioeconomic aspects of hospital costs might be involved as well. On the other hand, it would appear that there are definite trends toward increase in the relative importance of HBV in relationship to HCC in the United States. How much stems from immigration and from liberal use of inoculations, plasma, and transfusions a decade or more ago is unclear. Only time will tell whether the increase in clinically evident hepatitis beginning around 1965, undoubtedly associated with severalfold more subclinical infections, may similarly be followed by an increased incidence of HCC in another 5 to 10 years.

Cirrhosis is of variable morphology and

Table 7   Preneoplastic Conditions Previously Reported with HCC and Relative Incidence in Southern California

Preneoplastic or associated Condition (Reference)	Cirrhosis	Relative Frequency Reported [a]	Number of cases at LAC-USC-MC and JWCH
Alcoholic cirrhosis (26)	+	a	75 to 100
Chronic active viral hepatitis-B (20, 31)	+ (−)	a	75 to 100
Cryptogenic cirrhosis in adults	+	a	25 to 75
Hemochromatosis (32)	+	b	3
Throtrast induced (33)	0	b	0
Cirrhosis associated with chronic ulcerative colitis (34)	+	d	0
Androgens in Fanconi's anemia (35)	0	b, e	0
Estrogen therapy (36)	0	e	0
Phenobarbitone therapy > 10 years (37)	?	e	0
Following P[32] therapy for polycythemia (38)	0	d	0
Following renal transplant and immuno rx. (39, 40)	+, −	c	0
Aflatoxin contamination of foodstuff (41)	+	f	0
Hemihypertrophy (42)	−	b	0
Cystathioninuria (42)	−	b	0
Glycogenosis type I (43)	−	d	0
Familial (nonhepatitis B) (29, 30)	+	d	0
Congenital biliary atresia (44)	0	d	0
Alpha-1-antitrypsin (45–47)	+	c	11
Plant alkaloids (48)	+	f	0
Budd-Chiari's disease (49)	−	c	2
Congenital (50)	−	d	0
Porphyria cutanea tarda	+ or −	d	1

[a] Relative frequency: a, fairly common in common disease; b, fairly common in rare disease; c, uncommon in rare disease; d, one or occasional report; e, reported but questionable or doubtful interpretation; f, probably important in some geographic regions.

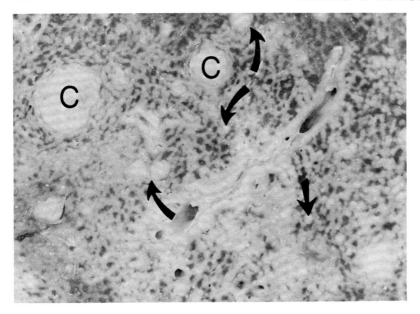

Figure 4 Cut surface of liver with multiple well-differentiated HCC (c) arising in a liver with idiopathic Budd-Chiari's disease with multiple smaller nodules of adenomatous hyperplasia (arrows). Courtesy of T. Starzl, University of Colorado School of Medicine (approximately X3).

etiology and is associated with different clinical patterns. It is undoubtedly premature to draw generalized conclusions about the worldwide cirrhosis-carcinoma relationship based on data from a few countries. However, one peculiarity is the lack of association of HCC with so-called "autoimmune" or "lupoid" hepatitis in spite of the histologic and clinical similarity of the hepatic disease to chronic active viral hepatitis type B. We have never found positive LE preparations or gamma G-type smooth muscle antibodies in patients with HCC. Although this may be because patients with lupoid hepatitis are predominantly women, it is possible that formation of HCC is associated with marked reduction of specific or generalized immune response. Thus Joske et al (27) reported occurrence of HCC in a patient with high familial incidence of chronic active hepatitis in which one-fourth of the family members affected had

positive lupus cell preparations. The patient with HCC had no HBsAg nor autoimmune features. Just as neoplasms are apparently more common in immunosuppressed patients (28), loss of autoimmunity features of chronic active hepatitis may be prerequisite to development of HCC.

Other Preexisting Diseases

The relationship of HCC to certain other preexisting cirrhotic conditions is reviewed in Chapter 4 (Shikata). Hepatic disorders underlying HCC recognized at LAC-USCMC and JWCH-USC are far less than anticipated from the number of predisposing conditions reported (Table 7, Fig. 4).

A relationship of recent concern regards the aberrations of alpha 1 antitrypsin and HCC. Early studies of Sharpe related a certain chronic liver disease in children who

Table 8 Protease Inhibitor Variations and HCC

	TOTAL CASES	MS (%)	MZ (%)	FE (%)	UNIDENTIFIED (%)	MV, MP, SS, ZZ, SZ
NORMAL	1051	6.2	3.1	< 0.1	< 0.1	0.9
HCC	74	2.7	6.8	2.7	< 0.1	

had alpha 1 antitrypsin (A1AT) homozygously aberrant genotype ZZ (29). The relationship of liver disease in adults to aberrant A1AT types (also called protease inhibitor or pi system) (45–47, 28, 51) is less frequently recognized. However, as early as 1967 Ganrot et al reported 20 adult patients with pi type ZZ who had no lung disease; 3 died, 2 with cirrhosis and 1 with HCC (45). Recently from the same medical center Berg et al described 14 adults with pi type ZZ, 8 had fibrosis or cirrhosis, and 3 patients also had HCC (46). Rawlings et al reported a patient with pi type MZ who had HCC arising in a cirrhotic liver (47). We have performed pi genotyping on sera of 74 patients with HCC in an attempt to see whether aberrant pi types are significantly associated with HCC more so than in a normal donor population (Table 8). Four different aberrant subtypes were found, an incidence that may not differ from that in the general population. On limited data, 13% of the patients with HCC had some abnormality of pi type, all were cirrhotic but 3.5% of the patients (or 1/4 of those with abnormal pi type) had other reasonable causes for cirrhosis, either alcoholic liver disease or B-viral cirrhosis as underlying conditions. Of the "normal" population 10.2% had aberrant pi genotypes. It would appear that the chronic liver disease occasionally associated with aberrant pi genotypes does not account for significant numbers of HCC in the southwestern United States. However, the incidence of pi associated cirrhosis is low, and our series of patients small. Our data do not preclude the possibility that such aberrant genotypes, when

they occur, may be associated with high incidence of cirrhosis and carcinoma, particularly MZ type which in 74 patients with HCC was twice as frequently encountered as in the normal population.

PARAPLASTIC CHANGE

Aside from the cirrhosis, histologic alterations that we might characterize as *paraplastic* (or what Farber calls initiated cell alterations, see Chapter 1) begin to become more prominent in conjunction with the development of carcinoma. The paraplastic changes are not prerequisite to the development of carcinoma and may be found, but usually in less striking fashion, in cirrhotic livers not bearing HCC.

Dysplastic Changes

Dysplasia is a pattern of cellular pleomorphism in which the nuclei are polyploid or multiple and often have folds. The cytoplasm is abundant and often polychromatophilic. Coarsely or megalonodular nonalcoholic cirrhotic livers in which HCC develops, tend to have the most striking liver cell dysplasia (Fig. 5). The dysplastic feature was emphasized by Anthony in his study of HCC in Ugandans. He found dysplastic cellular changes in livers of about 50% of patients with cirrhosis and HCC whereas only about 5% of patients with HCC developing in noncirrhotic livers had similar hepatocellular dysplastic changes (52). In the 225 patients with HCC from LAC-USCMC and USC-JWCH, only 22.7% of those with nonalcoholic cirrhosis had

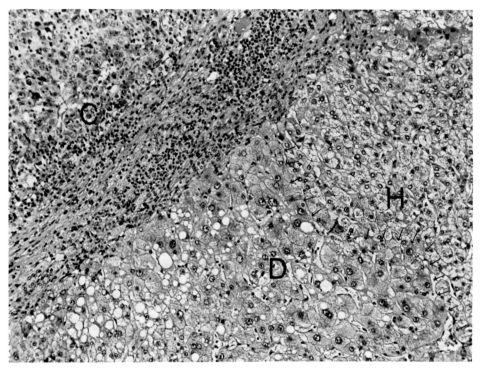

Figure 5   Photomicrograph of nonalcoholic cirrhotic liver with HCC *(c)* showing an area of
marked nuclear dysplasia *(d)* sharply set off (arrows) from a region of hydropic hepatocytes *(h)*
(2 methacrylate hematoxylin and eosin, X203.70; JWS5239ᴶ73). Courtesy of W. K. Bullock,
M. D.

dysplasia compared with only 5.3% of those with HCC developing in noncirrhotic liver.

Alcoholic cirrhotic livers (even those that are macronodular) and hemochromatotic livers in which HCC developed showed dysplastic changes in 14.4%. Thus in the United States, dysplasia seems less common in cirrhotic livers bearing HCC than it does in Uganda.

Adenomatous Regeneration

Although somewhat less obvious than cellular dysplasia, adenomatous regeneration within preexisting cirrhotic nodules is more common in our material. Precarcinomatous adenomatous change seems to develop in the tumor-involved alcoholic cirrhotic livers with at least as great a frequency as it does in nonalcoholic cirrhotic livers (Figs. 5 to 9).

Typically, HCC develops in the alcoholic cirrhotic liver after the nodule has become discrete and the cord pattern has become reestablished within the quiescent cirrhotic nodule. The morphologic transition between the adenomatous proliferative change and the orderly cord arrangement of the quiescent cirrhotic nodule is often subtle. The adenomatous area, on the other hand, may occasionally be difficult to distinguish from extremely well-differentiated trabecular carcinoma. The adenomatous foci appear as rounded but poorly defined areas within regenerative nodules (Fig. 9). The cord structure of the adenoma is often maintained in spite of its overall bulging character. The hepatocytes may become more regular (Fig. 9) or less

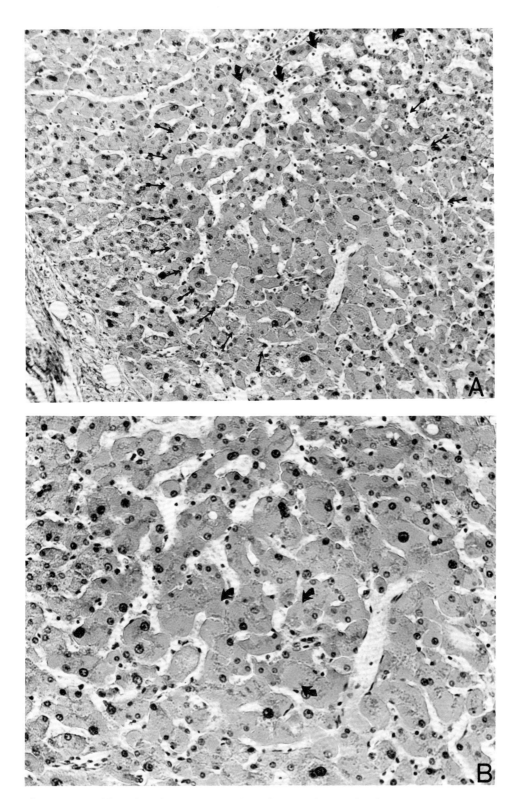

Figure 6 One of the earlier adenomatous paraplastic changes is shown in this photomicrograph (light arrows) occurring in an alcoholic cirrhotic liver. *(a)* Note the developing angiomatous pattern of sinusoids at the margin near top of figure (heavy arrows) (hematoxylin and eosin, 186.90X). *(b)* The deeply eosinophilic and regular reestablished hepatic cords develop a smooth homogenous cytoplasm resembling the ground glass cells of Hadziyannis but giving a negative reaction to the Shikata stain or Afroudakis technique (hematoxylin and eosin, X373.80).

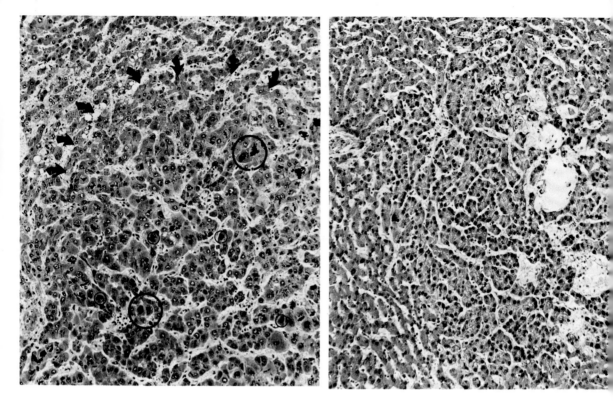

Figure 7 A more common change in a quiescent alcoholic cirrhotic liver is the bulging, poorly defined growth zone (arrows) within which the hepatocytes have become atypical and, in this instance, formed alcoholic hyalin (sample encircled) not present in the nontumor liver (hematoxylin and eosin, X105; JWA100-74).

Figure 8 On occasion the well-differentiated cords are transformed fairly abruptly into low-grade trabecular carcinoma. Note the vascular ectasia at the right margin of this early neoplastic region (hematoxylin and eosin, X105; JWA149-68). Courtesy of D. Tatter, M. D., LAC–USCMC 68759.[1]

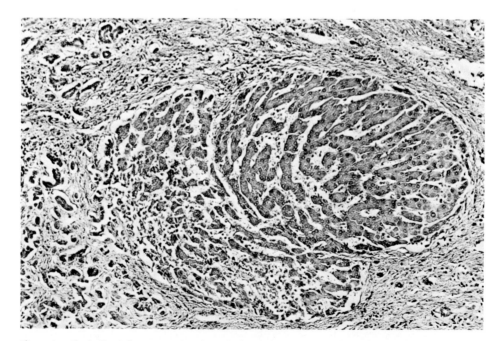

Figure 9 Alcoholic cirrhotic patient with HCC elsewhere. Note the bulging adenomatous portion of a quiescent cirrhotic nodule that may, in fact, be early carcinoma (hematoxylin and eosin, X102.06; JWA77-66).

organized (Fig. 8) but usually are more deeply eosinophilic and less affected by autolytic changes in autopsy. Since adenomatous areas occasionally subtly blend into early HCC multifocally, it would seem at least in our material, that HCC spread within a liver may have the appearance of multifocal origin rather than metastatic. However, Okuda has taken the opposite viewpoint in the study of HCC arising from cirrhotic livers in Japan (53), and admittedly, histologic appearances that suggest multiple foci may be deceiving.

MORPHOLOGY OF HCC

Gross

The most common gross classification of HCC arose from Eggel's manuscript of 1901, which related gross tumor pattern to underlying predisposing condition (2). Eggel designated one class representing 64.4% of the cases as *nodular* in which the tumor occurred in the form or shape of larger nodules *discretely delineated from normal liver.*

The second most common was designated as *massive*, making up to 23% of the cases. In the massive type the tumor formed a large mass that involved an entire lobe or most of it, and *infiltrated irregularly into the surrounding liver.*

Eggel's third group was the *diffuse* in which the entire liver was permeated by innumerable small tumor nodules surrounded by collagen resulting in a tumor-involved liver that was difficult to distinguish from cirrhosis by gross examination only. Patients with diffuse carcinomas made up 12.4% of Eggel's cases; all with diffuse HCC had cirrhosis.

Although there are many features of the gross pattern of HCC growth that might enter into descriptive terminology of the gross appearances of HCC, it is no small problem to decide whether the distinctions are meaningful in terms of etiology, patho-

genesis, and prognosis. However, it seems quite likely that the original descriptions as used (without photographs) by Eggel may not be applied in the same fashion today as he used them. Thus, although both Edmondson (3) and Nakashima (54) used "nodular" to describe the formation of nodular tumor masses as did Eggel, Eggel also emphasized the discrete character of the margin of the whole tumor delimiting it from nontumor liver; the latter was not necessarily a feature of the tumors described as "nodular" HCC shown by the later authors. As I interpret Eggel's description, many of the HCC seen in the United States today could somewhat uncomfortably be placed in either one or both of Eggel's "nodular" or "massive" categories, and some in none of his three.

Nakashima et al (54, 55) recently subdivided the gross pattern of HCC into eight more distinct and different patterns. Nakashima's classification tends to emphasize the differences in growth pattern and makes subdivisions in morphologic pattern of the tumor that are genuine and badly needed. However, as complete and detailed as Nakashima et al's description is, some of the features may be based more on the character of the underlying liver disease than on a true representation of a fundamentally different tumor growth, and the major emphasis is on the pattern of growth within the tumor, not in the relationship to nontumor liver. In addition, the term "massive" is still retained, an adjective that applies to size rather than relationship to surrounding structures. Essentially the same types of gross pattern are described in this chapter as those Nakashima recommended, but the effort is directed toward regrouping the tumor types into sets that may have similar etiologic and pathogenetic processes. The classification used in this chapter is compared with that proposed by Eggel and the expanded classification by Nakashima et al in Table 9. The relationship of each type to cirrhosis and alcoholic cirrhosis is indicated on

Table 9   Gross patterns of HCC growth

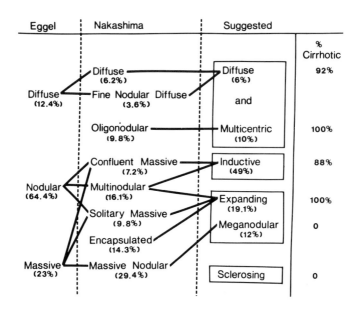

the right. Although correlation of each set with cirrhosis or noncirrhosis is high; that with specific kinds of cirrhosis is not.

Implicit in any communication dealing with the morphologic pattern of HCC is the inclusion of information dealing with the characteristics of the nontumor liver. The two more common growth patterns of carcinoma of the liver (Eggel's nodular and massive, our inductive and expanding), when they arise in cirrhotic livers, seem to reflect at their onset the fundamental growth characteristic of the cirrhotic liver in which they had their onset. Many continue to mimic the parent cirrhotic liver, but others begin to infiltrate the connective tissue compressed by the neoplastic nodules and efface the architectural pattern of original cirrhotomimetic growth. Thus at the time of autopsy, many tumors with a basically discrete multinodular configuration will have areas that are only poorly defined confluent lobalate. Conversely, the vascular invasion so characteristic to HCC, often results in portal veins packed with tumor that present as bulging nodules on cross section and may be confused with multinodular carcinoma.

The terminology suggested in this chapter deals with three different features of morphology: *(a)* the relationship of tumor to nontumor liver, *(b)* pattern of growth within the tumor (relationship of tumor to tumor), and *(c)* stromal reaction (relationship of tumor to stroma).

Relationship of Tumor to Nontumor Liver

There would appear to be differences in the fashion by which tumor has its genesis in the liver. Some writers including Okuda have emphasized the evidence that HCC arises from a single focus and metastasizes throughout the remainder of the organ whereas other investigators have defended a multifocal genesis. From the gross and microscopic appearances it seems possible that both mechanisms as well as diffuse simultaneous genesis may occur in specific instances. In addition, some neoplasms may be characterized by changes at the tumor margins or close to the main mass that resembles *in situ* neoplasia, as though those areas had neoplastic change induced by the adjacent neoplasm or affected by the same process but lagging behind in the development of frank cancer. Precise distinction of all types at autopsy may be infeasible in many instances because of the extensive intrahepatic spread and degree of involvement that may be present by the time of death. However, most tumors can be separated into broad groups: *(a)* those that are most clearly unifocal *(expanding, meganodular,* and *sclerosing)*; *(b)* those that have a morphologic pattern most suggestive of multifocal origin *(diffuse* and *multicentric)*; and *(c)* those that give the *appearance* of liver adjacent to the main mass in the process of undergoing malignant change *(inductive)*. With this third group it must be kept in mind that "all is not what seems," since the pattern of paraplastic and early neoplastic changes remote from the major tumor is sufficiently unusual in organ neoplasia that it seems worthy of characterization.

UNIFOCAL APPEARANCE.

Expanding HCC. Expanding HCC is the leading candidate for unifocal neoplastic genesis. Demarcation between tumor and nontumor is quite distinct, the nontumor liver is compressed by the expanding margin of the neoplasm (Fig. 10 to 12). Although it is common for the tumor to have metastasized to other parts of the liver by the time of autopsy, usually by invasion of the portal vein, the intrahepatic foci also tend to be discrete. Histologically one does not usually find the adenomatous paraplastic changes in the nontumor liver. Of the HCC that are well documented by gross photographs in our material, 19% could be characterized as expanding. In our material the expanding carcinomas arise in cirrhotic livers, about 1/2 of which are alcoholic type. However, the distinction between *expanding* HCC and the next category *meganodular* may be entirely related

to the background in which the tumor arises as the neoplastic pattern tends to simulate the nodularity in a cirrhotomimetic growth.

Although the expanding growth pattern has the demarcation of tumor growth that Eggel described under his term "nodular," the cut surface of the tumor may range from a confluent multinodular pattern (Fig. 10), to a bossilated soft bulging surface (Fig. 11) and often there are areas of both (Fig. 12). Rarely (3.6%), the expanding HCC has a capsule that encloses the grapelike mass of nodules to form a one or more sharply demarcated round masses (Fig. 13). Nakashima et al have stated that encapsulated multinodular HCC has a somewhat more favorable prognosis (54).

Meganodular. An additional growth pattern distinctive by virtue of the homogeneity of growth within a well-defined mass we have termed *meganodular.* Meganodular growth consists of tumor masses that are 3 to 15 cm in diameter and are unusually homogeneous within each nodular mass; some are solitary, a smaller number are confluent. The meganodular tumors arise predominantly in noncirrhotic livers (100% in our small group) and are found more frequently in women than men in a ratio of 5:1; in fact HCC arising in noncirrhotic livers in women fell into either meganodular or sclerosing stromal types (see below). Meganodular expanding carcinomas may be confluent (Fig. 12) or solitary (Fig. 14). Those with multiple foci at autopsy (Fig. 15) probably represent metastases. The figure shown represents a fatal case after early partial hepatectomy.

Sclerosing carcinoma. Certain tumors are characterized uniformly by dense fibrous reaction not just in some areas, but throughout the tumors (Fig. 16). Grossly they are almost invariably considered to be either metastatic carcinomas or cholangiocarcinomas. Many of these tumors are associated with pseudohyperparathyroidism. Microscopically they tend to be quite uni-

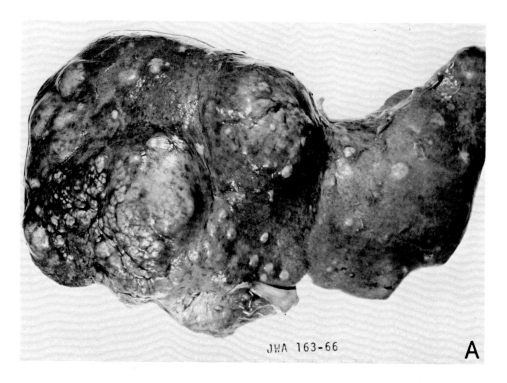

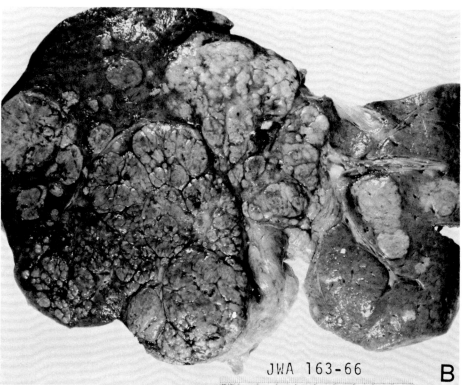

Figure 10 (a and b) Gross picture of noncirrhotic liver showing well-defined margins between expanding tumor masses. Microscopically there were not the paraplastic changes in the nonneoplastic liver. This suggested that the intrahepatic spread was by metastasis rather than induction (JWA163-66).

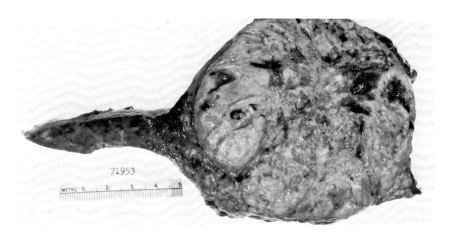

Figure 11 Expanding bossilated pattern in alcoholic cirrhotic liver. Courtesy D. Tatter, M. D., Lac-USCMC, 71953).

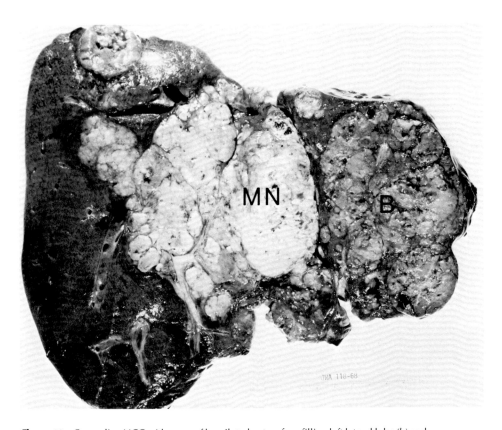

Figure 12 Expanding HCC with areas of bossilated cut surface filling left lateral lobe *(b)* and with confluent meganodular pattern in the medial aspect of the left lobe *(mn)* (JWA118-68).

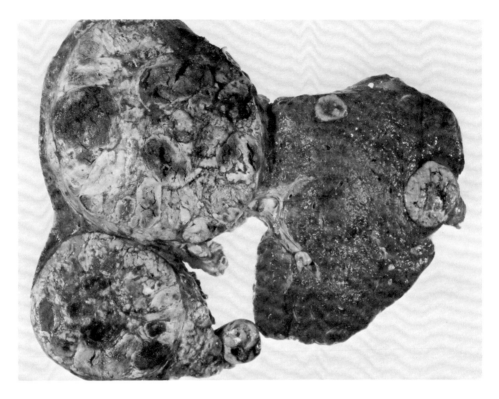

Figure 13 Encapsulated multinodular carcinoma arising in cirrhotic liver of a 55-year-old alcoholic cirrhotic Negro man (JWA176-71).

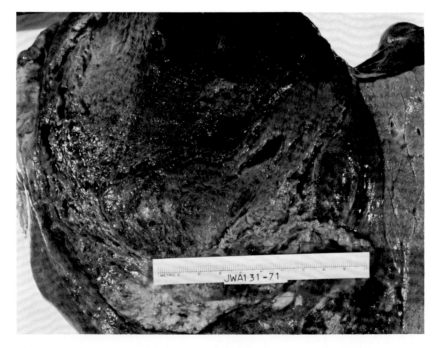

Figure 14 Solitary meganodular tumor in noncirrhotic liver of a 59-year-old Negro woman (JWA131-74).

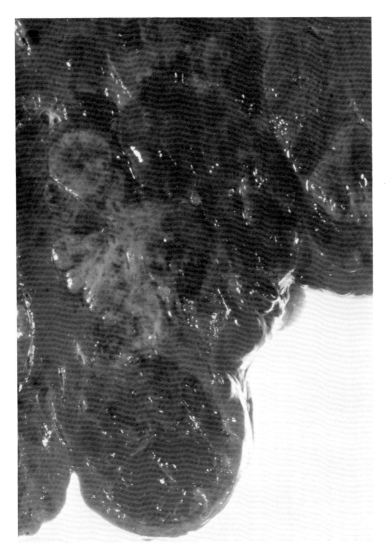

Figure 15 Cut surface of liver of a 35-year-old man with
multifocal meganodular expanding HCC (JWA8-74).

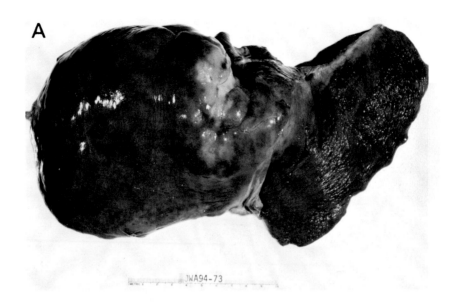

A

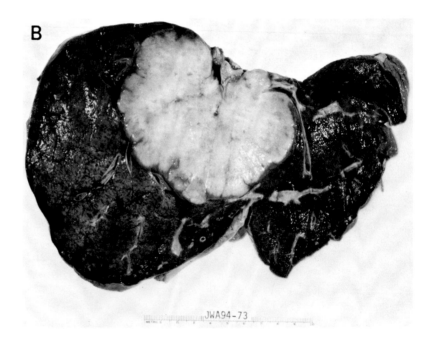

B

128

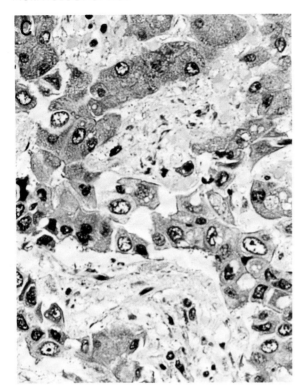

Figure 16 (a and b) Well-circumscribed sclerosing HCC arising in liver of a 46-year-old woman. Photomicrograph (c) shows that in spite of connective tissue, the histogenesis is hepatocellular. Arrow demarcates merge of hepatocytes into sclerosing HCC (hematoxylin and eosin, X420; JWA94-73).

form neoplasms from one area to another, although some are hepatocellular and others a variety of peripheral cholangiocarcinoma—a rare tumor that fits best into the intermediate class of *cholangiolocellular carcinoma*. In spite of the relatively uniform differentiation in any one tumor, it is possible that the histogenetic cell of all of the types is the cholangiole. All universally sclerosing carcinomas in our series have arisen in noncirrhotic livers. Some of the sclerosing carcinomas are solitary, well-defined tumor masses; others appear as multifocal, sclerotic areas with an invasive border. However, intrahe-patic spread appears metastatic. This group of sclerosing carcinomas, although including some hepatocellular, some cholangiolar, and some cholangiolocellular, includes only 50% of all of the cholangiocarcinoma; 50% of the cholangiolocellular were sclerosing. Of our total primary liver cancers 10 or 2.2% were sclerosing. Of these 10, 7 were HCC, 2 were cholangiocarcinoma, and 1 was cholangiolocellular.

MULTIPLE ORIGIN SUGGESTED

Diffuse and Multicentric. The diffuse and multicentric patterns are considered together since they both have the common

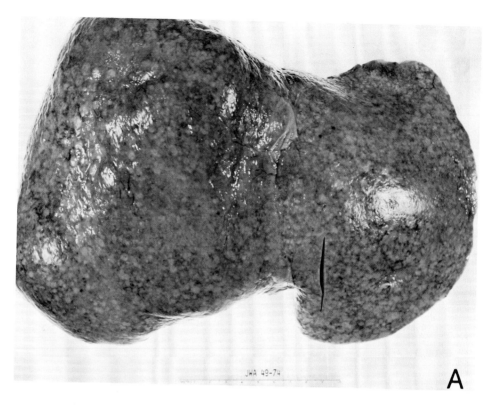

JWA 49-74

A

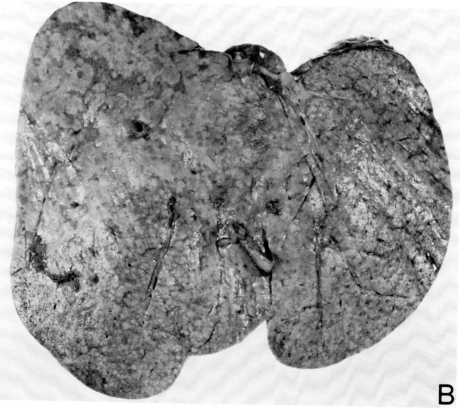

B

130

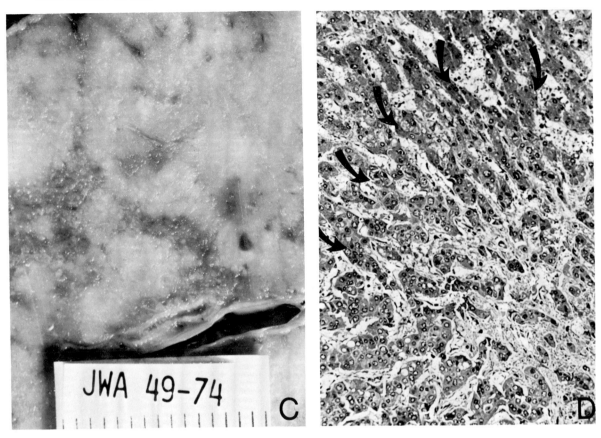

Figure 17   External surface of noncirrhotic liver with diffuse HCC shows uniform involve-ment *(a)* that is also seen on cut surface, both low power *(b)* and high *(c)*. Microscopically, the tumor is extremely well differentiated with nontumor liver blending into tumor (arrows) *(d)*. Tumor seemed to originate in each portal area (JWA49-74).

characteristic of multiple sites of apparent histogenesis with development occurring at all areas nearly simultaneously. In diffuse HCC, however, the tumor involves virtual-ly every functional unit of the liver. Most livers so involved are cirrhotic. We have studied one noncirrhotic liver with diffuse HCC (Fig. 17), but know of no other re-ported. When the liver is cirrhotic, the fact that it is also neoplastic may be overlooked because of the uniformity of involvement (Fig. 18 and 19). Only 6% of our patients with photographic documentation of gross HCC pattern have had diffuse HCC. This compares with 12.4% by Eggel and 9.8%

by Nakashima (Table 9). A characteristic of diffuse HCC is the extent of involve-ment that can occur without the develop-ment of symptoms.

Perhaps only representing an earlier stage of diffuse HCC is multicentric HCC in which scattered nodules are larger, soft-er, more bulging than the cirrhotic nod-ules, and are slightly discolored (Fig. 20). On microscopic examination many of these nodules will be neoplastic, others adeno-matous only. Although there may be some nodules larger and more obviously neo-plastic than others, in essence the appear-ance is of nearly simultaneous develop-

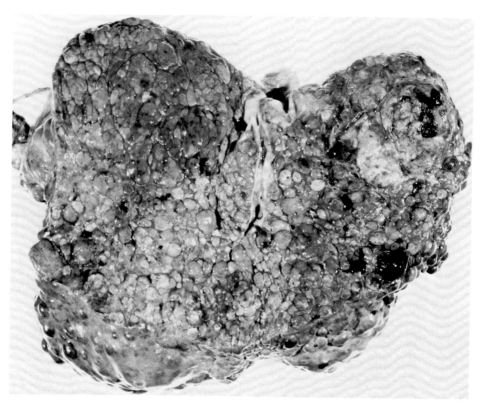

Figure 18 Diffuse HCC in coarsely nodular cirrhotic liver (JWA78-73).

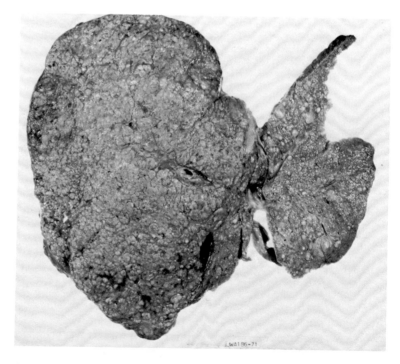

Figure 19 Diffuse HCC in micronodular cirrhotic liver (JWA186-71).

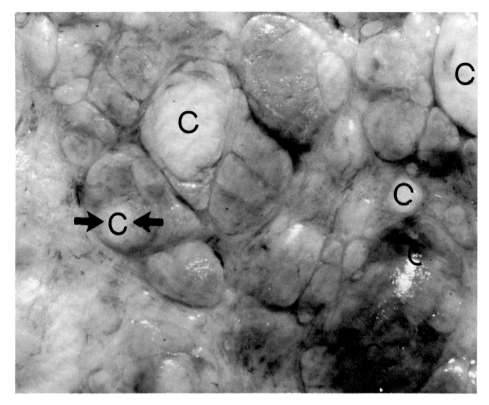

Figure 20 Early multifocal HCC, incidental autopsy finding (carcinoma indicated by c) (JWA59-65).

ment of neoplasia. In our material 10% of HCC were multicentric; all multicentric HCC were in cirrhotic livers, 80% in alcoholic cirrhotic livers. Most multicentric HCC are encountered as incidental autopsy findings.

PATTERN SUGGESTIVE OF INDUCTION OF TUMOR

Inductive Growth Pattern. The *inductive* pattern of HCC gives the appearance of the main neoplastic mass inducing neoplasia in adjacent liver or at least of *de novo* tumor arising in proximity to the main tumor mass (Fig. 6). Although it is quite true, particularly in advanced hepatic involvement, that the prime feature may be invasion rather than induction, some such

carcinomas are abounded by cirrhotic nodules much larger than those more remote, but not yet neoplastic (Fig. 21). Microscopically adjacent nodules often also have microscopic paraplastic adenomatous change. Again, in the advanced cases of HCC wherein most of the liver is involved, it may be impossible to distinguish spreading from expanding types (Fig. 22).

Developmental Pattern Within Tumor Mass (Relationship of Tumor to Tumor)

The developmental pattern within most HCC, as contrasted to its mode of encroachment on residual liver, ranges between the development of a well-circumscribed multinodular arrangement on one extreme (Figs. 21 and 23) and confluent, bossilated, fleshy tumor at the other

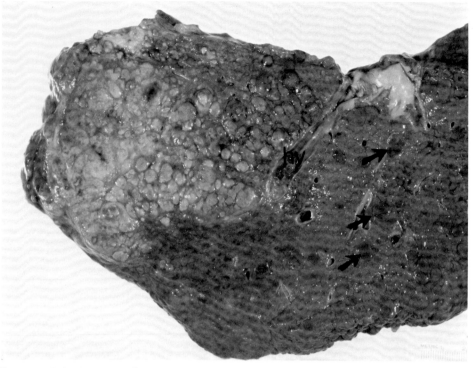

Figure 21 Inductive pattern of HCC with multinodular pattern of tumor growth. The margin of the tumor is poorly defined with scattered isolated nodules advancing into the nontumor liver. Note the tumor in the hepatic vein (h.v.) and the paraplastic adenomatous change of nodules in the nontumor liver (arrows). Courtesy D. Tatter, M. D., LAC–USCMC, 74459.

(Figs. 11 and 12). Although we have designated the first *multinodular* and the second *bossilated,* most HCC arising in cirrhotic livers have a mixed or an intermediate pattern (Fig. 24). Perhaps a major reason for designating descriptive features such as "bossilated" and "multinodular" when they both appear to arise in the same background liver disease is that reports that include photographs depicting studies of HCC undertaken in the Orient and Africa emphasize the multinodular pattern (56) whereas pure examples of multinodular HCC in our series are less common. One can frequently see an underlying multinodular pattern in which there has been a breakdown in integrity of the tumor nodules. This loss of distinctness of nodular

margins is the gross manifestation of invasion of the tumor into the internodular stroma. In our material the *expanding* relationship of tumor to nontumor liver tends to be associated with multinodular pattern within the tumor (although less than well defined) rather than bossilated. The spreading growth pattern is about equally often bossilated or multinodular, but again many have tumors that are a mixture or intermediate between nodular and bossilated.

MICROSCOPIC CHARACTERISTICS

There have been many terms applied to characterize the various histologic patterns

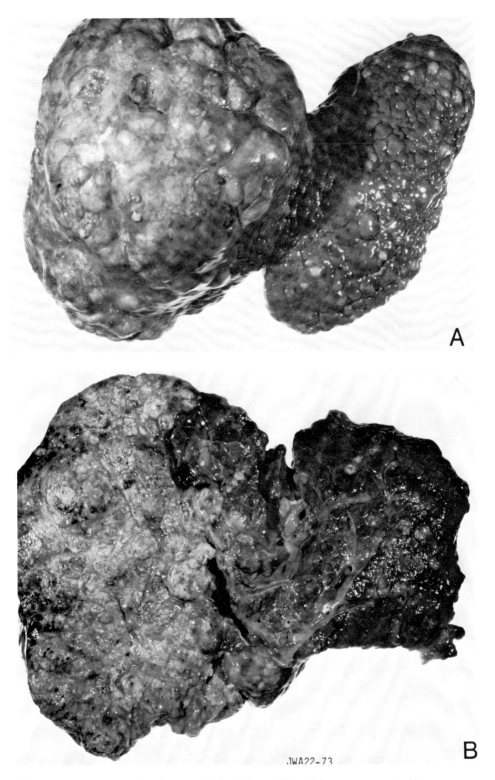

Figure 22 Extensive tumor involvement with breakdown of the nodular arrangement. At this late stage it is impossible to tell if the tumor started as an expanding or inductive lesion (JWA22-73).

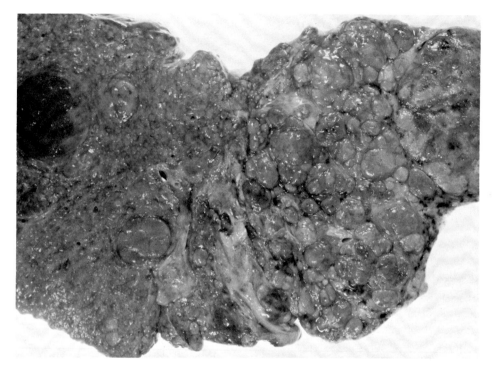

Figure 23 Multinodular developmental pattern of a carcinoma that has an inductive growth pattern.

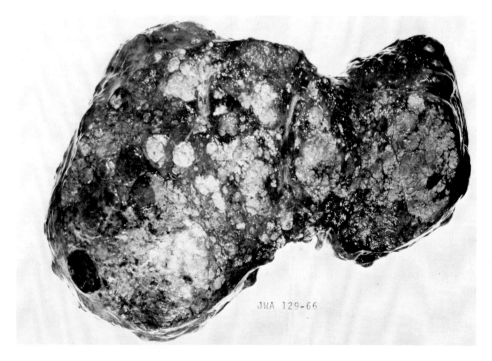

Figure 24 Mixed bossilated and multinodular pattern of tumor (JWA129-66).

assumed by HCC. At our present state of knowledge, it would seem that a major value in classifying many of these histologic types is to facilitate recognition of the primary tumor. Perhaps continued investigations will allow us to draw prognostic or clinical correlations at least from some of the less common histologic patterns.

The principal feature contributing to the morphologic appearance of a tumor can be broken down into *(a)* its *cytologic* differentiation, function, and degree of pleomorphism, *(b)* its *histologic* developmental pattern into cord, trabecular, or other structures, *(c)* the presence or absence of cirrhotomimetic tendencies to develop pseudolobular units, and *(d)* the stromal development. All of the above are intimately related and particularly the first two are studied in conjunction by the diagnostic pathologist. For descriptive purposes each component is discussed separately.

CYTOLOGIC DIFFERENTIATION

A characteristic feature of HCC is the cytologic similarity of the tumor cells to nonneoplastic liver. A discussion of the cytologic features of neoplasia of hepatocytes must include two frequently confused terms: *anaplasia* predominance of less differentiated forms (dedifferentiation), and *pleomorphism* development of varied (often bizarre) forms. Hepatocellular carcinomas develop some degree of either anaplastic or pleomorphic changes or both. The neoplastic hepatocyte usually retains the abundant eosinophilic cytoplasm with the polyhedral configuration; cohesiveness to adjacent hepatocytes is a highly consistent feature. The tumor cell nucleus is large and oval, with peripheralization of the chromatin forming a more prominent heterochromic membrane at the margin of the nucleus. Nucleoli are large and regular, and it is uncommon for nuclei of malignant hepatocytes to lack nucleoli. The

degree of anaplasia varies considerably, ranging from the tumor cells that seem indistinguishable from normal, recognizable as tumor only by growth pattern, to tumors in which cells resemble mesenchymal cells by virtue of less abundant cytoplasm with reduced eosinophilia, and larger, more primitive nuclei. With increasing anaplasia, cohesiveness is reduced. One may see the full range in the liver tumor of one patient (Figs. 25 to 28).

As one might anticipate, certain functional characteristics such as ability to form bile are inversely related in a rough fashion to the cellular anaplasia. Thus bile plugs are commonly found in well-differentiated HCC but become increasingly difficult to find in less well-differentiated tumors. As pointed out by Edmondson and Steiner (4), one early functional capacity to be lost in the neoplastic hepatocyte seems to be the ability to store hemosiderin. Even the well-differentiated HCC arising in a liver of a hemachromatosis patient is striking for its lack of iron. Such lack of incorporation could be partly related to rapid cell replication since it appears in the nontumor cirrhotic liver that the newer regenerative areas developing within the old have much less iron.

A reversion to a more primitive cell is reflected by the production of alpha fetoprotein (AFP) which appears in sera and is demonstrable in the cytoplasm of the tumor cell (Fig. 29). AFP is generally lacking in the extremely well-differentiated, slow growing tumor, and also in the undifferentiated cell that appears to be losing its morphologic and functional identity. Extremely anaplastic HCC usually are not associated with AFP in sera.

The prognosis of the patient does not appear to rest with the degree of anaplasia. This is probably because the symptoms do not develop until most of the liver has been replaced, irrespective of how rapidly the tumor has attained that state of re-

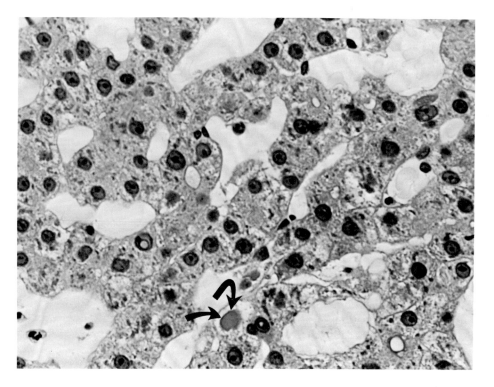

Figure 25 Photomicrograph of liver biopsy showing well-differentiated trabecular carcinoma. Note that the regular sized nuclei have prominent nucleoli, and that there are occasional hyaline bodies (arrow). Kupffer cells are sparse (hematoxylin and eosin, 531.20X; LACUSCMC #69-6669). Courtesy W. K. Bullock, M. D.

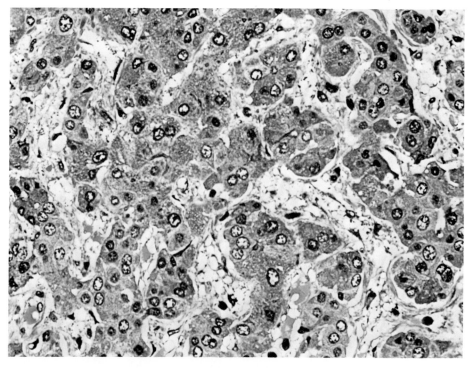

Figure 26 Segment of liver from a 61-year-old man showing slightly more pleomorphism than Fig. 25 but similar development (hematoxylin and eosin, 348.60X; JWA49-74).

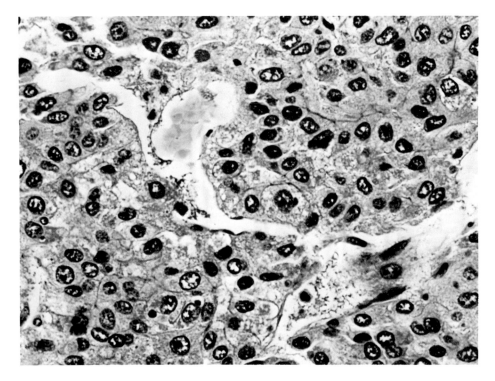

Figure 27 Photomicrograph of only moderately differentiated and moderately developed trabecular HCC (hematoxylin and eosin, X435.75; JWS3398-74).

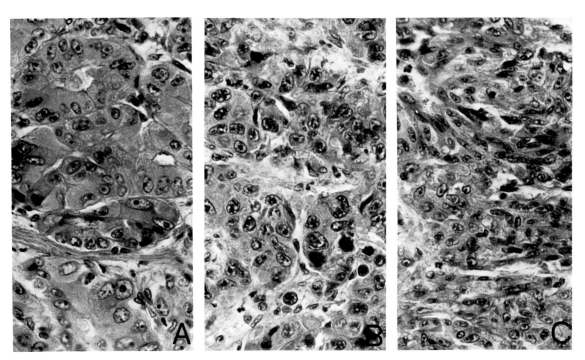

Figure 28 Photomicrographs from different parts of the same liver tumor studied at the time of autopsy. One area *(a)* shows some pleomorphism but relatively good cytologic differentiation. A second area *(b)* is quite pleomorphic and cytologically poorly differentiated, whereas *(c)* is undifferentiated but not pleomorphic. (hematoxylin and eosin, X420; JWA176-71).

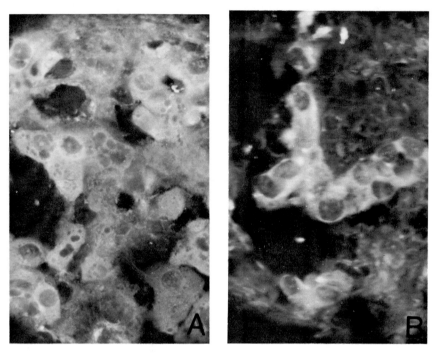

Figure 29 *(a)* Immunofluorescent stains for AFP in HCC show marked variation in content of this protein from one cell to the next. *(b)* Areas of liver invaded by tumor show fluorescence of tumor cells only (X400; JWA43-74).

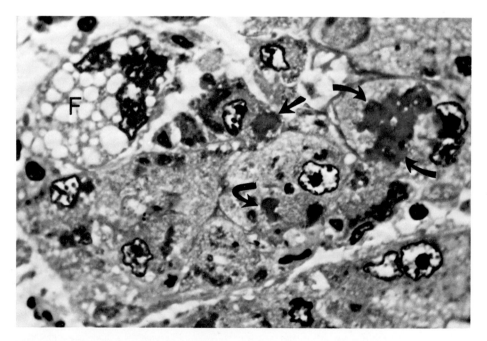

Figure 30 Alcoholic hyalin (Mallory bodies) are quite striking in this carcinoma in an alcoholic cirrhotic liver (arrows). Note also the foamy fatty change *(f)* (hematoxylin and eosin, X876.48; JWA77-66).

placement. Thus life expectancy is short once symptoms of hepatic disorder develop, irrespective of prior growth rate.

Pleomorphism, in the broad sense of the word, is common in HCC. The most common type of pleomorphic change is the acquisition of abnormal morphologic features not present in the neighboring nonneoplastic liver. Often such features will aid in the identification of the carcinoma. One very peculiar alteration is the development of *Mallory bodies* in tumor cells of a liver that has no such cytologic changes in the nontumor areas (Fig. 30). Mallory bodies, when they are found, seem to develop in the HCC of alcoholic patients long after the nontumor cirrhotic liver which no longer has Mallory bodies has become quiescent. We have seen it prominently in one HCC of a patient without cirrhosis about whom no information about prior alcoholic background was available and have found it in only one of the patients with confirmed nonalcoholism. Anthony, in his thorough review of hepatocellular carcinoma in Uganda (almost all nonalcoholic) did not mention alcoholic hyalin although he described other changes in hepatocytes that were more subtle (52). Thus we may presume that it is rare, although it does apparently occur, in the HCC arising in the nonalcoholic cirrhotic liver. In only one instance in our material were Mallory bodies found in metastases of HCC. Kelley et al described the electron microscopic features of Mallory bodies in HCC and showed evidence indicating that the reticular and the globular types may be of the same origin in spite of histologic dissimilarity (56). *Fat* may be found in tumor cells that are well differentiated. Since the fat is probably produced in the neoplastic cells but not released, the implication is that the hepatocytes are functioning, unlike normal hepatocytes but not like truly undifferentiated tumor cells (Figs. 30 and 31). Many otherwise well-differentiated HCC have striking numbers of round hyaline bodies in the tumor cell cytoplasm (Fig. 25) or as what appears to be a secretion product (Fig. 32).

Clear Cell

Occasionally a very striking feature of HCC will be the predominance of tumor clear cells to the extent that the distinction from clear cell carcinoma of kidney or of adrenal gland may be difficult. Some reviewers have considered such tumors to be of renal or adrenal rest origin. However, many have the macrotrabecular growth pattern (Fig. 33) or bile secretion so characteristic of HCC. Even more frequently, the clear cell pattern is only a characteristic of a part of the tumor (Fig. 34). Buchanan and Huvos (57) classified the HCC of 13 of 150 patients as clear cell type, but the percentage of the tumor that was made up of clear cells ranged between 30 and 100%. Clear cell carcinomas have been considered by some investigators to have a more favorable prognosis (3). Neither Buchanan and Huvos nor El-Domeiri et al (58) found improved survival in patients with clear cell carcinomas.

Giant Cell

Pure giant cell carcinoma of liver is uncommon, representing 1.8% of the HCC in our material. However 14% of HCC had some giant cell change. The tumor cells, in spite of their size and bizarre appearance, usually have many features of hepatocytes. They feature abundant eosinophilic cytoplasm and the nuclei have prominent nucleoli; however, the HCC made up entirely of pleomorphic giant cells usually lack the cohesive character that is such a characteristic of most HCC and are associated with greater amounts of stromal reaction (Fig. 35a). Occasionally the tumor cells arrange themselves radially about vascular structures (Fig. 35b). They generally fail to grow in the cirrhotomimetic pattern that characterizes a majority of cases of HCC,

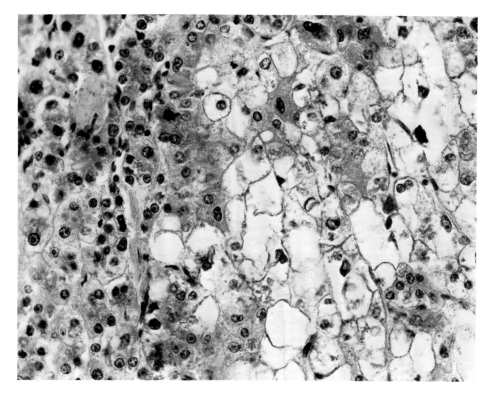

Figure 31 HCC in alcoholic cirrhotic liver of 73-year-old Caucasian man with an area of large fat droplet change (hematoxylin and eosin, X498; JWA5-62).

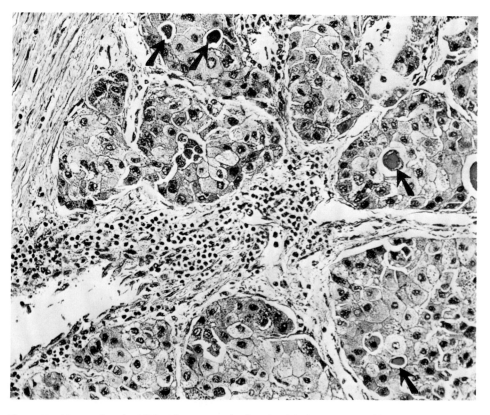

Figure 32 Macrotrabecular HCC with numerous hyaline droplets (hematoxylin and eosin, X357; JWA129-66).

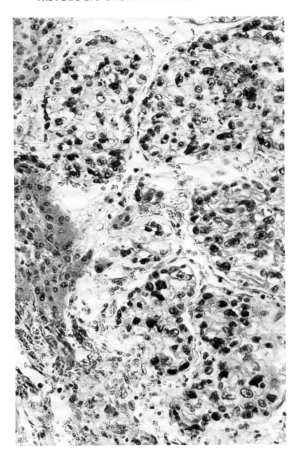

Figure 33 Clear cell area of HCC in macrotrabecular pattern (hematoxlyin and eosin, X210; JWS4957-74). Courtesy R. Rhoades, M. D.

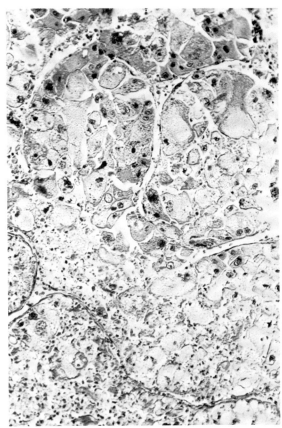

Figure 34 Pleomorphic clear cell HCC (hematoxylin and eosin, X210; JWA15-66).

although most (90%) arise from cirrhotic livers. The more common HCC with some giant cells usually either have organoid structures of HCC (Fig. 35c) or, cytologically, some parts of the tumor resemble hepatocytes elsewhere (Fig. 35d).

HISTOLOGIC GROWTH PATTERN

By histologic growth pattern, reference is made to the interrelationship between hepatocytes that result in, or fails to result in, an organoid arrangement. Similar to the cytologic characteristics, the histologic arrangement may be undeveloped, moder-

ately developed, or well developed.

The *microtrabecular* pattern of HCC is the most familiar and the most common, many variations of trabecular growth may occur to simulate other organoid patterns (acinar, adenoid, etc.) as parts of the tumors. Occasionally the growth may be such as to simulate normal liver (Fig. 25). The well-differentiated neoplastic trabecula is made up of a linear column of hepatocytes of one or more cells thick. The trabeculae are separated from blood sinusoid channels by widely spaced, flattened, and inconspicuous endothelial lining cells. Kupffer cells are not a usual component. Other than the endothelial cells, there is little ac-

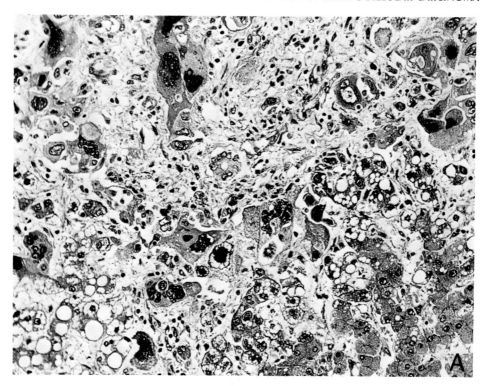

Figure 35 *(a)* Giant cell HCC arising in noncirrhotic liver of 46-year-old Caucasian man. Note, in addition to the bizarre cells, the loss of cohesiveness and the increase in loose connective tissue. (hematoxylin and eosin, X340.30; JWA187-68). *(b)* Giant cell HCC radially oriented toward vascular structure (hematoxylin and eosin, X350). Courtesy of J. Wolman, M. D., Los Angeles Veterans Administration Center, A435-71. *(c)* Other areas from *(b)* show scattered giant bizarre hepatocellular carcinoma cells in a predominately clear cell carcinoma with macrotrabecular pattern (hematoxylin and eosin, X210). *(d)* Multinucleated but otherwise well differentiated tumor cell. (hematoxylin and eosin, X420; JWA176-71).

companying stroma in the typical microtrabecular carcinoma and the orderly trabecula often give the impression of forming a mesh in clear space (Fig. 36). It is not rare, however, for the HCC with undifferentiated cytologic features to continue to grow in a trabecular fashion (Fig. 37). On occasion, when the canaliculus is retained, the five or six-cells arranged radially about it have an *acinar* appearance on cross section particularly when a greater stromal component is included in the tumor and cells have a clear zone at the base (Fig. 38). Many variations are produced if the canaliculus is greatly dilated. If the cellular proliferation about a prominent cana-

liculus is less, individual structures may appear ductal (Fig. 39). If an entire zone has this pattern, it may be easy to confuse it with a ductal carcinoma. Infrequently the tumor cells are elongated with basally placed nuclei to give a *pseudoglandular* appearance (Fig. 40). This appearance is accentuated more so when there has been secretion of mucinous material in localized areas resulting in neoplastic cystic areas (Fig. 41). A common variation is a pattern that has a marked accumulation of secretion to produce the *adenoid* pattern (Fig. 42) which sometimes is sufficiently extreme as to present with flattened cuboidal cells and sufficient uniformity as to resemble

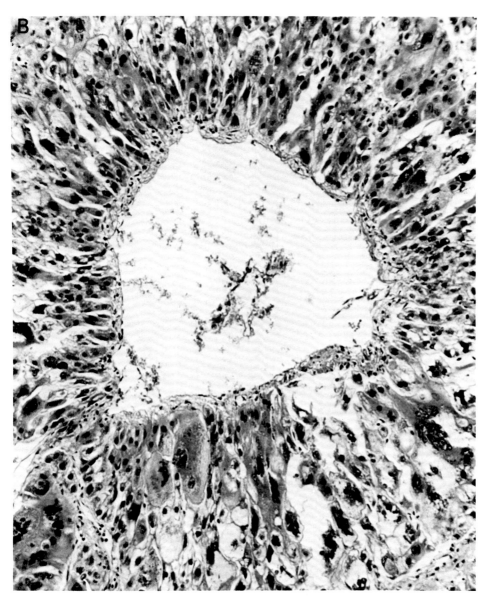

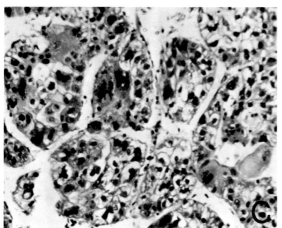

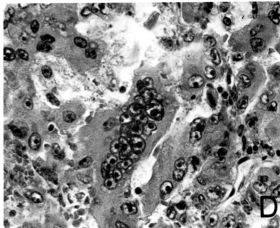

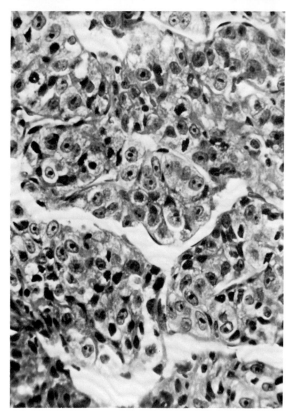

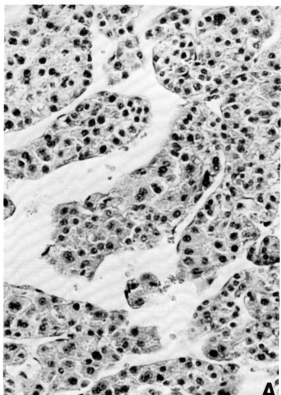

Figure 36 Fairly well-developed microtrabecular HCC in the noncirrhotic liver of an HBsAg positive 36-year-old Mexican man who did have some architectural distortion in the nontumor liver. Note the lack of supporting stroma. (hematoxylin and eosin, X420; LAC-USCMC 75-313). Courtesy of R. Terry, M. D.

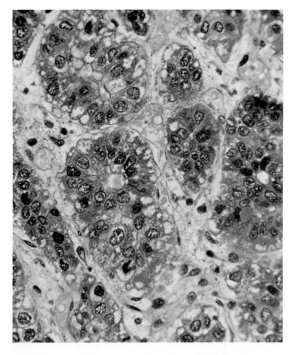

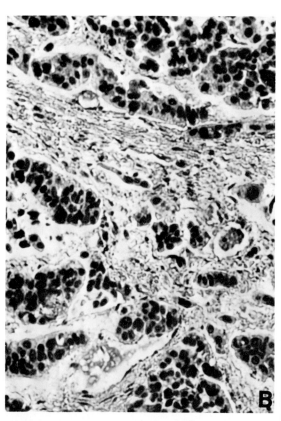

Figure 38 Acinar arrangement of hepatocytes in liver biopsy with trabecular, acinar, and adenoid areas (hematoxylin and eosin, X210; JWS843-75).

Figure 37 Microtrabecular carcinomas may include forms with cytologically less well-differentiated features (a) and others with undifferentiated features (b). [hematoxylin and eosin, X210; JWS3398-72 (a) and JWA131-71 (b)].

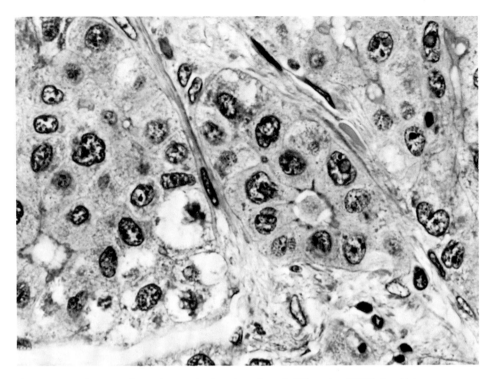

Figure 39 High power photomicrograph of moderately well-differentiated HCC, in which many areas feature tumor cells arranged radially about canaliculi, and impart a ductal arrangement to some areas. (hematoxylin and eosin, X892.50 JWS3012-74).

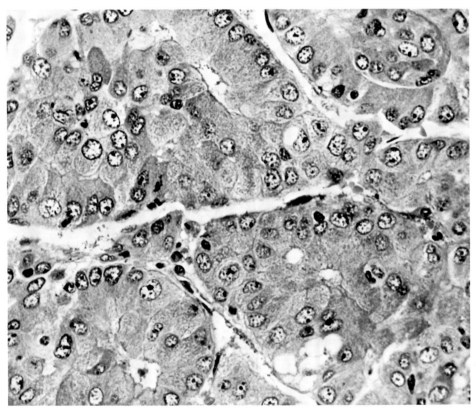

Figure 40 Area of pseudoglandular formation in otherwise trabecular HCC arising in silent, developing cirrhotic liver of an HBsAg+, AFP+, 60-year-old man. (hematoxylin and eosin, X892.50; JWA45-71).

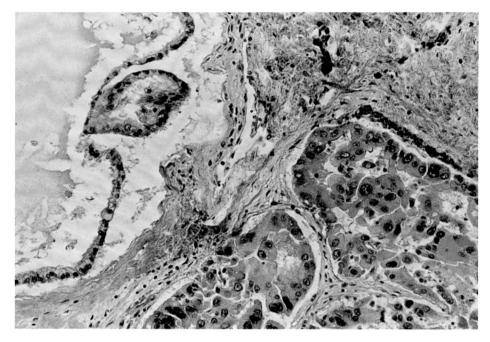

Figure 41 HCC with areas in which the tumor cells, although resembling hepatocytes, have begun to form glandlike structure with even areas in which neoplastic cuboidal cells line cystic structures (hematoxylin and eosin, X178.50; JWA2-72).

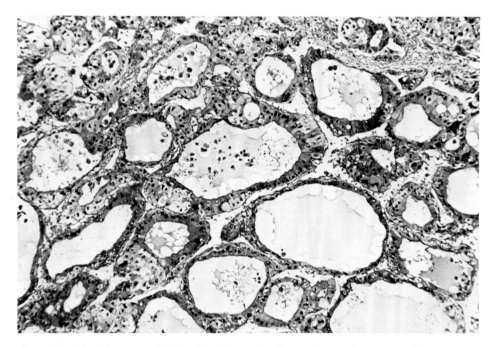

Figure 42 Adenoid pattern of HCC arising in a trabecular carcinoma of a 69-year-old Mexican alcoholic cirrhotic man (hematoxylin and eosin, X178.50; JWA172-68).

thyroid gland. The metastases from HCC with adenoid or pseudoglandular patterns tend not to feature the same glandular arrangement nor is the metastatic distribution, when it occurs, that of ductal carcinoma.

A variation of the microtrabecular pattern results when the trabecula are solid cores several cells thick. The pattern is characterized as *macrotrabecular* (Figs. 32 and 33). The tumor cells are not oriented toward a canalicular center but fit together like cobblestones. Often such thick fingers of tumor do have a hyaline secretory product, however, which looks as though it had replaced a previous dead cell, and indeed the hyaline bodies are often found extracellularly in HCC as well as intracellularly. Characteristically macrotrabecular HCC has very little stroma.

Often areas of tumor, particularly areas of macrotrabecular carcinoma, grow solidly without pattern creating whole fields of hepatocytes that are cohesive and fitted together to resemble cobblestones. In this regard the tumor is growing in a fashion similar to that of regenerating liver. We refer to the growth pattern as *cobblestone* (Fig. 43). Such tumor on needle biopsy, if cytologically well differentiated, may be difficult to distinguish from nontumor liver unless the tumor margin is included (Fig. 44). When such tumor develops in islands surrounded by collagen, it resembles squamous cell carcinoma, but lacks the basaloid cells marginating each islet that are so common in squamous cell carcinoma (Fig. 45).

In recent years, considerable comment has been made regarding the "peliosis hepatis" pattern in livers of patients receiving certain steroid hormones (see Chapter 7 by Johnson). This coincidence is described in the liver of adenoma-peliosis-contraceptive treated patients and of the benign-acting carcinoma-peliosis-androgen patients. The vascular changes in livers of such patients are predominantly in the nontumor liver, and actually appear to represent sinusoidal or vascular ectasia rather than the round, concise "flea bitten" pattern of the very rare peliosis hepatis. However, occasionally a highly vascularized pattern reminiscent of peliosis hepatis pattern may occur *within* a well-differentiated carcinoma (Fig. 46); such tumors are grossly spongy and seem hemorrhagic in areas because of the pooling of blood. This pattern is rare and the term *pelioid* is proposed. In 1915 L'Esperance described a variety of hemorrhagic tumor under the term *atypical hemorrhagic malignant hepatoma* (59). From the photomicrographs, L'Esperance's cases appear to be highly pleomorphic HCC but not the same pattern as pelioid HCC.

Rarely a microtrabecular pattern with its lack of supporting stroma may have sufficient proliferative activity to result in a well-defined papillary growth pattern. In a recent case from LAC-USCMC, only a search of many sections from the tumor revealed areas with bile-secreting, well-differentiated, and well-developed trabecular pattern (Fig. 47).

The histologic growth pattern of some tumors is best described only as undeveloped. Such tumors are less cohesive thus lacking the jigsaw close fit of the cobblestone arrangement. Usually such tumors will have a developed pattern in some areas but lack such development elsewhere. Although there is a rough direct relationship between cellular differentiation and development of histologic pattern, it is not rare to find areas of giant cell change (Fig. 35*b*) or undifferentiated carcinoma (Fig. 37*b*) arranged in trabecular fashion, nor is it uncommon to find a cytologically well differentiated HCC without a developed growth pattern (Fig. 44).

Other histologic patterns in the liver seem to be related to differences in stromal response or to development of lines of differentiation along more than one line (see mixed tumors below). The histologic types of tumor described above are most characteristic when supporting stroma is very

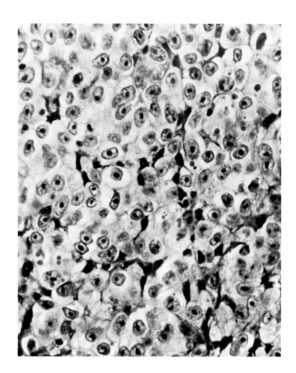

Figure 43 Cobblestone pattern of growth of HCC (hematoxylin and eosin; LAC-USCMC, 75-313). Courtesy of R. Terry, M. D.

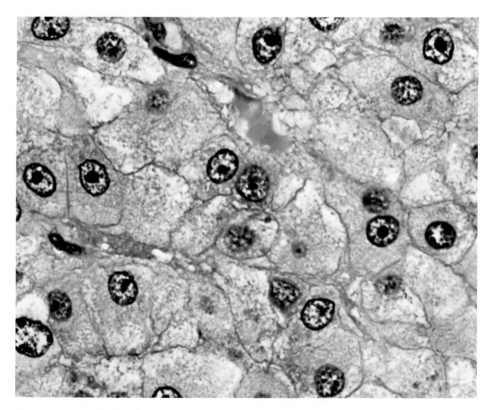

Figure 44 Area of well-differentiated HCC with cobblestone pattern, although one can see some residual cord structure. Diagnosis of HCC on such a limited area is not warranted. (hematoxylin and eosin, X850; JWS476-73).

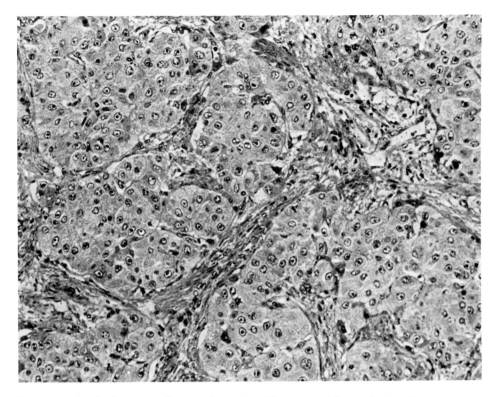

Figure 45 Islands of HCC in collagen with occasional features reminiscent of trabecular components but generally separated into clusters of cobblestone-type hepatocytes (hematoxylin and eosin, X178.50; JWA163-66).

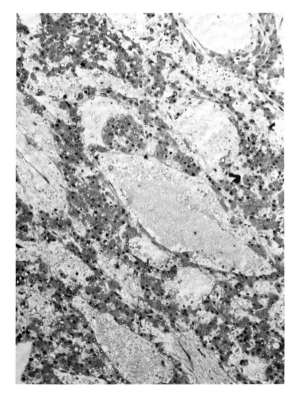

Figure 46 Highly vascularized, well-differentiated HCC with pelioid pattern (hematoxylin and eosin, X85; JWS4274-74).

scanty. Stromal connective tissue seems to inhibit free development of trabecular pattern; instead the cordlike structure is shortened to simulate a glandular or acinar arrangement (Figs. 26, 38, and 41) or islands of cobblestone pattern that resemble clusters of squamous cell carcinoma that may be found in the midst of dense stroma (Fig. 45). But most frequently, increase in fibrous stroma is associated with formation of ductlike arrangement of hepatocytes, often the deeply eosinophilic cytoplasm allows the identification of hepatocellular character of the tumor. As a rule regional variation of growth pattern is seen in an hepatocellular carcinoma (Figs. 47 and 48).

Calcification in HCC is described as an occasional radiologic finding (55). Both calcification and ossification are common in hepatoblastomas; calcium deposits were not encountered in the tumors of this series.

An uncommon pattern of fibrosis was found in four patients HCC studied from the autopsy series but was also seen in one submitted biopsy from a 16-year-old boy. This fibrosis might be characterized as *lamellar* since the relatively acellular connective tissue fibers are arranged in somewhat parallel dense layers of fine collagen fibers. In spite of the amount of fibrosis, the malignant hepatocytes are still recognizable as liver cells, although many look as though they were undergoing eosinophilic necrosis with deeply eosinophilic cytoplasm and pyknotic nuclei (Figs. 49 and 50). The term *eosinophilic hepatocellular carcinoma with lamellar fibrosis* is proposed for this small

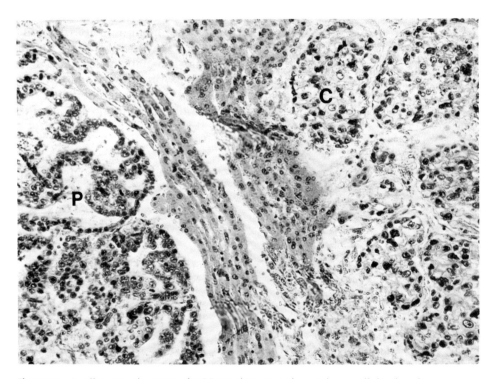

Figure 47   Papillary growth pattern of HCC *(p)* other areas of tumor have well-developed macrotrabecular clear cell areas *(c)* (hematoxylin and eosin, X178.50; LAC-USCMC, 87818). Courtesy of R. Rhoades, M. D.

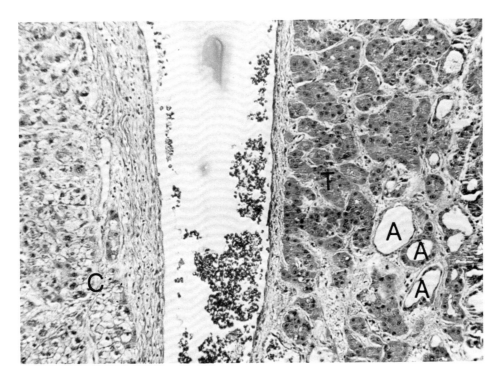

Figure 48 HCC with well-differentiated trabecular growth in spite of enveloping collagen *(t)* early adenoid development *(a)* and clear cell carcinoma *(cc)* (H & E X120).

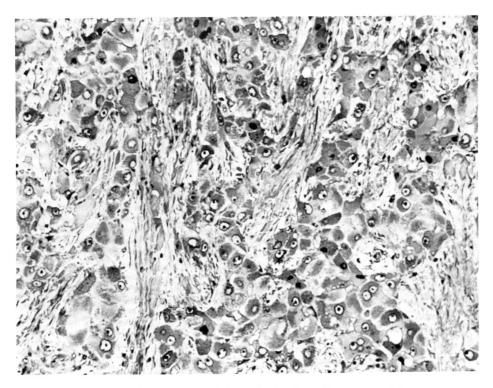

153

Figure 49 Lacy pattern of HCC with parallel strands of collagen fibers arranged about columns of cells. An uncommon pattern tentatively labeled *eosinophilic HCC with lamellar fibrosis* (H & E 178.50X).

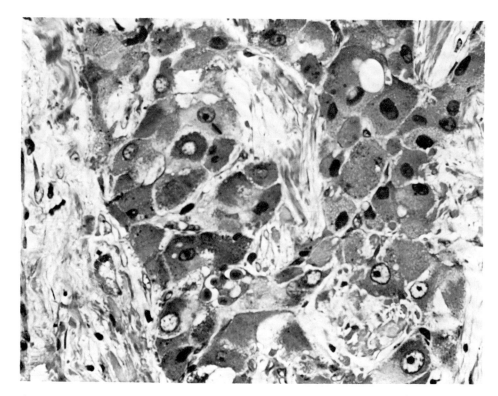

Figure 50 High power microphotograph of Fig. 49. It can be seen that there is no cord or trabecular arrangement, many nuclei appear pyknotic, and the cytoplasm usually eosinophilic, but there is little pleomorphism (hematoxylin and eosin, X357).

group. So far in our material the lamellar fibrosis pattern has principally been found in HCC arising in noncirrhotic livers (4 of 5) and has been associated with slightly improved survival time in those few patients. Although all of the patients in this series with eosinophilic hepatocellular carcinoma with lamellar fibrosis have been postpubertal, three of the five were under 30 years old. One was an asymptomatic HBsAg carrier but was a chronic drug user. The only other one tested for HBsAg was negative but did have protease inhibitor type MZ. Edmondson recorded a similar case in a 14-year-old white girl who has been found to be alive and well 10 years after local resection (3, 60, personal communication).

Sclerosing Liver Carcinomas

The group of sclerosing liver carcinoma,

made up of sclerosing peripheral cholangiocarcinomas, sclerosing hepatocellular carcinomas [liver cell carcinoma with dense stroma of Edmondson (3)], and sclerosing cholangiolocellular carcinomas, have much in common. They arise in noncirrhotic livers in about equal incidence in men or in women between the ages of 40 and 65 (average age 61.9). There is a high coincidence of pseudohyperparathyroidism associated with these tumors (61–63) in our material. Six of nine cases of otherwise unexplained hypercalcemia recognized among our 247 patients with HCC were associated with sclerosing liver carcinomas. Of the total number of 15 uniformly sclerosing carcinomas, many had no or only a cursory study of calcium and phosphorus dynamics. Many cholangiocarcinomas have areas of sclerosis; however, those placed into this class were rather uniformly charac-

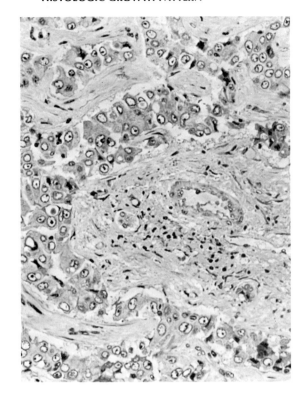

Figure 51 This 46-year-old Caucasian woman, who was admitted with Budd-Chiari's syndrome and pseudohyperparathyroidism, had an umbilicated sclerotic tumor (24a) which on section was glistening and well demarcated, obliterating hepatic veins (24b). Although the tumor was markedly sclerotic with ductlike arrangement of cells, the tumor cells retained their granularity and the characteristics of hepatocytes (Fig. 51) and could be seen to blend with the nonneoplastic hepatocytes at the margins (Fig. 24c) (hematoxylin and eosin, X210; JWA94-73).

terized by sclerosis that enveloped each cord, making the distinction of hepatocellular from cholangiolar and cholangiolocellular quite difficult.

The sclerosing hepatocellular carcinomas are often diagnosed as cholangiocarcinomas because of the ductlike pattern and the smaller size of individual tumor cells when compared to ordinary hepatocellular carcinoma. Unlike many hepatocellular carcinomas that feature ductal elements (Fig. 40 and 41), uniformly sclerosing carcinomas have tended not to be of mixed cellular types. The sclerosing HCC is made of shrunken hepatic cords which nonetheless have the granular eosinophilic cytoplasm and the large oval nuclei with prominent nucleoli so characteristic of the hepatocytes. There is no basement membrane about the tumor cords. The cells are, nonetheless, cohesive. Often there

is no lumen, but rather a solid core of cells surrounded by dense collagen (Fig. 51).

The sclerosing cholangiocarcinoma is made up of more cuboidal cells with scantier, clearer cytoplasm, a more well-defined lumen of the duct, and somewhat more precise alignment of the base of the cells where a basement membrane can usually be found. The nuclei are somewhat smaller with uniform nuclear chromatin rather than having peripherally located chromatin as in the HCC. Nucleoli are not prominent in cholangiocarcinomas (Figs. 52a and b).

A small number of sclerosing liver carcinomas can only be classified as cholangiolocellular in type (see cholangiolocellular). Cholangiolocellular carcinoma is a term used by Steiner in describing relatively rare carcinomas that resemble cholangioles (canal of Hering). Many of the tumors that Steiner placed in-

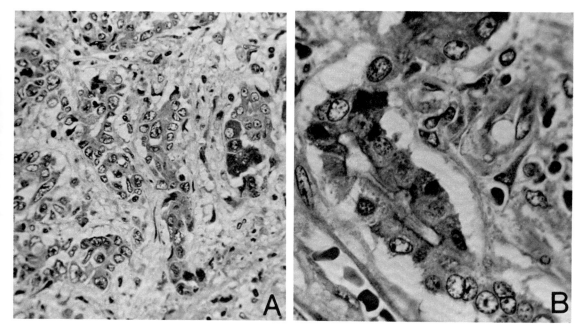

Figure 52 Comparison with sclerosing peripheral cholangiocarcinoma shows somewhat more cuboidal cells *(a)*, irregular nuclei with few nucleoli, and a basement membrane in some areas *(b)* (hematoxylin and eosin, X210 *(a)* and X420 *(b)*; JWS880-75).

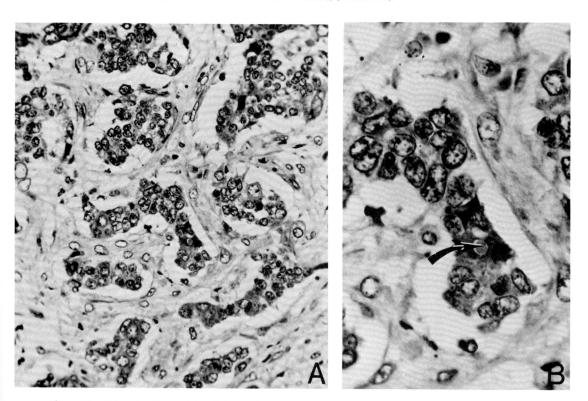

Figure 53 Sclerosing cholangiolocellular carcinoma. *(a)* Note the primitive cords of cuboidal cells with scanty cytoplasm and round, regular nuclei without nucleoli. *(b)* On higher power these cords have canaliculi with secretion at one point (arrow) (hematoxylin and eosin, X210 *(a)* and X420 *(b)*; JWA123-74).

to this class were sclerosing tumors judging from accompanying photomicrographs (43). Since the cholangiole occupies a morphologic and intermediate developmental position between the liver cell and the bile duct, it has been speculated that many tumors with elements of hepatocellular as well as ductal elements may have truly originated in cholangioles, differentiating along both ductal and hepatocellular liver. However, the cholangiolocellular carcinoma applies to tumors that retain the cuboidal cell morphology throughout the entire tumor, with very meager cytoplasm and similarity to the cholangiole. Whether the three tumors that constitute the sclerosing liver carcinoma group deserve to be placed in one related category is conjectural. Certainly the setting in which they arise and the syndrome they may produce is similar, and they tend to have fairly uniform morphologic features within any one case showing little or no mixture of hepatocellular with cholangiolar or cholangiolocellular.

Cholangiolocellular Carcinoma

The concept of this relatively rare carcinoma was introduced by Steiner (64) and Steiner and Higginson (65) to describe the tumors that arise from the canal of Hering or cholangiole. Such tumors have constituted only 0.8% of our primary liver carcinomas at LAC-USCMC. Steiner accumulated data to show that it represented about 1% of liver cancers. One of the two tumors classified in our series at LAC-USCMC and USC-JWCH as cholangiolocellular was a sclerosing carcinoma (see above). The neoplastic cells are fairly uniform, tending not to differentiate significantly into either hepatocellular or ductal tumors. They retain the configuration usually associated with cholangioles in that they form double layered cuboidal epithelial cell cords which do, on close inspection, have a tiny lumen. The cytoplasm is scanty and pale and forms a narrow clear zone around the dark oval nuclei which lack the prominent nucleoli usually found in hepatocellular carcinoma. The tumor structures resemble the proliferating "pseudoductules" or "cholangioles" one finds in areas of hepatic fibrosis (Fig. 53a and b). Steiner has emphasized the point that although these tumors resemble cholangioles, resemblance is not proof of histogenesis (64, 65). Nonetheless, the distinctive morphologic features of cholangiolocellular carcinoma combined with its *lack* of relationship with cirrhosis and its lack of sex predilection places the tumor in a class different from usual hepatocellular carcinoma.

Combined Carcinomas

Combined carcinomas of the liver may be separated into three classes: (a) glandular or ductal metaplasia in HCC (Figs. 38 to 40 and 42), (b) contiguous hepatocellular and ductal carcinoma wherein it appears that each may have arisen from a common origin, each differentiating along separate lines (Figs. 41 and 48); (c) hepatocellular and bile duct carcinomas may arise separately from different foci in the same liver.

Hepatocellular carcinomas with areas of ductal or glandular change are fairly common and are not usually referred to as combined. Trabecular carcinoma readily develops an acinar pattern (Fig. 38) which is only a step from a ductal character or conversely, an acinar arrangement of hepatocytes may undergo transition to high columnar cells resulting in a glandular configuration (Fig. 40). Trabecular carcinomas that have a supporting stroma seem particularly prone to develop larger nuclei and clearer, less abundant cytoplasm resulting in the appearance of an adenocarcinoma.

Hepatocellular and ductal carcinomas developing separately from what would appear to be a common source are much less common. One of the least often occurring

Table 10   Metastatic Patterns of HCC and Cholangiocarcinoma

	HCC Noncirrhotic (39 Cases)	HCC Cirrhotic (188 Cases)	Peripheral Cholangioca (18 Cases)
No metastases	33%	54.8%	25.0%
Single metastases	25.0	19.1	18.8
Lung	41.0	38.8	25.0
Lymph node (portal)	43.6	16.5	68.8
Portal vein	23.0	37.2	12.5
Hepatic vein	18.0	22.9	18.8
Skin	0	2.7	0
Serosa	23.1	7.4	25.0
Adrenal gland	3.0	6.9	18.0
Bone marrow	7.7	8.0	25.0
Heart	2.6	1.6	0
Spleen	7.7	2.1	6.3
Pancreas	0	1.1	0
CNS	2.6	1.1	0
Kidney	0	0	0
Diaphragm	2.6	3.7	6.3
Gallbladder	10.3	5.3	0
Other	5.1	3.2	6.3

pattern is that in which hepatocellular and bile duct carcinoma arise simultaneously in different sites in the liver. Such an occurrence may be no more frequent than anticipated by chance alone.

METASTATIC PATTERNS OF HCC

The metastatic pattern of HCC arising in cirrhotic liver is surprisingly uniform from case to case although there is a statistical relationship to the presence or absence of underlying cirrhosis and to the microscopic degree of differentiation or pleomorphism of the neoplasm. As shown in Table 10, nearly twice as many patients dying with HCC in a cirrhotic liver were free of metastases as when the HCC developed in a noncirrhotic liver. This may be because the patient with HCC and cirrhosis develops hepatic failure and dies sooner before metastases develop. There is also a slight relationship of metastases with degree of

cellular differentiation. Patients whose tumors were classified as well differentiated included 66% without metastases, those moderately differentiated totaled 46.9%, while poorly differentiated HCC had not metastasized in 33.8% of cases. Those classified as "variable differentiation" or "giant cell" had a metastatic pattern similar to moderately differentiated HCC.

There are greater differences between the metastatic pattern of cholangiocarcinomas and the commoner HCC arising in a cirrhotic liver (Table 10).

The most common site of spread of HCC is to lungs, occurring in 41% of noncirrhotic patients and in 38.8% of cirrhotics. Nearly equal is involvement of the portal vein with extension retrograde into the extrahepatic portion of that vessel (see Table 10 and Figs. 54, 55). Microscopically, many of the small vascular portal venous radicles are plugged with tumor and, to a lesser extent, microscopic radicles of the hepatic vein are involved. However, in-

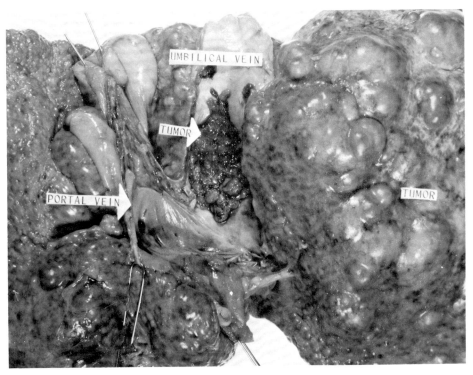

Figure 54 Gross photograph of alcoholic cirrhotic liver with HCC of left lobe. Note the tumor thrombotic material in the portal vein with a widely patent dilated umbilical vein (JWA48-62).

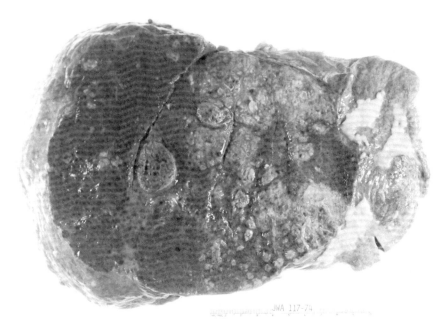

Figure 55 Intrahepatic portal vein spread in inductive HCC arising in alcoholic cirrhotic patient.

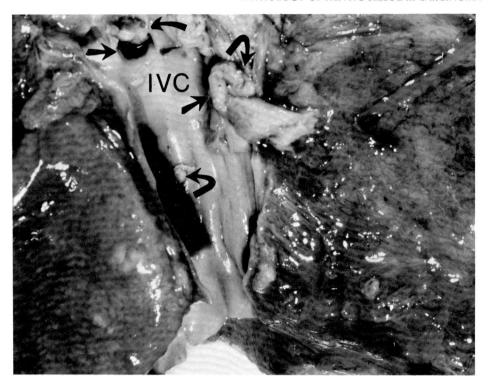

Figure 56   Gross photograph of posterior surface of liver showing opened inferior vena cava (IVC) with tumor extending out orifices of hepatic veins (arrows) (JWA69-67).

volvement of hepatic vein branches of a caliber allowing gross identification of that method of spread is less common, identified in 23% of HCC arising in cirrhotic livers and 18% of those involving noncirrhotic livers (Fig. 56). Of areas remote from the liver, the lung is by far the most commonly involved organ. Of the 225 patients with HCC in our autopsy series, 39% had lung involvement and in the 111 who had any metastases, the lung was involved in 80.2% (Fig. 57). Metastasis to the lungs is apparently by way of microemboli. In 55% of patients with lung metastases, the pulmonary involvement was only recognizable microscopically as showers or isolated, occasional intravascular foci. Apparently many such tumor emboli fail to survive the sudden trip to the pulmonary vascular bed and can be recognized as degenerating or

hyalinizing structures occluding the vessel lumen (Fig. 57b). Radiographic demonstration of HCC metastic to the lung is uncommon. The metastatic foci in the lung rarely attain a diameter as large as 1 cm. Occasionally, however, the tumor emboli may produce the syndrome of pulmonary hypertension. Apparently the vascularization of the growing emboli by the bronchial vasculature results in increased arterial shunting that may be mistaken clinically for the pulmonary vascular spiders occasionally found in the cirrhotic patient.

The next most common metastatic site of HCC arising in cirrhotic liver is the periportal lymph nodes; this site accounted for 43% of patients with HCC arising in noncirrhotic livers but in only 16.5% of patients with HCC arising in cirrhotic livers.

The other metastatic sites are much less

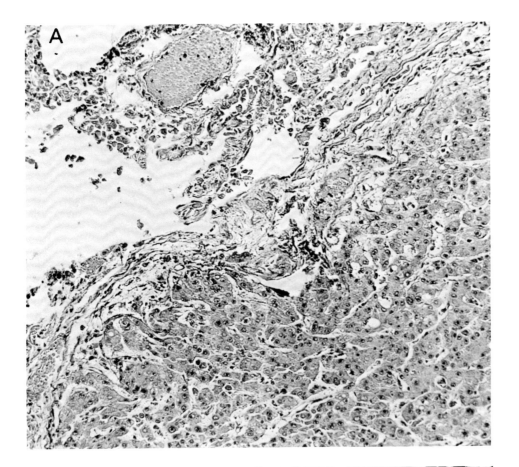

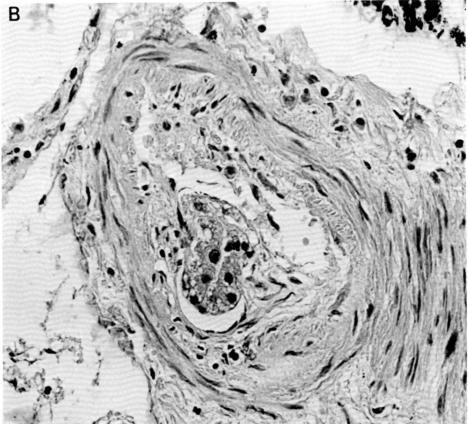

Figure 57 *(a)* Well-differentiated HCC in lung of patient with alcoholic cirrhosis (Figs. 9 and 30) and HCC (hematoxylin and eosin). *(b)* Other areas include vessels with organizing thrombic material and a well-differentiated trabecula of HCC with pyknotic nuclei (hematoxylin and eosin; reproduced at same size JWA77-66).

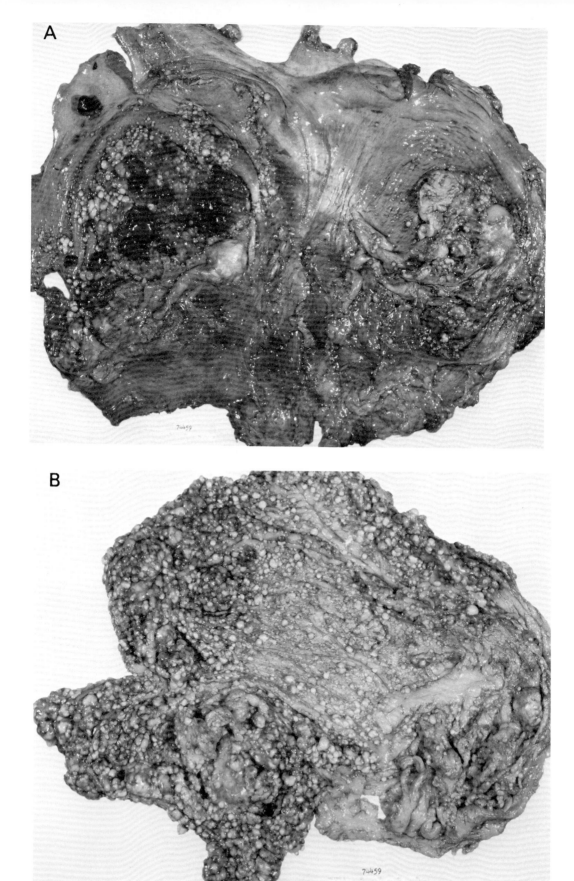

Figure 58 HCC may spread over the abdominal surface of the diaphragm (a) or to omentum (b) (LACUSCMC #74459). Courtesy of D. Tatter, M. D.

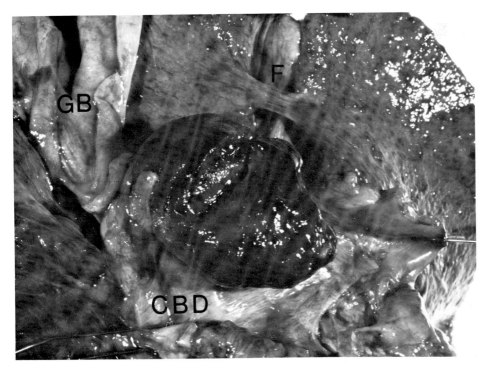

Figure 59 Tumor growth into the common bile duct (CBD) with obstruction is uncommon. This 47-year-old black man had asymptomatic HBsAg-positive chronic liver disease. His primary tumor was small but entered the duct system producing symptoms much earlier than would otherwise have occurred. F: ligamentumeres and falciform; GB: gallbladder (JWA31-70).

commonly recognized in HCC and are indicated in Table 10 (See also Fig. 58, 59, 60). Certain regions of metastatic spread were not identified in the autopsy series of 225 cases from a 20-year period but have been submitted from outside contributors, from surgical pathology, or found subsequent to the 20-year study.

Sclerosing liver carcinomas of hepatocellular, cholangiolar, or cholangiolocellular type have a metastatic pattern more closely akin to that seen with cholangiocarcinoma (see Table 10 and Chapter 11).

The duration of survival of patients after recognition of carcinoma is quite brief, generally under three months and apparently is unrelated to gross or microscopic morphology. A large number of our pa-

tients sought medical attention because of the development of signs of hepatic failure or of a expanding hepatic mass. There is no definitive way of knowing the length of time the patients had a neoplasm. In more recent years the recognition of the relationship of HCC to quiescent chronic active hepatitis type B and to the low titer of HBsAg in serum may permit prospective serial AFP analysis of more patients with low titer HBsAg in the fashion undertaken by Okuda (14). Whether more innovative techniques to purge hepatitis B by either exogenous or endogenous manipulations will be successful in reducing the incidence of carcinoma in such patients is unknown. It is conceivable, as in the alcoholic cirrhotic who discontinues his imbibition, that an irreversible pattern forward

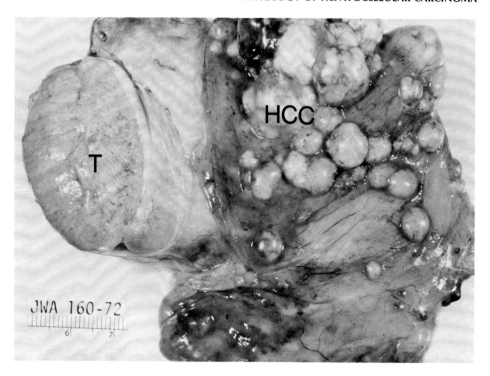

Figure 60   Metastases to the spermatic cord and epididymis occurred in this 63-year-old Mexican man with HCC arising in alcoholic cirrhosis. T: testis; HCC: hepatocellular carcinoma (JWA160-72).

neoplasia may be set early in the disease.

Paraneoplastic Syndrome

Hepatocellular carcinoma has been recognized to be associated with ever increasing numbers of extrahepatic abnormalities that follow development of the neoplasm. Many of the factors have a humeral activity (see Chapters 14 to 16), others are measurable serologic anomalies. These abnormalities have been referred to as "paraneoplastic syndromes," and the major ones are listed in Table 11 (66–91). Relatively few of the paraneoplastic syndromes were recognized among the 225 cases of HCC, but some of the anomalites are not associated with clinical symptoms and some factors, although sought liberally in testing today,

are found by methods not generally used or available five years ago. Since a majority of patients who died of HCC between 1954 to 1973 were not correctly diagnosed during life, prospective studies were infeasible.

Hypoglycemia, the paraneoplastic syndrome most commonly identified in the 20-year period from 1954 through 1973, has been reported to be associated with recognizable histologic types (83). In our material, no characteristic histologic features of HCC occurring in association with hypoglycemia could be recognized.

Hypercalcemia, in our material, was found in far greater association with sclerosing carcinomas than with more common types of HCC (see p 000).

Amyloidosis was found in five patients, three were with HCC superimposed on alcoholic cirrhosis, one man with cholangio-

Table 11 Paraneoplastic Syndromes Associated with HCC

Condition (Reference)	Cases	Condition (Reference)	Cases
Aldolase, abnormal type (66)		Gynecomastia (79)	
Amyloidosis	5	Hypercalcemia (80)	10
Carcinoembryonic		Hyperlipidemia (81)	
antigen (67, 68)		Hypoglycemia (82, 83)	15
Carcinoid, syndrome (69)		Osteoarthropathy,	
Cryofibrinogenemia (70)		hypertrophic (84)	
Dysfibrinogenemia (71)		Phosphatase, Alkaline,	
Eosinophilia (72)		abnormal (85)	
Fetoprotein (73–76)	70%	Polycythemia (82, 86)	9
Ferritin abnormality (77)		Porphyria cutanea	
Gonadotropin (78)	1	tarda (87)	1
		Thrombophlebitis (88)	
		Vitiligo (89)	

carcinoma in a noncirrhotic liver, and one woman with mixed ductal and hepatocellular carcinoma in a noncirrhotic liver. The youngest was 59, the oldest 63 years old.

SUMMARY

In summary, an attempt has been made to further characterize and classify the gross appearance of HCC and the background hepatic lesion on which it arises. The classification proposed is based on a presumed difference of histogenesis. The microscopic patterns have been described, but the relationship to biologic behavior for most tumors remains in a statistical category only and is of little prognostic value in individual cases. Exceptions might be made for a tumor pattern called *eosinophilic HCC with lamellar fibrosis* which has a somewhat more favorable prognosis, and for *sclerosing liver carcinomas* which have an increased relationship to pseudohyperparathyroidism.

REFERENCES

1. Hanot VC, Gilbert A: *Etudes sur les Maladies du Foie,* 1888. Quoted by Rolleston HD: *Disease of the Liver, Gall Bladder and Bile Ducts,* 2nd ed. MacMillan, New York, 1912, pp 474.
2. Eggel H: Uber das Primare Carcinom der Leber. *Beitr Z Pathol Anat Allg Pathol* **30**:506–604, 1901.
3. Edmondson HA: *Tumor of the Liver and Intrahepatic Bile Ducts,* Section VII fascicle 25, Armed Forces Institute of Pathology, 1958.
4. Edmondson HA, Steiner PE: Primary carcinoma of the liver. A study of 100 cases among 48,900 necropsies. *Cancer* **7**:462–503, 1954.
5. Hale White, I: *Diseases of the Liver, Pancreas, Ductless Glands and Kidneys.* Rolleston HD (eds.) 1908, IV part 215, Macmillan & Co. as quoted in Rolleston HD: *Diseases of the Liver, Gall Bladder, and Bile Ducts,* 2nd ed., Macmillan, New York, 1912.
6. Becker FF: Hepatoma—Nature's model tumor. A review. *Am J Pathol* **74**:179–200, 1974.
7. Shikata T: Studies on the relationship between hepatic cancer and liver cirrhosis. *Acta Pathol Jap* **9**:267–311, 1959.
8. Shikata T: Cirrhosis and hepatocellular carcinoma. In *Hepatocellular Carcinoma.* Okuda K, Peters RL (Eds). Wiley, New York, 1975, Chapter 4.
9. MacSween RNM: A clinicopathological review of 100 cases of primary malignant tumors of the liver. *J Clin Pathol* **27**:669–682, 1974.
10. Geddes EW, Falkson G: Malignant hepatoma in the Bantu. *Cancer* **25**:1271–1278, 1970.
11. Rolleston HD: *Diseases of the Liver, Gall Bladder and Bile Ducts,* 2nd ed. MacMillan and Co., New York, 1912.
12. Ihde DC, Sherlock P, Winower SJ, Fortner JG: Clinical manifestations of hepatoma—A review of 6 years experience at a cancer hospital. *Am J Med* **56**:83–91, 1974.
13. Gall EA: Post hepatitic, post necrotic and nutri-

tional cirrhosis: A pathologic analysis. *Am J Pathol* **36**:241, 1960.

14. Okuda K, Kotoda K, Obata H, et al: Clinical observations during a relatively early stage of hepatocellular carcinoma, with special reference to serum α-fetoprotein levels. *Gastroenterology,* **69**:226–234, 1975.

15. Ohta Y: Viral hepatitis and hepatocellular carcinoma. In *Hepatocellular Carcinoma.* Okuda K, Peters R (Eds). Wiley, New York, 1975, Chapter 5.

16. Karvountis GG, Redeker AG, Peters RL: Long term follow-up studies of patients surviving fulminant viral hepatitis. *Gastroenterology* **67**:870–877, 1974.

17. Rubin E, Kros S, Popper H: Pathogenesis of post necrotic cirrhosis in alcoholics. *Arch Pathol* **73**:288–299, 1962.

18. Gall EA: Primary and metastatic carcinoma of the liver. *AMA Arch Pathol* **70**:206–232, 1960.

19. Edmondson HA, Peters RL: Liver. In *Pathology,* 7th ed. Anderson WAD (Ed). Mosby, in press.

20. Edmondson HA, Peters RL, Reynolds TB, Kuzma OT: Sclerosing hyaline necrosis of the liver in the chronic alcoholic. *Ann Intern Med* **59**:646, 1963.

21. Edmondson HA, Peters RL, Frankel HH, Borowsky S: The early stage of liver injury in the alcoholic. *Medicine* **46**:119–129, 1967.

22. Reynolds TB, Hidemura R, Michel H, Peters RL: Portal hypertension without cirrhosis in alcoholic liver disease. *Ann Intern Med* **70**:449–506, 1969.

23. Lee FI: Cirrhosis and hepatoma in alcoholics. *Gut* **7**:77–95, 1966.

24. Leevy CM, Gallene R, Ning M: Primary liver cancer in cirrhosis of the alcoholics. *Ann N Y Acad Sci* **1026**:1026–1040.

25. Shikata T, Ozawa T, Yoshiwara N, Akatsuka T, Yamazaki S: Staining methods of Australia antigen in paraffin sections. *Jap J Exp Med* **44**:25–36, 1974.

26. Afroudakis A, Liew C, Peters RL: An immunoperoxidase technique for the demonstration of the hepatitis B surface antigen in human livers. *Am. J. Clinical Pathology,* in press.

27. Joske RA, Laurence BH: Familial cirrhosis with autoimmune features and raised immunoglobulin levels. *Gastroenterology* **59**:546–552, 1970.

28. Joske RA, Laurence BH, Matz LR: Familial active chronic hepatitis with hepatocellular carcinoma. Report of a case. *Gastroenterology* **63**:441–444, 1972.

29. Sharp HL, Bridges RA, Krivit W, et al: Cirrhosis associated with alpha 1 antitrypsin deficiency.

Scand J Lab Invest **73**:934–939, 1969.

30. Campra J, Craig JR, Peters RL, et al: Cirrhosis associated with partial deficiency of alpha 1 antitrypsin in an adult. *Ann Intern Med* **78**:233, 238, 1973.

31. Vogel CL, Anthony PP, Sadikall F, et al: Hepatitis-associated antigen and antibody in hepatocellular carcinoma. *J Natl Cancer Inst* **48**:1583–1588, 1972.

32. Warren S, Drake EL: Primary carcinoma of the liver in hemochromatosis. *Am J Pathol* **27**:573–609, 1951.

33. Battifora H: Thorotrast and tumors of the liver. In *Hepatocellular Carcinoma.* Okuda K, Peters RL (Eds). Wiley, New York, 1975, Chapter 7.

34. Smith PM: Hepatoma associated with ulcerative colitis. Report of a case. *Dis Colon Rectum* **17**:554–556, 1975.

35. Johnson L: Androgenic-anabolic steroids and hepatocellular carcinoma. Okuda K, Peters R (eds). Wiley, New York 1975, Chapter 8.

36. Herman RE, David TE: Spontaneous rupture of the liver caused by hepatomas. *Surgery* **74**:715–719, 1973.

37. Schneiderman MA: Phenobarbitone and liver tumors. *Lancet* **2**:1085, 1974.

38. Chudecki B: Primary cancer of the liver following treatment of polycythemia vera with radioactive phosphorus. *Brit J Radiol* **45**:770–774, 1972.

39. Pritzker K: Neoplasia in renal transplant recipients. *Can Med Assoc J* **107**:1059–1062, 1972.

40. Arbus GS, Hung RH: Hepatocarcinoma and myocardial fibrosis in 8¾ year-old renal transplant recipient. *Can Med Assoc J* **107**:431–432, 1972.

41. Wogan GN: Aflatoxins and their relationship to hepatocellular carcinoma. In *Hepatocellular Carcinoma.* Okuda K, Peters RL (Eds). Wiley, New York, 1975, Chapter 2.

42. Geiser CF, Baez A, Schindler AM, Shih VE: Epithelial hepatoblastoma associated with congenital hemihypertrophy and cystathioninuria: presentation of a case. *Pediatrics* **46**:66–73, 1970.

43. Zangeneh F, Limbeck GA, Brown BI, Emch JR, et al: Type I glycogenosis and carcinoma of the liver. *Pediatrics* **74**:73–83, 1969.

44. Deoras MP, Dicus W: Hepatocarcinomas associated with biliary cirrhosis. *Arch Pathol* **86**:338–341, 1968.

45. Ganrot PO, Laurell CB, Eriksson S: Obstructive lung disease and trypsin inhibitors in alpha 1 antitrypsin deficiency. *Scand J Clin Lab Invest* **19**:205–208, 1967.

46. Berg NO, Eriksson S: Liver disease in adults with

alpha 1 antitrypsin deficiency. *N Engl J Med* **287**:1264–1267, 1972.

47. Rawlings W, Moss J, Cooper HS, et al: Hepatocellular carcinoma and partial deficiency of alpha 1 antitrypsin. *Ann Intern Med* **81**:771–773, 1974.

48. Gibson JB, Chan WC: Primary carcinomas of the liver in Hong Kong—some possible etiological factors. *Cancer Res* **39**:107–118, 1972.

49. Simson IW, Middlecote BD: The Budd-Chiari syndrome in the Bantu. In *Liver*. Saunders SJ, Terblanche J (Eds). Pitman Medical, London, 1973.

50. Okayasu I, Mori W, Hatanaka M: An autopsy case of congenital hepatic cell tumor. *Acta Pathol Jap* **24**:387–392, 1974.

51. Craig J, Dunn AEG, Peters RL: Cirrhosis associated with partial deficiency of alpha-1-antitrypsin: A clinical and autopsy study. *Human Pathol* **6**:113–120, 1975.

52. Anthony PP: Primary carcinoma of the liver. A study of 282 cases in Ugandan Africans. *J. Pathol* **110**:37–48, 1973.

53. Okuda K: Clinical aspects of hepatocellular carcinoma-analysis of 134 cases. In *Hepatocellular Carcinoma*. Okuda K, Peters RL (Eds). Wiley, New York, 1975.

54. Nakashima T, Kojiro M, Sakamoto K, et al: Studies of primary liver carcinoma. I. Proposal of new gross anatomical classification of primary liver cell carcinoma. *Acta Hep Jap* **15**:279–291, 1974.

55. Nakashima T: Vascular changes and hemodynamics in hepatocellular carcinoma. In *Hepatocellular Carcinoma*. Okuda K, Peters RL (Eds). Wiley, New York, 1975, Chapter 9.

56. Keeley AF, Iseri OA, Gottlieb LS: Ultrastructure of hyaline cytoplasmic inclusions in a human hepatoma: relationship to Mallory's alcoholic hyalin. *Gastroenterology* **62**(2):280–293, 1972.

57. Buchanan TF, Huvos AG: Clear cell carcinoma of the liver. *Am J Clin Pathol* **61**:529–539, 1974.

58. El-Domeiri AA, Huvos AG, Goldsmith HS, Foote FW: Primary malignant tumors of the liver. *Cancer* **27**:7–11, 1971.

59. L'Esperance ES: Atypical hemorrhagic malignant hepatoma. *J Med Res* **32**:225–250, 1915.

60. Edmondson HA: Differential diagnosis of tumors and tumor-like lesions of liver in infancy and childhood. *AMA J Dis Child* **91**:168–186, 1956.

61. Samuelsson S, Werner I: Hepatic carcinoma simulating hyperparathyroidism. *Acta Med Scand* **73**:539–547, 1963.

62. Naide W, Matz R, Spear PW: Cholangiocarcinoma causing hypercalcemia and hypophosphatemia without skeletal metastases. *Am J Dig Dis* **13**:705–707, 1968.

63. Knill-Jones RP, Buckle RM, Parsons V, Calne RY, et al: Hypercalcemia and increased parathyroid-hormone activity in a primary hepatoma. *NEJM* **282**:704–708, 1970.

64. Steiner PE: Carcinoma of liver in the United States. *Acta Unio Int Contra Cancerum* **13**:628–645, 1957.

65. Steiner PE, Higginson J: Cholangiolocellular carcinoma of the liver. *Cancer* **12**(2):753–759, 1969.

66. Schapira F, Dreyfus JC, Shapira G: Anomaly of aldolase in primary liver cancer. *Nature* **200**:995–967, 1963.

67. LoGerfo P, Krupey J, Hansen HJ: Demonstration of an antigen common to several varieties of neoplasia. *NEJM* **285**:138–141, 1971.

68. Reynoso G, Tsann MC, Holyoke D, Cohen E, et al: Carcinoembryonic antigen in patients with different cancers. *JAMA* **220**:361–365, 1972.

69. Primack A, Wilson J, O'Connor GT: Hepatocellular carcinoma with the carcinoid syndrome. *Cancer* **27**:1182–1189, 1971.

70. Bell WR, Bahr R, Waldmen TA, Carbone PP: Cryofibrinogenemia, multiple dysproteinemias and hypervolemia in patients with primary hepatoma. *Ann Intern Med* **64**:658–664, 1966.

71. vonFelton A, Straub PW, Prick PG: Dysfibrinogenemia in a patient with primary hepatoma. *NEJM* **280**:405–409, 1969.

72. Rank E: Eosinophilia and hepatocellular carcinoma. *Am J Dig Dis* **10**:548–553, 1965.

73. Abelev GI: Production of embryonal serum alpha globulin by hepatoma: review of experimental and clinical data. *Cancer Res* **28**:1344–1350, 1968.

74. Alpert E, Hershberg R, Shur P, Isselbacher KJ: Alpha fetoprotein in human hepatoma: Improved detection in serum and quantitative studies using a new sensitive technique. *Gastroenterology* **61**:173–243, 1971.

75. Kithier K, Housetek J, Masopost J, Radl J: Occurrence of specific fetal protein in primary liver carcinoma. *Nature* **212**:414, 1966.

76. Alpert E: Human alpha-1 fetoprotein. In *Hepatocellular Carcinoma*. Okuda K, Peters RL (Eds). Wiley, New York, 1975, Chapter 15.

77. Alpert E: Presented to symposium of cancer immunology of National Institutes of Health, Woodshole, Mass., 1972.

78. Floyd WS, Facog MD, Cohn SL, Facog MD: Gonadotropin producing hepatoma. *Obstet Gynecol*

　　　　41:665–668, 1973.

79. Summerskill WHJ, Adson MA: Gynecomastia as a sign of hepatoma. *Am J Dig Dis* **7**:250–254, 1962.

80. Keller RT, Goldschneider I, Lafferty FW: Hypercalcemia secondary to a primary hepatoma. *JAMA* **192**:782–784, 1965.

81. Santer MA, Waldmann TA, Fallon HS: Erythrocytosis and hyperlipidemia as manifestations of hepatic carcinoma. *Arch Intern Med* **120**:735–739, 1967.

82. McFadzean AJS, Todd D, Tsang KC: Polycythemia in primary carcinoma of the liver. *Blood* **13**:427–435, 1958.

83. McFadzean AJS, Yeung RTT: Further observations on hypoglycemia in hepatocellular carcinoma. *Am J Med* **47**:220–235, 1969.

84. Morgan AG, Walker WC, Makson MK, Herlinger H, et al: A new syndrome associated with hepatocellular carcinoma. *Gastroenterology* **63**:340–345, 1972.

85. Portugal ML, Azevedo MS, Manso C: Serum alpha fetoprotein and variant alkaline phosphatase in human hepatocellular carcinoma. *Int J Cancer* **6**:383–387, 1970.

86. McFadzean AJS, Todd D, Tso SC: Erythrocytosis associated with hepatocellular carcinoma. *Blood* **29**:808–811, 1967.

87. Thompson RPH, Nicholson DC, Farnan T, Whistmore DN, et al: Cutaneous porphyria due to a malignant primary hepatoma. *Gastroenterology* **59**:779–783, 1970.

88. Nusbacher J: Migratory venous thrombosis and cancer. *NY State J Med* **64**:2166–2173, 1964.

89. Curth W: Vitiligo with hepatoma. *Arch Dermatol* **99**:374–375, 1969.

90. Gluckman JB, Turner MD: Systemic manifestations of tumors of the small gut and liver. *Ann NY Acad Sci* **230**:318–331, 1974.

91. Margolis S, Homcy C: Systemic manifestations of hepatoma. *Medicine* **31**:381–391, 1972.

CHAPTER 9

VASCULAR CHANGES AND HEMODYNAMICS IN HEPATOCELLULAR CARCINOMA

TOSHIRO NAKASHIMA, M.D.

INTRODUCTION

It is now well established that incidence of hepatocellular carcinoma (HCC) varies tremendously from country to country—it occurs most frequently in South Africa, and Japan is among the countries that rank much higher in incidence compared to Europe and the United States (1). The Japanese literature (2–4) abounds with excellent studies on HCC mostly dealing with necropsy materials because of an extremely short clinical course. Remarkable progress has recently been made in the diagnosis of hepatocellular carcinoma following the advent of hepatic angiography (5), scintigraphy (6), and more recently by the discovery of alpha-fetoprotein (AFP) (7–10) as a specific detective measure. With early diagnosis, complete surgical removal of this carcinoma has become a reality (11).

It has been shown by Bierman et al (12), Breedis et al (13), and others that malignant neoplasms of the liver, whether primary or secondary, receive their principle blood supply from arterial sources. The liver is an organ that is not superimposed by other vascular organs on films and hence is amenable to roentgenologic diagnosis. In 1967 Yü (14) described angiographic characteristics in 50 cases of hepatoma studied by selective celiac arteriography. Okuda et al (15) demonstrated frequent reversal of portal blood flow in HCC. More often than not, angiographic abnormalities can be detected in HCC before space-occupying lesions become apparent on the scan. Because of these developments, much interest has recently been focused on the vasculature and hemodynamic changes in livers involved by HCC.

INTRAHEPATIC VASCULAR ANATOMY

Microcirculation of the Liver

Normal vasculature of the liver has been elucidated by a number of anatomical investigations, notably the series by Elias (16—18). The afferent vascular system consists of the portal vein and hepatic artery. The portal vein continuously and regularly divides, finally to terminate in the conducting vein of several hundred micra in diameter. Each conducting vein supplies a certain area without mutual anastomoses. The conducting vein further divides into the distributing veins which course either in the middle (axial distributing vein) or along the edge (marginal distributing vein) of the portal canal. Both send off inlet venules into the lobule.

The hepatic artery tributaries run in the portal canal alongside the portal vein branches, and the zones of supply roughly correspond with those of the portal branches. Usually no vascular communications are seen between these zones of supply. Whereas there is only one portal vessel in the portal canal except for the marginal distributing veins, arterial branches keep dividing and communicating in the canal, forming a plexus around the portal branch (19).

Arteriovenous communications which shunt blood bypassing the sinusoid have not been demonstrated in normal liver of large mammalian species (20) as examined morphologically, although Wakim and Mann (21) described arteriovenous shunts as being of moderately frequent occurrence in mammalian liver.

The terminal arterial branches may be grouped into the following: (1) the plexus around the bile duct; (2) arterial capillaries running along the margin of the portal canal; and (3) the translobular artery. In order for the two vessel systems that have differing pressures to merge in the sinusoid, a sphincter mechanism must be operative at places along the arterial capillaries (17, 22), inlet venules, sinusoid, and terminal hepatic vein (central vein) (23). Within the lobule, the most common pattern of sinusoidal arrangement is of the candelabra type. Occasionally, a monopodial arrangement is seen (24). Sinusoids are divided into two types functionally: one connects the inlet venules and terminal

hepatic vein straight, and another connects the former crosswise. The blood flow in the sinusoid is very slow, suiting the purpose of expediting exchange of substances between the blood and hepatocyte.

The hepatic venous system, as the efferent route starts from the sinusoid, transports blood thereon into the terminal hepatic veins, the sublobular vein, the collecting vein, and finally into the hepatic vein that joins the inferior vena cava.

Hepatic Blood Flow

Since there is no ideal method currently available for the measurement of hepatic blood flow, the absolute value of the flow and its changes in various conditions have not accurately been assessed. The ratio of the arterial flow relative to the total hepatic flow is believed to be 20 to 40%, but the reported figures fluctuate widely because of the influences by the posture of the patient, arterial pressure (25), and other yet unknown factors.

VASCULAR CHANGES IN LIVER CIRRHOSIS ASSOCIATED WITH HEPATOMA

Miyake's B-Type Cirrhosis (26)

An interrelation between cirrhosis and HCC has long been recognized, but no agreement has as yet been reached as to the histopathological type of cirrhosis that is closely associated with this carcinoma (3, 27, 28). After a geopathological survey comparing primary liver carcinoma in Japan and in other countries, Miyaji (29) concluded that the cirrhosis, which frequently coexists with this carcinoma, is a macronodular thin stromal type (Fig. 1) and roughly corresponds to "posthepatitic" cirrhosis by Gall's nomenclature (30), or the B-type cirrhosis by Miyake's classification in Japan. "Postnecrotic" cirrhosis, as Gall used the term (30), is also associated with carcinoma but to a lesser extent.

Since the discovery by Blumberg (31) of HBAg and of Hepatitis B Surface Antigen

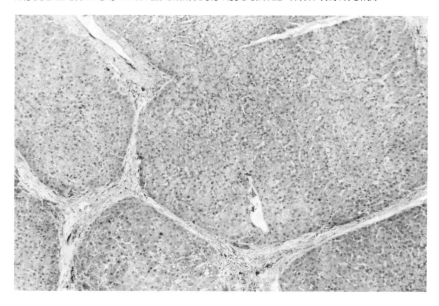

Figure 1   Histological findings of liver cirrhosis with HCC.

(HBsAg) and subsequent to the recognition of its relation to viral hepatitis B (32-34), a relationship of Hepatitis B agent has been suggested in cirrhosis and hepatoma as *a sequela* to viral hepatitis (35).

There is recent evidence that the incidence of HBsAg is high among the inhabitants in the areas where HCC is endemic (36–38) and that the patients have an extremely high positivity rate as detected by sensitive methods (38, 39). The histopathology of cirrhosis that is found in patient whose serum contains HBsAg is not necessarily uniform, however (40).

For the elucidation of vascular changes in the cirrhotic liver, various approaches and techniques have been employed, such as the injection-corrosion method, dye injection with gelatin, casting, tissue clearing, etc. Hemodynamic alterations may also be assessed indirectly by such studies. As a cause of portal hypertension, emphasis has been placed on the development of resistance along the hepatic vein tributaries resulting from compression and distortion by regenerative nodules (41). Similar changes

also occur in the intrahepatic portal branches. In addition, Miyake et al (42) observed diminution of portal venous bed, enlarged hepatic arterial bed, and shunt formation between the hepatic artery and the vein, occurring mostly within the vessels smaller than those of the eighth order. The pseudolobules of the liver of macronodular cirrhosis were seen densely surrounded and .penetrated by larger branches of the hepatic artery. It is highly probable that the transmitted pressure from the hepatic artery to the portal vein is one of the important causal factors of the portal hypertension.

Parasitic Cirrhosis

Schistosomiasis Japonica and Primary Liver Carcinoma

Hepatic fibrosis due to chronic schistosomiasis is not considered to be cirrhosis by most pathologists (43–45). It has been shown, however, that much greater numbers of ova are produced by *Schistosoma Japonicum* compared with *S. mansoni* and *S.*

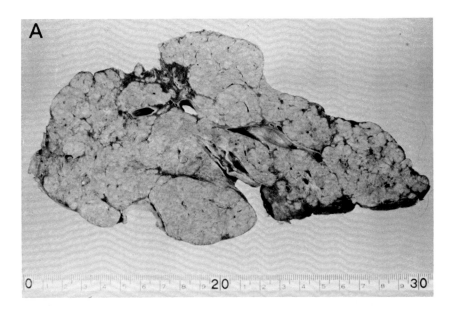

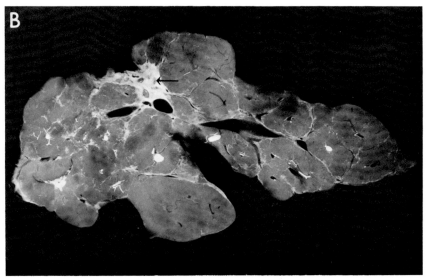

Figure 2 Gross appearance of parasitic liver cirrhosis. (a) Liver cirrhosis due to schistosomiasis japonica. Septal formation and large lobulation of the liver parenchyma. (b) Radiological findings (contrast medium injected). There is marked calcification (↑) around numerous ova in the portal tract.

haematobium (46), and that they are deposited in the terminal intrahepatic portal branches. In the acute stage of schistosomiasis japonica, the patient develops thrombopylephlebitis and peripylephlebitis. After the disease has become chronic by reinfections, cirrhosis eventually develops. Particularly, the farmers living in the endemic area are prone to repeated infections. In this type of cirrhosis, formation of regenerative nodules is minimal or absent, and the requirements for cirrhosis as defined by the Fifth Pan American Congress of Gastroenterology (47) are not met. However, we (48, 49) feel that advanced fibrosis in schistosomiasis japonica with marked gross anatomical alterations should be treated as a separate, special type of cirrhosis (Fig. 2a).

Angiological characteristics in this cirrhosis are the collapse of the terminal portal branches where numerous ova are seen deposited with disappearance of liver cells, accompanied by collagenization. The so-called pipe-stem fibrosis (50) which has been thought the typical hepatic fibrosis caused by *Schistosoma mansoni,* is rather infrequent in the liver of patients with schistosomiasis japonica, and formation of septa and gross lobulation of the liver paranchyma are much more common. Advanced calcification of numerous ova is sometimes seen as discrete densities on a plain roentgenogram (51) (Fig. 2b).

Working with a radiopaque gelatin-dye solution injected into the hepatic major vessel systems in schistosomiasis, Sakamoto in our department has made the gross and radiographic observation that the terminal portal branches are markedly collapsed permitting no further entrance of the dye beyond. Even medium-sized portal branches become flattened, tortuous, and monotonous with reduced ramifications. In large septa, arteries run serpiginous courses and then branches suddenly diminish in caliber and disappear abruptly with greater numbers of ova. In primary liver cancer the etiologic role of chronic hepatic

schistosomiasis has long been in dispute, and the weight of opinion seems against such possibility.

Gibson (46) recently reviewed the past studies made in Hong Kong, Africa (52), Taiwan and Brazil, and concluded that association between schistosomiasis and primary liver cancer is fortuitous and not significant. Steiner (43) reported that no schistosomal lesions were found within the liver cancer of African natives. Aside from the problem of whether hepatic schistosomal lesions are directly related to HCC, it is a common finding in the liver cancers of patients who also had schistosomiasis japonica, that egg nodules remain within the cancerous tissues showing an infiltrative growth (Fig. 3). Recent reports in Japan, notably of Iuchi et al (53), indicated some correlation between liver cancer and schistosomiasis japonica infestation. Our study (54) on a large series of necropsies including 227 cases of schistosomiasis and 146 cases of HCC, disclosed an incidence of this carcinoma of 10.6% in all schistosomiasis cases against 2.87% in nonschistosomiasis cases (54). Although the difference was statistically significant, in a large proportion of the cases with both schistosomiasis and liver carcinoma, Miyake's B-type cirrhosis was frequently superimposed on the changes of schistosomiasis (Fig. 4, 5a, 5b). HBsAg was positive in 27%, 10 times the positivity rate in the general population of this area, and the role of viral hepatitis cannot entirely be excluded.

Clonorchiasis and Hepatocellular Carcinoma

This disease is still endemic in South China along the coast, in Korea, and along the river of Chikugo, Kyushu, Japan, where our institute is located. Since its infection is accompanied by no acute clinical signs, less attention has been paid to this disease compared with schistosomiasis. The typical changes include adenomatous proliferation of the ductal epithelium and thickening of the duct wall as a result of chronic irrita-

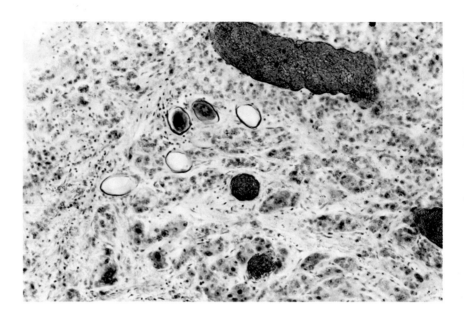

Figure 3 Hepatocellular carcinoma associated with schistosomal liver cirrhosis. Egg nodule remains within the cancerous focus. Vessel lumens contain barium used for vascular study.

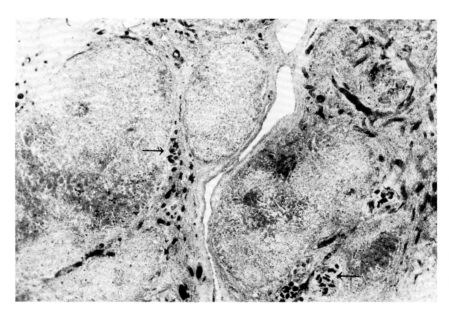

Figure 4 Hepatocellular carcinoma with Miyake's B-type cirrhosis and schistosomiasis japonica. (↑) Schistosome eggs.

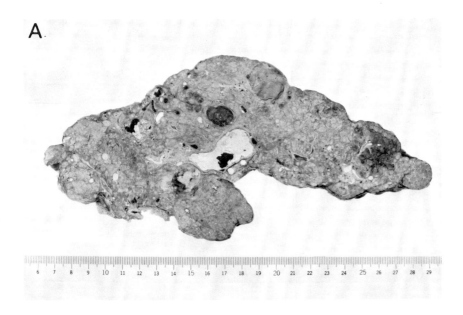

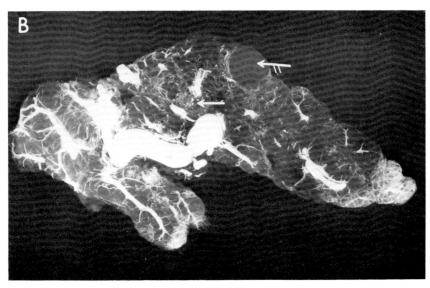

Figure 5 Gross pathological findings of parasitic liver cirrhosis with HCC. *(a)* Schistosomal liver cirrhosis with HCC. *(b)* Radiological findings of the same liver. A few carcinoma nodules are scattered in the liver. Some are hypervascular (↑) and some hypovascular (⇞).

tion by the flukes. In the liver containing more than 3000 to 4000 worms, ductal wall thickening is uniformly seen throughout the liver, affecting even the small bile ducts.

The so-called clonorchiasis cirrhosis has been refuted, and there is little evidence that cirrhosis in a strict sense develops even in the severest infection with this parasite (55). In advanced cases, however, the vascular alterations are marked throughout the liver with second parenchymal changes. Features of biliary tract disease and bacterial infection are often superimposed. The liver is diffusely affected with fibrosis, disorganization of the lobular architecture, and cell necrosis, but there is no evidence of nodular parenchymal regeneration (Fig. 6a, 6b). The vascular alterations in such livers are quite characteristic, showing marked dilatation and proliferation of arterial and portal branches that form capillary plexuses around the bile ducts. Probably because of the functional changes of these bile ducts, no involution of the capillary plexuses occurs (Figs. 7, 8).

It has long been thought that clonorchiasis is etiologically related to cholangiocarcinoma. In primary carcinomas of the liver seen in Hong Kong (56) and Canton (57), particularly in patients with cholangiocarcinoma, a high incidence of *Clonorchis sinensis* infection has been reported. Hou (56) thought that at least 15% of primary liver carcinoma in his material seen in Hong Kong were due to clonorchis infection. Such interpretation is disputable however.

VASCULAR CHANGES IN HEPATOCELLULAR CARCINOMA

Early detection of primary liver carcinoma has been and still is extremely difficult. The term "early" may have differing connotations, depending on the presence or absence of cirrhosis, and the degree of anaplasia of the tumor cell and tumor structure. In some cases, the tumor may grow rapidly soon after its evolution and form a large mass in a still early phase of the disease. In a liver with advanced cirrhosis, a small tumor may be discerned by celiac angiography; it remains unchanged or changes very little in size for a year or two. For this reason, we prefer the expression of "minimal" or "minute" hepatoma to "early" hepatoma, to denote a small carcinoma, and "advanced" hepatoma for a large tumor. It is more convenient to discuss hepatoma vasculature in these two sizes of the tumor.

Vasculature in Minimal Hepatoma

Hepatocellular carcinoma is sometimes not clearly differentiated from adenomatous proliferation or nodular hyperplasia that begins from liver cell regeneration. Since it has been thought that there is a transition from a "benign" to "malign" state, there is limitation to histological distinction of the two in the borderline changes. Furthermore, it is not infrequent to find individual cells in this carcinoma displaying characteristics of a benign tumor. One has necessarily to base the start of a study on the assumption that HCC is accompanied by abnormal proliferation of arterial capillaries.

"Minimal hepatoma" is used herein to define the neoplasm of the liver with one or a small number of tumor nodules less than 2 cm in diameter. "Minute nodule" is used for a nodule with a maximum diameter of 1.5 to 2.0 cm. This size has been chosen on the grounds that it is about the smallest detectable by hepatic angiography. And, since it is not very uncommon to find at the time of autopsy a minute nodule in a highly cirrhotic liver by chance, it seems a reasonable approach to study the vasculature of such small nodules for the elucidation of early vascular changes in HCC.

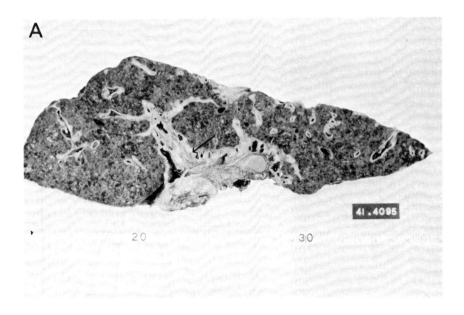

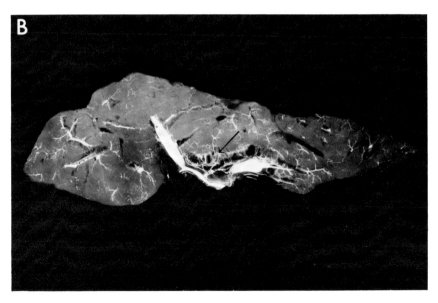

Figure 6 *(a)* Liver cirrhosis due to clonorchiasis. Ductal wall thickening (↑) is marked throughout the liver. *(b)* Radiological findings (contrast medium injected). Characteristic vascular alteration (↑) in the periductal areas.

177

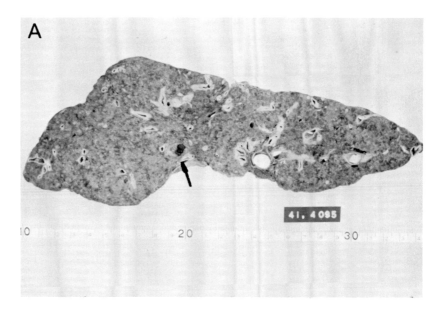

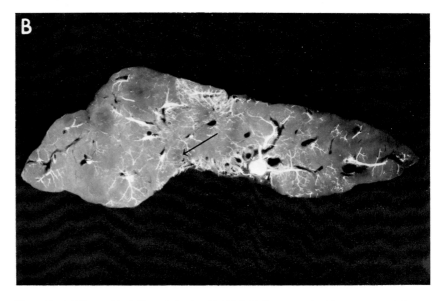

Figure 7 *(a)* Clonorchiasis liver cirrhosis with HCC. Only one minimal hepatoma nodule is seen (↑). *(b)* Radiological findings of the same. Tumor nodule is hypervascular (↑).

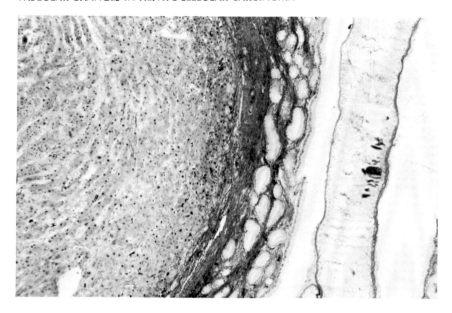

Figure 8 Minute hepatoma nodule adjacent to the bile duct showing adenomatous hyperplasia due to clonorchiasis.

Material for Study

We have seen 21 patients with cirrhosis in whom minute hepatoma nodules were found. In four of these, tumor vasculature was studied grossly as well as radiographically by injecting contrast medium mixed with dyed gelatin into the hepatic artery and portal vein at the time of autopsy. Table 1 lists these four cases. Case 4 does not fit the definition of minimal hepatoma just described, because it had about 30 minute hepatoma nodules throughout the liver. However, in order to compare the primary focus and metastatic lesions in the same liver, this case was added.

Structure and Vasculature of a Minute Hepatoma Nodule

A minute nodule may assume various structual patterns with a characteristic vasculature, depending on the manner of expansion.

EXPANSILE GROWTH OF MINUTE NODULES

Cases 1 and 3 represent this type of growth. The boundary between the tumor nodule and parenchyma is discrete. In most cases the primary tumor nodule presents this type of growth regardless of the pattern of subsequent growth. As it expands, the surrounding liver cells are atrophied by compression, reticulin fibers collapse, and collagenization and hyalinization ensue to form a pseudocapsule (Fig. 9a).

The portal vein elements are collapsed and flattened in the capsule, and never penetrate it to supply the nodule. In the surrounding area, however, many portal branches are seen crowding; they consist in the main of capillarized sinusoids (Fig. 10a–10d). Arterial branches run in and around the capsule in a fashion to surround the nodule and form a ring-shaped network (Fig. 10d). These gross vascular changes are seen in the hepatic arteriogram

Table 1   Cases with Minute Hepatoma

Case Number	Autopsy Number	Age	Sex	Pathological Diagnosis	Number of Tumor Nodules	Diameter of Largest Nodule (cm)	Degree of Anaplasia[a]
1	4095	67	M	Cirrhosis due to clonorchiasis; primary liver cell carcinoma	1	1.2	I
2	4159	53	M	Cirrhosis; primary liver cell carcinoma	1 (several coalescing)	1.5	II, III
3	4523	73	M	Cirrhosis due to clonorchiasis; primary liver cell carcinoma	1	0.7	I
4	4604	74	M	Cirrhosis, schistosomiasis Primary liver cell carcinoma	about 30	1.5	I, II

[a] According to Edmondson and Steiner.

as such indirect signs as "compression," "displacement," and "stretching." Although the tumor itself is hypervascular at the beginning, ramification is not extensive and it becomes hypovascular as it enlarges. The arterial capillaries that constitute the tumor vessels are derived from the capillary plexuses in the portal tract (Fig. 10a) and around the bile ducts. They enter the nodule through the capsule at one or two sites (case 3) (Fig. 10c) or several places (case 1) (Fig. 10a). In the former, arborization of the afferent vessel inside the nodule is more extensive.

One of the problems of interest is the venous channel to act as a vas efferens. Breedis and Young (13) suspect that the tumor stimulates only the proliferation of arteries during the formation of its stroma. Our study with transparent preparations demonstrated, however, that the tumor vessel consisted only of the arterial branches coming from the portal area and from the periductular capillary plexuses. Algire (58) theorized that tumor cells have

as a unique property a potential to stimulate continued growth of new capillary endothelium from the host. His hypothesis was supported by the experiments of Green (59). Greenblatt (60) and Ehrmann (61) observed that there was no need for the newly formed vessels to come in direct contact with the tumor cell. Folkman et al (62) succeeded in isolating a substance from tissues of human and animal tumors that induces proliferation of capillary endothelial cells, and named it "tumor angiogenesis factor" (TAF). With this factor they demonstrated an induction of mitosis in capillary endothelial cells as well as in pericytes. There is little doubt from these past studies that HCC cells elaborate a similar substance for angiogenesis, although experimental results do not always directly apply to human liver cancer.

MINIMAL HEPATOMA WITH SINUSOIDAL OF PERISINUSOIDAL GROWTH

This pattern of growth was seen in Case

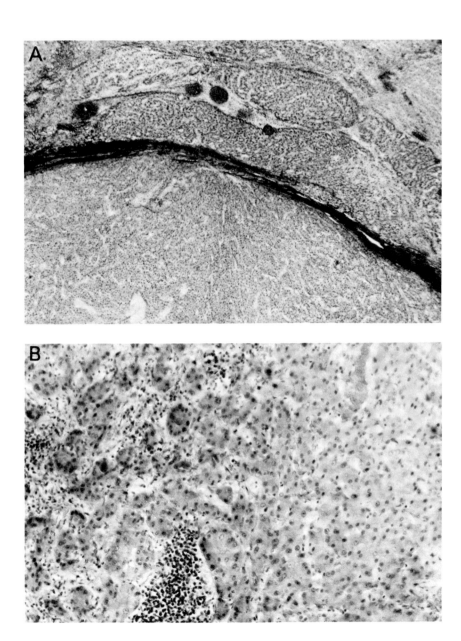

Figure 9 Structure of the minute hepatoma nodule. *(a)* Expansile growth of a minute nodule. Tumor nodule is clearly demarcated by a capsule. Tumor grows into the exterior in continuity, where it expands while forming a new capsule. *(b)* Perisinusoidal and sinusoidal growth. The growing front of the tumor tissue is ill-demarcated.

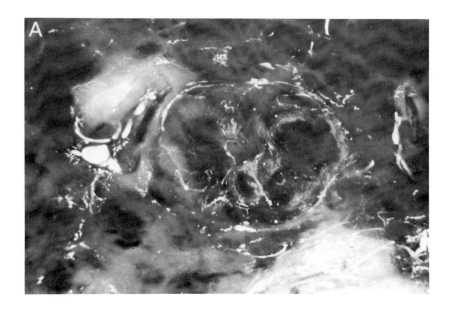

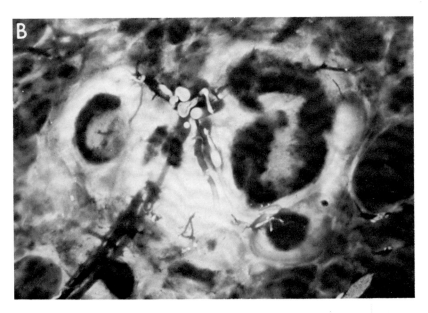

Figure 10 Vasculature in minimal hepatoma (transparent sections). *(a)* Case 1. Tumor vessels are derived from the capillary plexuses in the portal tract and around the bile ducts. *(b)* Case 2. Transformation of tumor nodule into a scar. Such an area is firm and has few tumor vessels.

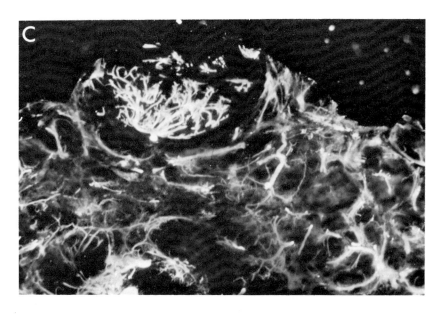

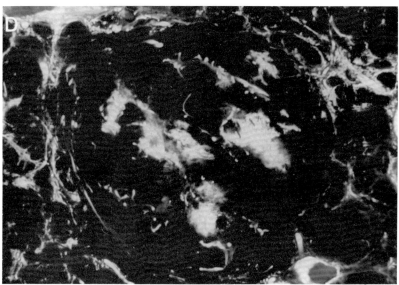

Figure 10 (cont.) *(c)* Case 3. Arborization of the afferent vessels in the nodule is more extensive. *(d)* Case 4. The tumor nodule is clearly demarcated by a capsule. Arterial branches run in and around the capsule in a fashion to surround the nodule, and constitute the tumor vessels.

4 and is typically seen in intrahepatic metastases. The tumor vessel in the interior of the nodule consists of only arterial capillaries (arterial tumor vessels), but the growing front of the tumor tissue is ill-demarcated and contains sinusoid and portal branches (Fig. 9b). When studied with transparent preparations, it is immediately apparent that these portal branches run around and adhere to the arterial tumor vessels, acting as efferent vasa. Portal vein branches acting as the efferent vessel for a hepatoma were described as early as 1937 by Wright (63).

Some investigators (64) have emphasized this finding of crowded portal branches, with inference that portal blood is required at the periphery of a rapidly growing tumor. However, we assume that these portal elements are a result of the replacement of hepatocytes by tumor cells after they have passed through the Disse's space or the sinusoid, and have inflicted damage on liver parenchyma. It explains the fact that the boundary between the tumor and parenchyma is not discrete, as well as the finding of liver cells remaining in the tumor at places. Yoshida (65) pointed out earlier, working with his experimental hepatoma system, that the vessels in the tumor do not necessarily represent newly formed ones; as the tumor infiltrates along a vessel, it may resemble at certain stage of the growth, one that is being neovascularized, or it looks as if a vessel was entering the tumor. He warned of the difficulty in the histological differentiation between tumor infiltration along a vessel and neovascularization. We have concluded in our study that arterial branches act as the afferent vessels and the capillarized sinusoids and portal branches act as the efferent channels.

MINIMAL HEPATOMA EXPANDING VIA VEINS

Hepatocellular carcinoma has a tendency to invade into portal branches (Fig. 11a), and this is considered one of the distinct characteristics of this carcinoma. It may oc-cur in an early stage of the disease. In the liver of case 2, there was marked subendothelial fibrosis of the tumor vessels and formation of a tumor thrombus in an adjacent portal branch. These changes are usually followed by local circulatory disturbances and, as a result, necrosis of liver parenchyma as well as tumor tissue itself ensues (Fig. 11b). The tumor will then shrink and sometimes disappear after resolution of the necrotic tissue. The supporting reticulin fibers collapse and become collagenized and hyalinized, turning a tumor nodule into a scar in some instances. Such an area is firm, looks gray, has few tumor vessels (Fig. 10b), and the disease progresses slowly in this region.

Consideration on the Histogenesis of HCC from the Viewpoint of Vascular Alterations

It has long been controversial as to whether HCC develops as a unicentric tumor or multicentrically. The multicentric genesis theory has been supported by the experimental observations in rats in which liver neoplasm develops multicentrically (66, 67). No conclusive evidence is available yet in man to decide on the histological mode of carcinogenesis. It has been the experience of the pathologist (68) that hepatocellular carcinoma arising in a cirrhotic liver is often multiple, and that it is usually solitary in a noncirrhotic liver. Such observations are not sufficient in determining the histogenesis in the early phase of the disease, nor are the opinions among the investigators in agreement. The author of this chapter favors the unicentric origin of HCC because of the following reasons. Considering that hepatocellular carcinoma is closely associated with cirrhosis and that the results of our study on vascular changes in cirrhosis and hepatoma, we had felt that careful examination of cirrhotic livers would reveal a minute early carcinoma which would have evaded detection at autopsy. Also, we had anticipated that roentgenologic examination of excised liv-

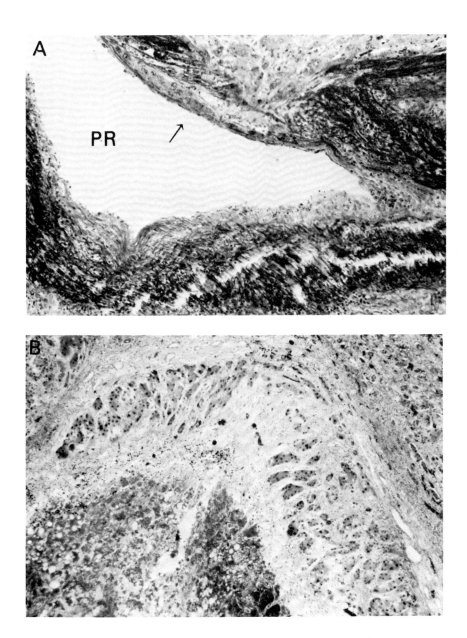

Figure 11 *(a)* Expanding via a vein. Carcinoma cells are invading the portal vein (↑). PV: portal vein. *(b)* Marked proliferation of the subepithelial fibrous tissue of the tumor vessels followed by necrosis of the tumor itself.

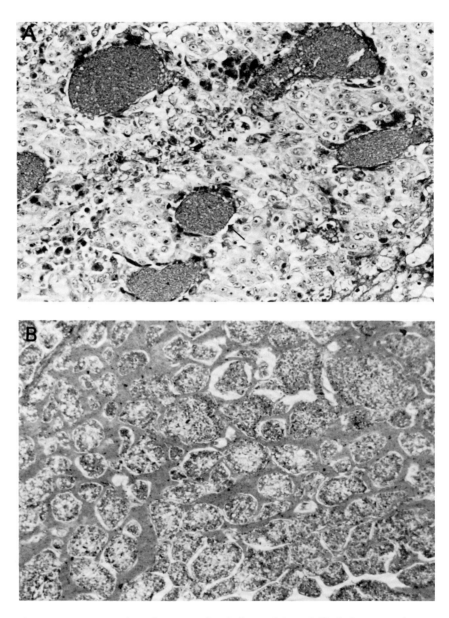

Figure 12 Tumor vessels. *(a)* Contrast medium in the arterial vessels (↑). *(b)* Contrast medium in blood spaces (↑).

ers should reveal minute nodules, even smaller than 1 cm in diameter. Employing the technique to inject contrast medium mixed with dye and gelatin from the hepatic artery and portal vein, and to examine a fixed and sliced liver, we found minute hepatocellular carcinoma in 4 cases of cirrhosis. In three of the four cases, the tumor was unicentric, and in one there were about 30 minute nodules. Although we could not decide whether the carcinoma developed multicentrically or unicentrically with early intrahepatic metastases in the latter, it cannot be denied that even a cirrhotic liver would develop hepatocellular carcinoma unicentrically. Berman expressed an opinion of unicentric origin in his monograph (1951). We observed in these minute nodules that the primary lesion would proliferate in most cases by the expansile growth pattern, making a discrete boundary with the parenchyma. It goes without saying that further investigation is required with a greater number of minute hepatoma before any conclusion is drawn.

Vasculature in Advanced Hepatocellular Carcinoma

According to Yü (1963), the major angiographic alterations in hepatoma are dilatation of the hepatic artery, displacement or stretching of the intrahepatic arteries, increased vascularity, tumor vessels, tumor stain or pooling of contrast medium, arteriovenous shunts within the tumor, and the findings related to coexisting cirrhosis such as coiling or tortuosity of the intrahepatic arteries. A classification of liver carcinoma based on vascular changes has been proposed by Honjo and his school in Japan (69). In this chapter, the blood vessels that form in accompaniment with tumor growth are discussed first.

Tumor Vessels

In hepatic arteriography, an indispensable procedure for the diagnosis of primary liver carcinoma, a large amount of contrast medium is usually distributed in the tumor in the arterial phase, demarcating it from the parenchyma. The contrast medium remains as a density through the venous phase. This latter phenomenon generally called "tumor stain" or "pooling of contrast medium" is to be distinguished from increased vascularity and tumor vessels. The angiographic abnormalities in the arterial phase are directly related to newly formed arterial tumor vessels, and the abnormalities in the venous phase to destroyed arterial tumor vessels, blood spaces and necrotic spaces of the tumor tissue.

ARTERIAL TUMOR VESSELS

Arterial tumor vessels are usually surrounded by tumor cells, are thin walled, and lack the muscular layer (Fig. 12a). Unlike normal arteries or arterioles that constrict by norepinephrine, a classical vasoconstrictor, tumor arteries lack normal neuromuscular and humoral response. They are different from normal arterial branches in that they do not divide in an orderly fashion with progressive and gradual diminution of caliber, and run tortuous courses with irregular diameters and localized saccular dilatations. Beside these angiographic differences, they also differ histologically from normal arteries. When studied by serial sectioning, they are seen communicating with arterial branches having a distinct muscle layer and lying outside the tumor nodule. This relation is more clearly seen in transparent preparations. Electronmicroscopically, basement membranes or a basement membranelike osmophilic layer is seen in the outer surface of the endothelial cells, a finding not seen in the normal sinusoid and suggestive of a closed circulation system. In some places, the endothelial cells are found to be arranged in multiple layers. Some of these vessels end in a necrotic tissue, but seem to contribute little to the angiographic finding of pooling or tumor stain.

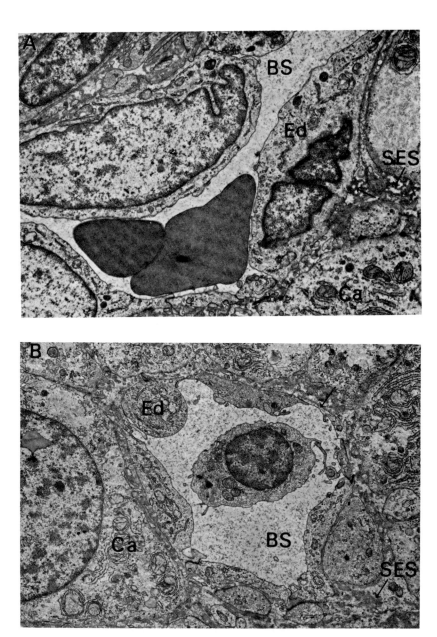

Figure 13 Transmission and scanning electron microscopic findings of tumor vessels. (a and b) Transmission electron micrograph. Endothelial cells are rather oval in shape and have a large nucleus. They contain abundant cytoplasmic organelles such as mitochondria and endoplasmic reticulums, but the paucity of pores is characteristic. The nuclear region of the cell body protrudes markedly into the lumen. They are separated from the cancerous liver cell layers by a considerable, wide subendothelial spaces. Dense filamentous materials, which are similar to the vascular basement membrane, exist just below the endothelial cells or in the subendothelial space. Ed: endothelial cell; BS: blood space; (↑): basement membranelike substance; SES: subepithlial space; Ca: carcinoma cell.

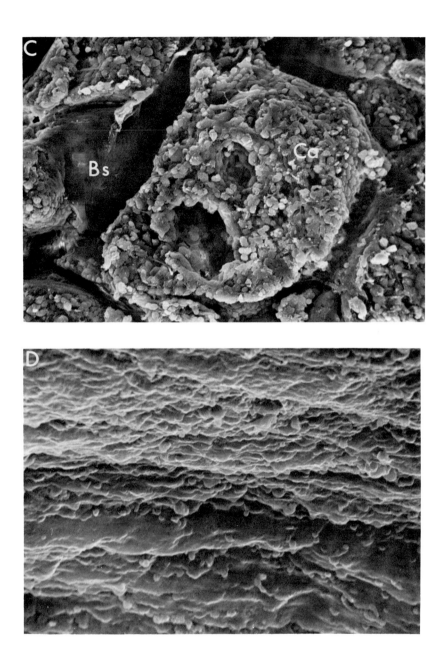

Figure 13 (c and d) scanning electron micrograph. The blood spaces vary in caliber and run in a very irregular fashion (c). Numerous microvilli of the endothelial surface of the blood space are seen, but the existence of pores is not evident (d).

BLOOD SPACES

One form of the tumor vessel is the so-called blood spaces that have formed during the proliferation of tumor cells mimicking the sinusoid in the normal liver (Fig. 12b). That it is lined by the endothelium as in the normal sinusoid and the Disse's spaces is readily seen by transmission and scanning electronmicroscopy (Fig. 13). It belongs to the "open circulation system." Recently Motta et al (70) described scanning electronmicroscopic findings of the wall of rat liver sinusoid under the title "Structure of Rat Liver Sinusoid and Associated Tissue Spaces as Revealed by Scanning Electronmicroscopy." Sakamoto (71) in our department reported scanning and transmission electronmicroscopic findings of the fenestrated endothelial lining of normal human liver sinusoid and blood spaces of hepatoma. By comparison of sections and angiograms, it has been found that tumor stain or pooling of contrast medium is more closely related to dilated and crowded blood spaces and necrotic spaces of the tumor tissue than to damaged arterial tumor vessels.

NECROTIC FOCI

Necrotic foci are frequently seen in advanced liver cell carcinoma, particularly in cases in which closed arterial tumor vessels predominate in vasculature (Fig. 14). In such nodules, blood spaces with an open circulation are scanty and the lumen is narrow probably because of the lack of communications with arterial tumor vessels and dilatation of the subepithelial spaces; they are not entered by the dye injected from the artery. More dye is found in the necrotic foci, the dye being seen sometimes in direct contact with tumor cells or tumor cells floating in it.

Gross Anatomical Classification of Primary Hepatocellular Carcinoma and Its Relationship to Tumor Vessels

Yü analyzed his angiographic findings in relation to the gross anatomical types of Eggel's classification (1901). However, we feel that the progress made in this field after Eggel has been such that his simple classification needs revision, with some consideration of clinical features if possible. Early diagnosis and early resection of hepatocellular carcinoma is no longer a dream, and resectability has to be assessed from more detailed anatomical or angiographic characteristics. Recently, Nakashima and Okuda (72) proposed a new classification that is based on the gross anatomical feature of the tumor in the cut surface, the appearance of the tumor-parenchyma boundary, and the mode of expansion, with angiographic characteristics in mind. Their classification and its relation to the previous classification (Eggel) is shown in Table 10 of Chapter 8, page 122).

Although this classification may seem too detailed and impractical, one of the significances is the separation of one distinct form from the rest. This particular type which we call "the encapsulated form" has clinically a distinct feature of slow progress and long survival. This form is defined as a liver containing one or several large tumor nodules that are clearly demonstrated from nontumorous tissue with a capsule. Angiographically, large vessels are displaced in a curvilinear fashion by the encapsulated nodule which has its own neovasculature. Histologically, it also has some characteristics. The following case is a typical example.

CASE 5. Autopsy No. 4402. 59-year-old male. Pathological diagnosis: Primary liver carcinoma, Miyake's B-type cirrhosis, and schistosomiasis. The cause of death was intraabdominal hemorrhage following rupture of a tumor nodule on the surface. The diagnosis of probable encapsulated form hepatoma had been made by hepatic angiography (Fig. 15a). Curvilinear displacement of arteries and a round stain in the venous phase with a thin radiolucent rim were the findings. At the time of autopsy, contrast medium with dye and gelatin was injected from the hepatic artery and the portal vein for roentgenologic and gross observations (Fig. 15b). It is apparent from Fig.

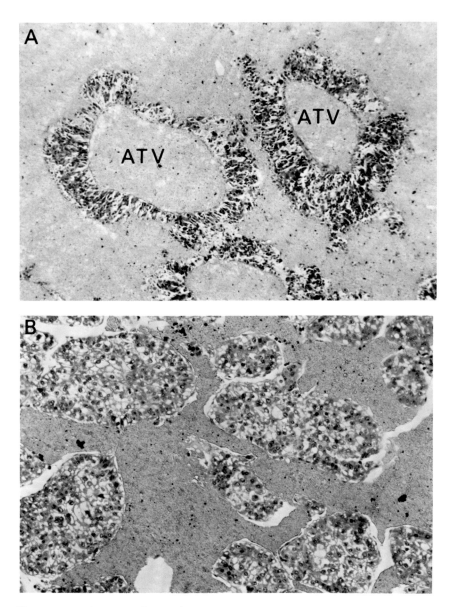

Figure 14 *(a)* Contrast medium in the arterial tumor vessels (ATV) and necrotic areas. *(b)* Contrast medium in the blood spaces and necrotic areas.

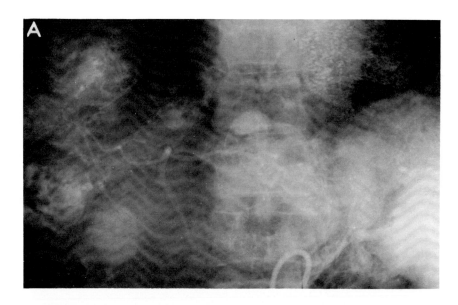

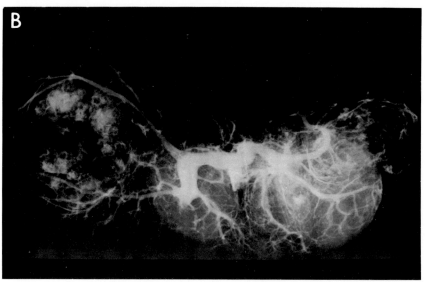

Figure 15 Gross anatomical classification of hepatocellular carcinoma. Encapsulated form: Case 5, No. 4402, 59-year-old male. *(a)* Sinusoidal phase of hepatic arteriography. *(b)* Radiological findings: at autopsy contrasted medium was injected from the hepatic artery and the portal vein.

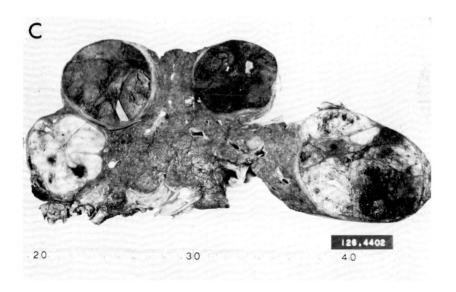

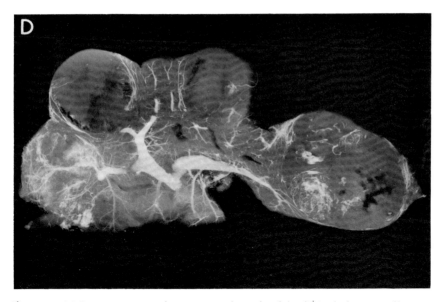

Figure 15 *(c)* Gross appearance: there are several round nodules distinctly demarcated by a capsule. *(d)* Radiological findings: soft X-ray film.

193

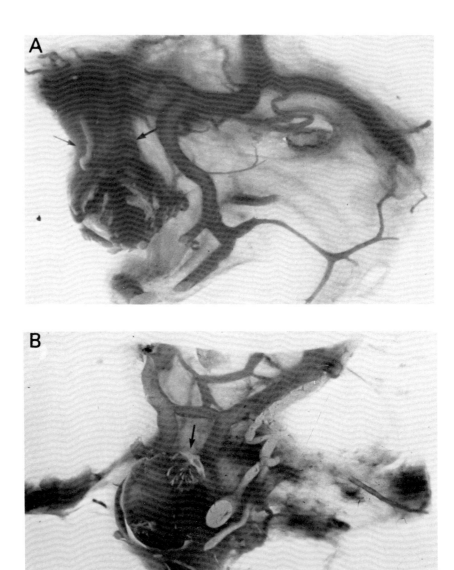

Figure 16   Tumor thrombus in the portal vein. *(a)* There are marked dilation and neovascularization taking place in the arterial capillaries surrounding the portal branch (↑). *(b)* Tumor vessels of the thrombus. Arterial tumor vessels are derived from the periportal artery (↑) (transparent preparation).

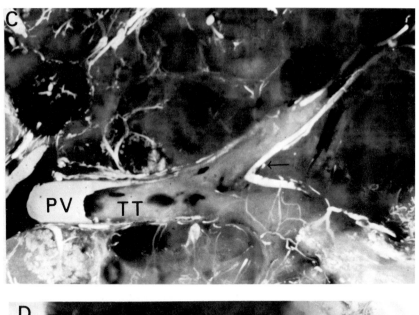

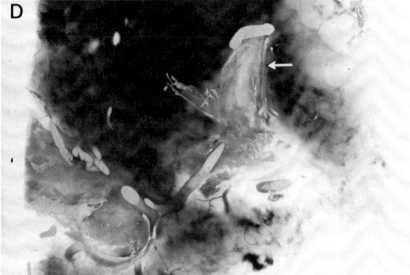

Figure 16 (c and d) Serial sections of the tumor thrombus. (↑): periportal artery.

15 that there are several round nodules distinctly demarcated with a capsule (Fig. 15c) and presenting typical radiographic changes. Soft X-ray films of the thin sections across the longest axis of the liver disclosed hypovascular tumor nodules (Fig. 15d). They were dark green, or the so-called green hepatoma. The capsule was the result of slow expansile growth. When seen in a transparent preparation, the portal branches were flattened by the capsule and no branch entered the tumor past it. The arteries which were also compressed run in the capsule in a ringlike course and send out thin branches into the nodule. No large efferent vessel was discernible, and the interior was necrotic, where no apparent tumor vessels were seen on the angiogram.

Growth of Tumor and Tumor Vessels

The tumor vessels in each of the four major patterns (68) of growth of liver cell carcinoma are now described separately.

Expansible Growth and Tumor Vessels

The tumor nodule is clearly bounded by a capsule composed of nontumorous tissues. Not only is this expansile mode the major growth pattern of minute hepatoma that arises in cirrhotic livers, but it is the growth pattern of the very primary lesion as well as of slow growing nodules in advanced carcinomas. Tumor grows into the exterior in continuity through the efferent vessels or by infiltrative invasion where it expands while forming a new capsule. Thus, old capsules remain embedded in a composite large tumor nodule to form septa and, grossly, the nodule seems as if it were produced by coalescence of several separate nodules. When studied by soft X-ray in slices made across the entire liver length, they are often seen to contain entirely different vasculatures. It is probably due to the fact that a nodule formed outside the major tumor develops its own tumor vessel system. The vessels in the septa are part of the tumor vessels and, unlike ordinary tumor vessels, sometimes contain a muscle layer.

Necrosis occurs commonly and extensively, presumably because of the presence of the thick capsule. Areas of necrosis are seen by angiography as poolings of contrast medium, but the tumor itself is rather hypovascular in general. Usually, only the capsule, the septa, and their adjacent areas are hypervascular.

Perisinusoidal and Sinusoidal Growths and Tumor Vessels

This pattern is seen at the growing front of intrahepatic metastases and a rapidly proliferating tumor nodule, the detail of which has already been given.

Intravenous Growths and Tumor Vessels

Intravenous growth is a characteristic tendency of the hepatocellular carcinoma. The tumor thrombi are more predominant in the portal vein, which is the draining vessel of the carcinoma, than the hepatic vein.

TUMOR THROMBUS IN THE PORTAL VEIN

One of the distinct features of primary hepatocellular carcinoma is its tendency to grow in the portal branches (68, 73). The carcinoma destroys the wall of a portal branch and invades into the lumen, but this phenomen may be explained by the following two anatomical events: (a) the arterial branches acting as afferent vasa of the tumor run in close approximation of or surround the portal branch and ramify the nutritional twigs to the wall of the portal vein and communicate with portal branches through the periductal capillary plexuses; and (b) the sphincter function normally operating in the arterial capillaries and other vessels are no more present in tumor vessels. Furthermore, there are increasing circulatory disturbances in the hepatic vein as a result of liver cirrhosis and associated HCC. The latter changes will disrupt the normal relationship between the arterial and portal pressures, causing a reversal of blood flow in the portal branches which now act as efferent vasa.

In case 4 with minute hepatoma nodules (Table 1), a tumor thrombus was found already in a portal branch draining a minute 1.5 cm tumor nodule. It is thus evident that formation of a tumor thrombus in a portal branch can be an early event. The tumor tissue entering the intrahepatic portal branches grows intraluminally in an expansile fashion as well as in continuous extension antegrade and retrograde while being supplied arterial blood from the arterial capillaries surrounding the portal branches and periductal capillary plexus. Furthermore, when it necrotizes, the necrotic fragments are sloughed off, lacking endothelial investment on the surface, and act as metastasizing seeds. In an old tumor thrombus, however, the endothelial cells cover its surface.

ARTERIAL CAPILLARIES AROUND THE PORTAL VEIN BRANCH CONTAINING A TUMOR THROMBUS

Marked dilatation and neovascularization takes place in the arterial capillaries surrounding the portal branch, on formation of a tumor thrombus; the portal branch is sheathed by numerous arterial branches (Fig. 16a), and distribution of arteries varies from place to place in the same liver, depending on the presence of thrombi. The documented angiographic characteristics, such as dilatation of the hepatic artery, may be a reflection of increased functional demand (14), but the thrombus-induced vascular changes are rather a local phenomenon.

VASCULATURE OF THE TUMOR THROMBUS IN THE PORTAL BRANCH

That a tumor thrombus in the portal vein is supplied by arteries like a tumor nodule in the parenchyma has been demonstrated by Hale (73) who studied with the injection-corrosion technique. Our study (74) with transparent preparations (Fig. 16b) and serial sections (Fig. 16c and d) have shown that the arterial blood supplying the thrombus is derived from the arterial capillaries surrounding the portal branch and periductal capillary plexuses. These are the two main arteriovenous shunts between hepatic arteries and portal

veins, and they lead to portal hypertention in liver cirrhosis associated with hepatocellular carcinoma. In the former type of anastomosis, arterial capillaries invade the tumor thrombus accompanied by scanty fibrous tissue, and gradually form septa by proliferation of fibrous tissue in the surrounding areas (Fig 17a and b). The latter sets up one type of arteriovenous shunt when disturbances of intrahepatic portal circulation due to extensive tumor thrombi become stronger (Fig. 17b and c).

Entrance of arterial blood into the portal vein is frequently observed angiographically in patients with extensive tumor thrombosis. Okuda and 1 (15) first described in detail the phenomenon of reversal of portal flow as visualized by contrast medium injected into the celiac artery in patients with hepatocellular carcinoma, in whom extensive tumor thrombi were found at autopsy.

ARTERIOVENOUS COMMUNICATIONS AT THE SITE OF HEPATIC VEIN THROMBUS

Tumor thrombosis in the hepatic vein is infrequent compared with portal thrombosis (73). Hepatic vein thrombosis is frequently accompanied by extensive portal thrombosis, and the former may be anticipated in patients in whom portal thrombosis has been clinically demonstrated. The hepatic vein thrombus is also supplied by arteries like portal vein thrombi, and there are possibilities of arteriovenous communications. We have seen a case with extensive portal thrombosis, in which an hepatic vein tumor thrombus was found to be extending into the inferior vena cava, right atrium, right ventricle, and further into the pulmonary arteries.

Distant Metastases and Tumor Vessels

Extrahepatic metastases histologically resemble the primary lesion, and the lung is the most frequent site of metastases. Contradicting the nature of HCC to be supplied by arterial blood, an injected dye enters lung metastases more often from

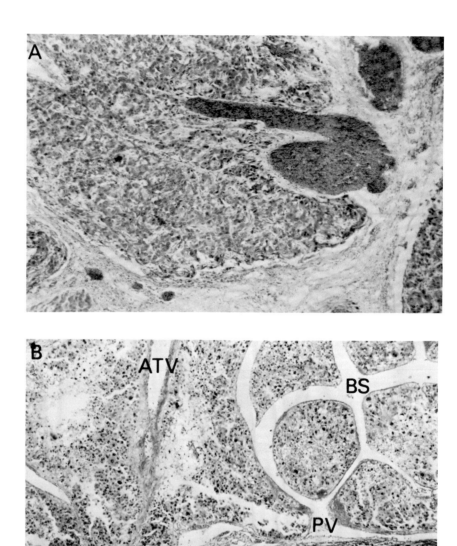

Figure 17 Tumor thrombus in the portal vein and esophageal varices. *(a)* Contrast medium is seen in the arterial tumor vessels of the tumor thrombus. *(b)* Arterial tumor vessel (ATV) is accompanied by fibrous tissues. Blood spaces (BS) of the tumor thrombus are connected with the portal vein lumen. (Okuda, K, et al: *Radiology* **117**: 303, 1975.)

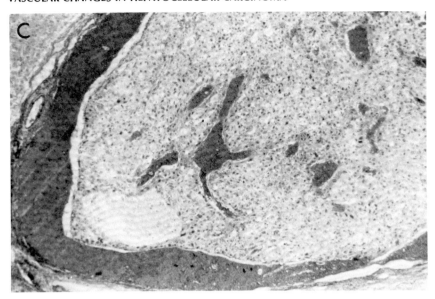

Figure 17 (c) The contrast medium injected from the hepatic artery is seen in the portal vein and tumor vessels of the tumor thrombus in the portal vein.

the pulmonary artery than from the bronchial. Although the former contains venous blood, it appears that metastatic lesions in the lung periphery can be nourished by the pulmonary vein.

EFFECTS OF HEPATOCELLULAR CARCINOMA ON PORTAL HYPERTENSION

Portal hypertension is caused by disturbances in portal blood flow, either intrahepatic or extrahepatic, subsequent to a block to the intrahepatic portal flow, an outflow block in the liver, and an increase in splachnic blood flow or hepatic arterial flow. Of the various diseases that give rise to portal hypertension, hepatic cirrhosis is the commonest and represents a typical example. Among the extrahepatic diseases, thrombosis of the portal trunk, superior mesentric vein, or the splenic vein is the most important; other causes include congenital stenosis of the portal vein and idiopathic portal hypertension. As to frequency, these extrahepatic diseases are less common compared with hepatic cirrhosis,

which is of prime importance as a cause of portal hypertension.

Inasmuch as HCC is a frequent complication of cirrhosis, its influence on the development and severity of portal hypertension is considerable. The most serious clinical complication of portal hypertension is varices in the esophagus and/or the cardia, and their rupture as a consequence. Splenomegaly is another manifestation (47) of portal hypertension accompanied by hematological abnormalities or the so-called hypersplenism of varying degrees.

Esophageal and Gastric Varices

Miyake et al emphasized as a cause of portal hypertension the arterioportal anastomoses that develop intrahepatically in cirrhosis, reasoning that hepatic arterial pressure is transmitted to the portal vein because of the pressure gradient. It is to be noted in this connection that about 75% of hepatocellular carcinomas are accompanied by hepatic cirrhosis and that tumor thrombi readily form in the portal branches. In advanced carcinoma, the tu-

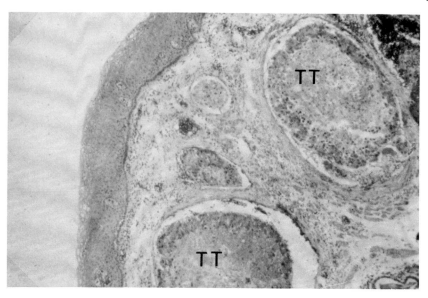

Figure 18   Tumor thrombi (TT) in esophagal varices.

mor thrombi further extend retrograde in the portal vein system causing severe circulatory disturbances. Arterial neovascularization in the tumor thrombus and arterioportal shunt through the periductal capillary plexus of the biliary tree, and hence increase in arterial inflow into the portal vein and give an impetus to the mounting portal pressure.

Incidence of Gastroesophageal Varices

Our survey (75, 76) of the *Annual of Pathological Autopsies in Japan* for a five-year period from 1966 to 1970, with respect to the incidences of gastroesophageal varices in cirrhosis, HCC associated with cirrhosis and HCC not associated with cirrhosis, disclosed that varices were most common in HCC with cirrhosis, being seen in 720 out of 1903 cases (37.8%); they were seen in 1253 of 3634 cases of cirrhosis (34.5%) and were least common in HCC without cirrhosis, being found in 75 of 918 (8.2%). A similar study made of the necropsies carried out in our department of pathology, revealed higher incidences of varices probably because of the more careful examina-

tions including sectioning of the materials for this particular purpose—varices are often overlooked during an autopsy because of their collapse. In our materials, varices were seen in 33 out of 46 patients who died of HCC with cirrhosis (71.5%), and in 15 of 27 (55.6%) dying of cirrhosis alone.

Tumor Thrombi in Gastroesophageal Varices

Formation of tumor thrombi in the gastroesophageal varices were rather infrequent (Fig. 18) being seen in 3 out of 46 cases studied, but the recognition would probably increase if varices were examined more carefully. This phenomen is a reflection of retrograde portal flow that frequently occurs in HCC associated with cirrhosis (15). Against our expectation (76), entrance of arterial tumor vessels from the variceal wall, as would occur in intrahepatic portal branches, was not demonstrated in tumor thrombi in the varices. It may be that formation of tumor thrombi in varices is a terminal event that will allow little time for neovascularization of the thrombus.

Hepatocellular Carcinoma and Splenomegaly

Our survey of the *Annual of Pathological Autopsies in Japan* for a recent five-year period (1966 to 1970) disclosed that splenomegaly was seen in 1395 out of 3634 cases of cirrhosis (43.9%), in 828 of 1903 cases of HCC with cirrhosis (43.5%), and 160 of 918 cases of HCC not associated with cirrhosis (17.4%). Thus, splenomegaly is more common in association with cirrhosis and in cases of HCC with cirrhosis compared to HCC alone. In most of our cases, the splenic artery was dilated and tortuous with a hardened wall.

To summarize the discussion on the influences of HCC on portal circulation, it may be said that hepatocellular carcinoma associated with cirrhosis often produces marked circulatory disturbances of the portal blood flow and arteriovenous anastomoses which lead to portal hypertension, splenomegaly, and formation of gastroesophageal varices.

REFERENCES

1. Berman C: *Primary Carcinoma of the Liver.* Lewis Co., London, 1951.

2. Kika G: Ueber das primäre Lebercarcinoma. *Cann Monogr.* **2**:906–1077; *Gann Monogr.* **3**:1–420, 1909 (in Japanese).

3. Yamagiwa K: Zur Kenntniss des primären parenchymatosen Lebercarcinoma (Hepatomas). *Virchows Arch* **206**:437–467, 1911.

4. Yamane S: Statistical and histological studies on 57 cases of primary hepatocellular carcinoma at Kyushu University School of Medicine (in Japanese). *Trans Soc Path Jap* **8**:544–549, 1919.

5. Seldinger SI: Catheter replacement of the needle in percutaneous arteriography: A new technique. *Acta Radiol* **39**:368–376, 1953.

6. Stirrett LA, Yuhl ET, Cassen B: Clinical applications of hepatic radioactivity surveys. *Am J Gastroenterol* **21**:310–317, 1954.

7. Bergstrand CG, Czar B: Demonstration of a new protein fraction in serum from the human fetus. *Scand J Clin Lab Invest* **8**:174, 1956.

8. Abelev GI: Production of embryonal serum α-globulin by hepatomas: Review of experimental and clinical data. *Cancer Res* **28**:1344–1350, 1968.

9. Tatarinov J: Detection of embryospecific α-globulin in the blood sera of patient with primary liver tumor. *Vop Med Khim* **10**:90–91, 1964 (Chem. Abstr.)

10. Watabe H, Hirai H: α f-globulin in rat (in Japanese). *Physio Chem Biol* **14**:218–221, 1969.

11. Lin T-Y: The results of hepatic lobectomy for primary carcinoma of the liver. *Surg Gynecol Obstet* **123**:289–294, 1966.

12. Bierman HR, Byron RL, Kelley KH, et al: Studies on the blood supply of tumors in man. III. Vascular patterns of the liver by hepatic arteriography in vivo. *J Natl Cancer Inst* **12**:107–131, 1951.

13. Breedis C, Young G: The blood supply of neoplasms in the liver. *Am J Path* **30**:969–985, 1954.

14. Yü C: Primary carcinoma of the liver (Hepatoma). Its diagnosis by selective celiac arteriography. *Am J Roentgenol* **99**:142–149, 1967.

15. Okuda K, Moriyama M, Yasumoto M, et al: Roentgenologic demonstration of spontaneous reversal of portal blood flow in cirrhosis and primary carcinoma of the liver. *Am J Roentgenol* **119**:419–428, 1973.

16. Elias H: A re-examination of the structure of the mammalian liver. I. Parenchymal architecture. *Am J Anat* **84**:311–333, 1949.

17. Elias H: A re-examination of the structure of the mammalian liver. II. The hepatic lobule and its relation to the vascular and biliary systems. *Am J Anat* **85**:379–456, 1949.

18. Elias H, Petty D: Terminal distribution of the hepatic artery. *Anat Rec* **116**:9–17, 1953.

19. Elias H: Observation on the general and regional anatomy of the human liver. *Anat Red* **117**:377–394, 1953.

20. Andrews WHH, Maegraith BG, Wenyon CEM: Studies on the liver circulation. II. The microanatomy of the hepatic circulation. *Ann Trop Med Parasit* **43**:229–237, 1949.

21. Wakim KG, Mann FC: The intrahepatic circulation of blood. *Anat Rec* **82**:233–253, 1942.

22. Märck W: Zur Kenntnis der sog. Arterienwülste beim Menschen und bei einigen Säugern. *Anat Nachr* **1**:305–318, 1951.

23. (a) Popper H: Über Drosselvorrichtungen an Lebervenen. *Klin Wschr* **10**:1693–1694, 1931.

    (b) Popper H: Über Drosselvorrichtungen an Lebervenen. *Klin Wschr* **10**:2129–2131, 1931.

24. Elias H, Sherrick JC: *Morphology of the Liver.* Academic Press, New York, 1969.

25. Grayson J, Mendel D: The role of the spleen and the hepatic artery in the regulation of liver blood flow. *J Physiol* **136**:60–79, 1957.

26. Miyake M: Pathology of the liver—liver cirrhosis. Tr Soc Path Jap **49**:589–632, 1960 (in Japanese).

27. Eggel H: Ueber das primäre Carcinoma der Leber. *Beitr Pathol Anat* **30**:506–604, 1901.

28. Nagayo M: Liver cirrhosis. II. Pathoanatomical studies (in Japanese). *Tr Soc Path* Jap **4**:31–72, 1914.

29. Miyaji T: Association of hepatocellular carcinoma with cirrhosis among autopsy cases in Japan (1958–1967). In *Alpha-fetoprotein and Hepatoma.* Hirai H, Miyaji T (Eds). University of Tokyo Press, Tokyo, 1973, pp 179–182.

30. Gall EA: Posthepatitic, postnecrotic, and nutritional cirrhosis: A pathologic analysis. *Am J Pathol* **36**:241–271, 1960.

31. Blumberg BS, Alter HJ, Visnich S: A "new" antigen in leukemia sera. *JAMA* **191**:541–546, 1965.

32. Blumberg BS, Gerstley BJS, Hungerford DA, et al: A serum antigen (Australia antigen) in Down's syndrome, leukemia, and hepatitis. *Ann Intern Med* **66**:924–931, 1967.

33. Prince AM: An antigen detected in the blood during the incubation period of serum hepatitis. *Proce Natl Acad Sci* **60**:814–821, 1968.

34. Okochi K, Murakami S: Observations on Australia antigen in Japanese. *Vox Sang* **15**:374–385, 1968.

35. Sherlock S, Fox RA, Niazi SP, et al: Chronic liver disease and primary liver-cell cancer with hepatitis-associated (Australia) antigen in serum. *Lancet* **i**:1243–1247, 1970.

36. Vogel CL, Anthony PP, Mody N, et al: Hepatitis-associated antigen in Ugandan patients with hepatocellular carcinoma. *Lancet* **ii**:621–624, 1970.

37. Nishioka K, Hirayama T, Sekine T, et al: Relationship between hepatocellular carcinoma and Australia antigen (in Japanese). *Jap J Clin* **30**:1154–1158, 1972.

38. Tong MJ, Sun S-C, Schaeffer BT, et al: Hepatitis associated antigen and hepatocellular carcinoma in Taiwan. *Ann Intern Med* **75**:687–691, 1971.

39. Kubo Y, Sawa Y, Hashimoto H, et al: Hepatitis B antigen and alphafetoprotein in primary liver cell carcinoma. *Hepatitis Scientific Memoranda H-598,* November 1973.

40. Buchner F: Die Pathologie der unkomplizierten reversible Virushepatitis. *Schweiz. Zschr. allg. path. Bakt* **16**:322–334, 1953.

41. Kelty RH, Baggenstoss AH, Butt HR: The relation of the regenerated liver nodule to the vascular bed in cirrhosis. *Gastroenterology* **15**:285–295, 1950.

42. Miyake M, Saito M, Okudaira M: Studies on intrahepatic vascular alterations in cirrhosis of the liver. *Jap Circ J* **28**:33–39, 1964.

43. Steiner PE: Cancer of the liver and cirrhosis in Trans-Saharan Africa and the United States of America. *Cancer* **13**:1085–1166, 1960.

44. Gelfand M: The diagnosis and prognosis of schistosomiasis. *Am J Trop Med* **29**:945–958, 1949.

45. Andrade ZA: Hepatic schistosomiasis: Morphological aspects. In *Progress in Liver Diseases,* Vol 2. Popper H, Schaffner F (Eds). 1965, pp 228–242.

46. Gibson JB: Parasites, liver disease and liver cancer. *International Agency for Research on Cancer Scientific Publications No. 1.* Liver Cancer. Proceedings of a working conference held at the Chester Beatty Research Institute, London, England, June 30 to July 3, 1969, Lyon, 1971, pp 42–50.

47. Fifth Pan-American Congress of Gastroenterology, La Habana, Cuba, January 20–27, 1956. Report of the board for classification and nomenclature of cirrhosis of the liver. *Gastroenterology,* **31**:213–216, 1956.

48. Nakashima T: Liver cirrhosis due to schistosomiasis japonica (I) (in Japanese). *Acta Hepat Jap* **10**:485–500, 1969.

49. Tsutsumi H, Nakashima T: Pathology of liver cirrhosis due to schistosoma japonicum. In *Research in Filariasis and Schistosomiasis,* Vol 2. M Yokogawa (Ed). Univ. Tokyo Press, Tokyo, 1972, pp 113–128.

50. Symmers WSC: Note on a new form of liver cirrhosis due to the presence of the ova of Bilharzia haematobia. *J Pathol Bact* **9**:237–239, 1904.

51. Okuda K, Jinnouchi S, Arakawa M, et al: Generalized calcification of the Acta in advanced schistosomiasis japonica—a case report. *Scta Hepato–Gastroenterol* **22**:98–102, 1975.

52. Higginson J, Oettlé AG: Cancer incidence in the Bantu and "Cape colored" races of South Africa: Report of a cancer survey in the Transvaal (1953–1955). *J Natl Cancer Inst* **24**:589–671, 1960.

53. Iuchi M, Hayakawa M, Kitani K, et al: Primary hepatocellular carcinoma in chronic schistosomiasis japonica (2) (in Japanese). *Acta Hepat Jap* **14**:249–252, 1973.

54. Nakashima T, Okuda K, Kojiro M, et al: Primary liver cancer coincidental with schistosomiasis japonica. A study of 24 cases. *Cancer,* **36**:1483–1489, 1975.

55. Hou P-C: The pathology of Clonorchis sinensis infestation of the liver. *J Pathol Bact* **70**:53–64, 1955.

56. Hou P-C: The relationship between primary carcinoma of the liver and infestation with Clonorchis sinensis. *J Pathol Bact* **72**:239–246, 1956.

57. Liang P-C, Tung, C: Morphologic study and etiology of primary liver carcinoma and its incidence in China. *Chin Med J* **79**:336–347, 1959.

58. Algire GH, Chalkley HW: Vascular reactions of normal and malignant tissues in vivo. I. Vascular reactions of mice to wounds and to normal and neoplastic transplants. *J Natl Cancer Inst* **6**:73–85, 1945.

59. Green HSN: Heterologous transplantation of mammalian tumors. *J Exp Med* **73**:461–473, 1961.

60. Greenblatt M, Shubik P: Tumor angiogenesis: Transfilter diffusion studies in the hamster by the transparent chamber technique. *J Natl Cancer Inst* **41**:111–124, 1968.

61. Ehrmann RL, Knoth M: Choriocarcinoma: Transfilter stimulation of vasoproliferation in the hamster cheek pouch—studied by light and electron microscopy. *J Natl Cancer Inst* **41**:1329–1341, 1968.

62. Folkman J, Merler E, Abernathy C, et al: Isolation of a tumor factor responsible for angiogenesis. *J Exp Med* **133**:275–288, 1971.

63. Wright RD: The blood supply of newly developed epithelial tissue in the liver. *J Pathol Bact* **45**:405–414, 1937.

64. Hayashi S, Sano H, Takemae T: Hepatic devascularisation in advanced stage of liver cancer—Ligation of the branches of the hepatic artery and portal vein (in Japanese). *Saishin-Igaku* **28**:511–521, 1973.

65. Yoshida T: *Yoshida Sarcoma* (in Japanese) Neiraku Shobo, Tokyo, 1949.

66. Kinoshita R: Studies on the cancerogenic chemical substances. *Trans Soc Pathol Jap* **27**:665–727, 1937.

67. Oota K, Matsumoto S: Collision of multicentric cancerous foci against each other in experimental rat liver cancer. *Gann Monogr* **45**:581–590, 1954.

68. Popper H, Schaffner F: *Liver: Structure and Function.* The Blakiston Division, McGraw-Hill, New York, 1957.

69. Honjo I, Suzuki T: Selective arteriography of the liver and pancreas (in Japanese). *Rinsho Geka* **24**:317–326, 1969.

70. Motta P, Porter KR: Structure of rat liver sinusoids and associated tissue spaces as revealed by scanning electron microscopy. *Cell Tissue Res* **148**:111–125, 1974.

71. Sakamoto K, Nakashima T, Kojiro M, et al: Vascular changes in advanced primary hepatocellular carcinoma. *Ninth Meeting of the Western Japan Society of Hepatologists,* Yonago, 1974.

72. Nakashima T, Kojiro M, Sakamoto K, et al: Studies on primary liver carcinoma. I. Proposal of new gross anatomical classification of primary liver cell carcinoma (in Japanese). *Acta Hepat Jap* **15**:278–291, 1974.

73. Edmondson HA: Tumors of the liver and intrahepatic bile ducts. Section VII, fascicle 25, Armed Forces Institute of Pathology, Washington, D. C., 1958, pp 32–109.

74. Kuratomi S, Sakamoto K: Vascular architecture in primary liver carcinoma (in Japanese). *Jap J Gastroenterol* **70**:1104–1105, 1973.

75. Nakashima T: Upper gastrointestinal bleeding (in Japanese). *Acta Hepat Jap* **14**:676, 1973.

76. Nakashima T: Esophageal varices (in Japanese). *Acta Hepat Jap* **15**:254–255, 1974.

CHAPTER 10 TUMORS OF THE LIVER IN CHILDHOOD

BENJAMIN H. LANDING, M.D.

This chapter is based on the pathologic features of 74 tumors or tumorlike lesions of the liver that were recorded in the autopsy and surgical pathology files of the Department of Pathology, Childrens Hospital of Los Angeles during the period 1926 to 1974. Patients whose diagnosis was based on clinical or radiologic findings only, or whose surgical or autopsy material could not be obtained from the institution where the studies were performed, were not included. The series presented is generally illustrative of the spectrum and relative frequency of hepatic tumors in children, with the exception that hemangiomas, large enough to cause hepatomegaly or cardiovascular symptoms but responsive to nonsurgical therapy, will be underrepresented.

CATEGORIES OF LIVER TUMORS IN CHILDREN

Gall (1) has divided the tumors of the liver into eight general categories based on the nature of the presumed cell of origin. His list and the appropriate tumor types observed in the material surveyed for this chapter are presented in Table 1.

ANGIOMATOUS TUMORS

Benign

Although some workers feel that hepatic hemangiomas form a single category of lesion, with the several possible microscopic patterns really being variations on a single basic theme (2), the clinical data presented in Table 2 and summarized in Table 3 would appear to justify division of the larger category of benign hemangiomas into at least the categories listed. For example, none of the patients with the pattern called diffuse sinusoid dilatation had clinically apparent disease, whereas approximately half with lesions called capillary or cavernous hemangioma had clinical manifestations of the tumor (congestive heart failure—2, abdominal mass—6, obstructive jaundice—1), and all three patients diagnosed as having fibrovascular hamartoma had significant symptoms (11). The terms

Table 1

Category of Tumor (Gall's Classification)	Types of Children's Hospital Los Angeles Series	Number of Cases
1. Primary epithelial neoplasm, parenchymal	Hepatoma (hepatocellular carcinoma)	1
	Hepatoma secondary to other liver disease	8
2. Primary epithelial neoplasm, ductal	None observed	
3. Hematopoietic neoplasm	Not included in study	
4. Supporting tissue neoplasm	Hemangiomas	17
	Fibrovascular hamartoma	3
	Simple cyst	3
5. Teratoid and embryonal neoplasms	Hepatoblastoma, cystic and solid, benign and malignant	34
	Rhabdomyosarcoma	5
6. Miscellaneous and uncertain neoplasms	Monotypic small celled tumor	3
7. Metastatic neoplasms	Not included in study	
		74

Table 2 Angiomatous Tumors

Patient	Sex	Age	Surgical/ Autopsy	Other features
Capillary hemangioma (benign hemangioendothelioma)				
1	m	2 months	A	Multiple small liver lesions, cirsoid aneurysm, brain and scalp
2	f	4 months	S	
3	m	4 months	A	Malformation of brain, aplastic anemia
4	m	1–3/12	A	*H. influenzae* meningitis
Sclerosing capillary hemangioma				
1	f	6 weeks	S	
Diffuse sinusoid dilatation				
1	f	12 days	A	Cystic fibrosis, meconium ileus, solitary renal cyst
2	m	4 months	A	Pneumococcus meningitis
3	m	5 months	A	Acute gastroenteritis
Cavernous hemangioma				
1	m	2 days	S	
2	m	3 weeks	A	Two liver lesions Tetralogy of Fallot with pulmonic atresia
3	f	2 months	A	Died, congestive heart failure
4	m	3 months	S	Probable congestive failure, died, postoperative peritonitis
5	f	2-8/12	A	Rupture, hemoperitoneum

206

Table 2 *(Cont.)*

6	f	4 years	S	
7	f	5-6/12	A	Transposition of great arteries
8	f	12-5/12	A	Multiple small liver lesions, transposition of great arteries, vertebral hemangioma
9	m	18 years	S	Membranoproliferative glomerulonephritis, renal transplant, incidental removal of liver lesion
Fibrovascular hamartoma				
1	f	1 days	A	Died, congestive heart failure
2	f	2 weeks	A	Abdominal mass, obstructive jaundice
3	m	1-9/12	S	

Table 3   Clinical Behavior of Angiomatous Tumors of Liver in Children

	Total in Group	Clinically Apparent	Clinically Inapparent
Capillary hemangioma	4	1	3
Sclerosing capillary hemangioma	1	1	0
Diffuse sinusoid dilatation	3	0	3
Cavernous hemangioma	9	4	5
Fibrovascular hamartoma	3	3	0

diffuse sinusoid dilation and cavernous hemangioma do not appear to need elaboration (see Figs. 2 to 6), and the term capillary hemangioma (benign hemangioendothelioma) also has a generally accepted microscopic counterpart (see Fig. 1). Sclerosing hemangioma, in the liver as in the skin and other loci, appears to be a stage in the involutionary process commonly seen in capillary hemangiomas, whether spontaneously occurring or assisted by steroid therapy, local radiation, or other means.

The term fibrovascular hamartoma has been retained in this study, partly for historic reasons, to include relatively large tumors, with definite capillary or cavernous vascular component, but also with large areas of myxoid fibrous tissue which often shows cystic foci (2, 9), "pseudolymphangioma," resembling changes which can be seen in myxoid connective tissue of nasal polyps, for example. Lesions with these features may show, especially peripherally, septa containing bile ductules. The separate term fibrovascular hamartoma has been retained to indicate that there can be a pathologic and perhaps a true continuum between fibrovascular hamartoma and the lesion (q.v.) called benign hepatoblastoma (Figs 7–10). That a hamartoma of the liver (with hamartoma defined as a benign tumorlike lesion composed of cell types normally found in the site, whether during fetal life or later) might contain both epithelial and stromal components is not surprising, since the hepatic primordium has both mesodermal and endodermal components; restriction of the term hamartoma to a "one-sided" lesion containing chiefly stromal components, versus the use of benign hepatoblastoma

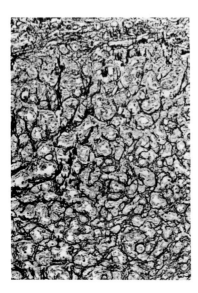

Figure 1 Capillary hemangioma (reticulum stain) showing small interconnecting vascular channels, which tend to be larger with thicker layers of lining endothelial cells on the periphery of the lesion (Table 2, capillary hemangioma, patient 2) (X 77).

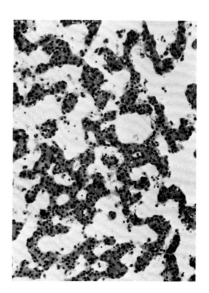

Figure 2 Diffuse sinusoid dilatation pattern of hemangioma (Table 2, diffuse sinusoid dilatation, patient 1). Atrophy of hepatocytes in the parenchymal cords between the dilated sinusoids appears to be the mechanism of progression from this pattern to that called cavernous hemangioma (X 77).

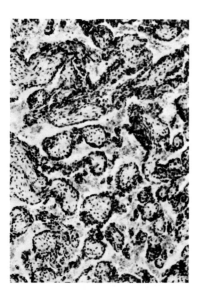

Figure 3 Cavernous hemangioma in 3-month-old male with congestive heart failure (Table 2, cavernous hemangioma, patient 4). The appearance suggests that conversion of the parenchymal cords of hemangioma with the diffuse sinusoid dilatation pattern to fibrous cords is the origin of this pattern (X 77).

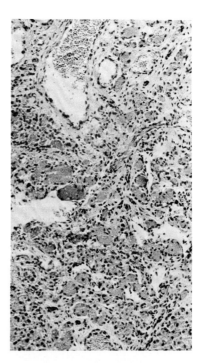

Figure 4 Area of mixed capillary and cavernous hemangioma patterns in predominantly cavernous hemangioma (Table 2, cavernous hemangioma, patient 8). The pattern suggests that progression from capillary to cavernous hemangioma is a result from enlargement of the channels between "feeding vessels" (X 77).

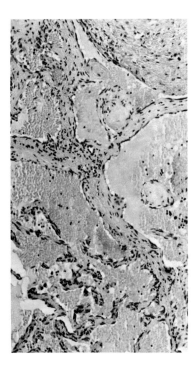

Figure 5 Cavernous hemangioma (Table 2, cavernous hemangioma, patient 9), showing organizing thrombus in a large channel (X 77).

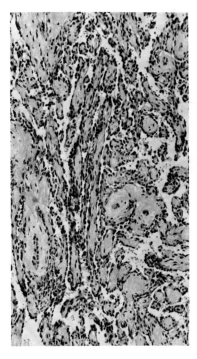

Figure 6 Cavernous hemangioma in a 2-month-old female with congestive heart failure (Table 2, cavernous hemangioma, patient 3). Persistent bile ductules can be seen in some of the fibrous septa (X 77).

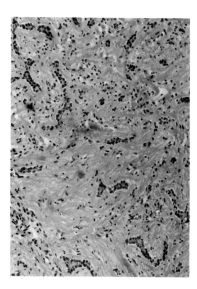

Figure 7 Solid fibrous area in predominantly cavernous hemangioma (Table 2, cavernous hemangioma, patient 6). Such areas provide a morphologic transition between some hemangiomas and the lesion called benign hepatoblastoma (X 77).

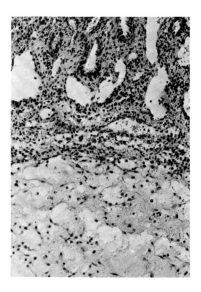

Figure 8 Fibrovascular hamartoma (Table 2, fibrovascular hamartoma, patient 3), showing central myxoid "pseudolymphangiomatous" area, with angiomatous peripheral zone containing residual bile ductules. The occurrence of congestive heart failure in some patients with fibrovascular hamartoma indicates the basically angiomatous nature of the lesion, but this slide illustrates the possibility of progression to a "mixed tumor" or benign hepatoblastoma pattern (X 77).

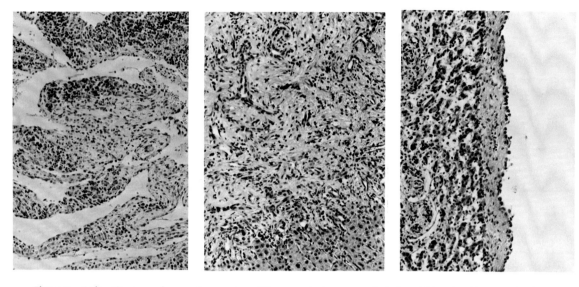

Figure 9 *(Left)* Cavernous hemangioma region of fibrovascular hamartoma in 1-day-old female with congestive heart failure present at birth (Table 2, fibrovascular hamartoma, patient 1). The very prominent extramedullary erythropoiesis suggests that intrauterine hypoxia due to obstruction of umbilical vein return to the liver may be important in some infants with large congenital hepatic tumors (X 77).

Figure 10 *(Center)* Margin of lesion coded as benign hepatoblastoma (Table 5, benign hepatoblastoma, patient 2) showing admixture of fibrous tissue, bile ductules, and small vascular channels. Note the similarity of the lesion to that of Fig. 7. However, in this patient no areas of apparent hemangioma were demonstrated (X 77).

Figure 11 *(Right)* Simple (mesothelial) cyst in liver of a 1-day-old girl with omphalocele, congenital heart disease, and deficiency of the pericardial portion of the diaphragm (X 77).

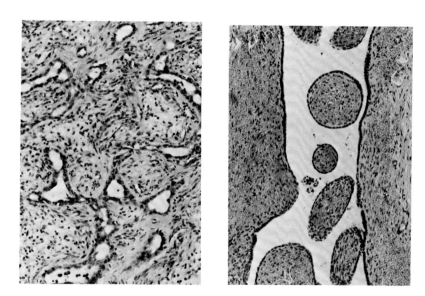

Figure 12a *(Left)* Benign solid hepatoblastoma (Table 5, benign hepatoblastoma, patient 1) showing mixture of bile ductules and connective tissues (X 77).

Figure 12b *(Right)* Benign cystic hepatoblastoma, or multilocular cyst (Table 5, benign cystic hepatoblastoma, patient 1), showing large epithelium-lined spaces with fibrous walls (X 77).

for what could reasonably be considered a "mixed hamartoma," results from an effort to assign as precise an anatomic picture as possible to each term in the vocabulary employed. In short, whether separation of fibrovascular hamartoma from benign hepatoblastoma by the criteria used in this chapter is etiologically or pathogenetically justified remains to be established. The reported age peak in the second year of life, and male preponderance (8), are not seen in the short series of this study.

PARENCHYMAL TUMORS

One can propose analogy of the embryonic tumors of the liver to those of the kidney, as follows:

Benign hepatoblastoma
    = Mesoblastic nephroma
Benign cystic hepatoblastoma (multilocular cyst) = Benign cystic nephroma (multilocular cyst)
Malignant cystic hepatoblastoma = ?
Malignant hepatoblastoma
    = Wilms' tumor (nephroblastoma)

Simple Cyst of the Liver

In the series reviewed, three infants had, as incidental findings at the time of autopsy, simple cysts of the liver with fibrous capsule and lining of large "epitheloid" cells with opaque acidophilic cytoplasm. Whether these should be considered to be mesothelial cysts or cysts lined by cells derived from hepatic or biliary tract epithelium is uncertain. The fact that all these infants had omphalocele, and the known association of the Beckwith syndrome (Wiedemann-Beckwith, hyperplastic fetal visceromegaly, or EMG—for exomphalos, macroglossia, gigantism-syndrome) with malignant hepatoblastoma raises the possibility that such lesions represent "hepatoblastoma in situ," despite the lack, to date, of histologic support for such an hypothesis. This is in contrast to the histologic si-

milarity of nodular renal blastoma (Wilms' tumor in situ) to true nephroblastoma. The abnormal development of the abdominal wall and the presence, in at least one of the infants, of a diaphragmatic defect (abnormality of the septum transversum), however, suggests that these cysts are of coelomic (mesothelial) origin (Fig. 11).

Benign Cystic Hepatoblastoma (Multilocular Cyst of the Liver)

The three patients with this lesion were all two years of age or less. All presented with abdominal mass and have done well following surgical excision of the lesion. Possible male preponderance is of interest, since malignant hepatoblastoma shows female preponderance (4 males/6 females) for patients with onset of clinical disease during the first year of life, despite more marked male preponderance (6 males/0 females) for patients with onset between 1 and 2.5 years (see Table 4, Fig. 12a, 12b). The possibility that malignant change can occur in benign cystic hepatoblastomas is illustrated in Fig. 13, 14.

Benign Hepatoblastoma

Only one patient, a 3-year old boy with abdominal mass, fell into this category. The concept differs from that of benign cystic hepatoblastoma in specifying that the tumor mass is solid; justification for the distinction may be the apparent lack of transition between the possibly comparable renal lesions, mesoblastic nephroma, and cystic nephroma. Willis (6) has suggested that "adenoma" of the liver might arise by maturation of malignant hepatoblastoma. No evidence to support this proposal has been observed in this study. If such maturation does occur, benign hepatoblastoma would seem the expected pattern. Because of its typically large size and range of age in young adulthood, the lesion, focal nodular hyperplasia (also called adenoma of the liver by some workers (7), might appear a suspect for "matured hepatoblastoma," but

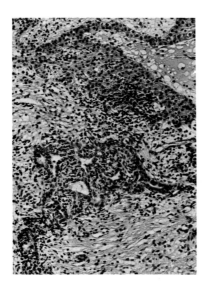

Figure 13 Area of epithelial proliferation in marginal zone of benign cystic hepatoblastoma (Table 5, benign cystic hepatoblastoma, patient 2), perhaps illustrating an early stage of transition from benign to malignant cystic hepatoblastoma (X 77).

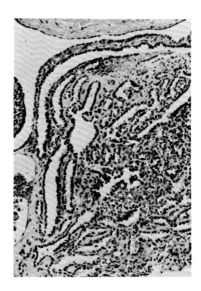

Figure 14 Trabecular and papillary intracystic growth pattern of malignant cystic hepatoblastoma (Table 5, patient 2). Areas of cyst with simple epithelial lining are also seen, and the pattern suggests that this highly malignant tumor can arise in the lesion called benign cystic hepatoblastoma or multilocular cyst (X 77).

the lack of observation of transitional phases speaks against this.

Malignant Cystic Hepatoblastoma

This entity emphasizes that not all cystic "mixed" tumors of the liver of young children are benign. The two patients in this series, one male and one female, had short courses after initial surgical treatment.

Malignant Hepatoblastoma

The single most common liver tumor in children is the highly malignant hepatoblastoma (4, 5, 10)—22 of the 27 patients in this study are known to have died, 2 with rupture of the tumor and hemoperitoneum, 2 others of the primary tumor, and 4 of operative complications. Of the 22 who died, 14 had metastic disease (lungs 12, lymph nodes 6, central nervous system 3, etc.). The series shows most peculiar sex ratios, with female preponder-

ance (6/4) for patients presenting under one year of age, male preponderance (6/0) in patients presenting beyond one year but under 2.5 years, and female preponderance again (7/3) in those over 2.5 years, so that the overall ratio is 14 females to 13 males.

Hepatoblastoma has been divided into epithelial and mixed (epithelial and stromal components) categories, but the data of Table 4 may not support this distinction. Definitely mixed hepatoblastomas were concentrated in infants under 18 months of age (6 of 12), and in children over 10 years (2 of 4), but, if the "broad septal" pattern of hepatoblastoma is included with the mixed pattern, no age-related distribution is apparent. Whether this is the correct assignment, whether the "broad septal" pattern should be considered a variation of epithelial hepatoblastoma, and whether the mixed hepatoblastomas of infants and those of adolescents

Table 4 Parenchymal Tumors

	Sex	Age	Surgical/Autopsy	Other Features
Benign (solid) hepatoblastoma				
1	m	9 months	S	
2	m	3 years	S	
Benign cystic hepatoblastoma (multilocular cyst)				
1	f	5 months	S	
2	m	7 months	S	
3	m	2 years	S	
Malignant cystic hepatoblastoma				
1	m	8 months	S	Survived 3 months
2	f	2-6/12	S	Known to have died

	Sex	Age Onset	Duration Survival	Epithelial	Mixed	Broad Septal Pattern	Osteoid	Other features
Malignant hepatoblastoma								
1	f	1 month	4 months		+	+	+	Lipid histiocytosis of RE system
2	f	5 months	0	+			+	Postoperative hemorrhage
3	f	5 months	1 month	+		+	+	Infection, postoperative biliary fistula
4	f	8 months	1 month		+			Peritonitis, lung metastases
5	m	8 months	3 months	+			+	Initial radiation, postoperative hemorrhage
6	m	9 months	3 months		+			Rupture, hemoperitoneum
7	f	10 months	2 weeks	+				Probable Beckwith syndrome, metastases lungs, falx
8	m	10 months	3 months		+			Metastases lungs, nodes
9	m	1 year	?	+		+		No follow-up data
10	f	1 year	3 months		+			No follow-up data
11	m	1-1/12	11/12		+		+	Metastases brain, spinal cord, orbit

213

Table 4 Parenchymal Tumors (*Cont.*)

	Sex	Age								
12	m	1 yr, 5 months	?			+			Known to have died	
13	m	1 yr, 7 months	1 yr, 2 months	+	+	+			Metastases lungs, mesentery, stomach, small intestine	
14	m	1 yr, 11 months	5 months	+		+			Metastases lungs, nodes, brain; sexual precocity	
15	m	2 years	?	+		+			No followup data	
16	m	2 yr, 11 months	6 months	+	+				Metastases lungs	
17	f	2 yr, 6 months	3 months	+	+	+			Metastases lungs, nodes	
18	f	3 yr, 6 months	0	+	+	+			Metastases lungs, adrenals, pancreas	
19	m	3 yr, 8 months	0	+	+				Postoperative hemoperitoneum, metastases lungs	
20	f	4 yr, 10 months	8 months	+					Metastases lungs, bones, kidneys	
21	f	5 years	?	+					Recurrence after 14 months	
22	f	5 yr, 3 months	2 yr, 10 months	+	+	+			Metastases lungs, nodes, ? thymic deficiency	
23	f	10 years	?	+	+				No followup data	
24	f	10 yr, 8 months	?				+		Known to have died	
25	m	13 years	11 months				+		Metastases lungs, nodes peritoneum	
26	m	13 yr, 6 months	?	+	+				No followup data	
27	f	?	0	+		+			Died, no clinical data available	

Hepatoma, primary

	m	4 yr, 6 months	3 months						Metastases, lungs	

	Sex	Age Onset of Tumor	Alive/Dead
Hepatoma secondary			
Primary Disorder			
Biliary atresia	m	3-2/12	D
Chronic hepatitis with cirrhosis	f	14-10/12	A
Familial cholestatic disorder, ? Byler's disease	m	13-1/12	D
Glycogen storage disease (von Gierke)	f	3-4/12	D
		20 years	D

214

Table 4 Parenchymal Tumors (Cont.)

	Sex	Age Onset	Duration Survival		Other Features
Soto's syndrome (cerebral gigantism)					
Tyrosinosis	m		15-8/12	D	
	f		4-3/12	D	
	m		8 years	D	
Sarcomas					
Monotypic small-celled tumors, ? sarcomas					
1	f	6 years	?		No follow-up data
2	m	8 years	?		No follow-up data
3	m	14 years	7/12		Metastases lungs, kidneys, bones, spinal cord, nodes, intestine "Meningioma-in-situ", left choroid plexus
Rhabdomyosarcomas					
Apparently intrahepatic					
1	m	6 months	3 weeks		Metastases lungs, nodes
2	f	10-8/12	2-3/12		Died of infection
Of extrahepatic bile ducts					
1	f	4-11/12	?		Known to have died
2	f	6-10/12	9/12		Died with radiation nephritis
3	f	7-6/12	6/12		Died with postoperative shock

	Sex	Age	Surgical/Autopsy	Other Features
Simple (mesothelial cyst)				
1	f	1 day	A	Omphalocele, congenital heart disease
2	m	1 day	A	Omphalocele, congenital heart disease
3	f	3 day	A	Omphalocele, congenital heart disease

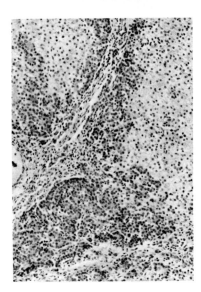

Figure 15 Malignant hepatoblastoma, epithelial type (Table 5, malignant hepatoblastoma patient 3) showing typical pattern of lobular growth, with larger more hepatocytic cells centrally in the lobules and smaller darker cells peripherally (X 77).

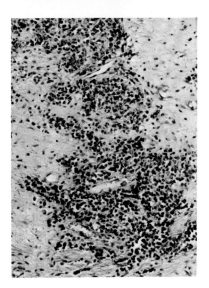

Figure 16 Malignant hepatoblastoma, mixed type (Table 5, malignant hepatoblastoma, patient 1), showing area of admixture of connective tissue and small dark epithelial component cells, and emphasizing similarity of appearance of such areas to patterns seen in mixed tumors in other sites (X 77).

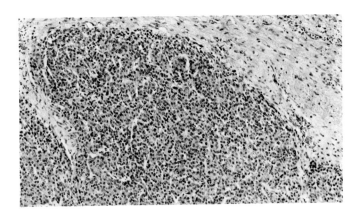

Figure 17 Malignant hepatoblastoma, showing area of "broad septal pattern," without apparent transition or intermingling of stromal tissue and epithelial component, suggesting that the broad septal pattern does not, in itself, warrant the interpretation of malignant hepatoblastoma, mixed type (Table 5, malignant hepatoblastoma, patient 9) (X 77).

should be considered basically different, albeit similar, tumors remain to be established (Figs. 15–17). In Table 4 the presence of osteoid, a classical microscopic criterion of hepatoblastoma, is tabulated separately. Osteoid is not treated as a stromal component justifying inclusion of tumors containing osteoid in the mixed hepatoblastoma category, because of the evidence, illustrated in Figs. 18 to 21, that

osteoid formation is a secondary lesion resulting from thrombosis. The mechanism of such osteoid transformation of organizing thrombi is not known, but one is reminded of the high incidence of phleboliths in venous hemangiomas. The osteoid in hepatoblastomas often calcifies and can be demonstrated radiologically. Calcification visible in X-rays, or bone seen microscopically, are thus not diagnostic of teratoma

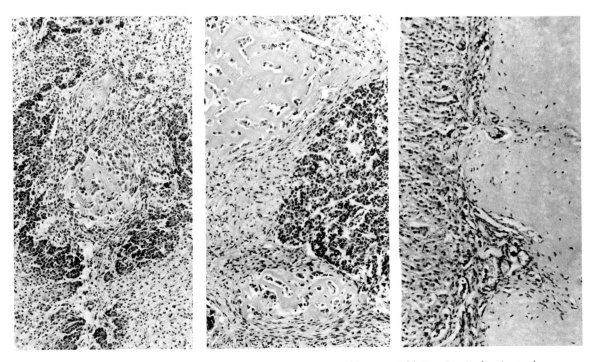

Figure 18 *(Left)* Small areas of osteoid formation in malignant hepatoblastoma (Table 5, patient 3), showing tendency of osteoid to be associated with small dark-celled epithelial component, and to be in septa between epithelial lobules (X 77).

Figure 19 *(Center)* Larger areas of osteoid formation in malignant hepatoblastoma (Table 5, patient 2) (X 77).

Figure 20 *(Right)* Very large osteoid area, adjoining apparently normal hepatic parenchyma, on margin of malignant hepatoblastoma (Table 5, patient 9) (X 77).

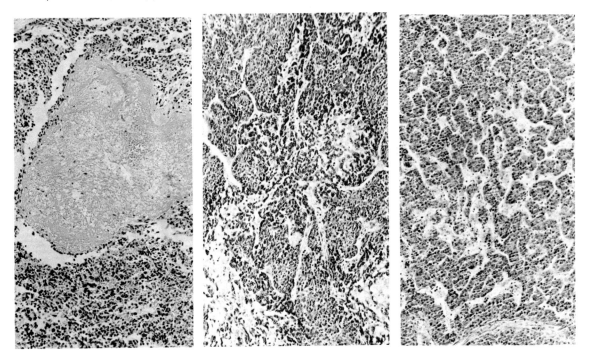

Figure 21 *(Left)* Thrombus in small-celled area of malignant hepatoblastoma (Table 5, patient 13). The appearance suggests that such thrombi form the sites of development of osteoid (X 77).

Figure 22 *(Center)* Malignant hepatoblastoma (Table 5, patient 24), showing typical mixed growth pattern, with mingling of small dark epithelial, cell component and stroma in narrokw septa (X 77).

Figure 23 *(Right)* Unusually trabecular area of growth in malignant hepatoblastoma (Table 5, patient 14). The cords of tumor cells are narrower than those typically seen in true hepatoma (X 77).

217

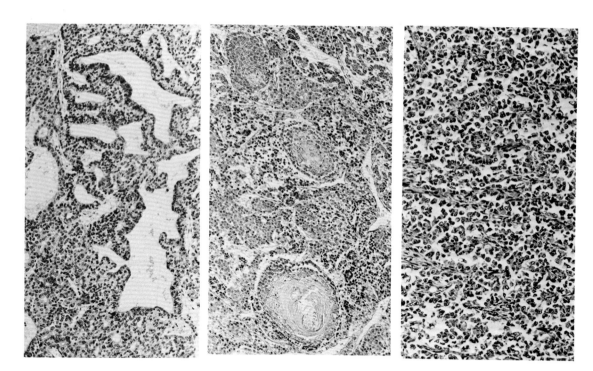

Figure 24 *(Left)* Area of unusually lacunar pattern in malignant hepatoblastoma (Table 5, patient 22). Such patterns suggest that the small dark-celled epithelial component of malignant hepatoblastomas demonstrates partial differentiation toward ductular (? Hering duct) epithelium (X 77).

Figure 25 *(Center)* Squamous epithelial pearls, a relatively rare pattern of differentiation (or ? metaplasia) in malignant hepatoblastoma (Table 5, patient 14) (X 77).

Figure 26 *(Right)* Area of "sickle-form" cells in malignant hepatoblastoma (Table 5, patient 5). Whether this cell type is derived from epithelial cells or from stromal cells, in the latter case perhaps reflecting a Kupffer-cell component, is uncertain (X 77).

nor of osteogenic sarcoma, two tumors that have been reported to arise in the liver, and it is possible that some reports of these tumors arising in the liver reflect misinterpretations of hepatoblastomas with calcifying osteoid. As Ishak and Glunz (5) have pointed out, metastases of hepatoblastomas essentially never contain osteoid, supporting the position that osteoid is not a basic, but a secondary, component of these tumors. Foci of squamous epithelium are also found, relatively rarely, in malignant hepatoblastomas (Fig. 25). Squamous carcinoma has been repotted to arise in nonparasitic cysts of the liver (presumably in the tumors here called cystic hepatoblastomas), but apparently no instance of this phenomenon has been reported in a child.

The basic microscopic feature of malignant hepatoblastoma, the presence of a population of larger cells resembling hepa-

tocytes, and of a smaller more embryonic cell population, is well illustrated in Figs. 15 to 27. Most often, the smaller cells are peripheral in the lobules of malignant epithelial cells, but the proportion of the two populations varies widely. Rarely, the hepatocytic cells contain large fat vacuoles, so that at the extreme they resemble mesodermal fat cells. Whether this form of tumor merits a separate name will require further study, as does the possibility that some reports of primary lipoma or liposarcoma of the liver reflect misinterpretation of the nature of these tumors. As implied above, an important microscopic criterion distinguishing epithelial hepatoblastoma from true hepatoma (hepatocellular carcinoma) is the commonly trabecular pattern of the latter (cf. Figs. 28 to 33).

Malignant hepatoblastoma has been observed in siblings (12), but no instances of

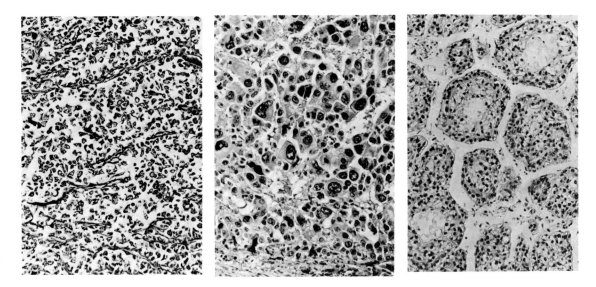

Figure 27 *(Left)* Reticulum stain of same specimen shown in Fig. 26. Slender stromal bands are separated by broad strands of poorly cohesive "sickle-form" cells (X 77).

Figure 28 *(Center)* Marked cellular atypia in primary hepatoma, the only instance of true hepatoma in this series not apparently arising in an abnormal liver (X 77).

Figure 29 *(Right)* Secondary malignant hepatoma in 3 year, 2 month old boy with biliary atresia. Cytoplasmic swelling of cells in the centers of the trabecula may reflect the hypercholesterolemia of chronic biliary cirrhosis. Note that the cells are larger, and the trabecular cords typically broader, in true hepatoma as compared to trabecular areas in hepatoblastoma (cf. Fig. 23) (X 77).

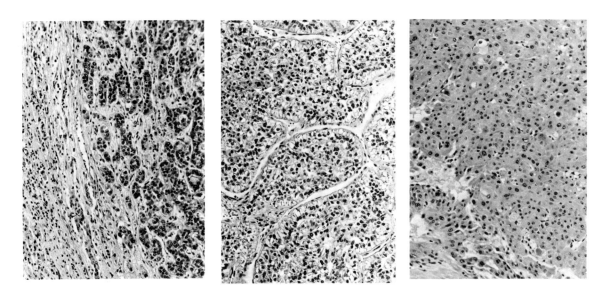

Figure 30 *(Left)* Trabecular cord pattern in hepatoma in a 13-year-old boy with familial chronic cholestatic disease and cirrhosis (X 77).

Figure 31 *(Center)* Broad trabecular cord pattern in area of same hepatoma shown in Fig. 30 (X 77).

Figure 32 *(Right)* Hepatoma in 15 year 8 month-old boy with Sotos' cerebral gigantism. The cells of this tumor contained an unusual number of hyaline cytoplasmic globules (X 77).

familial behavior were observed in this series. The occurence of this tumor in patients with the Beckwith syndrome can explain some such observations. As Sotelo-Avila has proposed (13), probably all patients with hemihypertrophy and hepatoblastoma (or other appropriate tumors) should be considered to have the Beckwith syndrome. Patients with this disease have been observed to have malignant hepatoblastoma, Wilms' tumor, adrenal cortical carcinoma, umbilical myxoma, and orbital rhabdomyosarcoma, among other tumors, so that the occasional occurrence of these tumors in patients who also have hepatoblastoma can be expected.

In contrast to Wilms' tumor, rhabdomyoblasts occur very rarely, if at all, in malignant hepatoblastomas, and their demonstration in a "mixed" malignant tumor of the liver in a child should suggest metastatic Wilms' tumor. In this study, monotypic rhabdomyosarcomas of either intrahepatic or major bile duct origin have been separated from the category of malignant hepatoblastoma.

Typically, malignant hepatoblastoma forms a large solitary liver tumor; occasionally patients do show multiple nodules of tumor in the liver, but intrahepatic metastases seems the most probable explanation of this finding, although there seems no obvious reason why multicentric origin could not occur in patients with the Beckwith syndrome, for example.

In a number of the malignant hepatoblastomas listed in Table 4, larger or smaller areas of angulate ("sickle-form") cells suggesting the malignant histiocytic cells of "Kupfferoma"—malignant histiocytoma, reticulum cell sarcoma, hemangioendothelial sarcoma or angioblastic reticuloendothelioma of the liver—have been observed (Figs. 26 and 27). In the absence of tissue culture or other functional and histochemical studies, a definite conclusion as to whether the "sickle-form" cell appearance is a permissible variation of malignant hepatic epithelial cells, or whether it reflects

Kupffer cell differentiation of the stromal component of mixed hepatoblastoma is not possible. The mesenchymal component in the hepatic anlage would suggest that the latter possibility is not unreasonable.

HEPATOMA (HEPATOCELLULAR CARCINOMA)

As Table 4 shows, this appears to be a very rare primary liver tumor of children, the data of many previous authors (e.g., (3)) being confused by failure to distinguish epithelial hepatoblastoma from true hepatoma. Most helpful criteria are the typical "broad cord" trabecular pattern of hepatoma (Figs. 29 to 33), and the presence of the larger hepatocellular and smaller embryonic cell epithelial components in epithelial hepatoblastoma (Figs. 15 to 18). Biologically, true hepatoma does not appear to differ significantly from hepatoblastoma.

Hepatoma secondary to underlying liver disease has been, in the series studied, much more common than true primary hepatoma (8 patients with secondary versus one with primary hepatoma). The occurrence of hepatoma as a complication of biliary atresia, chronic hepatitis, von Gierke's disease, tyrosinosis, and possibly in familial cholestasis (Byler's disease) has been reported by others, but association with Sotos' cerebral gigantism apparently has not. Whether the occurrence is meaningful or coincidental cannot be stated. Of the primary liver diseases predisposing to hepatoma, tyrosinosis, appears to be the most dangerous in this regard—two of three patients with tyrosinosis in the population from which the material was drawn died with hepatoma, and material from another suggestive patient was not available for study. Von Gierke's glycogen storage disease (glucose-6-phosphatase deficiency) also causes hepatoma—not in association with antecedent cirrhosis—with significant frequency (two of four patients in the source population). Type 4 glycogen stor-

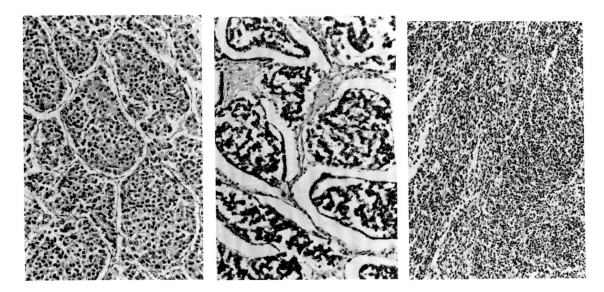

Figure 33 *(Left)* Hepatoma in 4 year 3 month-old girl with tyrosinosis (X 77).

Figure 34 *(Center)* Monotypic tumor, of uncertain nature, in a 14-year-old boy. Angiosarcoma and Ewing's tumor primary in the liver are possible interpretations (X 77).

Figure 35 *(Right)* Apparently intrahepatic small-celled rhabdomyosarcoma of a 6-year-month-old boy. A very poorly defined interlacing "herring-bone" pattern is discernable (X 77).

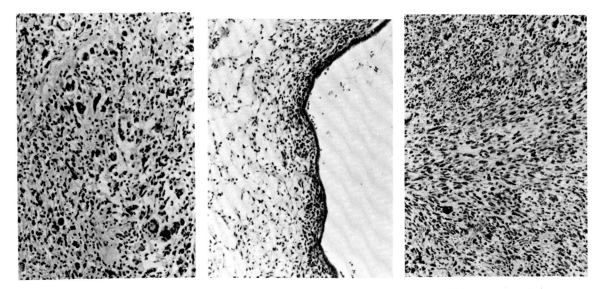

Figure 36 *(Left)* Intrahepatic rhabdomyosarcoma in 10-8/12 year-old girl. Residual tumor was present in the liver, despite several resections, but death was the result of infection (X 77).

Figure 37 *(Center)* Botryoid rhabdomyosarcoma of extrahepatic bile ducts in 6-10/12 year-old girl, showing "rind" or "cambium-layer" of small tumor cells surrounding the central myxoid zones in the polypoid masses of sarcoma botryoides (X 77).

Figure 38 *(Right)* Solid area in rhabdomyosarcoma of extrahepatic bile ducts in 7-6/12 year-old girl, showing herring-bone pattern and scattered large atypical rhabdomyoblasts (X 77).

age disease (brancher enzyme deficiency) can possibly lead to hepatoma, but this did not occur in the patient with type 4 glycogen storage disease in the base population. The association of hepatoma with antecedent cirrhosis is not general, or, at least, the risk is not apparently equal for different causes of cirrhosis, since hepatoma was not observed in the base population in patients with the following causes of cirrhosis in childhood (see also Table 5).

Alpha-1-antitrypsin deficiency.
Congenital hepatic fibrosis.
Cystinosis.
Focal biliary cirrhosis of fibrocystic disease.
Galactosemia.
Gaucher's disease.
Hurler's disease.
Infantile polycystic disease.
Thalassemia.
Wilson's disease.

SARCOMAS OF THE LIVER

MONOTYPIC SMALL-CELLED SARCOMAS.

The liver tumors of three patients have been placed in this presumably nonhomogeneous descriptive category because of inability to assign them to any other entity included in the vocabulary employed. One of these tumors is illustrated in Fig. 34. This tumor in a 14-year-old boy may well be a true angiosarcoma, although Ewing's tumor primary in the liver probably cannot be disproved. Intrahepatic primitive rhabdomyosarcoma may be the most probable explanation of some tumors falling in this category, but more definitive study of their nature is necessary.

RHABDOMYOSARCOMA. Both intrahepatic primary rhabdomyosarcoma and botryoid rhabdomyosarcoma of the larger (extrahepatic) bile ducts are known entities (Figs. 35–39). Except for differences in clinical picture (tumor mass versus obstructive jaundice) the distinction in primary sites does not seem very fundamental. The series shown in Table 3 illustrates the older age group and female preponderance of sarcoma botryoides of the extrahepatic bile ducts. Although all five patients with intra- or extrahepatic rhabdomyosarcoma are known to have died, it is of interest that only one, the only infant and only male in the group, had extraabdominal metastasis, so that curability of these rhabdomyosarcomas with newer methods of treatment, including appropriate chemotherapy, may well be significantly better than past data would suggest.

OTHER TUMORS OF THE LIVER

Table 5 presents a list, probably incomplete, of reported liver tumors, examples of which were not observed in this series of liver tumors in children. Several of the entities in this list merit comment:

ANGIOSARCOMA. One patient whose tumor may really have been an angiosarcoma is discussed above under the heading, "monotypic small-celled sarcoma." Industrial exposure to vinyl chloride has been reported to cause angiosarcoma of the liver in adults. The possibility that plastic umbilical vein catheters can induce angiomatous tumors of the liver in children has been raised but no supportive cases were found in this study.

CYSTADENOCARCINOMA. This term should be employed, as regards children, to designate apparent origin of an epithelial malignancy in a preexistent benign cystic hepatoblastoma (multilocular cyst). In the two patients listed in Table 4 under the heading "malignant cystic hepatoblastoma," the malignant component was stromal, not epithelial.

HEPATOMAS WITH APLASTIC ANEMIA AND FANCONI'S ANEMIA. Whether the occurrence of hepatomas in patients with bone marrow hypofunction results from treatment with androgenic steroids is uncertain.

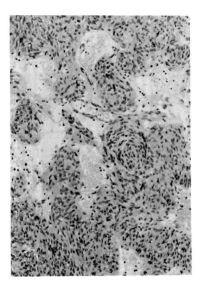

Figure 39 Gastric leiomyosarcoma metastatic to the liver in 12-3/12 year-old boy, showing the difference between the pattern of leiomyosarcoma, and that of rhabdomyosarcoma (cf. Figs. 35 and 38) (X 77).

Table 5   Reported Liver Tumors Not Observed in CHLA Series

Ameloblastoma, malignant
Angioma in Rendu-Osler-Weber disease
Angiosarcoma (see also Kupffer cell sarcoma)
   With vinyl chloride exposure
   With renal polycystosis
Bile duct adenoma
Carcinoid
Bile duct carcinoma (cholangiocarcinoma)
Choriocarcinoma
Cystadenocarcinoma
Fibroma
Fibromatosis
Fibrosarcoma
Follicular lymphoma
Ganglioneuroma
Hemangiopericytoma
Hepatoma with aplastic anemia
   With choledochal cyst
   Following neonatal hepatitis
   With Fanconi's anemia
   With hepatic veno-occlusive disease
   In renal transplant recipient
Kupffer cell sarcoma (hemangioendothelial sarcoma, angioblastic reticuloendothelioma, reticulum cell sarcoma; cf. similar tumors following thorotrast)
Leiomyoma
Leiomyosarcoma

Leiomyosarcoma of hepatic vein
  Of ligamentum teres
Lipoma
Liposarcoma
Malignant tumor with tuberose sclerosis
Melanoma, malignant
Mesothelioma
Mucoepidermoid carcinoma
Myelolipoma
Myxoma
Myxosarcoma
Neurofibroma
Osteogenic sarcoma
Plasmacytoma
Pseudocyst, traumatic
Pseudolipoma
Pseudotumoral granulomatous hepatitis (pseudotumoral sarcoidosis)
Squamous carcinoma arising in nonparasitic cyst
Teratoma, benign and malignant
Xanthofibrogranuloma

Interestingly, hepatoma has apparently not been observed in patients with chronic endogenous androgen overproduction from the adrenogenital syndrome.

HEPATOMAS WITH CHOLEDOCHAL CYST AND FOLLOWING NEONATAL HEPATITIS. If the suggestion that neonatal hepatitis, biliary atresia, and choledochal cyst are usually outcomes of the same basic process, "infantile obstructive cholangiopathy," is valid, occurrence of hepatoma in patients who survive long enough with or following any of these three disorders may be expected. One patient with biliary atresia who developed hepatoma is listed in Table 4.

KUPFFER CELL SARCOMA. The possibility that some malignant hepatoblastomas have a Kupffer cell component is discussed above. Other than this unproved possibility, no instance of definite hepatic origin of histiocytic lymphoma has been observed in the base population of this study.

LIPOMA AND LIPOSARCOMA. That some reports of these tumors may be based on hepatomas or hepatoblastomas with exceptionally high lipid content is mentioned above. Histochemical and ultrastructural

studies of such tumors are needed. The term pseudolipoma has been applied to masses of fatty tissue (omentum, appendix epiploica) adherent to the surface of the liver.

OSTEOGENIC SARCOMA. The frequent occurrence of osteoid, calcified or not, in malignant hepatoblastomas necessitates careful analysis of the cellular composition of any liver tumor before a definite diagnosis of osteogenic sarcoma can be maintained. The rarity of osteoid formation in metastases of osteoid-containing malignant hepatoblastomas suggests that the histologic features of metastatic lesions could be decisive.

TERATOMAS. As for osteogenic sarcoma, the presence of osteoid or bone in a liver tumor is not diagnostic of teratoma, and the presence of neural, respiratory tract, or other components seems necessary to establish the diagnosis of true teratoma primary in the liver.

Secondary manifestations of hepatic tumors are summarized in Table 6.

Congestive heart failure due to arterio-

Table 6   Reported Syndromes Secondary to Liver Tumor

With angiomas
  Afibrinogenemia
  Congestive heart failure
  Microangiopathic hemolytic anemia
  Triad syndrome

With hepatoblastomas, hepatomas, etc.
  Amenorrhea-galactorrhea
  Cystathioninuria
  Hypercalcemia
  Hypercholesterolemia
  Hyperlipemia
  Hypoglycemia
  Osteomalacia
  Polycythemia
  Sexual precocity (gonadotropin-producing
    tumors with virilization = hepatogenital
    syndrome)

venous shunting in angiomatous tumors is probably the most common secondary manifestation of liver tumors in children (three patients in the series reviewed). Hyperconsumption of blood cellular and clotting factor components by thrombosis in hemangiomas, with thrombocytopenia, angiopathic hemolytic anemia, hypofibrinogenemia, or combinations thereof, with or without bleeding tendency, can also be threats to life, or cause difficulty at surgery.

Cystathioninuria is not specific for hepatoblastomas, and is also relatively common in neuroblastoma, for instance. The mechanism of hyperlipemia and/or hypercholesterolemia, with lipid histiocytosis of the reticuloendothelial system, in some patients with hepatoblastoma is not known. Since the only patient with this phenomenon in the present series was the youngest, the idea that the lipidosis is not simply secondary to the tumor, but somehow the result of an independent primary property of the patients, seems tenable. Some patients reported as having Niemann-Pick disease in association with hepatic tumor appear to be examples of this phenomenon, and there is clearly no regular association of liver tumor with true Niemann-Pick disease.

Sexual precocity due to gonadotropin secretion by hepatoblastomas has been called the hepatogenital syndrome. The apparent limitation of this sexual precocity to males [4] recalls the pattern of precocity seen also with pineal tumors.

REFERENCES

1. Gall EA, Schiff L: *Tumors of the Liver.* In *Diseases of the Liver,* 2nd ed. Lippincott, Philadelphia and Montreal, 1963; Chapter 23, (pp 702–727).
2. Kidd P, Rosenberg HS: Vascular tumors of the liver. Abstracts, Interim Meeting of Pediatric Pathology Club, Houston, Texas Sept. 21-23, 1973.
3. Edmondson HA: Tumors of the liver and intrahepatic bile ducts. *Atlas of Tumor Pathology,* Section 7, fascicle 25. Armed Forces Institute of Pathology, Washington, D.C., 1958.
4. McArthur JW, Toll GD, Russfield AB, Reiss AM, Quinby WC, Baker WH: Sexual precocity attributable to ectopic gonadotropin secretion by hepatoblastoma. *Am J Med* **54**:390–403, 1973.
5. Ishak KG, Glunz PR: Hepatoblastoma and hepatocarcinoma in infancy and childhood. Report of 47 cases. *Cancer* **20**:396–422, 1967.

6. Willis RA: *The Pathology of the Tumours of Children.* Charles C. Thomas, Springfield, Ill., 1962, 200 pp (see especially p 59).

7. Garancis JC, Tang T, Panares R, Jurevics I: Hepatic adenoma. Biochemical and electron microscopic study. *Cancer* **24**:560–568, 1969.

8. Kissane JM, Smith MG: *Pathology of Infancy and Childhood.* CV Mosby Co., St. Louis, 1967, 1082 pp (see especially pp 279–284).

9. Sutton CA, Eller JL: Mesenchymal hamartoma of the liver. *Cancer* **22**:29–34, 1968.

10. Carter R: Hepatoblastoma in the adult. *Cancer* **23**:191–197, 1969.

11. Blumenfeld TA, Fleming ID, Johnson WW: Juvenile hemangioendothelioma of the liver. Report of a case and review of the literature. *Cancer* **24**:853–857, 1969.

12. Fraumeni JF, Rosen PJ, Hull EW, Barth FR, Shapiro SR, O'Connor JF: Hepatoblastoma in infant sisters. *Cancer* **24**:1086–1090, 1969.

13. Sotelo-Avila C, Gooch WM, III, Castro R: Neoplasms associated with Beckwith's syndrome. *Am J Pathol.* **78**:41a, 1975.

CHAPTER 11 CHOLANGIOCARCINOMA AND RELATED LESIONS

WATARU MORI, M.D.

KOU NAGASAKO, M.D.

Carcinomas of the biliary system, beginning at the bile ductule and ending at the papilla of Vater, can be classified into four large categories pathologically as well as clinically: (1) cholangiocarcinomas that arise from small radicles of intrahepatic bile ducts (peripheral type of bile-duct-cell carcinoma of Edmondson); (2) cholangiocarcinomas of the major intrahepatic bile ducts (including hilar type); (3) carcinomas of the extrahepatic bile duct (bile duct carcinoma); and (4) carcinomas of the papilla of Vater.

The first, peripheral cholangiocarcinoma, is a true primary hepatic cancer and occasionally resembles hepatocellular carcinoma (HCC) both in clinical signs produced and gross morphologic pattern to some extent. The second, the large duct or hilar cholangiocarcinoma, is also considered as a primary hepatic cancer by most workers; however, its character, especially clinically, is quite different if it arises at the hilum. The second, third, and fourth types, although relatively small carcinomas, cause symptoms early in the course of their

development because of their special or strategic location. Clinically the latter three show the same symptoms represented by biliary obstruction, jaundice. Hence cholangiocarcinomas of major intrahepatic bile ducts and carcinomas of extrahepatic bile ducts including that of Vater's papilla are often considered as peripapillary tumors in a broad sense of the word. Consequently some of these lesions are quite minute when found during operation or autopsy. In Thorbjarnarson's series the smallest lesion was 3×2 mm and was found in the main hepatic duct (1).

Histologically, there is no fundamental difference among carcinomas arising from the biliary tracts from intrahepatic small ducts to the papilla of Vater. Almost all of them are adenocarcinoma made up of cuboidal or columnar epithelium.

In the following description, we call the above numbered classification as follows: (1) peripheral and (2) large duct or hilar cholangiocarcinoma (often called cholangiocellular carcinoma in the past) and (3) peripapillary and (4) other extrahepatic bile duct carcinoma, or simply, bile duct carcinoma. Carcinomas arising from the gallbladder are omitted in this discussion, although carcinoma of the neck of the gallbladder often produces initial symptoms that result from spread of the tumor along the cystic artery to involve and occlude the hepatic ducts at the bifurcation. Rare carcinomas of the cystic duct may occlude the common bile duct. A subclass of the intrahepatic cholangiocarcinoma is a variously disputed carcinoma arising from the canal of Hering called cholangiolocellular carcinoma by Steiner and in the proposed classification of the World Health Organization (WHO).

Since the introduction of direct cholangiography (percutaneous transhepatic cholangiography and transendoscopic cholangiography) carcinomas along the biliary tract have become diagnosed rather easily, since the contrast agent comes in direct contact with the tumor. However, unfortunately, Renshaw's statement that "surgical treatment of malignant conditions of the biliary tract has not advanced proportionately with that of other parts of the upper abdomen" (2), made in 1922, still holds true today.

HISTORICAL REMARKS AND DEFINITION

Hanot and Gilbert (1888) originally expressed the opinion that primary liver cancer could be divided into carcinoma of the hepatic cells (cancer trabéculaire) and carcinoma of the bile duct (cancer alvéolaire) (3). In 1901 Eggel collected 162 cases of primary liver cancer from the literature and divided them into "carcinoma solidum" and "carcinoma adenomatosum" (4). In 1911 Goldzieher suggested that tumors that arise from hepatocytes be called "carcinoma hepatocellulaire" and that those that arise from epithelium of the smaller bile ducts be called "carcinoma cholangiocellulaire" (5). In the same year Yamagiwa described detailed morphology of primary hepatic carcinoma and advo-

cated the terms hepatoma and cholangioma (6). Since that time, these terms have been widely used throughout the world, especially in Japan. While many tumors fall into one or the other of these two classes, tumors of mixed structure also occur. Thus, while the distinction between hepatocellular carcinoma and cholangiocarcinoma is useful, it is not always an absolutely sharp one. Köhn considered all liver carcinomas to originate from a common pluripotential undifferentiated liver cell, and the morphology of the tumors is dependent on the influence of the environment (7). Observations in embryos revealed that cholangioles (canal of Hering) and ducts are both derived from the hepatic cells. Popper stresses, therefore, that all carcinomas revealing some hepatic cells can be considered a single entity, regardless of the presence of cholangiolar elements (8).

There is also confusion in terminology as to the relationship of cholangiocarcinoma with extrahepatic bile duct carcinoma. Hoyne excluded any tumors arising from the common hepatic duct, either external to the liver, at the porta hepatis, or in the short course of this duct within the anatomic confines of the liver itself, from the class of primary carcinomas of the liver. He believes that such tumors properly should be classified as "primary carcinoma of the hepatic duct." According to Hoyne, only carcinomas arising from bile ductules are called cholangiocarcinomas (9).

However, most workers define cholangiocarcinoma as a primary cancer of the liver originating from intrahepatic bile duct, including both small radicles and major branches. It usually has glandular structure, of cuboidal or columnar cells, and is often equipped with abundant stroma of connective tissue. Usually, cholangiocarcinomas have relatively little in common with hepatocellular carcinomas. They have far less definite association with cirrhosis (10–13), they do not have differences in frequency based on sex nor geographic ori-

Table 1   Incidence of Cholangiocarcinoma Among Primary Liver Cancer

Author	Autopsies Taken From	Total		Hepatoma	Cholangiocarcinoma		Others
		Number	%		Number	%	
Miyaji (18)	36,380	410	1.75	373	29	7.1	8
Cruickshank (19)		108		80	21	20.0	7
San Jose (16)		80		73	6	7.5	1
Edmondson (10)	48,900	100		75	25	25.0	
Tull (20)		134		102	32	24.0	
Hoye (9)	16,303	31	0.19	20	11		
MacDonald (12)	23,114	108	0.47	84	24		
Patton (21)	12,980	60	0.46	47	13		
Mori (13)	5,118	113	2.21				

gin, and they seem to arise from a single focus.

Cholangiocarcinomas resemble other glandular carcinomas of tubular origin in macro- and microscopic appearance. Cholangiocarcinoma should be diagnosed after careful exclusion of carcinoma arising in other parts of the body, especially in the extrahepatic bile ducts and gallbladder since almost 90% of the cancer involving the liver at the time of autopsy is metastatic (13). The chief distinguishing features of primary and metastic carcinoma are the nature of the tumor cells themselves, arrangement of tumor cells, and stromal pattern.

It has been found by critical study that intrahepatic bile duct carcinomas in pure form are less common than usually believed (8, 14–16). Carcinoma of the extrahepatic bile ducts is uncommon but not rare. The course of such carcinoma is rapid and dramatic because even a small lesion may completely obstruct the bile duct. Carcinomas of the extrahepatic bile ducts and the gallbladder are of common embryonic origin and have similar anatomic structure. Carcinoma of the papilla of Vater is sometimes excluded in reviews of statistics of carcinoma of the extrahepatic bile duct because of the difficulty of determining with certainty the exact site of origin (17).

CHOLANGIOCARCINOMA

Cholangiocarcinoma can also be termed cholangioma, intrahepatic bile duct carcinoma, and cholangiocellular carcinoma.

Incidence, Sex, and Age

The relative incidence of cholangiocarcinoma among primary liver cancer reported among autopsy cases ranges from about 5 to 30% (Table 1).

Like hepatocellular carcinoma, cholangiocarcinoma is a disease of older individuals. In Hoyne's series the average age of patients who died with cholangiocarcinoma was 56.9 years (9). In MacDonald's 24 cases of cholangiocarcinoma, the average age was 67 years (12). Patients with the disease under the age of 40 are rare.

Hepatocellular carcinoma seems to be predominantly a disease of men. In cholangiocarcinoma, however, no sex difference is stressed as in HCC. In Eggel's series, 57.1% of the cancers of the bile ducts (carcinoma adenomatosum) occurred in women (4). Six of the 11 cholangiocarcinomas of Hoyne's series (9) and 9 of 21 cholangiocarcinomas of Cruickshank's series (19) were found in women (Table 2).

Table 2
Sex Distribution of Cholangiocarcinoma

Author	Cholangiocarcinoma	Male	Female
Hoyne (9)	11	5	6
Cruickshank (19)	21	12	9
MacDonald (12)	24	13	11
Meyerowitz (22)	22	12	10

Pathogenesis

The etiology of cholangiocarcinoma is unknown. *Clonorchis sinensis* was proposed as influential in the genesis of cholangiocarcinoma by Hou (23). However, as Berman concluded, the significance of parasitic infection in the development of primary carcinoma of the liver is questionable (24). Certain pathologic conditions of the biliary tract are sometimes quoted to be responsible for the development of cholangiocarcinoma. Sane reported two cases in which cholangiocarcinoma was associated with hepatolithiasis, cholangitis, and cholelithiasis (25). Fried has suggested that the increased tendency toward formation of cholangiocarcinomas in women may be caused by the prevalence of infection of bile ducts followed by inflammatory hyperplasia of the smaller bile ducts (26). In Cruickshank's series, congenital cysts of the liver were found to be associated with cholangiocarcinomas in two women (19). Here again, the true causal relationship, if any, is obscure. Cholangiocarcinoma is only occasionally associated with cirrhosis. Even when accompanied by cirrhosis, it is often the obstructive (biliary) form (11). It is suspected that usually the fibrosis or "cirrhosis" follows rather than precedes the development of cholangiocarcinoma. The relationship of thorotrast to cholangiocarcinoma is discussed in Chapter 6 by Battifora.

Symptoms and Diagnosis

From the standpoint of symptoms, cholangiocarcinomas should be considered in terms of location—the peripheral form (bile-duct-cell carcinoma, Edmondson), which arises from small ducts, and the hilar form, which arises from larger ducts. Peripherally located cholangiocarcinomas lack early symptoms. They resemble HCC in many respects and preoperative, nonhistological differentiation from HCC or metastatic carcinoma may be impossible.

The symptoms of the peripheral cholangiocarcinoma are abdominal swelling and pain, weight loss, and jaundice. All these symptoms appear after the tumor has become enlarged. Jaundice was not noticed in five patients of Meyerowitz's series, in which the tumors were peripherally situated (22). Therefore, early diagnosis except by chance is nearly impossible. On the contrary, the main signs and symptoms of hilar cholangiocarcinoma are similar to those of extrahepatic bile duct carcinomas. Jaundice is usually the first sign and if not, it begins shortly after the onset of pain in the right upper quadrant. If cholangiocarcinomas exist at the junction of the right and left hepatic ducts within the liver, the appearance of jaundice is early. In such instances even a small tumor may cause jaundice and death of the patient (22). Hence the surgical exploration may be carried out early in the course of the disease (27). Later in the course of the disease, symptoms of malignancy such as anorexia, weight loss, fatigue, and weakness appear.

Cholangiography and, less often, hepatic angiography are helpful for diagnosis. Alpha fetoprotein (AFP) is not detectable in serum of patients with cholangiocarcinoma, and a positive correlation has not been found so far between hepatitis B surface antigen (HBsAg) and cholangiocarcinoma.

Gross appearance

Grossly, the livers involved by cholangiocarcinoma are usually enlarged

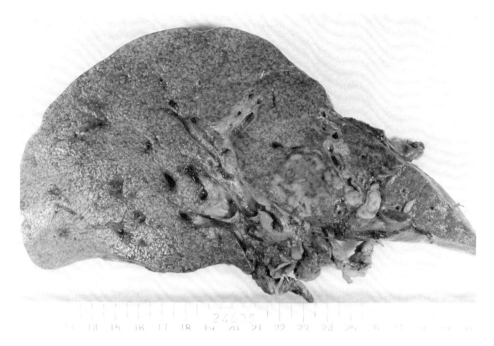

Figure 1 A nodular cholangiocarcinoma located at the root of the left hepatic lobe.

partly due to the tumor itself and partly due to hydrohepatosis or to associated cholangitis with or without abscess formation (Figs. 1 to 6). In Patton's data the average liver weight of a patient with a cholangiocarcinoma was 2677 g whereas a liver bearing HCC averages 2884 g (21). However, in some instances, especially in hilar cholangiocarcinomas, there may be no increase in the weight of the liver. The gross appearance of primary liver cancers was described by Eggel (1901) as massive, nodular, and diffuse. That classification has been applied both to HCC and peripheral cholangiocarcinomas.

Usually, cholangiocarcinomas are grayish white, firm, solid, and fibrous (Figs. 1 to 4). Cut surfaces usually are sclerotic, gray white or pale white tumor, with dense fibrous stranding. Sclerosis is frequently most marked in the central part of the tumors (Fig. 4). On occasion, when located in the hilar region, tumor fans out widely into the hepatic substance (Fig. 3). Sometimes daughter nodules are irregularly distributed throughout the liver. This form of tumor is not highly vascularized and hemorrhage from it is not a common event. Vessels are far less frequently invaded than in HCC, and portal thrombosis, when it does appear, is usually a result of secondary cholangitis and not tumor thrombosis. However, it is occasionally impossible to distinguish grossly between the two types of primary liver cancers, HCC, and peripheral cholangiocarcinoma, especially when there is no invasion of veins and no obvious bile secretion by the tumor (19).

Edmondson divided cholangiocarcinoma into bile-duct-cell carcinoma and hilar carcinoma on the basis of their gross appearances and location. Edmondson's concept of bile-duct-cell carcinomas was that they arose from smaller intrahepatic bile ducts. They were simply described as gray, white,

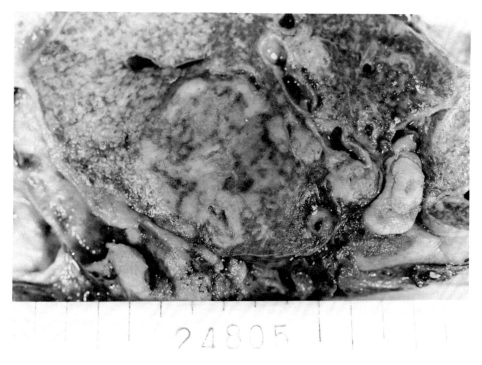

Figure 2 Higher magnification of the mass in Fig. 1, about 3 cm in diameter, showing early infiltration.

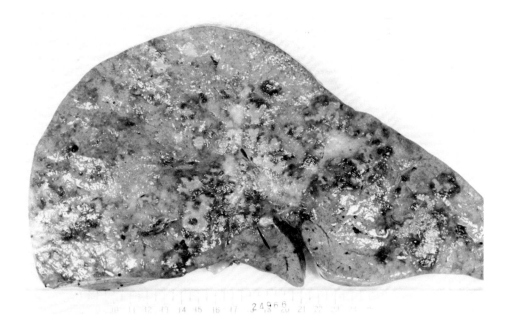

Figure 3 Cholangiocarcinoma arising at the hepatic hilum and infiltrating diffusely and rather extensively.

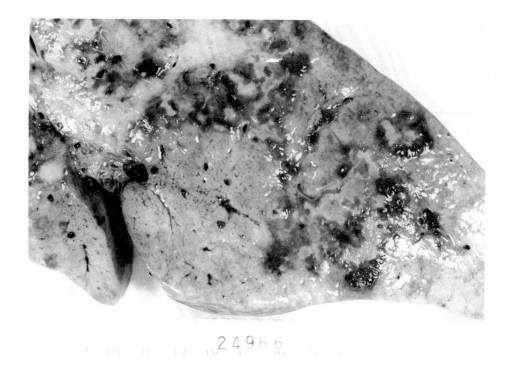

24966

Figure 4 Higher magnification of Fig. 3. Necrotizing tendency of the tumor is remarkable.

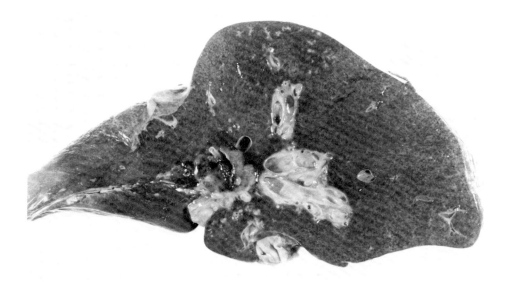

Figure 5 A walnut-sized, centrally necrotic cholangiocarcinoma at the junction of the right and left main bile ducts, causing marked dilatation of the intrahepatic bile ducts.

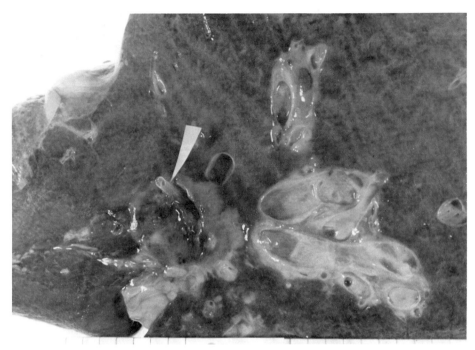

Figure 6   Higher magnification of Fig. 5. Cannula for drainage is indicated by the arrow.

or yellowish white and were usually firm. On the other hand, in hilar carcinomas, the bile ducts were obstructed at the hilum by a carcinoma and the intrahepatic branches were notably dilated. Biliary type of cirrhosis was present in six among seven in Edmondson's series. The growth of the carcinoma often obstructed the portal vein by constriction, but in no cases was the portal vein thrombosed (10). Many of the adenocarcinomas that involve the bifurcation of the hepatic duct resemble scars both grossly and microscopically, so that even if the tumor is found it may be mistaken for a benign stricture or localized form of sclerosing cholangitis (27).

Klatskin further divided hilar cholangiocarcinomas into three types: (1) a firm, intramural, annular fibrous collar or nodules encircling and constricting the hepatic duct; (2) a bulky hard mass, centered on and extending deep into the parenchyma; and (3) a spongy, friable mass within the bile duct lumen (27).

The surrounding liver is smooth and usually noncirrhotic but may be deeply stained with bile, a feature contrasting with the tumor itself which is not pigmented. Bile stasis of this order occurs only when the tumor, by reason of its location, obstructs major ducts, and sometimes results in biliary type of cirrhosis. Signs of cholangitis may accompany the tumor.

Histology and Differential Diagnosis

Cholangiocarcinomas have a tubular (Figs. 7 and 8) or acinar structure resembling those of adenocarcinomas of the extrahepatic bile ducts. The cell type is cuboidal or columnar as a rule. The nucleus is smaller and less variable in size than those of HCC. The cytoplasm is usually clear but sometimes granular. Mucus secretion is sometimes found (Fig. 9), but there is no

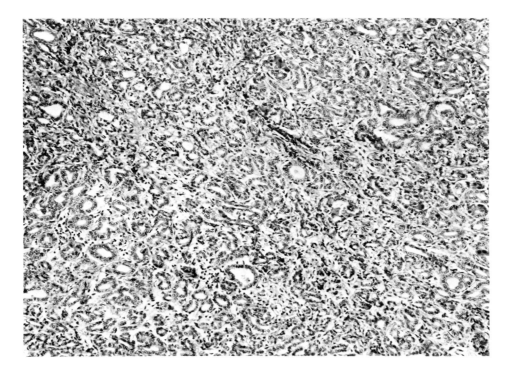

Figure 7 Cholangiocarcinoma (histologically tubular adenocarcinoma). The cells are low cuboidal in type. The stroma is rather meager for this type of carcinoma.

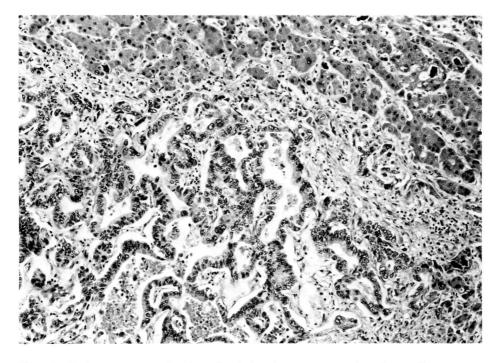

Figure 8 Cholangiocarcinoma (histologically tubular adenocarcinoma). The cells are tall columnar. Normal hepatic tissue with bile thrombi is seen in the upper part of the photo.

235

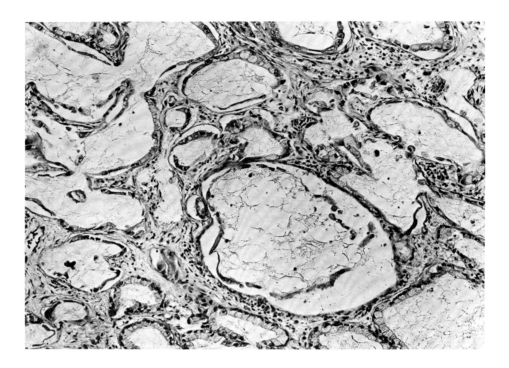

Figure 9 Cholangiocarcinoma (histologically scirrhous adenocarcinoma) with a large amount of fibrous stroma.

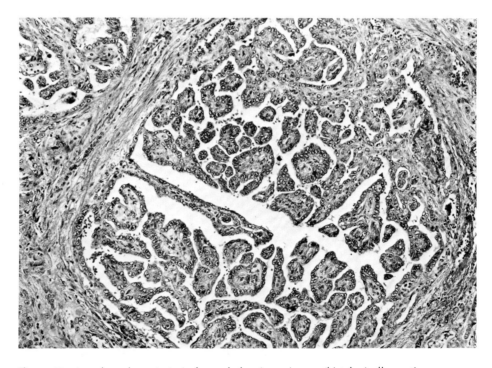

Figure 10 Lymph node metastasis from cholangiocarcinoma (histologically cystic adenocarcinoma). The cells are mucin-producing clear type and the glands are filled with mucin.

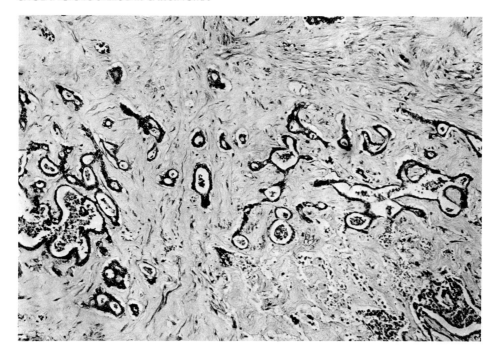

Figure 11   Cholangiocarcinoma (histologically papillary adenocarcinoma).

bile production. Occasionally cholangiocarcinoma of larger hepatic duct branches are papillary (Fig. 10).

The tumor cells provoke a variable desmoplastic reaction. The tumor masses, therefore, most often lie in a connective tissue stroma, giving much more scirrhous features than does HCC. But the degree of desmoplastic reaction among the cholangiocarcinomas varies considerably (Figs. 7 and 11), as among HCC. Most cholangiocarcinomas are well differentiated adenocarcinomas, but undifferentiated forms do occur (Figs. 12 and 13). It is often impossible to histologically distinguish cholangiocarcinomas from carcinomas of the extrahepatic bile ducts and other adenocarcinomas that have metastasized to the liver; thus it is always necessary to exclude the possibility of extrahepatic point of origin.

The liver bearing a hilar cholangiocarcinoma shows typical appearance of biliary obstruction, the predominant features being moderate to marked bile stasis, portal fibrosis, ductal proliferation, and a periportal inflammatory reaction with varying proportions of neutrophils, eosinophils, and mononuclear cells. It is not rare to see signs of chronic inflammation along the intrahepatic bile ducts, particularly in hilar carcinomas, but also in cholangiocarcinomas.

CHOLANGIOLOCELLULAR CARCINOMA (STEINER, HIGGINS, WORLD HEALTH ORGANIZATION)

Cholangioles (canal of Hering) are the terminal ramifications of the bile duct tree that connect the interlobular ducts, which are the smallest elements still within the portal areas at the lobular level, and the

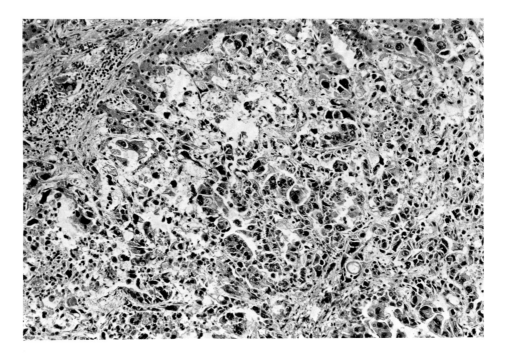

Figure 12 Cholangiocarcinoma (histologically poorly differentiated adenocarcinoma). Pleomorphism of tumor cells is marked. Atrophic hepatic cords are noted at the margin of the tumor.

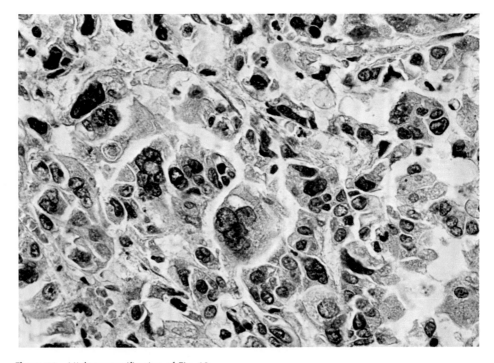

Figure 13 Higher magnification of Fig. 12.

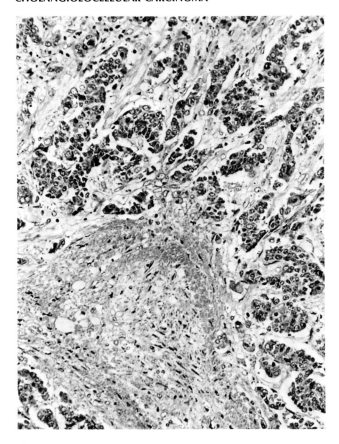

Figure 14 Cholangiolocellular carcinoma. Note the solid cords of primitive cells resembling cholangioles. Courtesy of Dr. R. L. Peters.

canaliculi of the hepatic cords. Cholangioles may be recognized as rare rosettes of 3 to 4 ductlike cells, each with scanty clear cyoplasm but with small oval nuclei. They are located just outside or at the level of the limiting plate of the portal area. One may hunt through several sections to find a single cholangiole. Embryologically the cholangioles develop from the same anlage as the hepatic cells, but they show cytologic differences from the liver cells as well as from the cells of the interlobular bile ducts (8). Steiner and Higgins proposed the term cholangiolocellular carcinoma as a special type of primary liver carcinoma arising from cholangioles (14). The

tumor is noncharacteristic in its gross appearance. The most characteristic microscopic feature of cholangiolocellular carcinoma, according to Steiner, is the tendency for the neoplastic cells to be arranged in small cords (Fig. 14). The individual tumor cells resemble strikingly the epithelial cells of the cholangioles.

Cholangiolocellular carcinomas might be considered as a subgroup of the HCC (8, 18), and it seems evident that they are not actually different from the cholangiomatous part of the mixed type. Histogenesis cannot be stated with certainty, and it would be unwise to regard them as necessarily arising from the cholangioles simply

Table 3   Microscopic differences between hepatocellular carcinoma and cholangiocarcinoma

	Hepatocellular Carcinoma	Cholangiocarcinoma
Arrangement of cells	Arranged in cords (simulate lobules of hepatic tissue); sometimes rosettelike structure	Tubuloalveolar structure
Cells		
Shape	Polygonal and polyhedral	Cuboidal or columnar
Cytoplasm	Acidophilic	Clear, somewhat basophilic
Nucleus	Large, round, vesicular; often contain multiple nucleoli	Small and hyperchromatic
Stroma	Capillary stroma	Connective tissue stroma
Bile secretion	+	−

because of their morphologic similarity.

Mixed types of primary hepatic carcinoma

Primary hepatic carcinomas containing elements of both HCC and cholangiocarcinoma constitute about 4% of primary carcinomas of the liver (28). Popper, however, has maintained that careful study will reveal some ductule forms in most HCC and some hepatic type of cells in most of the cholangiocarcinomas (8). Not only do liver cells and small bile ducts have a common origin, but the ability of each type of cell to form the other is maintained and is exhibited in hepatic regeneration as well as neoplasia. Allen and Lisa noted that three patterns of mixed types of primary hepatic carcinoma may occur: (1) separate tumors, each of which is composed of only one type of cell; (2) contiguous tumors, each of which is a different cell type and which may mingle as they grow; and (3) individual lesions that have both types of cells so intimately associated that they can only be interpreted as arising from the same site (29). Edmondson suggested that hepatobiliary carcinoma was a fitting name for this group (10).

Differential Diagnosis

Grossly, distinction between HCC and cholangiocarcinoma is sometimes difficult, and final diagnosis must be made histologically. Findings of the surrounding liver parenchyma, including an association of hepatic cirrhosis, the degree of portal vein invasion by the tumor, and alpha fetoprotein test even with the serum collected at the time of autopsy are helpful in such instances. According to Hoyne, four important features are pointed out for distinguishing between cholangiocarcinoma and HCC microscopically (Table 3) (9).

Since the histologic resemblance to tumors of extrahepatic bile duct, gallbladder, or pancreatic origin, and indeed to those arising in other portions of the alimentary tract may be striking, a distinction between cholangiocarcinoma and tumors metastatic from one of the above extrahepatic sites often cannot be made on histologic grounds alone. Very careful gross examination of the rest of the body may provide best assurance of the diagnosis of peripheral cholangiocarcinoma.

Metastasis

Peripheral cholangiocarcinomas as a rule metastasize earlier and more frequently than do HCC (9). Intrahepatic metastases and secondary growth to the extrahepatic biliary tracts often occur. Cholangiocarcinomas often spread towards the bed of the gallbladder. In some cases it may be very difficult to differentiate between cholangiocarcinoma and primary cancer of the gallbladder. Metastasis through the lymphatics to the hilar and peripancreatic nodes occur in about one-half of the cases, and this is the usual method of spread. Blood stream spread is rare compared with that of HCC.

In Cruickshank's 17 patients, lymph node involvement was noted in 9. Other organs involved are as follows: adrenals in 7, lungs in 3, diaphragm in 2, pleura in 2, peritoneum in 2, bone in 2, and kidney in 1 (19). In Patton's 13 cases lymph nodes were involved in 9 cases, lungs in 7, bones in 6, peritoneum in 6, spleen in 5, adrenals in 4, and kidneys in 2.

Prognosis

Early diagnosis of peripheral cholangiocarcinoma is difficult, and its prognosis is poor. If there is jaundice, cure by surgery is most unlikely. The proximity of the vital structures permits the tumors to grow to an inoperable state in a short period of time, usually before the onset of symptoms. Occasionally patients diagnosed while still preicteric can undergo resection of the tumor successfully.

The average survival after appearance of jaundice, in Meyerowitz's series, was 11 months, ranging from 1 to 43 months (22). Some of the patients with cholangiocarcinoma are said to have survived for as long as 5 years (30), but such survivals are principally in patients with hilar cholangiocarcinoma. The prognosis depends, largely, on whether the tumor is hilar and remains localized in the form of a stricture producing biliary obstruction and liver failure over a long period, or whether it is peripheral, spreads diffusely along the bile duct with rapid dissemination via the blood stream, and causes fatal carcinomatosis (22).

CARCINOMA OF THE EXTRAHEPATIC BILE DUCT

Incidence, Age, and Sex

Sako (31) quoted an incidence of 0.012% (32) to 0.458% (33) in autopsy material collected from the literature. Operative incidence has been reported as 0.5% (34) to 1.4% (33) of all operation on the biliary tree.

The majority of patients are between 50 and 70 years of age (31, 36). The age ranged from 70 to 89 in reported series. Gray recorded an average age incidence of 59.2 years (37), and Sako reported 59.2 years (31).

Men are slightly more often affected than women. The incidence was 58% in Judd's series, 61% in Gray's series, and about 60% in Sako's series. This is almost the same sex distribution as that of cholangiocarcinoma, and in marked contrast to carcinoma of the gallbladder, which occurs in women far more frequently than men (Table 4).

Table 4   Sex incidence of extrahepatic bile duct carcinomas

	Male	Female	Total
Judd (35)	58	42	100
Rolleston (38)	55	35	90
Devic (31)	30	16	46
Sako (36)	106	75	181

However, considering the much greater prevalance of other cancers from the gastrointestinal tract in men, carcinoma of the extrahepatic bile duct could still be called a cancer with considerably relative predilection to develop in women.

Pathogenesis

Cholelithiasis and associated chronic inflammation are most frequently referred to as causative factors of extrahepatic bile duct carcinoma. The rate of concommitant occurrence of cholelithiasis is 20.2% in Stewart's series (39), 38.7% in Sako's series (31), and 41.3% in Kuwayti's series (17). However, correlation at the level seen between gall stones and gallbladder carcinomas (64.6%) (40) is not evident with extrahepatic bile duct malignancies.

Clonorchis sinensis was thought to be an important etiologic agent. Under certain conditions, secretion of carcinogenic agents into the bile has been considered too, but definite proof is lacking so far (41).

The relation to benign papilloma or papillomatosis of the bile duct, sometimes with the possibility of multicentricity of cancer development, has also been discussed (42, 43).

Clinical Feature and Diagnosis

The diagnosis of carcinoma of the extrahepatic biliary tract is rarely confirmed during life without surgical exploration (46, 47); thus the diagnosis is seldom made prior to the onset of jaundice.

Due to the location of tumor, jaundice is of early onset and is progressive. The degree and rapidity of onset of the jaundice depend on the rate at which the bile ducts are occluded. Thus the typical and essential symptom of carcinoma of the biliary tract is gradually increasing and unremitting obstructive jaundice, associated with acholic stools, dark urine, and pruritus. Jaundice may or may not be accompanied by epigastric pain. In patients with long-standing disease, hepatomegaly ensues together with dilatation of bile duct and, in the carcinoma of the distal duct, the gallbladder may become markedly dilated (Courvoisier's sign). Later many nonspecific symptoms appear that are attributable to carcinoma.

Brunschwig, however, points out that carcinoma arising in the extrahepatic bile ducts may infiltrate along the wall of the ducts and not form a localized obstructing mass; consequently, an advanced stage of the disease may be attained before jaundice is found (44).

Laboratory tests are the reflection of obstructive jaundice, such as high serum levels of bilirubin and alkaline phosphatase activity. Nonspecific hepatic injury can also be detected.

Recently, accurate clinical diagnosis using radiological methods has become possible. Percutaneous transhepatic cholangiography and endoscopic cholangiography point out exactly the site and nature of the obstructive jaundice.

Site of Origin

The most frequent primary site for carcinomas of extrahepatic bile ducts is the common hepatic or common bile duct. However, because of extensive growth involving adjacent structures, the exact site of origin of the tumor in many instances cannot be identified (51), especially in advanced cases (Table 5 and Fig. 15).

Table 5   Relative frequency of primary sites of extrahepatic bile duct carcinoma

| | Total Cases | Location Distribution* | | | | |
		A	B	C	D	E
Kuwayti (17)	63	6	15	8	11	23
Thorbjarnarson (48)	31	2	9	3	7	10
Clement (50)	37	1	16	3	8	9
Van Heerden (36)	78	11	26	4		24
Kasai	27	0	8	0	5	14
Total	236	20	74	18	44	80
Incidence (%)		8.5	31.4	7.6	18.6	33.9

*See Fig. 15.

Gross findings

In general, the carcinomas arising proximally in the biliary tract are said to grow rather slowly. The gross pathologic findings of the tumor can be classified as follows: (*a*) nodular lesion (Figs. 5 and 6);

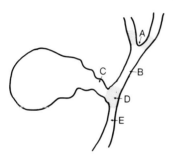

Figure 15 Diagram of the extrahepatic biliary tree to indicate areas of relative frequency of carcinoma. (See Table 5.)

(*b*) papillary lesion (Fig. 10); and (*c*) diffusely infiltrating lesion (Figs. 3 and 4) (51).

Most commonly, the lesion is a circumscribed, firm, grayish tan nodule (31), namely, a nodular lesion. The growth usually involves the whole thickness of the wall. In some cases the carcinomas encircle the wall, forming an annular stricture. Stenosis of varying degrees or complete obstruction of the lumen eventually occurs. Below the tumor the ducts are collapsed and the mucosa lacks the usual bile stain. Above the obstructing tumor the ducts are dilated, sometimes to several times normal diameter.

Less commonly, a papillomatous growth is observed (Fig. 10). Papillary lesions generally invade the wall only superficially. The patient may be asymptomatic for a considerable period, and sometimes the tumor may cause intermittent symptoms of obstruction. There is no particular segment of the ducts that is specifically selective for a single type of tumor (35).

Histology

Almost all the carcinomas of the extrahepatic biliary passage are adenocarcinoma. Some are papillary adenocarcinomas. Squamous cell carcinoma has been reported by some (31), and a rare mixed form is called adenoacanthoma. The lining cells of tubules of adenocarcinoma are cuboidal of columnar and are in various stages of differentiation, but usually are moderately well differentiated. The numbers of mitotic figures correlates with the degree of anaplasia. Desmoplastic reaction and formation of scirrhous lesion are the rule. The amount of fibrous stroma, however, varies greatly from case to case.

Metastasis

Early metastasis occurs mainly in bulky medullary-type lesions of papillary tumor. The small scirrhous tumors tend to metastasize late (50). Ordinarily, generalized extensive spread is rare (39, 52). The most common site of metastasis is the liver, followed by the regional lymph nodes, the pancreas, and the peritoneum. Invasion of nerves and perineural lymphatics is stressed (1, 17, 10, 34), as often seen with carcinoma of the pancreas.

Sometimes, the pattern of the tumor spread reflects no tendency to spread locally before metastasizing to the regional lymph nodes. In three of Judd's cases there were metastases in the regional lymph nodes and to the peritoneum, with no evidence of the involvement of the structures immediately adjacent to the bile ducts. Thorbjarnarson (1) found no metastases at the time of operation or autopsy in 57% of his cases; however, there is an opinion that there is no difference in the survival time between patients with and without metastases (35).

The incidence of metastasis is roughly proportionate to the degree of anaplasia. Neither of Kuwayti's two patients with grade 1 carcinoma had any metastasis while the two with grade 4 carcinoma did have metastases (17).

CARCINOMA OF THE AMPULLA OF VATER (PERIPAPILLARY TUMOR IN THE STRICT SENSE)

In most instances it is impossible to determine accurately the origin of the carcinoma of and around the ampulla. Cooper reported that in early cases the site of origin may be one of the following tissues (53).

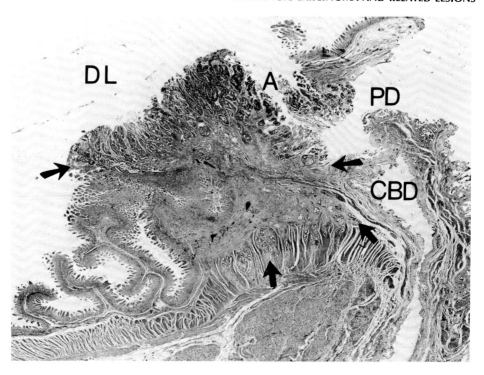

Figure 16 Carcinoma of the ampulla of Vater. Even though small, it is difficult to be certain of origin. This appears to arise from ampullary epithelium (type 1). CBD, common bile duct entrance; PD, pancreatic duct entrance; A, ampulla; DL, duodenal lumen; arrows, margins of tumor infiltration. Courtesy of Dr. R. L. Peters.

1. Epithelium lining the ampulla of Vater (when an ampulla is present).

2. Duodenal epithelium of the periampullary region or the duodenal papilla.

3. Epithelium of the terminal common duct.

4. Epithelium of the terminal pancreatic duct.

5. Aberrant pancreatic tissue.

Of the above, 1, 3, and 4 might be considered as extrahepatic bile duct carcinomas from the viewpoint of histogenesis. However, as mentioned above, it is difficult to determine the exact site of origin in many cases (Fig. 16). Therefore, they are usually gathered together and discussed as peripapillary tumors.

Duodenal epithelium of the periampullary region is probably the most common site of origin. Half the cases in the literature were believed to have arisen from this point. Carcinomas of the ampulla of Vater may be divided grossly into papillary and ulcerating tumors with variations between two extremes; papillary tumors are rather predominant (53). Pancreatic invasion was present in 13 among 37 cases, and it had an excellent correlation to tumor size (54).

Clinically, obstructive jaundice occurs early in the course of illness, when a decision is required whether to do a laparotomy. Recently, it has become possible to observe the ampulla of Vater directly by duodenal endoscopy, so that even a small carcinoma of that area can be observed and confirmed histologically by biopsy.

REFERENCES

1. Thorbjarnarson B: Carcinoma of the bile duct. *Cancer* **12**:708–713, 1959.

2. Renshaw K: Malignant neoplasms of the extrahepatic biliary ducts. *Ann Surg* **76**:205–221, 1922.

3. Hanot VC, Gilbert A: *Etudes sur les Maladies du Foie; Cancer (Epitheliome), Sarcome; Melanomes; Ystes Non Parasitaires; Angiomes.* Asselin & Houzeau, Paris, 1888.

4. Eggel H: Ueber das primäre Carcinoma der Leber. *Beitr Pathol Anat Allg Pathol* **30**:506–604, 1901.

5. Goldzieher M, ven Bokay Z: Der primäre Leberkrebs. *Virchows Arch Pathol Anat* **203**:75–131, 1911.

6. Yamagiwa K. Zur Kenntnis des primären parenchymatösen Leberkarzinoms (Hepatoma). *Virchows Arch Pathol Anat* **206**:437–467, 1911.

7. Köhn K: *Der primäre Leberkrebs.* Springer, Berlin, 1955.

8. Popper H, Schaffner F: Primary hepatic carcinoma. In *Liver: Structure and Function.* Popper H, Schaffner F (Eds). Blakiston, New York, 1957, pp 593–612.

9. Hoyne RM, Kernohan JW: Primary carcinoma of the liver: A study of 31 cases. *Arch Intern Med* **79**:532–554, 1947.

10. Edmondson HA, Steiner PE: Primary carcinoma of the liver: A study of 100 cases among 48,900 necropsies. *Cancer* **7**:462–503, 1954.

11. Gall A: Primary and metastatic carcinoma of the liver. Relationship to hepatic cirrhosis. *Arch Pathol* **70**:226–232, 1960.

12. MacDonald RA: Cirrhosis and primary carcinoma of the liver: Changes in their occurrence at the Boston City Hospital 1897–1954. *New Engl J Med* **255**:1179–1183, 1956.

13. Mori W: Cirrhosis and primary cancer of the liver-comparative study in Tokyo and Cincinnati. *Cancer* **20**:627–631, 1967.

14. Steiner PE, Higginson J: Cholangiolocellular carcinoma of the liver. *Cancer* **12**:753–759, 1959.

15. Ohlsson EG, Norden JG: Primary carcinoma of the liver. A study of 121 cases. *Acta Pathol Microbiol Scand* **64**:430–440, 1965.

16. San Jose D, Cady A, West M, et al: Primary carcinoma of the liver, analysis of clinical and biochemical features of 80 cases. *Am J Dig Dis* **10**:657–673, 1965.

17. Kuwayti K, Baggenstoss AH, Stauffer MH, et al: Carcinoma of major intrahepatic and extrahepatic bile ducts exclusive of papilla of Vater. *Surg Gynecol Obstet* **104**:657–673, 1965.

18. Miyaji T, Imai S: Pathological studies on 639 cases of hepatoma autopsies in Japan during the 10 years from 1946 to 1955 inclusive. *Acta Hepatol Jap* **1**:100–102, 1960.

19. Cruickshank AH: The pathology of 111 cases of primary hepatic malignancy collected in the Liverpool region. *J Clin Pathol* **14**:120–131, 1961.

20. Tull JC: Primary carcinoma of the liver: A study of one hundred and thirty-four cases. *J Pathol Bact* **35**:557–562, 1932.

21. Patton RB, Horn RC Jr: Primary liver carcinoma. Autopsy study of 60 cases. *Cancer* **17**:757–768, 1964.

22. Meyerowitz BR, Aird I: Carcinoma of the hepatic ducts within the liver. *Brit J Surg* **50**:178, 184, 1962.

23. Hou PC: The relationship between primary carcinoma of the liver and infestation with *Clonorchis sinensis. J Pathol Bact* **72**:239–246, 1956.

24. Berman C: *Primary Carcinoma of the Liver.* Lewis, London, 1951.

25. Sane S, MacCallum JD: Primary carcinoma of the liver: Cholangioma in hepatolithiasis. *Am J Pathol* **18**:675–687, 1942.

26. Fried BM: Primary carcinoma of the liver. *Am J Med Sci* **168**:241–267, 1924.

27. Klatskin GK: Adenocarcinoma of the hepatic duct at its bifurcation within the porta hepatis. *Am J Med* **38**:241–256, 1965.

28. Higgins GK: The pathologic anatomy of primary hepatic tumors. In: Recent Results in Cancer Research: Tumors of the liver. Springer, Berlin, 1970.

29. Allen RA, Lisa JR: Combined liver cell and bile duct carcinoma. *Am J Pathol* **25**:647–655, 1949.

30. Altemeier WA, Gall EA, Zinninger MM, et al: Sclerosing carcinoma of the major intrahepatic bile ducts. *Arch Surg* **75**:450–460, 1957.

31. Sako K, Seitzinger GL, Garside E: Carcinoma of extrahepatic bile ducts; review of literature and report of 6 cases. *Surgery* **41**:416–437, 1957.

32. Bolli C: Per 1 anatomia patologica delle vie biliari estraepatiche. *Lav Ist Anat Istol Pathol Perugia* **5**:5–45, 1946.

33. Masuda KI: Ueber extrahepatale primäre Krebs der Gallengänge mit besonderer Berücksichtigung ihrer Infiltration in die Nervenzweige. *Trans Soc Pathol Jap* **25**:753–756, 1935.

34. Neibling HA, Dockerty MB, Wargh JM: Carcinoma of extrahepatic ducts. *Surg Gynecol Obstet* **89**:429–438, 1949.

35. Judd ES, Gray HK: Carcinoma of the gall bladder and bile ducts. *Surg Gynecol Obstet* **55**:308–315, 1932.

36. van Heerden JA, Judd ES, Dockerty MB: Carcinoma of the extrahepatic bile ducts. *Am J Surg* **13**:49–55, 1967.

37. Gray HK, Sharpe WS: Carcinoma of the gall bladder, extrahepatic bile ducts, and major duo-

denal papilla. *S Clin North Am* **21**:1117–1127, 1941.

38. Rolleston H, McNee JW: *Diseases of the Liver, Gall-Bladder and Bile-Ducts*, 3rd ed. Macmillan, London, 1929, pp 489–504.

39. Stewart HL, Lieber MM, Morgan DR: Carcinoma of the extrahepatic bile ducts. *Arch Surg* **41**:662–713, 1940.

40. Jones CJ: Carcinoma of the gallbladder, a clinical and pathologic analysis of fifty cases. *Ann Surg* **132**:110–120, 1950.

41. Steiner PE: A carcinogenic extract from human bile and gallbladders. *Proc Soc Exp Biol Med* **51**:362–383, 1942.

42. Dick JC: Carcinoma of the lower end of the common bile duct. *Brit J Surg* **26**:757–763, 1939.

43. Zenker H: Der primäre Krebs der Gallenblase und seine Beziehung zu Gallensteinen und Gallenblasennarben. *Dtsch Arch Klin Med* **44**:159–184, 1888.

44. Okinaka S, Nakao K, Ibayashi H, et al: A case report of the development of biliary tract carcinoma 11 years after the injection of Thorotrast. *Am J Roentgenol* **78**:812–818, 1957.

45. Roberts JC Jr, Carlson KF: Hepatic duct carcino-

ma 17 years after the injection of thorium dioxide. *AMA Arch Pathol* **62**:1–7, 1956.

46. Jackson CE, Caylor HD: Adenocarcinoma of the common bile duct with resection, anastomosis of the hepatic to the cystic duct and cholecystogastrostomy. *Am J Surg* **71**:696–701, 1946.

47. Thorbjarnarson B: Carcinoma of the intrahepatic bile ducts. *Arch Surg* **77**:908–917, 1958.

48. Thorbjarnarson B, Glenn F: Carcinoma of the gallbladder. *Cancer* **12**:1009–1015, 1959.

49. Brunschwig A, Bigelow RR: Advanced carcinoma of the extrahepatic bile ducts. *Ann Surg* **122**:522–528, 1945.

50. Clemett AR: Carcinoma of the major bile duct. *Radiology* **84**:894–903, 1965.

51. Cohn EM: *Tumors of the Gallbladder and Bile Duct*. In *Gastroenterology*, Vol 3. Bockus HL (Ed). Saunders, Philadelphia, 1965, pp 811–826.

52. Redmond AD, Majeranowski JF: Systemic spread of cystic duct carcinoma. *Ann Intern Med* **40**:632–640, 1954.

53. Cooper WA: Carcinoma of the ampulla of Vater. *Ann Surg* **106**:1009–1034, 1937.

54. Moody F, Thorbjarnarson B: Carcinoma of the ampulla of Vater. *Am J Surg* **107**:572–579, 1964.

CHAPTER 12 MESENCHYMAL TUMORS OF THE LIVER

KAMAL G. ISHAK, M.D., Ph.D.

INTRODUCTION

With the exception of the cavernous hemangioma, mesenchymal tumors of the liver are exceptionally rare. Many are discovered incidentally at autopsy or at the time of exploration of the abdomen for an unrelated condition. Some lead to an acute abdomen from rupture, others produce symptoms due to pressure on adjacent organs and viscera while still others may be manifested by signs and symptoms related to complicating factors (e.g., hypoglycemia, congestive heart failure, blood coagulation abnormalities, etc.). Only one tumor, the malignant hemangioendothelioma (angiosarcoma), often produces signs and symptoms (e.g., jaundice, hepatomegaly, ascites, abnormalities of tests of hepatic function, etc.) pointing to the liver as the seat of the patient's illness. While the majority of the mesenchymal tumors of the liver in the past have remained undiagnosed until the time of laparatomy or necropsy, improve-

ments and refinements of diagnostic (particularly radiographic) technics now facilitate earlier and more accurate diagnoses.

The following account of mesenchymal tumors of the liver is based on a review of the literature and the experience of the author with examples in the files of the Armed Forces Institute of Pathology (AFIP). The methodology for the special stains referred to in the text or legends to the illustrations follows that of the "Manual of Histologic Staining Methods of the Armed Forces Institute of Pathology"(1).

CLASSIFICATION

The following classification of mesenchymal tumors of the liver is based on the World Health Organization monograph "Histological Typing of Soft Tissue Tumours" published in 1969(2).

I. TUMORS OF FIBROUS TISSUE
   A. Benign
      1. Fibroma
   B. Malignant
      1. Fibrosarcoma

The opinions and assertions contained herein are the private views of the author and are not to be construed as official or as reflecting the views of the Department of the Army or of Defense.

II. TUMORS OF ADIPOSE TISSUE
   A. Benign
      1. Lipoma
      2. Myelolipoma
      3. Angiomyolipoma
      4. Hibernoma
   B. Malignant
      1. Liposarcoma

III. TUMORS OF MUSCLE TISSUE
   A. Benign
      1. Leiomyoma
      2. Epithelioid leiomyoma
   B. Malignant
      1. Leiomyosarcoma
      2. Rhabdomyosarcoma

IV. TUMORS OF BLOOD VESSELS
   A. Benign
      1. Hemangioma
      2. Infantile hemangioendothelioma
   B. Malignant
      1. Malignant hemangioendothelioma

V. TUMORS AND TUMORLIKE LESIONS OF LYMPH VESSELS

VI. TUMORS OF MESOTHELIAL TISSUES
   A. Benign
      1. Benign mesothelioma
   B. Malignant
      1. Malignant mesothelioma

VII. TUMORS OF PLURIPOTENTIAL MESENCHYME (MESENCHYMOMAS)
   A. Benign
      1. Benign mesenchymoma
   B. Malignant
      1. Malignant mesenchymoma

VIII. TUMORS OF DISPUTED OR UNCERTAIN HISTOGENESIS
   A. Benign
      1. Granular cell tumor
      2. Myxoma
   B. Malignant

TUMORS OF FIBROUS TISSUE

Benign

Fibroma

Edmondson(3) discusses fibrous tumors of the liver under the category of "fibromatosis." Both cases illustrated in the Armed Forces Institute of Pathology Fascicle "Tumors of the Liver and Intrahepatic Bile Ducts" appear to represent low-grade fibrosarcomas. Reference is made by Edmondson to three fibromas published in the literature, but I have not had an opportunity of reviewing them.

There are two fibromas of the liver in the AFIP files. One occurred in a 62-year-old male patient whose only complaint was that of progressive enlargement of the abdomen. At the time of laparotomy a large tumor was shelled out of the left lobe of the liver. It measured 24 cm in diameter and weighed 2280 g. Grossly the tumor had a knobby surface and was encapsulated (Fig. 1). It was very firm in consistency and showed a bulging ivory-white cut surface which was roughly textured with occasional whorls. Microscopically the tumor consisted largely of interlacing bundles of fibroblasts and collagen (Figs. 2 and 3): the latter stained intensely blue with the Masson trichrome. Silver stains showed a prominent pattern of reticulin fibers generally running parallel to the cells and collagen bundles. Nuclei of the fibroblasts were elongated with tapered ends and showed no pleomorphism; no mitotic figures were seen in multiple sections examined from different parts of the tumor (Fig. 2).

The second patient was a 62-year-old Caucasian female who complained of abdominal enlargement and occasional fleeting abdominal pain. By palpation a large mass was found occupying the right upper and lower quadrants of the abdomen. A cholecystogram revealed a large homogeneous soft tissue tumor density in the right half of the abdomen. At the time of lapar-

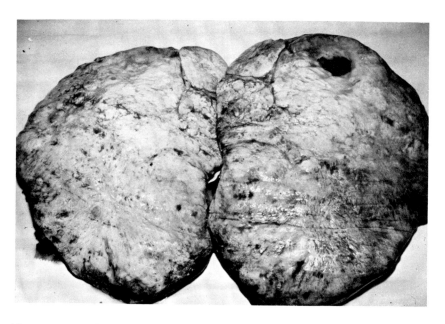

Figure 1   Gross photograph of transected fibroma of liver (AFIP Neg 74-12902).

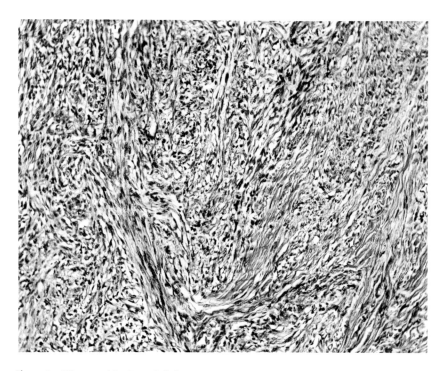

Figure 2   Fibroma of the liver. Cellular area shows elongated cells arranged in bundles (AFIP Neg 74-10824; hematoxylin and eosin, X120).

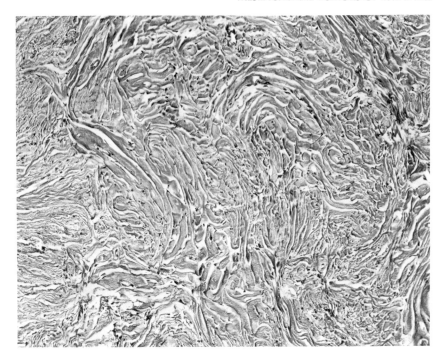

Figure 3 Fibroma of the liver. Acellular area is composed of thick interlacing bundles of collagen (AFIP Neg 74-10827; hematoxylin and eosin, X110).

otomy a large tumor mass occupied the entire right upper quadrant, and had displaced the right kidney, pancreas, duodenum, and stomach to the left. The tumor was attached to the liver and covered by Glisson's capsule but did not infiltrate the substance of the liver. Following dissection of the tumor from the liver the patient died from cardiac arrest. The resected tumor was irregularly ovoid and measured 23 × 20 × 13 cm; it weighed 3850 g. The cut surface was lobulated and tan with an occasional pale yellow soft area, one cystic area, and one partially calcified focus. Microscopically this tumor resembled the one described above.

Malignant

Fibrosarcoma

Several published cases which have been reviewed by the author(4-14) together with two cases on file at AFIP are summarized in Table 1. This tumor is extremely rare judging by the necropsy incidence from the Mayo Clinic(5) and Cook County Hospital, Chicago(14). There was only one case of fibrosarcoma of the liver in a total of 24,196 necropsies at the Mayo Clinic from 1914 to 1953; in this period of time there were 45 cases of primary carcinoma of the liver(5). At Cook County Hospital there was one fibrosarcoma in 37,819 autopsies performed from 1951 to 1970(14).

As is evident from Table 1, all cases have occurred in middle-aged or elderly persons. There is a preponderance of this tumor in males (11 of 13 patients). The majority of patients presented with abdominal enlargement with or without a palpable mass. One of the patients had symptoms and signs of an acute abdominal crisis re-

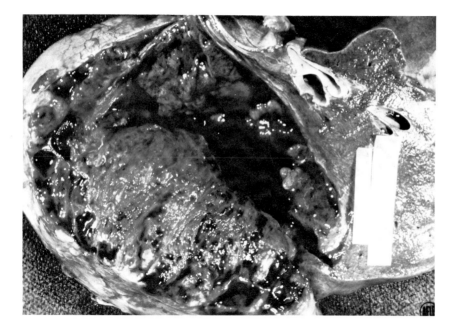

Figure 4 Gross photograph of fibrosarcoma of the liver showing foci of hemorrhage and cavitary necrosis (AFIP Neg 74-12872-2).

sulting from hemoperitoneum due to rupture of the neoplasm. Two patients had had recurrent episodes of hypoglycemia, while a third case with hypoglycemia is briefly alluded to by Edmondson(3). Hypoglycemia is a recognized feature of nonpancreatic fibrogenic tumors(15–18). In this context it is worthwhile noting that hypoglycemia has also been reported in fibrosarcoma metastatic to the liver (17–19). Four patients with primary fibrosarcoma of the liver had weight loss. Other symptoms were probably related to pressure on adjacent viscera and organs. Two patients were clinically jaundiced at the onset of their illness(5, 11). In no case was the diagnosis established prior to surgical exploration and biopsy or necropsy. Needless to say once a hepatic tumor is diagnosed by biopsy as a fibrosarcoma a complete work-up of the patient is necessary to rule out a primary tumor at some other site. It should be borne in mind that metastases to the liver may occur many years after resection of a fibrosarcoma in another organ(20).

In the 10 cases in which the location is stated (Table 1), 8 had arisen in the right and 2 in the left lobe of the liver. The liver of one patient had two tumors, smaller satellite nodules were present about the main tumor in two other patients. Fibrosarcomas can attain a large size judging by the weights of the resected tumor or of the liver at necropsy. One of the surgical specimens weighed 5200 g(4) while one of the necropsied livers weighed 7232 g(12). Cirrhosis of the liver was an associated finding in only 2 of the 13 cases(9, 14). In 2 of the reported cases(8, 14) there was neoplastic invasion of the portal vein, whereas in 2 other cases there was direct extension of the tumor into the duodenum or jejunum (AFIP Case 1)(8). Intraabdominal metastases (regional lymph nodes, omentum, peritoneum) were found in 3 cases (AFIP Case 2(5, 9), while in 1 case there were multiple metastases to the lungs(8).

Grossly, fibrosarcomas of the liver resemble similar tumors arising in other sites (Fig. 4). Microscopically, these tumors are well-circumscribed and usually nonencapsulated (Fig. 5). They are composed of spindle-shaped cells arranged in interlacing bundles (Fig. 5), and may form a "herring-bone" pattern. Varying amounts of collagen fibers are seen to arise from the neoplastic cells and to lie between them. A network of reticulin fibers sur-

Table 1   Fibrosarcoma

Author(s) (Reference)	Age/Sex	Clinical	Location	Pathology	Course
Shallow and Wagner (4)	60/M	Abdominal enlargement. Anorexia. Weight loss. Round, firm, smooth upper abdominal mass.	Left lobe	Firm, smooth tumor with few necrotic foci. Weight 5200 g	Tumor resected; Died 11 days P.O.[a] from ? pulmonary embolism. No autopsy.
Simpson et al (5)	66/M	R.U.Q.[b] pain. Anorexia. Weakness. Weight loss. Jaundice. Hepatomegaly.	Right lobe	Grayish cystic tumor, 18 cm in diameter, with necrotic center. Metastases to regional nodes and omentum.	Died 18 days P.O.[a] from peritonitis secondary to perforation of jejunum.
Steiner (6)	45/M	N.S.[c]	N.S.[c]	Liver weighed 4000	Clinical course lasted 1 year.
Ojima et al (7)	62/M	Abdominal distension. Edema of legs. Hemoptysis.	Right lobe	Liver weighed 3190 g. Tumor ("size of child's head").	Died 4 months after onset from gastrointestinal hemorrhage.
Snapper et al (8)	55/M	Recurrent hypoglycemia. R.U.Q.[b] mass. Cafe-au-lait spots. Multiple skin papillomas.	Right lobe Satellite nodules Left lobe	Tumor white, firm, homogeneous to whorly surface. Invasion of portal vein. Multiple pulmonary metastases.	Died 5 years after onset. Treated with repeated courses of X-irradiation.
Totzke and Hutcheson (9)	56/F	Abdominal distension. R.U.Q.[b] and left flank pain. Anorexia. Occasional nausea. Dyspnea. Ascites and pretibial edema.	Right lobe	Solid, soft, pink-yellow mass, 8 cm in diameter. Several smaller satellite nodules. Postnecrotic cirrhosis. Metastases to paraaortic nodes.	N.S.[c]
Balouet and Destombes (10)	38/M	N.S.[c]	N.S.[c]	N.S.[c]	N.S.[c]
Cavallo et al (11)	30/F	Epigastric pain and vomiting, 3 months'	Right lobe	Liver weighed 2800 g Two nodules, 8 and 5	Died P.O.[a] following cholecystectomy.

Source	Age/Sex	Clinical features	Lobe	Pathology	Outcome
		duration. Hemoperitoneum, cause undetermined, at laparotomy.		cm in diameter—solid, yellowish-white with with central necrosis in larger tumor.	
Smith and Rele (12)	37/M	Pain right chest and shoulder. Hepatomegaly.	Right lobe	Liver weighed 7325 g Massive, solid, fleshy, tan to cream-colored tumor. No cirrhosis.	Died shortly after exploratory laparotomy. No autopsy.
Walter et al (13)	66/M	Epigastric fullness. Mass below right costal margin. Weight loss. Mass ("size of child's head") extending from right costal margin to umbilicus. Hepatomegaly. Hepatic scan—defect in right lobe.	Right lobe	Tumor weighed 2780 g Multinodular, solid, elastic tumor.	Alive and well 1 year after excision.
Alrenga (14)	51/M	Intermittent abdominal pain and distension. R.U.Q.[b] mass. Weight loss. Cachexia.	Right lobe	Liver weighed 1200 g Grayish-white firm tumor 17 cm in diameter. Micronodular cirrhosis. Tumor invasion of portal vein.	Died shortly after administration.
AFIP Case 1	45/M	Recurrent hypoglycemia. R.U.Q.[b] mass. Liver biopsy—fibrosarcoma.	Left lobe	Liver weighed 5400 g. Tumor firm, pearly white with areas of necrosis and hemorrhage. Invasion of duodenum.	Died 3 years after onset.
AFIP Case 2	73/M	Dyspnea. Right shoulder pain. Weight loss. Chest X-ray—elevated right hemidiaphragm.	Right lobe	Tumor had ruptured with hemoperitoneum (1500 ml). Peritoneal metastases.	Died shortly after administration.

[a] P.O.: Postoperative.
[b] R.U.Q.: Right upper quadrant.
[c] N.S.: not stated.

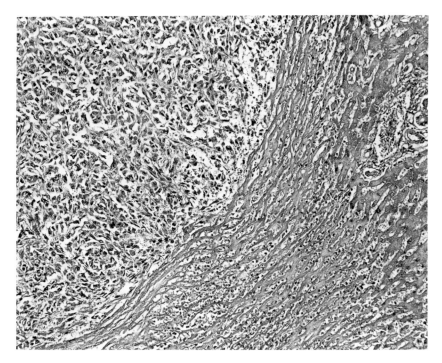

Figure 5 Fibrosarcoma of the liver. A segment of the tumor is sharply demarcated from the adjacent liver (right) (AFIP Neg 74-10799; hematoxylin and eosin, X100).

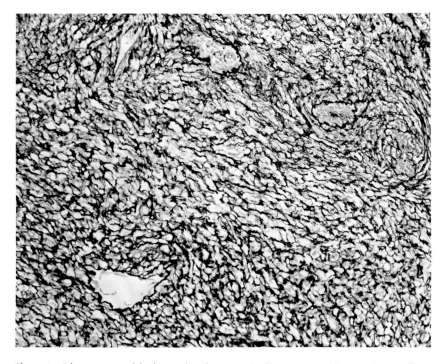

Figure 6 Fibrosarcoma of the liver. Abundant reticulin fibers surround the neoplastic cells (AFIP Neg 74-10805; Wilder's reticulum, X100).

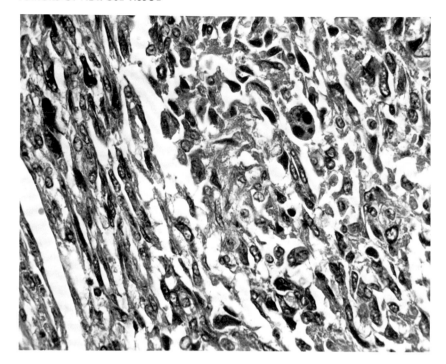

Figure 7 Fibrosarcoma of the liver. Note nuclear pleomorphism and hyperchromasia (AFIP Neg 74-10803; hematoxylin and eosin, X395).

rounds the neoplastic cells (Fig. 6). The nuclei have pointed ends and show varying degrees of pleomorphism, hyperchromasia, and mitotic activity (Fig. 7). Areas of mecrosis may be present particularly in the more central portions of the tumor.

The behavior of these tumors is difficult to predict because of their rarity. Most of the reported patients have died in less than one year from the time of diagnosis, although in a number of them, death was not directly related to the tumor. The patient reported by Walter et al(13) was alive and well for one year after excision of his tumor. Another patient (AFIP Case 1) lived for three years after the diagnosis was established by exploration and biopsy. A third patient who had been treated with several courses of X-irradiation lived for five years(8).

TUMORS OF ADIPOSE TISSUE

Benign

Although these tumors have been subtyped in the Classification and examples of all the types have been studied at AFIP, the number of cases in each group, including those which have been published(21–24) is too small to justify separate consideration. They are therefore all summarized together in Table 2.

With the exception of one patient, all of the tumors occurred in patients in the fourth decade or later. Six of the seven patients were female. Four of the eight patients were obese and two of them also had diabetes mellitus. One patient(23) had tuberous sclerosis while another (AFIP Case 4) was suspected of having this disease but the diagnosis was not verified.

Table 2 Lipomatous Tumors

Author(s) (Reference)	Age/Sex	Clinical	Location	Pathology	Course
Simon (21)	70/F	N.S.[c]	Left lobe	Spherical, yellow nodule, 2 cm in diameter. Lipoma (?hibernomalike cells).	Died following drainage of gallbladder. Autopsy showed adenocarcinoma of gallbladder with metastases.
Young (22)	54/F	Obesity, diabetes mellitus, hypertension. Precordial pain. Pericardial friction rub.	Right lobe	Round, well-demarcated yellow nodule, 2 cm in diameter. Lipoma.	Died 12 days after admission from renal failure and pericarditis.
Ramchand et al (23)	24/M	Tuberous sclerosis. Intestinal obstruction.	Right lobe	Soft, yellow, nonencapsulated nodule, 1 cm in diameter. Lipoma.	Died 2 days after enterostomy for relief of intestinal obstruction.
Grosdidier et al (24)	63/F	Obesity, diabetes mellitus, gout. Slight hepatomegaly. Hepatic scan—defect.	Right lobe	Yellow, nonencapsulated nodule, 12–13 cm in diameter. Myelolipoma.	Right lobectomy. No distant follow-up.
AFIP Case 1	53/F	Obesity, Arteriosclerotic heart disease. Hypertension.	Left lobe	Yellow circumscribed nodule, 2 cm in diameter. Myelolipoma.	Died from multiple infarcts in kidneys, adrenals, and spleen. Also had a papillary carcinoma of thyroid gland.

Case	Age/Sex	Clinical and radiologic findings	Location	Gross and microscopic findings	Outcome
AFIP Case 2	66/F	Obesity. Arteriosclerotic heart disease. Hypertension. Myocardial infarction.	Right lobe	Pale yellow nodule, 2 cm in diameter. Angiomyolipoma.	Died from myocardial infarction.
AFIP Case 3	57/M	Hepatic failure due to alcoholic liver disease.	Right lobe	Yellow nodule 1 cm in diameter. Angiomyolipoma.	Died from hepatic failure due to alcoholic liver disease with early micronodular cirrhosis. Also had a perforated duodenal ulcer and acute pancreatitis.
AFIP Case 4	39/F	Mass in R.U.Q.[b] Upper G.I. series—calcified mass in R.U.Q.[b] and radiolucent mass in upper abdomen. Hepatic scan—diminished activity in medial part of left lobe and right lobe. Intravenous pyelogram—normal. Bone survey—multiple irregular sclerotic defects in vertebrae, ileum, and lower rib cage.	Right lobe	Pedunculated encapsulated mass 8 × 6 × 5 cm in diameter. Cut with gritty sensation. Grey glistening cut surface. Angiolipoma with hibernomalike cells.	Both tumors excised. Uneventful postoperative recovery.
			Central part of liver	Encapsulated light yellow tumor 8 × 6 × 6 cm in diameter. Cut surface yellow, greasy, and homogeneous. Lipoma.	

[a] P.O.: Postoperative.
[b] R.U.Q.: Right upper quadrant.
[c] N.S.: Not stated.

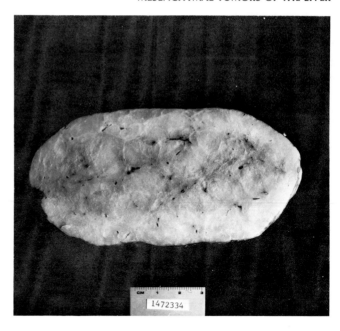

Figure 8 Gross photograph of well-encapsulated lipoma (AFIP Neg 74-12901).

With the exception of two cases, the lipomatous tumors summarized in Table 2 were incidental findings at the time of autopsy. The patient reported by Grosdidier et al(24) had hepatomegaly and an hepatic scan showed a defect which at the time of laparotomy was found to correspond to a myelolipoma (12 to 13 cm in diameter) in the right lobe of the liver; a right hepatic lobectomy was performed. AFIP Case 4 was a 39-year-old white female who complained of a mass in the right upper quadrant (RUQ). An upper gastrointestinal radiographic series showed a calcified mass in the RUQ. An hepatic scan showed diminished activity in the medial left lobe and in the right lobe. At the time of laparotomy two lipomatous tumors were removed from the liver (Table 2).

Five of the nine tumors listed in Table 2 were located in or arose from the right lobe of the liver, two were in the left lobe, and 1 involved both lobes of the liver. Only

two tumors (AFIP Case 4) had a pedicle. All the tumors were well circumscribed and yellow in color (Fig. 8) with the exception of the pedunculated tumor which was grossly calcified and gray-tan in color. The two patients whose symptoms and signs ultimately led to exploration had tumors that were between 8 and 13 cm in diameter. The lipomatous tumors found incidentally at the time of autopsy were all quite small (1 to 2 cm in diameter).

Microscopically the major component of this group of tumors is mature adipose tissue. Three of the published tumors(21–23) and one of the AFIP tumors (AFIP Case 4) were classified as *lipomas*. The case reported by Grosdidier et al(24) and AFIP Case 1 had multiple foci of hematopoiesis within the lipoma, justifying the use of the term *myelolipoma* (Figs. 9 and 10). Both of these tumors closely resembled adrenal myelolipomas(25). It is also of interest that myelolipomas have been reported in the

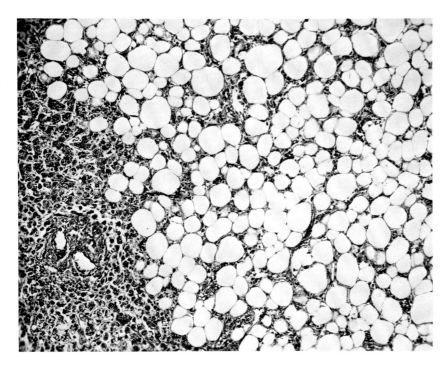

Figure 9 Myelolipoma of the liver. Tumor is composed of large adipose cells and abuts directly on the hepatic parenchyma on the left (AFIP Neg 79-9773; hematoxylin and eosin, X80).

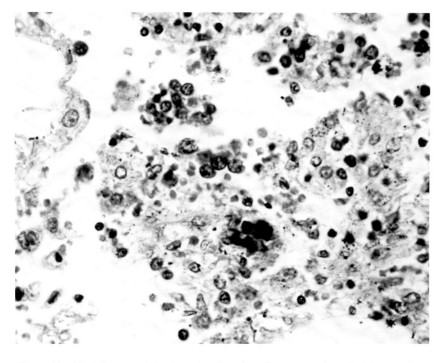

Figure 10 Myelolipoma of the liver. Nucleated erythrocytes and erythroblasts and a megakaryocyte in sinusoidal vessels (AFIP Neg 72-9770; hematoxylin and eosin, X530).

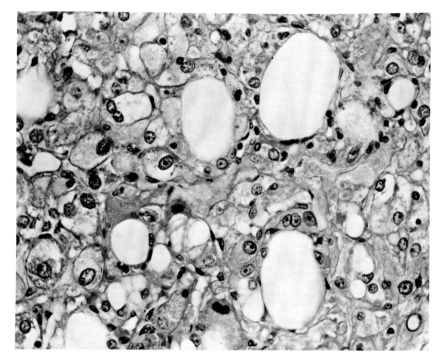

Figure 11 Angiolipoma of the liver. Hibernomalike cells with granular cytoplasm, as well as mature lipocytes (AFIP Neg 74-8023; hematoxylin and eosin, X300).

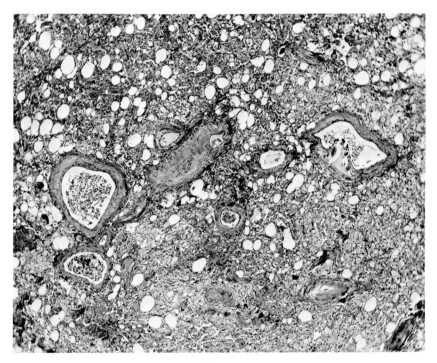

Figure 12 Angiolipoma of the liver. The tumor is composed of adipose tissue and many thick-walled vessels showing calcification (AFIP Neg 74-8021; hematoxylin and eosin, X50).

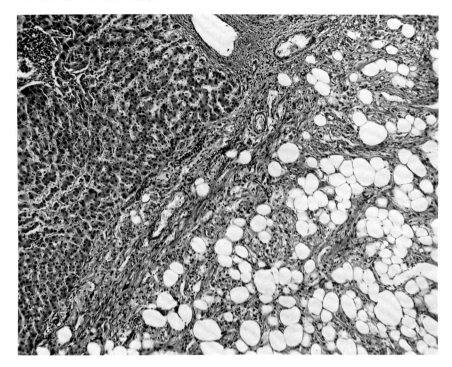

Figure 13   Angiolipoma of the liver. A segment of the tumor (right) is separated from the liver by a pseudocapsule. The tumor is composed of fat cells intermingled with collagenous tissue and blood vessels (AFIP Neg 73-11849; hematoxylin and eosin, X70).

livers of seven captive wild Felidae(26).

One of the tumors studied by the author (AFIP Case 4) was classified as an *angiolipoma*. This was a pedunculated tumor arising from the right lobe of the liver which cut with an extremely gritty sensation. In addition to mature fat cells, there were many cells that had a granular eosinophilic cytoplasm suggesting immature lipocytes or hibernomalike cells (Fig. 11). Multiple thick-walled vessels were scattered throughout the tumor (Fig. 12). The majority of these vessels were densely calcified (usually concentrically but sometimes segmentally); some were also encrusted with hemosiderin. The appearance of these vessels, together with the demonstration of remnants of an internal elastic lamina in some of them, suggested that most of them were arteries. Additionally, noncalcified thin-walled veins were also scattered throughout the tumor.

Two tumors studied by the author were classified as *angiomyolipomas* (AFIP Cases 2 and 3). These consisted of an admixture of adipose tissue, thick-walled arteries, veins, bundles of smooth muscle admixed with fibrous tissue, and occasional nerve fibers (Figs. 13–16). Both tumors were microscopically indistinguishable from similar benign mixed mesodermal tumors arising in the kidney(27) or uterus(28).

Lipomas of the liver must be distinguished from *pseudolipomas*. Three such cases have been reported(29) and there are five examples of this entity in the AFIP files. Like the published cases all five pseudotumors occurred in males who were 44, 49, 53, 63, and 81 years of age. All patients had generalized arteriosclerosis and four

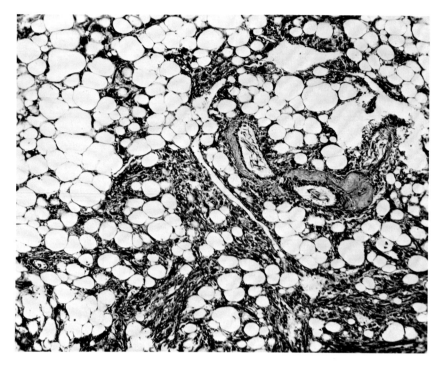

Figure 14 Angiolipoma of the liver. Admixture of adipose tissue with collagen and smooth muscle bundles. Note two thick-walled vessels (AFIP Neg 73-11848; Masson trichrome, X75).

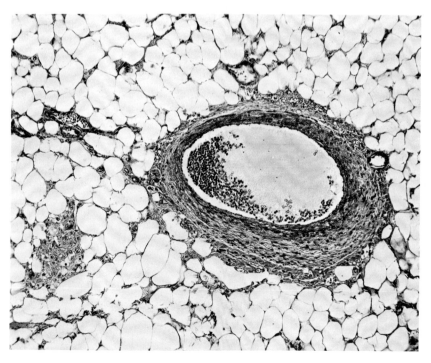

Figure 15 Angiomyolipoma of the liver. Thick-walled vessel is surrounded by adipose tissue (AFIP Neg 74-8016; hematoxylin and eosin, X100).

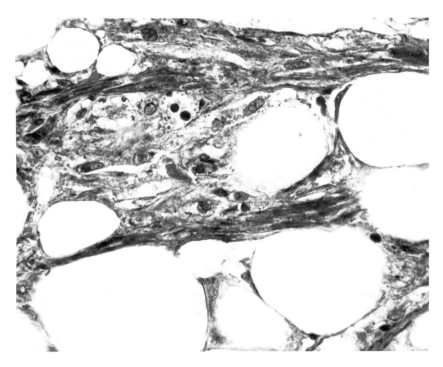

Figure 16 Angiomyolipoma of the liver. The lesion is encapsulated and embedded in a concavity on the surface of the liver (AFIP Neg 74-9533; Masson trichrome, X14).

died in congestive heart failure; the fifth patient died from bronchopneumonia. Associated conditions included multiple benign adenomatous polyps of the colon in one patient, and bilateral adrenal cortical hyperplasia and a large benign fibrous mesothelioma of right pleura in another patient. Three of the patients were obese. Two of the patients had had appendectomies many years previously, but the other three patients had not had previous abdominal surgery. It is of interest in this regard that the patient reported by Persaud(29) had also undergone appendectomy 24 years before his cholecystectomy for cholelithiasis. Two of the pseudolipomas in the AFIP files were located on the surface of the right and one was located on the surface of the left lobe of the liver; the location of the other two was not known. Their size varied from 0.4 to 1.5 cm in diameter.

Grossly these pseudoneoplasms all lay on the surface of the liver partially embedded in a concavity lined by a focally thickened Glisson's capsule. They were quite firm and three cut with a gritty sensation. Two had a yellow cut surface while three were pearly white. In one case a nodule similar to the one in the liver was found on the serosa of the greater curvature of the stomach, but unfortunately it was not submitted to microscopic examination.

Microscopically the pseudolipomas are encapsulated oval or spherical masses of mature adipose tissue undergoing degenerative changes (Figs. 17 and 18). Three of the five lesions showed diffuse or focal calcification and in one there was also osseous metaplasia (Fig. 19) as was the case in the lesion reported by Persaud(29). A few cholesterol clefts were seen in one of the lesions. The livers of the AFIP cases with pseudolipomas showed no histologic abnormalities except for moderate fatty

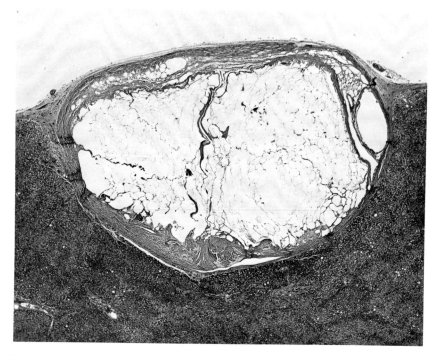

Figure 17 Pseudolipoma of the liver. The lesion is encapsulated and embedded in a concavity on the surface of the liver (AFIP Neg 74-9533; Masson trichrome, X14).

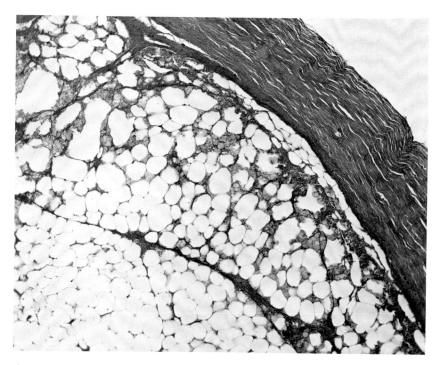

Figure 18 Pseudolipoma of the liver. A segment of the lesion is surrounded by a thick capsule. Fat cells are degenerated and lack nuclei (AFIP Neg 74-9535; hematoxylin and eosin, X35).

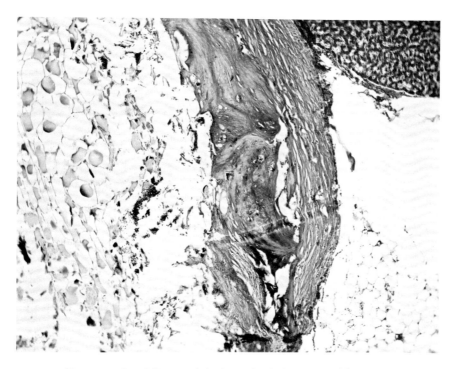

Figure 19 Pseudolipoma of the liver. Ossified segment of lesion (AFIP Neg 69-6466; hematoxylin and eosin, X50).

metamorphosis in two cases.

The pathogenesis of pseudolipoma of the liver is uncertain. According to Rolleston and McNee(30) it is thought to represent an imprisoned or encapsulated appendix epiploica that had lost its moorings to the large bowel and had migrated and become attached to Glisson's capsule. The history of previous intraabdominal surgery in some of the patients and the occurrence of a similar nodule on the serosa of the stomach in one of the AFIP cases lend some support to this hypothesis.

Malignant

To the author's knowledge there are no cases of primary liposarcoma of the liver published in the literature.

TUMORS OF MUSCLE TISSUE

Benign

Leiomyoma

Two cases of leiomyoma of the liver have

been reported(31, 32). One patient was a 42-year-old woman who gave a five-month history of a slowly growing mass in the RUQ. At the time of laparotomy a 10 × 12 cm firm multinodular mass was excised from the liver. It was grayish-white with a homogeneous cut surface in which were scattered multiple small cystic spaces(31). The second patient was an 87-year-old woman who presented with sudden hematemesis, pain in the epigastrium, hypotension, and fever. On physical examination almost the entire abdomen was filled with a firm and slightly tender mass. The patient died shortly after admission to a hospital. At the time of autopsy there was a large, lobulated, and encapsulated mass arising from the left lobe of the liver; it weighed 3750 g. The cut surface was yellowish-white and coarsely trabeculated, with occasional soft and red areas. There were numerous gastric erosions and the lumen of the stomach contained 1 liter of clotted blood. Other autopsy findings included cholelithiasis and reduplication of

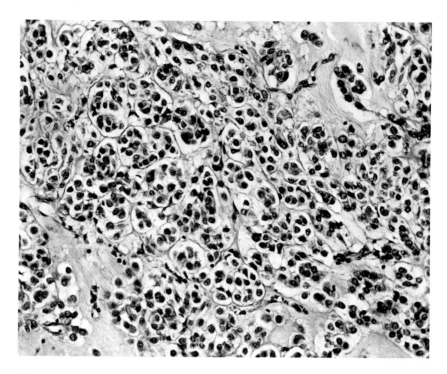

Figure 20   Epithelioid leiomyoma of the liver. Uniform round-polygonal cells are arranged in small nests (AFIP Neg 74-7349; hematoxylin and eosin, X195).

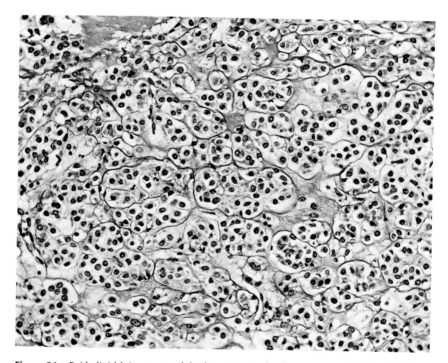

Figure 21   Epithelioid leiomyoma of the liver. Nests of cells are surrounded by reticulin fibers (AFIP Neg 74-7348; Wilder's reticulum, X180).

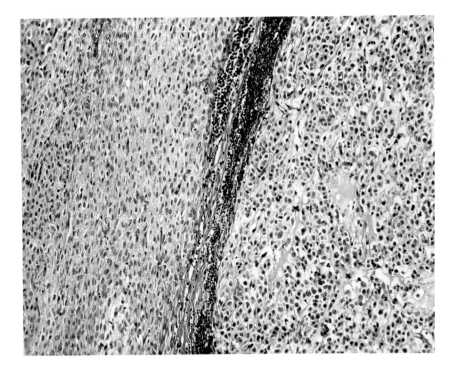

Figure 22 Epithelioid leiomyoma of the liver. Portion of the tumor with epithelioid pattern (right) is sharply demarcated from another portion (left) showing typical elongated leiomyomatous cells (AFIP Neg 74-7346; hematoxylin and eosin, X110).

the right renal pelvis and ureter(32). Both cases were described as typical leiomyomas on histologic examination.

Epithelioid Leiomyoma (Leiomyoblastoma, Bizarre Leiomyoma)

One example of this type of tumor was studied by the author. This occurred in a 64-year-old male who presented with a mass in the epigastrium and anemia of undetermined type and etiology. At the time of laparotomy an oval hemorrhagic and cystic mass, 15 cm in diameter, was found to be attached by a pedicle to the right lobe of the liver, inferior to the insertion of the round ligament. All other abdominal organs and viscera were normal to inspection and palpation. The tumor was removed by division of the pedicle, and the patient made an uneventful postoperative recovery and was alive and well at least 19 months later at the time of his most recent clinical visit.

Microscopically the tumor was quite cellular and was predominantly composed of round or polygonal cells arranged in small nests bounded by reticulin fibers (Figs. 20 and 21). The cells appeared empty or had a scanty amount of a faintly eosinophilic cytoplasm. Nuclei were centrally placed, were quite uniform in size and shape, and were moderately chromatic; no mitoses were present. In the more peripheral areas the tumor was composed of parallel bundles of elongated smooth muscle cells. In some areas the two patterns were sharply demarcated (Fig. 22) but in other areas there was a transition from the leiomyomatous to the "leiomyoblastomatous" cells. In all respects this tumor was similar to others which arise in the stomach, mesentery, or omentum(33–35).

Malignant

Leiomyosarcoma

This is a rare tumor of the liver and thus there are no published figures on its incidence in relation to other primary hepatic malignancies.

Leiomyosarcomas may arise within the liver or from the ligamentum teres. Published examples of the former together with one case from the AFIP files are summarized in Table 3. Like fibrosarcoma of the liver these tumors seem to occur in middle-age or later. Four occurred in males and three in females. Five of the seven patients had a mass in the RUQ or epigastrium. The remaining two patients had hepatomegaly and in one of them the liver was nodular to palpation. Two of the patients had experienced weight loss prior to their seeking medical attention and one patient was emaciated when first examined. Three of the patients had ascites. Tests of hepatic function in four of the patients showed a normal total serum bilirubin level, and normal or slightly elevated transaminase values. Elevated alkaline phosphatase values were reported in three patients (less than a threefold elevation in two and a sevenfold elevation in one). Gastrointestinal radiographic series showed displacement of the stomach and/or colon in two patients. Hepatic scan revealed a defect or defects in the livers of four patients (37–40) Angiographic studies in one patient showed a relatively avascular tumor(39). The diagnosis of leiomyosarcoma was established by percutaneous hepatic biopsy in three patients(36, 40) and AFIP Case 1. In three others the diagnosis was made at the time of laparotomy(38, 39).

In three of the patients the leiomyosarcoma formed a single mass, which was in the right lobe in two cases and in the left in one case. In another patient there was one large mass in the right lobe and multiple small satellite nodules in the remainder of the liver. One patient had two nodules located in the left lobe, while another patient had multiple nodules of varying size throughout the liver. (In one patient the location of the tumor was not stated.) The nodules varied from 2 to 15 cm in maximum diameter. The heaviest necropsied liver with leiomyosarcoma weighed 11,200 g and an estimated 95% of the organ was replaced by tumor(40). In the three patients who were autopsied there were widespread metastases in two and a single pulmonary metastasis in the third. There was no associated cirrhosis in any of the cases listed in Table 3.

Grossly and microscopically, leiomyosarcoma of the liver resembles similar tumors arising in other organs and tissues (Fig. 23). The tumors are nonencapsulated and have an infiltrating periphery (Fig. 24). They are composed of elongated spindle-shaped cells arranged in sharply intersecting bundles (Fig. 25). The cytoplasm is acidophilic and may exhibit longitudinal myofibrils. The nuclei are elongated, usually have blunt ends, are hyperchromatic, and show considerable variation in size. Typical and atypical mitoses are frequent (one or more per high power field). Areas of necrosis are frequently seen, particularly in the more central regions of the tumor.

The prognosis in primary leiomyosarcoma of the liver is poor though probably somewhat better than that of hepatocellular carcinoma. Three of the patients had their tumors surgically excised. One died 4 months postoperatively and had widespread metastases at the time of autopsy(39); the other patients were alive and well 8 and 12 months after surgery(38, 39). One patient was treated with chemotherapeutic agents but no follow-up was given(36). The remaining patients whose neoplasms were not surgically or otherwise treated died; one died shortly after admission to the hospital(37) while the other two patients died 21 and 24 months after onset of their illness (AFIP Case 1) (40).

Leiomyosarcomas arising from the liga-

Table 3 Leiomyosarcoma

Author(s) (Reference)	Age/Sex	Clinical	Location	Pathology	Course
Watanuki and Kusama (36)	55/M	R.U.Q.[b] mass "size of child's head." Liver biopsy—leiomyosarcoma.	N.S.[c]	N.S.[c]	Treated with anitcancer drugs. No follow-up.
Yamaguchi et al (37)	63/F	R.U.Q.[b] mass—firm, nodular, felt to be part of liver. Ascites. Peripheral edema. Hepatic scan—defect.	Left lobe	Liver weighed 3400 g Large, firm, "fibrous" tumor with central necrosis. Several smaller satellite nodules. No metastases.	Died shortly after admission.
Meinikov and Jakharov (38)	32/F	Epigastric mass 7–8 cm in diameter. Hepatomegaly 5–6 cm. below right costal margin. Upper G.I. series—stomach displaced to left and anteriorly. Hepatic scan—defect in left lobe.	Left lobe	Two tumors. Larger one elastic, dark red. and 9 × 10 cm in diameter. Smaller ore rubbery, gray-white and 4.5 × 6 cm in diameter.	Left lobectomy. Patient alive and well 1 year later.
Wilson et al (39)	Case 1 54/M	R.U.Q.[b] mass. Upper and lower G.I. series—displacement of stomach and colon. Hepatic scan—space-occupying lesion. Angiogram—relatively avascular tumor	Right lobe	Large nodular mass weighing 2300 g.	Alive 8 months after excision.
	Case 2 49/F	Malaise, weakness, easy fatigability. Weight loss. R.U.Q.[b] mass.	Right lobe	Multinodular mass.	Died 4 months after excision. Widespread metastases at autopsy.

(continued on next page)

Table 3 (continued)

Author(s) (Reference)	Age/Sex	Clinical	Location	Pathology	Course
Fong and Ruebner (40)	62/M	Abdominal swelling. Weight loss. Subsequent edema and ascites. Enlarged nodular liver. Hepatic scan—multiple defects. Liver biopsy—leiomyosarcoma.	Both lobes	Liver weighed 11,200 g. Multiple nodules 2–15 cm in diameter scattered throughout liver.	Died 21 months after onset. Widespread metastases at autopsy.
AFIP Case 1	40/M	Hematemesis. Melena. Emaciation. Pleural effusion, bilateral. Ascites. Hepatomegaly. Liver biopsy (2 years before death)—leiomyosarcoma.	Right lobe	Large tumor mass 10 × 15 cm in diameter with necrotic center. Several small (1.5–2 cm satellite nodules in remainder of liver.	Died shortly after admission. One small pulmonary metastasis at autopsy.

[a] P.O.: Postoperative.
[b] R.U.Q.: Right upper quadrant.
[c] Not stated.

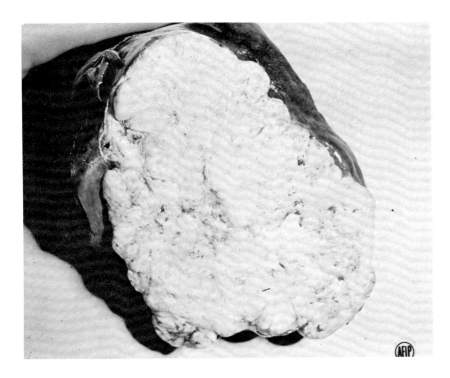

Figure 23 Gross photograph of well-circumscribed lobulated leiomyosarcoma (AFIP Neg 74-12869).

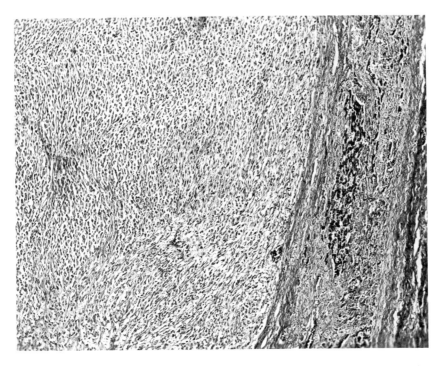

Figure 24 Leiomyosarcoma of the liver. The tumor is sharply circumscribed and separated from the hepatic parenchyma (right) by a pseudocapsule (AFIP Neg 73-12439; hematoxylin and eosin, X35).

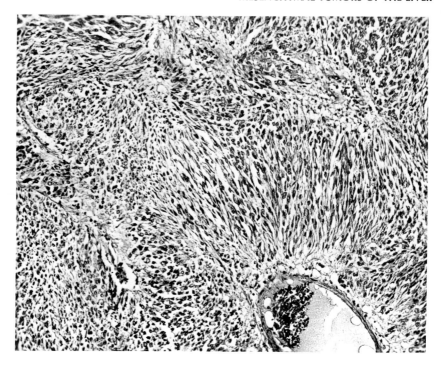

Figure 25 Leiomyosarcoma of the liver. Neoplastic cells are arranged in intersecting bundles (AFIP Neg 73-12441; hematoxylin and eosin, X90).

mentum teres of the liver are summarized in Table 4. They have been separated from the other leiomyosarcomas in Table 3 because of their unique location and because the prognosis appears to be better in this group than in the leiomyosarcomas located elsewhere in the liver. Two of the four patients were male and two female. The ages ranged from 11 to 29 years. All of the patients presented with an upper abdominal mass usually accompanied by discomfort or pain. All patients were explored and found to have encapsulated tumors that were described as arising from or attached to the round ligament of the liver. These tumors were quite large with maximum diameters varying from 8.5 to 35 cm. The gross and microscopic features of these leiomyosarcomas of the round ligament do not differ significantly from those arising elsewhere

in the liver. The histology of AFIP Case 1 (Table 4) is illustrated in Figures 26 to 28.

One of the patients with leiomyosarcoma of the ligamentum teres, an 11-year-old girl, is alive and well four years after resection of her tumor (AFIP Case 2, Table 4). Another patient (AFIP Case 3) is alive and well two years following surgery. The patient reported by Mital and Bazaz-Malik(41) died in the immediate postoperative period. AFIP Case 1 died seven months following exploration and biopsy of his tumor and postoperative x-irradiation; the cause of death was said to be coronary thrombosis but no autopsy was performed.

In addition to leiomyosarcomas arising from the liver or the ligamentum teres two cases of malignant smooth muscle tumors

Table 4 Leiomyosarcoma of Ligamentum Teres

Author(s) (Reference No.)		Clinical	Pathology	(Reference) Course
Mital and Bazaz-Malik (41)	45/M	Progressive abdominal swelling and discomfort. History of supraumbilical mass 22 years previously. Two excisions 10 and 5 years before final admission. Intraabdominal mass 35 × 25 cm in size, with uneven surface.	Firm, oval-encapsulated greyish-white mass 35 × 20 × 15 cm in diameter. Cut surface had whorled appearance.	Left lobectomy. Patient died P.O.[a] from shock. No autopsy.
AFIP Case 1	29/M	Left upper quadrant pain. Nausea. Vomiting. Movable, nontender supraumbilical mass. Liver biopsy—spindle-cell sarcoma.	Pedunculated, irregularly ovoid mass, 20 × 12 × 10 cm in diameter. Pale yellow cut surface with central necrosis.	Patient died 7 months after excision of tumor from coronary thrombosis. No autopsy.
AFIP Case 2	11/F	Upper abdominal discomfort. Nausea. R.U.Q.[b] mass.	Vascular encapsulated mass 8 × 6 × 6 cm in diameter. Rubbery consistency. Yellow cut surface.	Tumor excised. Patient alive and well 4 years later.
AFIP Case 3	21/F	Epigastric mass discovered on routine physical examination.	Pedunculated encapsulated mass 8.5 × 6 × 3.5 cm in diameter.	Tumor excised. Patient alive and well 2 years later.

[a] P.O.: Postoperative.
[b] R.U.Q.: Right upper quadrant.

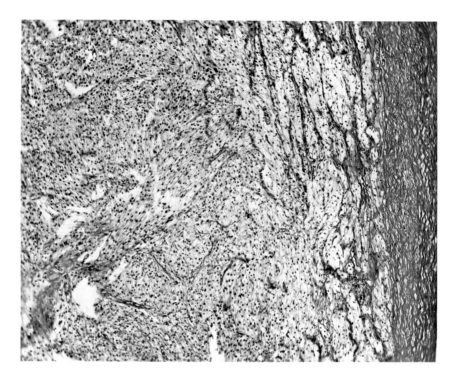

Figure 26 Leiomyosarcoma of ligamentum teres. The tumor is surrounded by a thick capsule (right). Bundles of neoplastic cells are randomly oriented (AFIP Neg 74-7333; hematoxylin and eosin, X35).

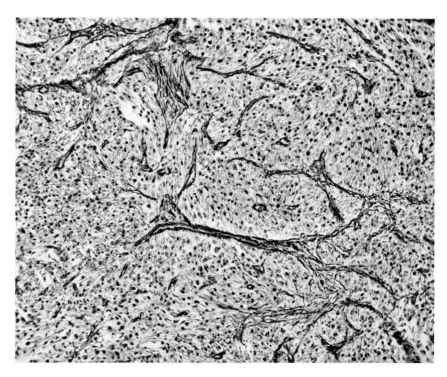

Figure 27 Leiomyosarcoma of ligamentum teres. Neoplastic cells show no associated reticulin fibers (AFIP Neg 74-7648; Wilder's reticulum, X100).

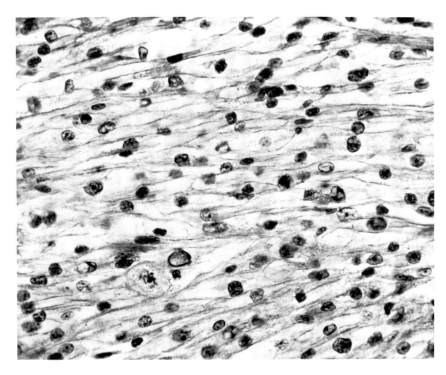

Figure 28 Leiomyosarcoma of ligamentum teres. High power photomicrograph showing nuclear details and mitotic figure in lower part of field (AFIP Neg 74-7336; hematoxylin and eosin, X300).

arising from a hepatic vein have been reported(42, 43). These occurred in males aged 33 and 64 years. Both patients died in hepatic coma secondary to a fulminating form of the Budd-Chiari syndrome. In the case reported by MacMahon and Ball(43) there was direct invasion of the adjacent right lobe of the liber with formation of a mass measuring 8 × 5 × 4 cm.

Leiomyosarcomas of the inferior vena cava may also extend into a hepatic vein, directly invade the liver, or metastasize to it. An extensive review of primary leiomyosarcomas of the inferior vena cava (and other large veins and arteries) has recently been published by Kevorkian and Cento(44).

Rhabdomyosarcoma

These primary tumors of the liver are discussed in Chapter 10, which is a study of tumors of the liver in children.

TUMORS OF BLOOD VESSELS

Benign

Hemangioma

The cavernous hemangioma is the most common benign hepatic tumor of the liver. In a series of 570 hemangiomas from all sites recorded at the Johns Hopkins Hospital up to 1935 there were 109 in the liver, an incidence of about 19%(45). The liver was by far the commonest site for hemangiomas located in internal viscera and organs. Figures on the incidence from necrospsy series of cases include those of O'Donoghue(46), Edmondson(3), Ochsner and Halpert(47), and Feldman(48). O'Donoghue(46) mentions that there were 140 patients with hemangiomas in 20,029 autopsies at Cook County Hospital, Chicago, Illinois. In a series of 50,000 autopsies at the Los Angeles County Hospital, Los Angeles, California, there were 176 hemangiomas of the liver(3). At the Veterans Administration Hospital, Houston, Texas, 55 patients had cavernous hemangiomas of the liver in a series of 2400 necropsies(47). Feldman(48) found 96 examples of hemangioma of the liver in 1319 autopsies in adult persons.

Hemangiomas of the liver occur at all ages and in both sexes. They are uncommon in the pediatric age group but data on their incidence in childhood are difficult to ascertain because of their frequent confusion with infantile hemangioendothelioma(49). An idea of their relative frequency in relation to infantile hemangioendothelioma can be gathered from a series at AFIP in which there were 4 hemangiomas and 26 hemangioendotheliomas in children(49). Hemangiomas in the pediatric age group are covered in the chapter on tumors of the liver in children (Chapter 10); further discussion in this chapter is therefore limited to hemangiomas in the adult.

There is general agreement that hemangiomas occur more frequently in women than in men. Ratios of females to males in various reports are 4.5 to 1(50), 6 to 1(46), and 1.3 to 1(3). Differences in these ratios are probably reflections of the type of population under study. Thus Schumacker's ratio is based on a review of surgically treated patients(50) whereas Edmondson's ratio is based on an autopsy series(3). Edmondson has pointed out that hemangiomas appear to develop in women at an earlier age and are more prone to become clinically manifest. This is borne out by the series of 35 hemangiomas reported from the Mayo Clinic, Rochester, Minnesota from 1907 to 1954 inclusive (51). In this series 11 patients were explored because of signs and symptoms produced by the hemangioma; 10 of these patients were women. In 24 patients in whom the hemangiomas were found incidentally at operation, there were 19 women and 5

men. Ninard(52) has drawn attention to the number of cases of hemangiomas which have been reported in multiparous women. Edmondson(3) has raised the possibility of a role of the female sex hormones in the development of hemangiomas of the liver, especially since it is known that angiomatous lesions of the gingiva and skin do develop during pregnancy. Morley et al(53) have recently reported rapid enlargement of a cavernous hemangioma of the liver in a 57-year-old woman who had been on estrogen preparation, Premarin, for 18 months.

The majority of hemangiomas of the liver are asymptomatic and are found incidentally at the time of laparotomy or autopsy. In a series of 89 cases at Memorial Hospital for Cancer and Allied Diseases, New York, only 12 (13.5%) had symptoms referable to the hemangioma; in 77 (86.5%) cases the hemangioma was an incidental finding at the time laparotomy or autopsy(54). The patients who had had symptoms leading to surgical exploration have been the subject of a number of reviews(50, 52, 55–57). In those cases in which the patients seek medical attention because of the hemangioma about half present with swelling of the abdomen or an upper abdominal mass. The other half have pain or symptoms referable to the gastrointestinal tract, which are most probably related to pressure on or displacement of adjacent viscera or organs. The symptoms may be of a few months to many years duration. Episodes of sudden pain may be due to thrombosis in the hemangioma. A smaller number of patients may present with an acute abdominal crisis due to hemoperitoneum from rupture of the hemangioma. In the series of 66 cases reviewed by Schumacker(50) 3 patients (4.5%) had spontaneous rupture of the hemangioma. Fourteen cases with rupture were reported in the series of 71 operated cases reviewed by D'Errico(56), an incidence of 19.7%. A detailed analysis of 11 patients with ruptured hemangiomas culled from the literature, together with a case report, was published by Sewell and Weiss in 1961(58). The patient reported by these authors was four months pregnant when her hemangioma ruptured. A unique case of a large pedunculated hemangioma causing obstetric difficulty was described by Rubin(59); the patient, a 33-year-old woman, had had 13 children before her last pregnancy.

A number of hematologic complications have been reported in association with hemangioma of the liver in adults. These have included thrombocytopenia and hypofibrinogenemia(60–62). The patient reported by Behar et al(61) had hypofibrinogenemia that was associated with increased fibrinogenolysis and an intermittent hemorrhagic tendency, which finally proved to be fatal. The patient's hemangioma had a diameter of 20 cm and microscopically showed massive deposition of fibrin within its vascular spaces. In the well-studied patient reported by Martinez et al(62) there was, in addition to the hypofibrinogenemia, a short englobulin lysis time, a prolonged thrombin time, and an increase of fibrinogen-fibrin split products. These and other coagulation studies suggested to the authors that their patients' hypofibrinogenemia might have been due to a fibrinolytic process unrelated to intravascular coagulation. Although a microangiopathic hemolytic anemia has been reported in patients with infantile hemangioendothelioma and in adults with angiosarcoma of the liver (see below), the author is not aware of a published example of this complication in a patient with cavernous hemangioma of the liver.

The diagnosis of hemangioma is rarely made before exploratory laparotomy or autopsy(50, 56). The majority of patients who are symptomatic have a palpable mass in the upper abdomen. In one patient with multiple hemangiomas a venous hum was heard in the region of the umbilicus(63), and reference is made by Shumacker(50)

to another patient in whom a murmur was auscultated. Few of the reports on hemangioma contain results of tests of hepatic function. In the series reported by Henson et al(51) tests were reported in 6 of 11 patients who were explored because of symptoms referable to the hemangioma. The bromosulfophthalein retention test was normal in all 6. Three patients had very slight increases in values for the serum bilirubin. Results of other liver function tests done less frequently were all within normal limits. Of the 2 patients with multiple hemangiomas reported by Levitt et al(63) 1 had repeatedly normal tests of hepatic function. The other patient had an icterus index of 14.8 units and a 1:1 ratio of serum albumin to globulin. Because of the danger of fatal bleeding from percutaneous hepatic biopsy this technic is contraindicated in the diagnosis of hemangioma of the liver.

Scout roentgenograms of the abdomen may reveal hepatomegaly or calcification(61, 64, 65). As pointed out by Pantoja(66) the calcification must be a late manifestation of the tumor. All 13 of Plachta's patients(65) and Aspray's patients(64) were between the ages of 67 and 86. In the case reported by Aspray streaks of calcification radiated from the center of the hemangioma. A calcified phlebolith 0.5 cm in diameter was found in one of the cases reported by McLaughlin(67). Hemangiomas that attain a large size may compress adjacent hollow viscera and organs, as can be demonstrated by upper and lower gastrointestinal radiographic series, intravenous pyelography, and so on(50,51). The stomach is the organ most frequently displaced. The diaphragm was elevated in two of the cases reported by Henson et al and the kidney was displaced in one(51). Liver scan in cavernous hemangioma of the liver reveals an area or areas of decreased uptake(62, 66).

By far the most useful radiographic technique for the preoperative diagnosis of hemangioma of the liver is arterio-graphy (66–68). Cavernous hemangio-mas show large feeding vessels which, al-though displaced, are crowded together, as well as large dilated varixlike spaces that are rapidly filled with contrast medium and remain densely opacified throughout the entire angiographic examination(68). According to McLaughlin(67) the tendency of the vascular spaces to be arranged in rings or to be C-shaped, due to fibrous obliteration of the centers of the lesions, is probably pathognomonic for hemangio-ma of the liver.

Hemangiomas of the liver may occasion-ally be associated with similar tumors in other tissues and organs. A number of ex-amples published in the literature up to 1950 are cited by Ninard(52). Feldman(48) has drawn attention to the frequent asso-ciation of hemangiomas of the liver with benign cysts. Eighteen (19%) of 96 patients with hemangioma of the liver had cysts, 11 of which were located in the liver and 6 in the pancreas. Other published examples of this association are also reviewed by this author. Chung(69) has recently reported two hemangiomas in a liver with multiple von Meyenburg complexes (bile duct ha-martomas); the patient also had polycystic disease of the kidneys. The frequent occur-rence of single or multiple cavernous hemangiomas (20.6%) with focal nodular hyperplasia has been noted by Benz and Baggenstoss(70). Calculi of the bilary tract were found in 13% of the patients re-ported by Feldman(48) and in 45.7% of those reported by Henson et al(51). The differences may again reflect the patient populations studied. Thus the former ser-ies(48) is drawn from autopsied cases whereas the latter(51) is composed of pa-tients who were explored either for symp-toms related to the hemangioma or for other abdominal surgery.

Grossly, hemangiomas of the liver may be single or multiple and are located in either the right or left lobe, or much less frequently in other lobes. On the basis of figures from three reports, about 10% of the livers with hemangioma will contain more than one tumor(47, 48, 50). Al-though Shumacker(50) in his review of the literature found the left lobe to be the more frequent site for a hemangioma, subsequent series have shown the right lobe to be more often involved(3, 47, 48, 51). Hemangiomas of the liver may be pe-dunculated. In the series of operated cases reported by Schumacker(50) and D'Erri-co(56) 15.2 and 19.7%, respectively, of the hemangiomas were pedunculated. In two of the autopsy series no pedunculated tu-mors were found(47, 48). It would appear that the hemangioma that has grown to a sufficiently large size to become symptoma-tic is more likely to become pedunculated than the small tumor that is found inciden-tally at the time of autopsy or laparatomy.

Hemangiomas of the liver may vary in size from a few millimeters to tumors with a maximum diameter of over 30 cm. The majority of those found incidentally are leass than 5 cm in diameter(45, 47, 51). Other than those that are pedunculated, most of the hemangiomas will present as reddish-purple or blue masses beneath Glisson's capsule but they may be deeply located in the substance of the liver. They are well circumscribed but generally non-encapsulated. When palpated they are fluc-tuant and compressible unless they have undergone regressive changes such as thrombosis, fibrosis, or calcification. When sectioned they partially collapse due to the escape of blood and present a spongy sur-face. Grossly visible, recent, or organized thrombi may be present in the vascular spaces of the tumor, and calcification can be detected by the gritty sensation im-parted to the knife. Fibrosis usually begins centrally(3) but the entire hemangioma may appear as a firm gray-white nodule due to diffuse sclerosis (Fig. 29).

Microscopically the typical hemangioma is a well-demarcated tumor composed of

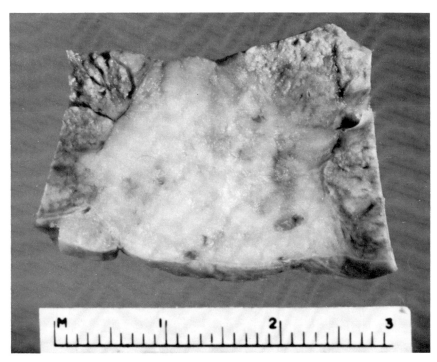

Figure 29 Sclerosed hemangioma of the liver. Gross photograph showing well-circumscribed subcapsular tumor with a homogeneous grey-white cut surface (AFIP Neg 68-4663).

multiple vascular channels of varying size lined by a single layer of flattened endothelial cells (Figs. 30–32). These are supported by a scanty amount of collagenous tissue, but the stroma may be very compact and hyalinized—sclerosed hemangioma (Figs. 33 and 34). Calcification of the hyalinized fibrous tissue may be spotty and dustlike or may be very dense with occasional ossification (Fig. 35); phleboliths may rarely be found in the lumen of the vascular channels. Partially or completely organized thrombi are often present in the lumen of some or many of the vascular compartments of the lesion (Fig. 36). Most hemangiomas do not contain hepatic parenchymal elements or bile ducts.

The gross and microscopic differential diagnosis of cavernous hemangioma include peliosis hepatis, hereditary hemorrhagic telangiectasia, infantile hemangioendothelioma, and malignant hemangioendothelioma. Vascular and hemorrhagic primary tumors (e.g., hepatoblastoma, hepatocellular carcinoma) or metastatic tumors can be readily distinguished by microscopic examination. Infantile hemangioendothelioma is covered in the Chapter 10 and malignant hemangioendothelioma is discussed in the next section of this chapter.

Peliosis hepatis is a disorder of the liver usually characterized grossly by multiple vascular spaces of varying size filled with blood (Fig. 37). In most cases the ragged margins of the cavities are not lined by endothelium (Fig. 37). The condition has been reported in association with a number of diseases (tuberculosis, various malignant tumors, etc.) as well as in patients receiving

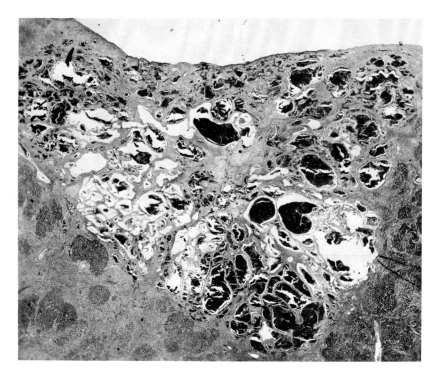

Figure 30 Cavernous hemangioma of the liver. Tumor is well-circumscribed and is located immediately subjacent to the Glisson's capsule. Surrounding liver shows a micronodular (Laennec's) cirrhosis (AFIP Neg 64-4137; hematoxylin and eosin, X9.5).

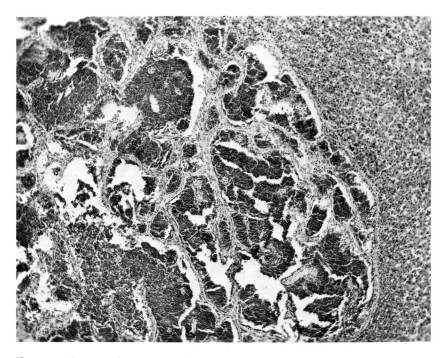

Figure 31 Cavernous hemingioma of the liver. The tumor was one of many similar tumors scattered in a liver that also contained multiple von Meyenburg complexes (biliary microhamartomas) (AFIP Neg 66-490; hematoxylin and eosin, X55).

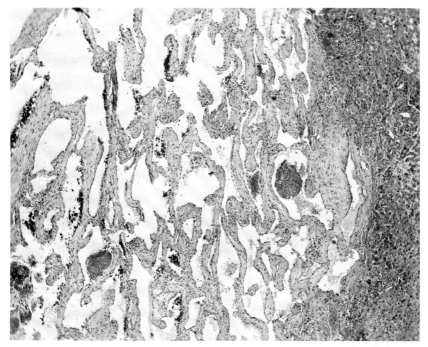

Figure 32   Cavernous hemangioma of the liver. A segment of the tumor is sharply demarcated from the adjacent liver (right) but is nonencapsulated. Cavernous spaces intercommunicate and are lined by a single layer of flat endothelial cells (AFIP Neg 65-12313; hematoxylin and eosin, X50).

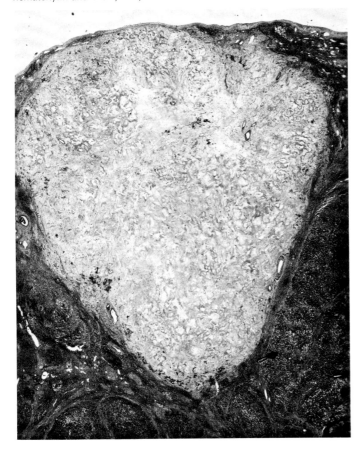

Figure 33   Sclerosed hemangioma of the liver. Wedge-shaped tumor abuts on Glisson's capsule. The tumor is characterized by a large amount of fibrous tissue replacing the cavernous spaces (AFIP Neg 70-9703; Masson's trichrome, X10).

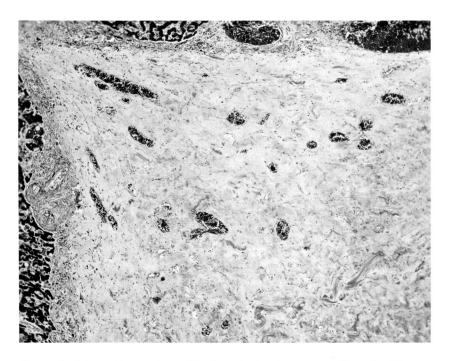

Figure 34   Sclerosed hemangioma of the liver. An abundant amount of hyalinized fibrous tissue surrounds the small and partially obliterated vascular channels (AFIP Neg 68-8445; hematoxylin and eosin, X50).

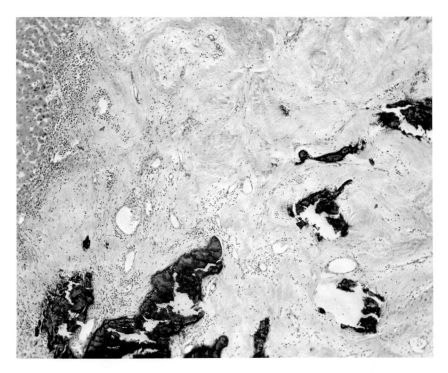

Figure 35   Sclerosed hemangioma of the liver with extensive calcification (AFIP Neg 74-8027; hematoxylin and eosin, X55).

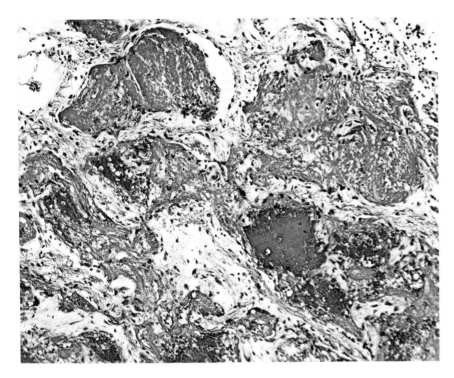

Figure 36 Cavernous hemangioma of the liver. Vascular lumina are completely occluded by thrombi (AFIP Neg 74-9528; hematoxylin and eosin, X90).

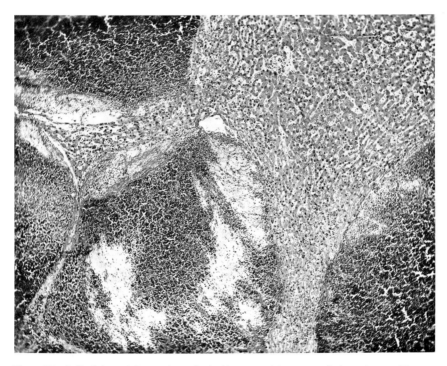

Figure 37 Peliosis hepatis in a patient who had been receiving oxymetholone therapy. The large blood-filled cavities are not lined by endothelium (AFIP Neg 72-8402; hematoxylin and eosin, X50).

283

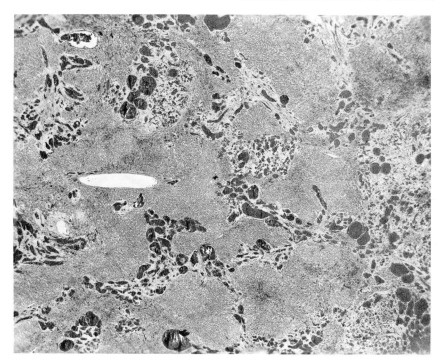

Figure 38 Hereditary hemorrhagic telangiectasia. Extensive involvement of the liver by telangiectases extending periportally and perilobularly (AFIP Neg 73-5551; hematoxylin and eosin, X12).

anabolic steroids (71–74). In the past peliosis hepatis was considered a terminal disorder not associated with any significant morbidity. In a recent series of seven patients who developed peliosis hepatis while receiving androgenic-anabolic steroids, two patients had intraperitoneal hemorrhages while three patients died because of liver failure(74).

Hereditary hemorrhagic telangiectasia (Rendu-Osler-Weber syndrome) may involve the liver(75-77). According to Martini(76), 55 patients with this disease had been reported up to 1959 in whom hepatic involvement was suspected clinically and who had had hepatosplenomegaly. In addition, there were 15 cases in which the clinical diagnosis was verified by biopsy and/or autopsy. Six patients personally observed by that author had multiple telangiectases in the liver as well as cirrhosis. Not all cases of hereditary hemorrhagic tel-

angiectasia with liver involvement have cirrhosis; whether or not it predisposes to cirrhosis is not known and in fact is doubted by some workers(75). Hepatic involvement in this disease is characterized by multiple telangiectatic foci of varying size composed of veins and occasional small capillaries (Figs. 38–40). The smaller lesions are often seen periportally but an abnormal number of vessels may also be present within the portal connective tissue (Fig. 40). As they grow larger they encroach more and more on the hepatic lobule, and eventually multiple lobules may be replaced by the telangiectases (Fig. 39). The larger lesions may show considerable fibrosis probably secondary to thrombosis. In advanced cases, such as the one reported by Zelman(77), large regenerative nodules of hepatic parenchyma may be present.

The treatment of cavernous hemangio-

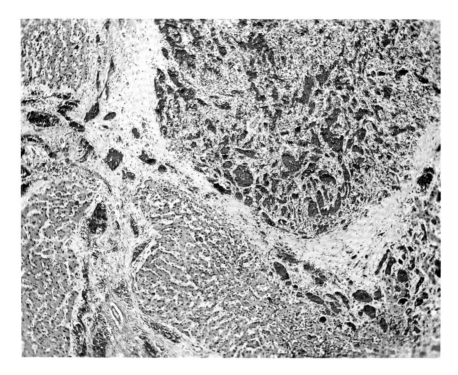

Figure 39 Hereditary hemorrhagic telangiectasia. A large lesion is present in the upper right quarter of the field. Other lesions are linked by their supporting fibrous base (AFIP Neg 73-5546; hematoxylin and eosin, X50).

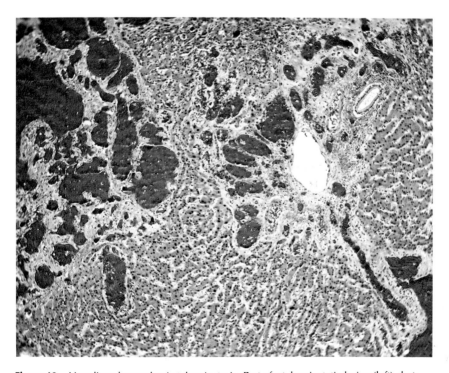

Figure 40 Hereditary hemorrhagic telangiectasia. Part of a telangiectatic lesion (left) abuts on a central vein (lower left). Portal area to the right contains an abnormal number of dilated veins (AFIP Neg 73-5547; hematoxylin and eosin, X55).

ma is surgical when the tumor is resectable. Detailed analyses of surgically treated cases reported in the literature are to be found in the reports of Shumacker(50) and D'Errico(56). Long-term follow-up studies have shown no evidence of recurrence in the series reported by Henson et al(51). Good results have been reported following radiation therapy when resection is not feasible such as in cases with massive or multiple tumors. The role of radiation therapy in the treatment of hemangiomas of the liver is extensively discussed in the publications of Issa(76) and Park and Phillips(54). With reference to this mode of therapy, note should be made of a case of hepatocellular carcinoma that occurred two decades after therapeutic radiation for a hepatic hemangioma(79). Although success has been reported in following treatment of hepatic hemangiomas and hemangioendotheliomas in children with corticosteroids and/or hepatic ligation(80–84), such modalities of therapy have not to the author's knowledge been used in treating hemangiomas in the adult.

Infantile Hemangioendothelioma

This tumor is discussed in Chapter 10.

Malignant

Malignant Hemangioendothelioma (Angiosarcoma)

Angiosarcoma is a rare tumor of the liver which is of much less frequent occurrence than hepatocellular or cholangiocellular carcinoma. It is, however, the most common malignant mesenchymal tumor of the liver. It is estimated that only about 25 cases of angiosarcoma occur each year in the United States(85). An idea regarding the incidence of this tumor relative to other malignant tumors of the liver can be gathered from autopsy series published from large hospitals in this country. Edmondson(3) had one angiosarcoma in his

series of 50,000 autopsies at the Los Angeles County Hospital, Los Angeles, California from 1918 to 1954. The ratio of angiosarcoma to hepatocellular carcinoma and cholangiocellular carcinoma was 1:81 and 1:26, respectively. In a series of 39,700 autopsies at Cook County Hospital, Chicago, Illinois from 1951 to 1973, there were five angiosarcomas of the liver(86). The ratio of angiosarcoma to hepatocellular carcinoma in this series was about 1:30.

The data on angiosarcoma of the liver presented in the succeeding paragraphs is based mainly on a review of 55 cases studied at AFIP(87). Of the cases studied, 85% occurred in males. The youngest patient was 24 while the oldest was 93 years of age. The largest number of cases occurred in the sixth and seventh decades of life.

About two-thirds of the patients (61.8%) presented with signs and symptoms indicative of liver disease. These included abdominal enlargement due to hepatomegaly and/or ascites, abdominal pain, anorexia, nausea and occasional vomiting, and jaundice. Of the 37 patients with hepatomegaly, 5 had an irregular or nodular liver, while a definite mass was palpated in 8. Tenderness over the liver was elicited in 12 patients. Twenty of the patients had weight loss and 14 complained of weakness. On admission to hospital 12 of the patients were febrile. One of the patients was already in hepatic coma when he first came to medical attention.

Eight of the patients (14.5%) had signs and symptoms indicative of an acute abdomen due to hemoperitoneum from rupture of the angiosarcoma. One patient presented with signs of a generalized hemorrhagic diathesis. In 3 of the patients (5.5%) splenomegaly, with or without pancytopenia, was the initial mode of presentation. Five of the patients (9.1%) had symptoms and signs referable to metastasis to the skeleton or lungs.

Upper and lower gastrointestinal radiographic studies revealed displacement and

/or compression or distortion of the colon, stomach, or duodenum in 9 of 23 cases. There were areas of diminished uptake, usually multiple, in hepatic scans from 6 to 8 patients. Elevation of the right hemidiaphragm was found in 8 of 21 patients. Radiologic evidence of skeletal or pulmonary metastases was present in 7 of 25 patients.

Leukocytosis, usually with a shift to the left, was found in 65.6% and leukopenia in 21.9% of the patients. There was thrombocytopenia in 62.5% of the patients. The hematocrits and hemoglobins were low in about two-thirds of the cases. A prolonged prothrombin time was found in 16 of 22 patients in whom values were available. With references to hematologic abnormalities, there are several reports of a microangiopathic hemolytic anemia(88–90) or a consumption coagulopathy(91, 92) associated with angiosarcoma of the liver.

The total serum bilirubin value was elevated in about 60% of the cases; in the majority the levels remained below 10 mg/100 ml. Serum alkaline phosphatase values were increased in about 64% of the patients. There was bromosulfophthalein retention (greater than 5% at 45 minutes) in all 12 patients on whom the test was performed. Serum glutamic oxaloacetic transaminase values were normal in almost half the patients; values greater than 200 Karmen units were detected in only two of the sera tested. One-third of the patients had hypoproteinemia. Eight of 20 patients had hypoalbuminemia. A 1:1 or reversed albumin/globulin ratio was found in half the patients.

The total duration of the illness in the AFIP series was very brief. Of the 55 patients 25 died within 3 months of the onset of their illness. Nine others died within 6 months while the remainder died in less than 12 months of the onset. The patients with ruptured neoplasms generally died from exsanguination within hours or days. The majority of the other patients died in liver failure or from malignant cachexia.

Of the patients who were necropsied, 23 of 33 had ascites. Pleural effusions were present in 12 of 34 patients. Peripheral edema was noted in about one-third of the cases. The liver was heavier than normal in over 84% of the cases; in about half of these the weight was greater than 3000 g.

In 39 of the 55 cases the angiosarcoma was multicentric and involved both lobes of the liver. In 8 cases, the tumor consisted of a single mass in the right lobe. (No information was available regarding the type of involvement of the liver in the remaining 8 cases.) Grossly the tumor nodules varied from pinpoint foci to large nodules measuring several centimeters in diameter. In many of the cases the larger masses bulged beneath Glisson's capsule giving the liver a knobby surface. The cut sections showed small ill-defined hemorrhagic foci or large fairly well circumscribed but nonencapsulated nodules having a dark red-brown color (Fig. 41). The larger nodules either had a spongy cut section or consisted of large cavities with a shaggy lining and a content of clotted and/or liquid blood.

Microscopically the patterns of growth of angiosarcoma consist of varying combinations of sinusoidal, cavernous, or solid foci. The latter type of growth is never seen in the absence of either a sinusoidal or a cavernous pattern. The earliest recognizable pattern of angiosarcoma is the appearance of hypertrophied sinusoidal endothelial lining cells with hyperchromatic nuclei that can be detected even on low power magnification (Fig. 42). These cells are usually seen in ill-defined foci which may be less than the size of a hepatic lobule. Occasionally, however, this change is diffuse throughout the liver or alternatively, only one or two such cells may be found in a lobule. Initially the hepatic plates are intact although sinusoids partly or completely lined by the neoplastic endothelial cells are dilated. Progression

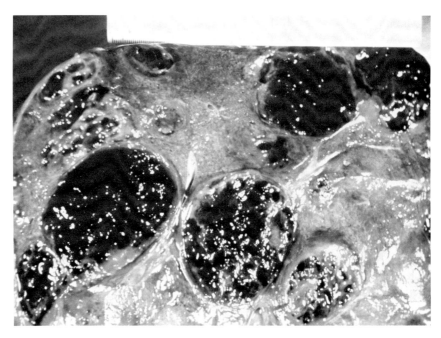

Figure 41 Gross photograph of angiosarcoma of the liver showing multiple hemorrhagic tumor nodules (AFIP Neg 74-12871).

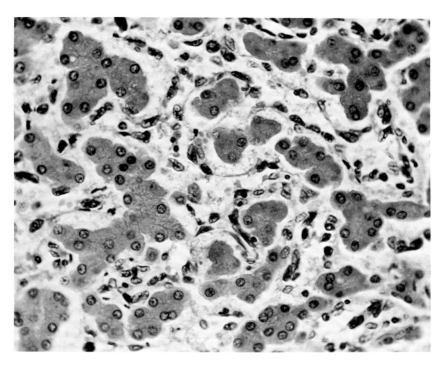

Figure 42 Angiosarcoma of the liver. Sinusoids are lined by prominent Kupffer cells with hyperchromatic nuclei. Hepatic plates are disrupted (AFIP Neg 64-3769; hematoxylin and eosin, X350).

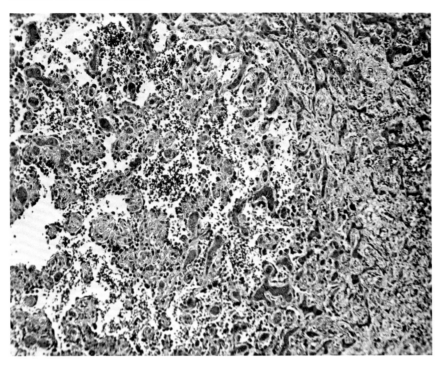

Figure 43 Angiosarcoma of the liver. Vasoformative nodule shows sinusoidal pattern of growth (AFIP Neg 74-7090; hematoxylin and eosin, X90).

involves increase in the size and nuclear hyperchromasia of these cells, greater sinusoidal dilatation, and disruption of the hepatic plate pattern (Fig. 43). As the hepatic plates become separated by the malignant endothelial cells, larger sinusoidal spaces, which vary greatly in size and complexity of shape, are formed (Fig. 44). Because of the peculiarities of sectioning, hepatic plates surrounded by the malignant cells often appear suspended in the larger spaces. The liver cells surrounded by the angiosarcoma cells undergo progressive atrophy and sometimes resemble small bile ducts but can be distinguished by their content of glycogen and lipofuscin pigment. Initially the malignant endothelial cells are supported by a single layer of reticulin fibers (Fig. 45) but as the nodules

grow there is an increase in the number of fibers, as well as progressive deposition of collagen bundles (Fig. 46). The collagen eventually completely replaces the space previously occupied by the atrophied hepatocytes.

With disappearance of liver cells and progressive enlargement of the vascular spaces lined by the neoplastic cells, the tumor nodules assume the cavernous pattern of growth (Fig. 47). The cells lining these spaces may consist of a single layer but more frequently they are multilayered or project into the cavity in intricate fronds and tufts supported by fibrous tissue (Fig. 48).

The malignant endothelial cells, whether lining sinusoidal or cavernous spaces, are usually elongated and have ill-defined cell

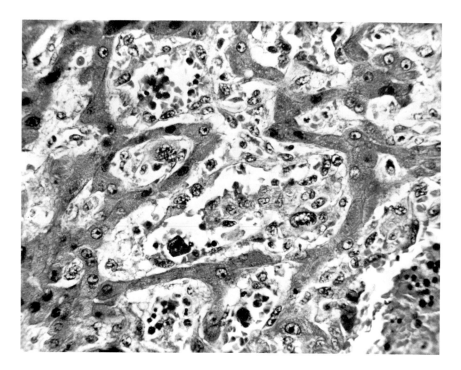

Figure 44 Angiosarcoma of the liver. Malignant endothelial cells line intercommunicating sinusoidal spaces. Note disruption of hepatic plates and atrophy of hepatocytes (AFIP Neg 71-11599; hematoxylin and eosin, X300).

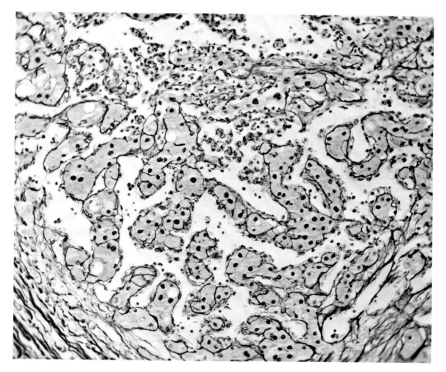

Figure 45 Angiosarcoma of the liver. A single layer of reticulin fibers separates the liver plates from the malignant endothelial cells lining the sinusoids (AFIP Neg 73-9016; Wilder's reticulum, X180).

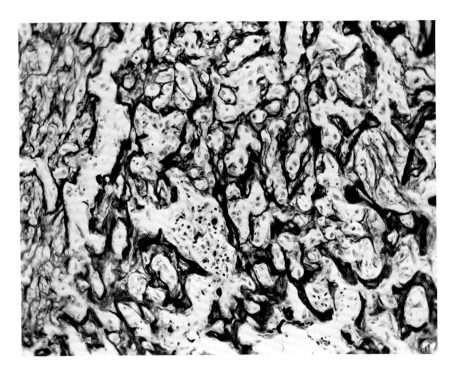

Figure 46 Angiosarcoma of the liver. There is a marked increase in the number and argentaphilia of reticulin fibers supporting malignant cells (AFIP Neg 66-382; Wilder's reticulum, X115).

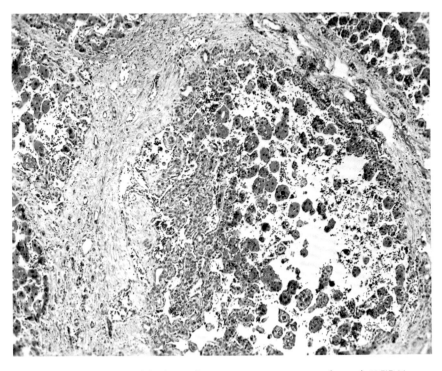

Figure 47 Angiosarcoma of the liver. There is a cavernous pattern of growth (AFIP Neg 73-8846; hematoxylin and eosin, XX70).

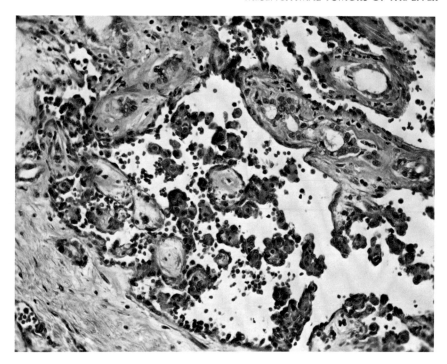

Figure 48   Angiosarcoma of the liver. Papillary formations of malignant endothelial cells project into cavernous space (AFIP Neg 73-8848; hematoxylin and eosin, X195).

borders. The cytoplasm is faintly eosinophilic and clear. No evidence of phagocytosis has been noted in any of the cases studied at AFIP. The nuclei are hyperchromatic and vary greatly in size and shape, but are generally longer in one axis. The chromatin granules are fine and the nucleoli small and amphophilic. The number of mitotic figures varies greatly from one case to another; thus there may be one mitosis in several high-power fields or several per high-power field (Fig. 49). Bizarre cells with irregular intensely hyperchromatic nuclei or multinucleated cells may be present in some of the cases (Fig. 50).

"Solid" tumor nodules are noted in a little over half the cases of angiosarcoma. These consist of closely packed elongated or fusiform cells resembling fibrosarcoma (Fig. 51). While slitlike vascular spaces are

scattered in these nodules, spaces lined by malignant endothelial cells are not visible. Very few reticulin fibers are present. As noted previously these nodules are not present in the absence of vasoformative tumor elements elsewhere in the same liver.

Neoplastic involvement of portal vein branches or central and sublobular veins is seen in the majority of cases of angiosarcoma (Fig. 52). In material examined at AFIP three out of every four cases showed malignant endothelial cells lining these veins and sometimes completely obliterating the lumen. These changes were seen both within well-defined tumor nodules and in nearby or, less frequently, in distant hepatic lobules.

Foci of extramedullary hematopoiesis are seen in the majority of cases of angiosarcoma of the liver (Fig. 53). Most of

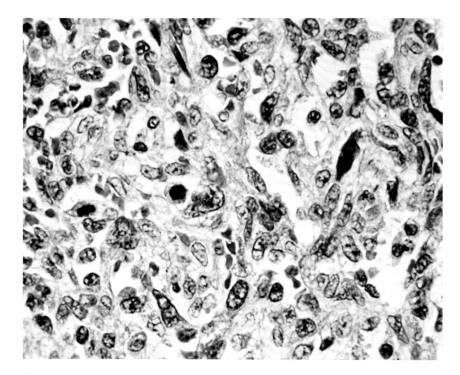

Figure 49 Angiosarcoma of the liver. There are marked nuclear pleomorphism and several mitotic figures (AFIP Neg 74-8651; hematoxylin and eosin, X530).

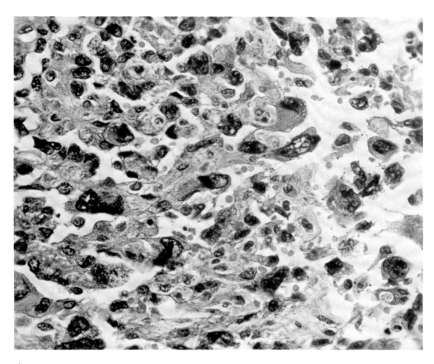

Figure 50 Angiosarcoma of the liver. Malignant cells have an irregular shape and bizarre, intensely staining nuclei (AFIP Neg 64-376; hematoxylin and eosin, X350).

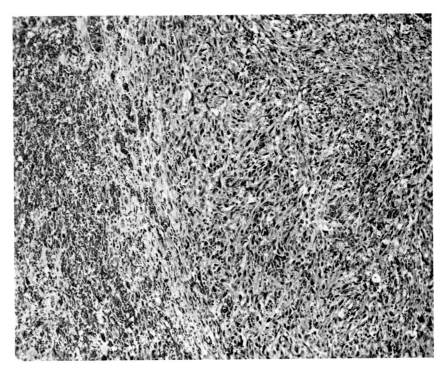

Figure 51 Angiosarcoma of the liver. Solid nodule composed of spindle-shaped cells (AFIP Neg 74-7091; hematoxylin and eosin, X90).

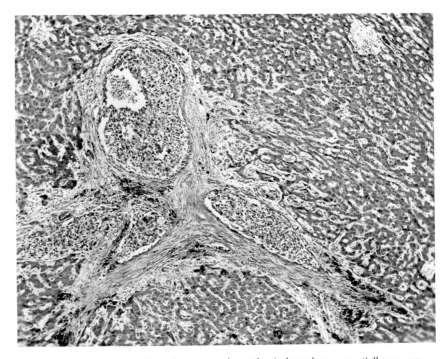

Figure 52 Angiosarcoma of the liver. Several portal vein branches are partially or completely occluded by proliferating endothelial cells. Black granules are thorotrast deposits (AFIP Neg 71-11583; hematoxylin and eosin, X50).

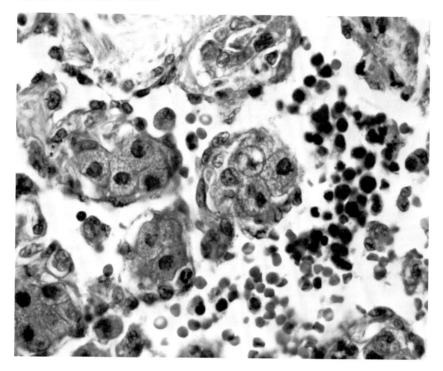

Figure 53 Angiosarcoma of the liver. Focus of nucleated erythrocytes and erythroblasts (AFIP Neg 73-8852; hematoxylin and eosin, X575).

these consist of nucleated erythrocytes and erythroblasts but occasional cases show megakaryocytes and precursors of the white blood series of cells. In about half the cases showing hematopoietic foci within the neoplasm similar cells are also present in the nonneoplastic lines.

Secondary changes in angiosarcoma include areas of hemorrhage, infarction, recent (or less often old) thrombosis, and varying degrees of fibrosis. No gross or microscopic evidence of calcification was noted in any of the cases studied at AFIP.

The nonneoplastic liver in angiosarcoma shows a variety of changes none of which are consistently seen in any one case. In the series of 55 cases studied at AFIP, there was only 1 case of a mixed micronodular and macronodular cirrhosis in a syphilitic patient who had been treated with arsenical drugs, induced malaria, and penicillin. In 43 cases on which enough tissue was available for evaluation of the nonneoplastic liver, there was no periportal fibrosis in 12 cases. There was minimal patchy periportal fibrosis in 13 cases and moderate fibrosis in 15 cases. Only 3 cases showed marked periportal fibrosis, and these were all in livers with thorotrast deposits. Capsular fibrosis was an infrequent finding and, when present, was usually in relation to thorotrast deposits or in areas overlying tumor nodules. Cholestasis of varying degrees of intensity was present in all livers in patients who died of liver failure. Other nonspecific changes, such as fatty metamorphosis and hemosiderosis, were seen in a few of the livers.

In 20 of the necropsied cases studied at AFIP, the liver was the only site of angiosarcoma. In autopsies with "metastases" the spleen was involved in 16 cases, the lungs

the liver and exposure to polyvinyl chloride (PVC) was first reported by Creech et al(128). The first three cases together with another case were subsequently reviewed in the weekly report "Morbidity and Mortality" of the Center for Disease Control, Atlanta, Georgia(85). All four male patients had worked continuously in the PVC polymerization section of a plant in Louisville, Kentucky for at least 14 years prior to the onset of their illness. In each case, in addition to the angiosarcoma, there was extensive cirrhosis of the nonalcoholic type. Other cases of angiosarcoma related to exposure to polyvinyl chloride have subsequently been reported in the United States and other countries(129–136).

Other than the development of angiosarcoma, workers exposed to PVC may have abnormalities of tests of hepatic function as well as evidence of portal hypertension. In a group of 13 workers reported by Lange et al(137), 12 patients had splenomegaly, 4 patients had esophageal varices, and 11 patients had increased bromosulfophthalein retention. Liver biopsy specimens from 5 of these workers revealed marked portal fibrosis. Creech et al(135) biopsied the liver of 32 biochemically abnormal but asymptomatic employees of a PVC production plant. Of the biopsy specimens 14 had varying degrees of fibrosis; 8 had marked portal fibrosis, dilated sinusoids, atypical sinusoidal living cells, and diffuse subcapsular fibrosis. Two patients had angiosarcoma. Angiographic studies were performed on 30 patients, half of whom had evidence of portal hypertension. Martin et al(138) have recently shown that PVC-associated hepatic fibrosis may progress despite cessation of exposure.

The oncogenic potential of vinyl chloride has been known since the work of Viola et al in 1971(139). These investigators showed that rats exposed 12 months to vapors of vinyl chloride developed tumors of the skin, lungs, and bones. Maltoni(140) subsequently produced angiosar-

comas of the liver in rats exposed to atmospheric vinyl chloride for a year in concentrations as low as 250 ppm. Gordon et al(136) have recently reported that mice develop angiosarcomas six to eight months after exposure to 2500, 200, and 50 ppm vinyl chloride in a closed inhalation system for seven hours, five times per week. Comparison of these experimentally produced angiosarcomas with those in human workers exposed to PVC has shown that the basic evolution of the angiosarcoma is the same in both.

In addition to angiosarcomas produced experimentally by thorotrast and vinyl chloride, a number of other chemicals and naturally occurring compounds have been shown in the past to induce such tumors. Hepatic angiosarcomas have been induced in rats fed cycad nut meal(141), in Syrian golden hamsters treated with methylhydrazine(142), in mice treated with urethan(143), and in rats treated with diethylnitrosamine(144) or dimethylnitrosamine(145).

TUMORS AND TUMORLIKE LESIONS OF LYMPH VESSELS

Lymphangiomas, if they do occur in the liver, must be excessively rare. The term "lymphangioma" or "cavernous lymphangiomatoid lesion" has been used as a synonym for mesenchymal hamartoma of the liver(3). Hepatic and splenic lymphangiomatosis may be part of the syndrome of skeletal lymphangiomatosis. Asch et al(142) recently reported a case and reviewed 12 previously published cases. The liver biopsy specimen from a 10-year-old girl reported by these authors showed multiple small and medium-sized vascular channels lined by endothelium and containing eosinophilic fluid and occasional erythrocytes. The fibrous walls of some of the larger cysts were calcified.

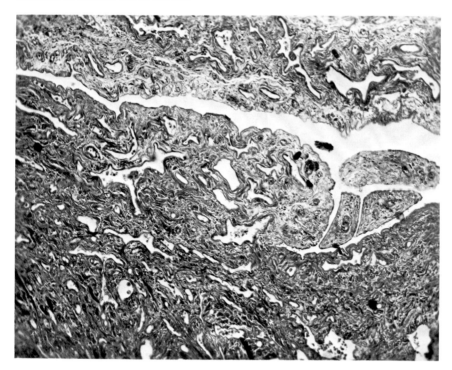

Figure 55   Benign mesothelioma of the liver. Multiple spaces lined by flat mesothelial cells are surrounded by fibrous tissue (AFIP Neg 73-12617; Masson's trichrome, X50).

TUMORS OF MESOTHELIAL TISSUES
Benign
Benign Mesothelioma

Only one benign mesothelioma of the liver has been reported in the literature(3). This was a firm fibrous tumor attached to Glisson's capsule by a broad base. Microscopically it was composed of moderately cellular tissue indented by deep clefts lined with mesothelial cells. Another example is on file at AFIP. An incidental autopsy finding in a 34-year-old Negro female who died of massive pulmonary embolism of uncertain etiology showed a history of hypertension and myocardial infarction four years before her demise. The liver at necropsy weighed 1400 g and showed two well-circumscribed yellowish-tan nodules protruding from the surface of the right lobe; one was 2.0 cm and the other was 0.5 cm

in diameter. Both tumors had a similar microscopic appearance with multiple cystically dilated spaces lined by cuboidal or flat endothelial cells with occasional papillary projections (Fig. 55–57). These were supported by fibrous tissue in which cords of liver cells and an occasional portal area were trapped. The hepatic parenchyma away from the nodules was essentially normal. Both tumors were classified as benign mixed tubular and fibrous mesotheliomas.

It is possible that the benign fibromas discussed in a previous section of the chapter actually represent fibrous mesotheliomas. Multiple sections from both tumors, however, failed to reveal any mesothelial cell component. In the absence of definite proof of their origin from mesothelium, such as tissue culture methods, the author would prefer to classify them as fibromas.

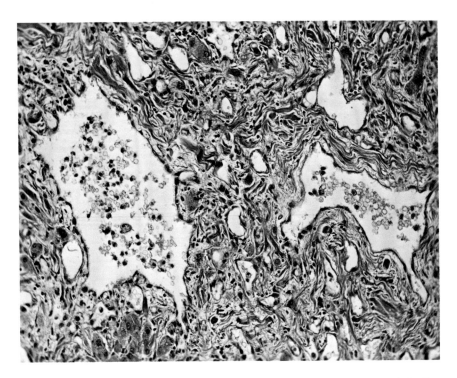

Figure 56 Benign mesothelioma of the liver. Varying-sized spaces lined by mesothelial cells are separated by randomly oriented collagen bundles (AFIP Neg 73-12612; hematoxylin and eosin, X100).

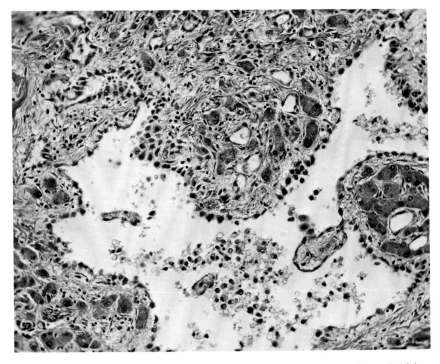

Figure 57 Benign mesothelioma of the liver. Cystically dilated space is lined by cuboidal mesothelial cells. Note papillary projection to the right and groups of darkly staining hepatocytes in the surrounding fibrous tissue (AFIP Neg 73-12611; hematoxylin and eosin, X115).

Malignant Mesothelioma

To the author's knowledge there are no published examples of primary malignant mesotheliomas of the liver.

TUMORS OF PLURIPOTENTIAL MESENCHYME (MESENCHYMOMAS)

Benign

Benign Mesenchymoma

As originally used by Stout(147) the term refers to benign tumors made up of two or more mesenchymal elements other than fibrous tissue. Although some of the benign mixed tumors of mesodermal origin, such as the angiomyolipoma described in the section on tumors of adipose tissue, would come under this designation, no purpose is served by introducing another term to describe them.

Malignant Mesenchymoma

These tumors are extremely rare and the author has not had the opportunity of studying any. A case of a bizarre tumor composed of an admixture of osteosarcoma, chondrosarcoma, and fibrosarcoma was reported by Sumiyoshi and Niho(148). This was a huge yellowish-gray multinodular mass in the right lobe of a cirrhotic liver of a 52-year-old male, The tumor had invaded branches of the portal vein and had grown into the inferior vena cava. There was one metastasis in the right atrium of the heart and several metastases to the small bowel. The authors reviewed four other cases of mixed malignant mesodermal tumors, all of which were also published from Japan.

It should be noted at this juncture that the term "malignant mesenchymoma" has been used to designate undifferentiated sarcoma of the liver occurring mainly in children(3, 149). In the author's experience these tumors do not show evidencee

of differentiation and therefore do not fit Stout's original meaning of the term malignant mesenchymoma(147).

TUMORS OF DISPUTED OR UNCERTAIN HISTOGENESIS

Benign

Granular Cell Tumor

To date, no granular tumor of the liver has been reported. At least 12 such tumors involving the extrahepatic biliary system have been published. These have occurred in the common hepatic duct, common bile duct, and the cystic duct and have been the subject of a recent review by LiVolsi et al(150). A more recent case was reported by Whisnant et al(151). An example of a granular cell tumor involving the common hepatic duct is illustrated in Figs. 58 to 60.

Myxoma

To the author's knowledge there is only one example of a myxoma of the liver published in the literature(3, 152). This occurred in a 58-year-old Caucasian male who developed sudden abdominal pain and had a palpable epigastric mass on physical examination. At the time of laparotomy a large tumor mass was found in the left lobe of the liver; the mass contained a large cyst that had ruptured. The cyst was evacuated and a biopsy was taken from the cyst wall. The patient died four months postoperatively. At the time of necropsy the liver weighed 2875 g. The left lobe was almost entirely replaced by a soft, lobulated, pale gray mass. Although the case was published as a "myxosarcoma" the authors(152) felt it was benign, an opinion shared by Edmondson(3) who reviewed the sections from the tumor.

Malignant

No examples of malignant granular cell tu-

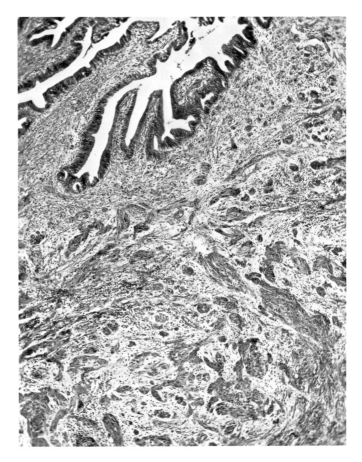

Figure 58 Granular cell tumor of the common hepatic duct. Nests of granular cells are infiltrating the wall of the duct, the mucosa of which is seen in the upper part of the field (AFIP Neg 74-9537; Masson's trichrome, X35).

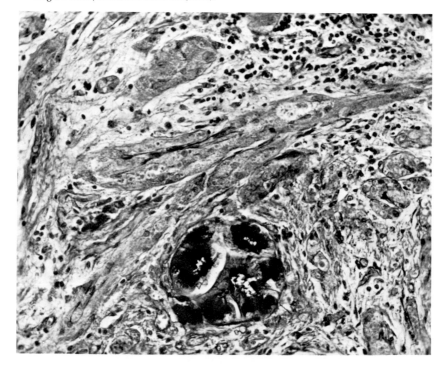

Figure 59 Granular cell tumor of the common hepatic duct. Elongated and polygonal granular cells surround a darkly staining mucous gland (AFIP Neg 74-9147; PAS, X245).

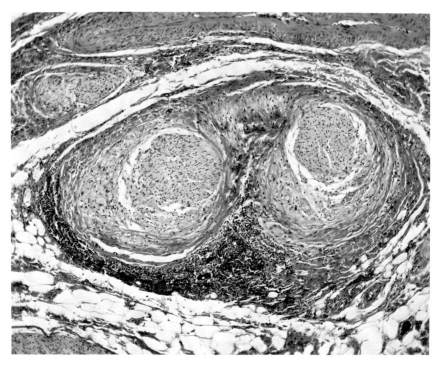

Figure 60   Granular cell tumor of the common hepatic duct. Granular cells grow between nerve bundles and their sheath in the wall of the duct (AFIP Neg 74-9142; hematoxylin and eosin, X75).

mor or myxosarcoma of the liver are known to the author.

REFERENCES

1. Luna LG (Ed): *Manual of Histologic Staining Methods of the Armed Forces Institute of Pathology,* 3rd ed. McGraw-Hill, New York, 1968.

2. Enzinger FM: *Histological Typing of Soft Tissue Tumours.* International Histological Classification of Tumours No. 3, World Health Organization, Geneva, 1969.

3. Edmondson HA: *Tumors of the Liver and Intrahepatic Bile Ducts, Atlas of Tumor Pathology,* Section VII, fascicle 25, Armed Forces Institute of Pathology, Washington, D. C.

4. Shallow TA, Wagner FB: Primary fibrosarcoma of the liver. *Ann Surg* **125**:439–446, 1947.

5. Simpson HM, Baggenstoss AH, Stauffer MH: Primary sarcoma of the liver. A report of three cases. *South Med J* **48**:1177–1182, 1955.

6. Steiner PE: Cancer of the liver and cirrhosis in Trans-Saharan Africa and the United States of America. *Cancer* **13**:1085–1149, 1960.

7. Ojima A, Sugiyama T, Takeda J, et al: Six cases of rare malignant tumors of the liver. *Acta Pathol Jap* **14**:95–102, 1964.

8. Snapper L, Schraft WC, Ginsberg DM: Severe hypoglycemia due to fibrosarcoma of the liver. *Maandschr Kindergeneeskd* **32**:337–347, 1964.

9. Totzke HA, Hutcheson JB: Primary fibrosarcoma of the liver. *South Med J* **58**:236–238, 1965.

10. Balouet G, Destombes P: A propos de quelques tumeurs mesenchymateuses hepatiques d'apparence primitive. *Ann Anat Pathol (Paris)* **12**:273–286, 1967.

11. Cavallo T, Lichewitz B, Rozov T: Primary fibrosarcoma of the liver. Report of a case. *Rev Hosp Clin Fac Med Sao Paulo* **23**:44–49, 1968.

12. Smith D, Rele SR: A case of primary fibrosarcoma of the liver. *Postgrad Med J* **48**:62–63, 1972.

13. Walter VE, Bodner E, Lederer B: Primäres Fibrosarkom der Leber. *Wien Klin Wochenschr* **84**:808–810, 1972.

14. Alrenga DP: Primary fibrosarcoma of the liver. Case report and review of the literature. *Cancer,* in press.

15. Lowbeer L: Hypoglycemia producing extrahepatic neoplasms. *Am J Clin Pathol* **35**:233–243, 1961.

16. Bower BF, Gordan GS: Hormonal effects of nonendocrine tumors. *Am Rev Med* **16**:83–118, 1965.

17. Volpe R, Evans J, Clarke DW, et al: Evidence favoring the sarcomatous origin of an insulin-like substance in a case of fibrosarcoma with hypoglycemia. *Am J Med* **38**:540–553, 1965.

18. Sneed SM, Fine G, Horn RC: Hypoglycemia associated with extrapancreatic tumors. *Cancer* **24**:158–166, 1969.

19. Bousvaros GA: Hypoglycemia in metastatic fibrosarcoma of the liver. *Brit Med J* **1**:836–838, 1960.

20. Cavallaro A, Ziparo V, Palestini M, et al: A case of extended right hepatic lobectomy for fibrosarcoma. *Panminerva Med* **15**:216–218, 1973.

21. Simon MA: Focal fat infiltration in the liver. *Am J Pathol* **10**:799–804, 1934.

22. Young S: A case of lipoma of the liver. *J Pathol Bact* **63**:336–337, 1951.

23. Ramchand S, Ahmed Y, Baskerville L: Lipoma of the liver. *Arch Pathol* **90**:331–333, 1970.

24. Grosdidier J, Boissel P, Macinot C, et al: Myelolipome hepatique. A propos d'une observation. *Nov Presse Med* **2**:1777–1779, 1973.

25. Plaut A: Myelolipoma in the adrenal cortex. *Am J Pathol* **24**:487–515, 1958.

26. Lombard LS, Garner FM, Brynjolfsson G: Myelolipomas of the liver in captive wild felidae. *Pathol Vet* **5**:127–134, 1968.

27. Lucke B, Schlumberger HG: *Tumors of the Kidney, Renal Pelvis and Ureter, Atlas of Tumor Pathology,* Section VIII, fasicle 30, Armed Forces Institute of Pathology, Washington, D. C.

28. Demopoulos RI, Denarvaez F, Kaji V: Benign mixed mesodermal tumors of the uterus. A histogenetic study. *Am J Clin Pathol* **60**:377–383, 1973.

29. Persaud V: Pseudolipoma of Glisson's capsule. *Arch Pathol* **88**:555–556, 1969.

30. Rolleston H, McNee JW: *Diseases of the Liver, Gall Bladder and Bile Ducts.* MacMillan, London, 1929, p 487.

31. Demel P: Ein Operierter Fall von Leber-Myom. *Virch Arch* **281**:881–884, 1926.

32. Rios-Dalenz JL: Leiomyoma of the liver. *Arch Pathol* **79**:54–56, 1965.

33. Stout AP: Bizarre smooth muscle tumors of the stomach. *Cancer* **15**:400–409, 1962.

34. Richman R, Meranze DR, Zibelman CS, et al: Malignant leiomyoblastoma. *Am J Clin Pathol* **49**:556–561, 1968.

35. Smithwick W, Biesecker JL, Leand PM: Leiomyoblastoma. Behaviour and prognosis. *Cancer* **24**:996–1003, 1969.

36. Watanuki K, Kusama K: A case of leiomyosarcoma of the liver. *Nippon Ika Diagn Z* **22**:552, 1955.

37. Yamaguchi T, Yanagisawa M, Ootori M, et al: Case of primary leiomyosarcoma of the liver. *Naika* **22**:1495–1497, 1968.

38. Meinikov RA, Jukharov VF: Leiomyosarcoma of the liver. *Vopr Onkol* **16**:73–75, 1970.

39. Wilson SE, Braitman H, Plested WG, et al: Primary leiomyosarcoma of the liver. *Ann Surg* **174**:232–237, 1971.

40. Fong JA, Ruebner BH: Primary leiomyosarcoma of the liver. *Human Pathol* **5**:115–119, 1974.

41. Mital RN, Bazaz-Malik G: Leiomyosarcoma of *Ligamentum teres* of the liver. *Am J Gastroenterol* **56**:48–51, 1971.

42. Koberle F, Pfleger R: Lebervenengeschwulst mit dem Symptomenbild einer Endophlebitis obliterans hepatica. *Wien Arch Intern Med* **34**:73–85, 1940.

43. MacMahon HE, Ball HG: Leiomyosarcoma of hepatic vein and the Budd-Chiari syndrome. *Gastroenterology* **61**:239–243, 1971.

44. Kevorkian J, Cento DP: Leiomyosarcoma of large arteries and veins. *Surgery* **73**:390–399, 1973.

45. Geschickter CF, Keasbey LE: Tumors of blood vessels. *Am J Cancer* **23**:568–591, 1935.

46. O'Donoghue JB, Nicosia AJ: Cavernous hemangioma of the liver. *Ill Med J* **98**:15–17, 1950.

47. Ochsner JL, Halpert B: Cavernous hemangioma of the liver. *Surgery* **43**:577–582, 1958.

48. Feldman M: Hemangioma of the liver. Special reference to its association with cysts of the liver and pancreas. *Am J Clin Pathol* **29**:160–162, 1958.

49. Dehner LP, Ishak KG: Vascular tumors of the liver in infants and children. A study of 30 cases and review of the literature. *Arch Pathol* **92**:101–111, 1971.

50. Shumacker HB: Hemangioma of the liver. Discussion of symptomatology and report of patient treated by operation. *Surgery* **11**:209–222, 1942.

51. Henson SW, Gray HK, Dockerty MB: Benign tumors of the liver. II. Hemangiomas. *Surg Gynecol Obstet* **103**:327–331, 1956.

52. Ninard B: *Tumeurs du Foie.* Librairie le Francois, Paris, 1950.

53. Morley JE, Myers JB, Sack FS, Kalk F, Epstein EE, Lannon J: Enlargement of cavernous haemangioma associated with exogenous administration of oestrogens. *S A Med J* 1:695–697, 1974.

54. Park WC, Phillips, R: The role of radiation therapy in the management of hemangiomas of the liver. *JAMA* 212:1496–1498, 1970.

55. Pozzi G: Angioma cavernosa del fegato. *Clin Chir* 8:625–650, 1932.

56. D'Errico G: I cavernomi del fegato di interesse chirurgico. Revista critica della letterature: 71 casi operati. *Ital Chir* 2:267–284, 1946.

57. Wilson H, Tyson WT: Massive hemangiomas of the liver. *Ann Surg* 135:765–770, 1952.

58. Sewell JH, Weiss K: Spontaneous rupture of hemangioma of the liver. *Arch Surg* 83:729–733, 1961.

59. Rubin IC: Large pedunculated angioma of the liver reaching down into the pelvis and causing obstetric difficulty. *Am J Obstet* 77:273–276, 1918.

60. Cooper WH, Martin JF: Hemangioma of the liver with thrombocytopenia. *Am J Roengenol Radiat Ther* 88:751–755, 1962.

61. Behar A, Moran E, Izak G: Acquired hypofibrinogenemia associated with a giant cavernous hemangioma of the liver. *Am J Clin Pathol* 40:78–82, 1963.

62. Martinez J, Shapiro SS, Holburn RR, et al: Hypofibrinogenemia associated with hemangioma of the liver. *Am J Clin Pathol* 59:192–197, 1973.

63. Levitt LM, Coleman M, Jarvis J: Multiple large hemangiomas of the liver. *New Engl J Med* 252:854–855, 1955.

64. Aspray M: Calcified hemangiomas of the liver. *Am J Roentgenol Radiat Ther* 53:446–453, 1945.

65. Plachta A: Calcified cavernous hemangioma of liver. Review of literature and report of 13 cases. *Radiology* 79:783–788, 1962.

66. Pantoja E: Angiography in liver hemangioma. *Am J Roentgenol Radiat Ther* 104:874–879, 1968.

67. McLaughlin MJ: Angiography in cavernous hemangioma of the liver. *Am J Roentgenol Radiat Ther* 113:50–55, 1971.

68. Abrams RM, Beranbaum ER, Santos JS, et al: Angiographic features of cavernous hemangioma of liver. *Radiology* 92:308–312, 1969.

69. Chung EB: Multiple bile duct hamartomas. *Cancer* 26:287–296, 1970.

70. Benz EJ, Baggenstoss AH: Focal cirrhosis of the liver: its relation to the so-called hamartoma (adenoma, benign hepatoma). *Cancer* 6:743–755, 1953.

71. Kent G, Thompson JR: Peliosis hepatis. *Arch Pathol* 72:658–664, 1961.

72. Yanoff M, Rawson AJ: Peliosis hepatis. *Arch Pathol* 77:159–165, 1964.

73. Nacim F, Copper PH, Semion AA: Peliosis hepatis. Possible etiologic role of anabolic steroids. *Arch Pathol* 95:284–285, 1973.

74. Baghieri SA, Boyer JL: Peliosis hepatis associated with androgenic-anabolic steroid therapy. *Ann Intern Med* 81:610–618, 1974.

75. Smith JL, Lineback ML: Hereditary hemorrhagic telangiectasia. Nine cases in one Negro family, with special reference to hepatic lesions. *Am J Med* 17:41–49, 1954.

76. Martini GA: Cirrhosis of the liver in hereditary hemorrhagic telangiectasia. *Proceedings of the First World Congress on Gastroenterology*, Vol 2. Williams and Wilkins, Baltimore, 1959, pp 857–858.

77. Zelman NS: Liver fibrosis in hereditary hemorrhagic telangiectasia. *Arch Pathol* 74:66–72, 1962.

78. Issa P: Cavernous haemangioma of the liver. The role of radiotherapy. *Brit J Radiol* 41:26–32, 1968.

79. Moore TA, Ferrante WA: Hepatoma two decades after radiation for hepatic hemangioma (Abstract). Meeting of American Association for the Study of Liver Diseases, San Francisco, Calif., May 19–25, 1974.

80. Goldberg SJ: Successful treatment of hepatic hemangioma with corticosteroids. *JAMA* 208:2473–2474, 1969.

81. Touloukian RJ: Hepatic hemangioendothelioma during infancy. Pathology, diagnosis and treatment with prednisone. *Pediatrics* 45:71–76, 1970.

82. Brown SH, Neerhout RC, Fonkalsrud EW: Prednisone therapy in the management of large hemangiomas in infants and children. *Surgery* 71:168–173, 1971.

83. DeLorimier AA, Simpson EB, Baum, RS, et al: Hepatic-artery ligation for hepatic hemangiomatosis. *New Engl J Med* 277:333–337, 1967.

84. Rake MO, Liberman MM, Dawson JL, et al: Ligation of hepatic artery on the treatment of heart failure due to hepatic hemangiomatosis. *Gut* 11:512–515, 1970.

85. Center for Disease Control: Angiosarcoma of the liver among polyvinyl chloride workers—Kentucky. *Morb Mortal Wkly Rep* 23:49–50, 1974.

86. Szanto PB, Alrenga DP, Khin U: Primary malignant neoplasms of the liver. Exhibit presented at the Joint Meeting of the American Association of Pathologists and Bacteriologists and the

International Academy of Pathology, San Francisco, Calif., March 9–16, 1974.

87. Ishak KG, McAllister HA: Angiosarcoma of the liver. Presented at Joint Meeting of College of American Pathologists and American Society of Clinical Pathologists, Washington, D. C., October 4–11, 1974.

88. Alpert LI, Benisch B: Hemangioendothelioma of the liver associated with microangiopathic hemolytic anemia. *Am J Med* **48**:624–628, 1970.

89. Donald D, Dawson AA: Microangiopathic haemolytic anaemia associated with haemangioendothelioma. *J Clin Pathol* **24**:456–459, 1971.

90. Pollard SM, Millward-Sadler GH: Malignant haemangioendothelioma involving the liver. *J Clin Pathol* **27**:214–221, 1974.

91. Case Record Massachusetts General Hospital. *New Engl J Med* **285**:279–287, 1971.

92. Truell JE, Peck SD, Reiquam CW: Hemangiosarcoma of the liver complicated by disseminated intravascular coagulation. *Gastroenterology* **65**:936–942, 1973.

93. Baker H deC, Paget GE, Daveson J: Haemangio-endothelioma (Kupffer-cell sarcoma) of the liver. *J Pathol Bact* **72**:173–182, 1956.

94. Kwittken J, Tartow LR: Haemochromatosis and Kupffer-cell sarcoma with unusual localisation of iron. *J Pathol* **92**:571–573, 1966.

95. Sussman EB, Nydick I, Gray GF: Hemangioendothelial sarcoma of the liver and hemochromatosis. *Arch Pathol* **97**:39–42, 1974.

96. MacMahon HE, Murphy AS, Bates MI: Endothelial cell sarcoma of the liver following thorotrast injections. *Am J Pathol* **23**:585–611, 1947.

97. Looney WB: An investigation of the late clinical findings following thorotrast (thorium dioxide) administration. *Am J Roentgenol* **83**:163–185, 1960.

98. Nettleship A, Fink WJ: Neoplasms of the liver following injection of thorotrast. *Am J Clin Pathol* **35**:422–426, 1961.

99. Suckow EE, Henegar GC, Baserga R: Tumors of the liver following administration of thorotrast. *Am J Pathol* **38**:663–677, 1961.

100. Rakov HL, Smalldon TR, Derman H: Hepatic hemangioendotheliosarcoma. Report of a case due to thorium. *Arch Intern Med* **112**:173–178, 1963.

101. da Silva Horta J: Late lesions in man caused by colloidal thorium dioxide (thorotrast). *Arch Pathol* **62**:403–418, 1965.

102. Wenz W, Ott G: Aktuelle Thorotrast probleme: Ein Lebersarkom mit intraperitoneale Blutung. *Strahlentherapie* **127**:463–469, 1965.

103. da Silva Horta J, Abbott JD, da Motta LC, Roriz ML: Malignancy and other late effects following administration of thorotrast. *Lancet* **2**:201–205, 1965.

104. da Silva Horta J: Late effects of thorotrast on the liver and spleen, and their efferent lymph nodes. *Ann NY Acad Sci* **145**:676–699, 1967.

105. Dahlgren S: Late effects of thorium dioxide on the liver of patients in Sweden. *Ann NY Acad Sci* **145**:718–723, 1967.

106. da Silva Horta J, da Motta LC: Follow-up study of thorium dioxide patients in Portugal. *Ann NY Acad Sci* **145**:830–842, 1967.

107. Mori T, Sakai T, Nozue Y, et al: Malignancy and other injuries following thorotrast administration. Follow-up study of 147 cases in Japan. *Strahlentherapie* **134**:229–254, 1967.

108. Boyd JT, Langlands AO, MacCabe JJ: Long-term hazards of thorotrast. *Brit Med J* **1**:517–521, 1968.

109. Ansari A, Weigent CE: Hemangioendothelial sarcoma of the liver. A clinicopathological study of an 81-year-old male veteran. *Am J Gastroenterol* **56**:420–427, 1971.

110. Baserga R, Yokoo H, Henegar GC: Thorotrast-induced cancer in man. *Cancer* **13**:1021–1031, 1960.

111. Becker Von V, Busscher K: Uber das Hamangioendotheliom der Leber. *Acta Hepatosplenol (Stuttgart)* **8**:356–379, 1961.

112. Dahlgren S: Thorotrast tumours. A review of the literature and report of two cases. *Acta Pathol Microbiol Scand* **53**:147–161, 1961.

113. Grampa G: Radiation injury with particular reference to thorotrast. In *Pathology Annual*, Vol 6. Appleton-Century-Crofts, New York, 1971, pp 147–169.

114. Smoron GL, Battifora HA: Thorotrast-induced hepatoma. *Cancer* **30**:1252–1259, 1972.

115. Teller NC: Follow-up of thorium dioxide patients in the United States. *Ann NY Acad Sci* **145**:674–675, 1967.

116. Tessmer CF, Chang JP: Thorotrast localization by light and electron microscopy. *Ann NY Acad Sci* **145**:545–575, 1967.

117. Terzakis JA, Sommers SC, Snyder RW, et al: X-ray microanalysis of hepatic thorium depositions. *Arch Pathol* **98**:241–242, 1974.

118. Guimaraes JP, Lamerton LF: Further experimental observations in the late effects of thorotrast administration. *Brit J Cancer* **10**:527–532, 1956.

119. Swarm RL, Miller E, Michelitch HJ: Malignant vascular tumors in rabbits injected intravenously with colloidal thorium dioxide. *Pathol Microbiol* **25**:27–44, 1962.

120. Johansen C: Tumors in rabbits after injection of various amounts of thorium dioxide. *Ann NY*

Acad Sci **145**:724–727, 1967.

121. Regelson W, Kim U, Ospina J, et al: Hemangioendothelial sarcoma of liver from chronic arsenic intoxication by Fowler's solution. *Cancer* **21**:514–522, 1968.

122. Morris JS, Schmid M, Newman S, et al: Arsenic and noncirrhotic portal hypertension. *Gastroenterology* **64**:86–94, 1974.

123. Roth F: The sequelae of chronic arsenic poisoning in Moselle vintners. *Ger Med Mon* **2**:211–217, 1957.

124. Denk R, Holzmann H, Lange HJ, et al: Uber Arsenspatschaden bei obduzierten Mosel Winzern. *Med Welt* **11**:557–567, 1969.

125. Franklin M, Bean WB, Hardin RC: Fowler's solution as an etiologic agent in cirrhosis. *Am J Med Sci* **219**:589–596, 1950.

126. Rosenberg HG: Systemic arterial disease and chronic arsenicism in infants. *Arch Pathol* **97**:360–365, 1974.

127. Rennke H, Prat GA, Etcheverry RB, et al: Hemangioendothelioma maligno del higado y arsenicismo chronica. *Rev Med Chil* **99**:664–668, 1971.

128. Creech JL, Johnson ML: Angiosarcoma of liver in the manufacture of polyvinyl chloride. *J Occup Med* **16**:150–151, 1974.

129. Center for Disease Control: Angiosarcoma of the liver—Connecticut. *Morb Mortal Wkly Rep* **23**:210, 216, 1974.

130. Block JB: Angiosarcoma of the liver following vinyl chloride exposure. *JAMA* **229**:53–54, 1974.

131. Lee FI, Harry DS: Angiosarcoma of the liver in a vinyl-chloride worker. *Lancet* **1**:1316–1318, 1974.

132. Monson RR, Peters JM: Proportional mortality among vinyl-chloride workers. *Lancet* **2**:397–398, 1974.

133. Falk H, Greech JL, Heath CW, et al: Hepatic disease among workers at a vinyl chloride polymerization plant. *JAMA* **230**:59–63, 1974.

134. Makk L, Creech JL, Whelan JG, et al: Liver damage and angiosarcoma in vinyl chloride workers. *JAMA* **230**:64–68, 1974.

135. Creech JL, Makk L, Whelan JG, et al: Hepatotoxicity among polyvinyl chloride (PVC) production workers during the first year of surveillance program (Abstract). American Association for the Study of Liver Diseases, Twenty-fifth Anniversary Meeting, Chicago, Illinois, October 29–30, 1974.

136. Gordon DE, Thomas LB, Kent G, et al: Hepatic angiosarcoma in man and rodents following prolonged exposure to vinyl chloride (Abstract). American Association for the Study of Liver Diseases, Twenty-fifth Anniversary Meeting, Chicago, Ill., October 29–30, 1974.

137. Lange CE, Juhe S, Stein G, Veltman G: Die sogenannte Vinylchlorid-Krankheit eine berufsbedingte Systemklerose? *Gut Arch Arbeitsmed* **32**:1–32, 1974.

138. Martin JF, Waggoner JG, Berk PD: Persistence of vinyl chloride (VC) induced hepatic injury after cessation of exposure (Abstract). American Association for the Study of Liver Diseases, Twenty-fifth Anniversary Meeting, Chicago, Ill., October 29–30, 1974.

139. Viola PL, Bigotti A, Caputo A: Oncogenic response of rat skin, lungs, and bones to vinyl chloride. *Cancer Res* **31**:516–522, 1971.

140. Maltoni C: Cited by FI Lee and DS Harry (131).

141. Laqueur GL, Mickelsen O, Whiting MG, et al: Carcinogenic properties of nuts from *Cycas circinalis L. indiginous* to Guam. *J Natl Cancer Inst* **31**:919–951, 1963.

142. Toth B, Shimizu H: Methylhydrazine tumorigenesis in Syrian golden hamsters and the morphology of malignant histiocytomas. *Cancer Res* **33**:2744–2753, 1973.

143. Deringer MK: Response of strain DBA/2eBDe mice to treatment with urethan. *J Natl Cancer Inst* **34**:841–847, 1965.

144. Hadjiolov D: Hemangioendothelial sarcomas of the liver in rats induced by diethylnitrosamine. *Neoplasma* **19**:111–114, 1972.

145. Hadjiolov D, Markow D: Fine structures of hemangioendothelial sarcomas in the rat liver induced with N-nitrosodimethylamine. *Arch Geschwulstforsch* **42**:120–126, 1973.

146. Asch MJ, Cohen AH, Moore TC: Hepatic and splenic lymphangiomatosis with skeletal involvement. Report of a case and review of the literature. *Surgery* **76**:334–339, 1974.

147. Stout AP: *Tumors of the Soft Tissues, Atlas of Tumor Pathology*. Section II, fascile 5, Armed Forces Institute of Pathology, Washington, D.C.

148. Sumiyoshi A, Niho Y: Primary osteogenic sarcoma of the liver—Report of an autopsy case. *Acta Pathol Jap* **21**:305–312, 1971.

149. Stanley RJ, Dehner LP, Hesker AE: Primary malignant mesenchymal tumors (mesenchymoma) of the liver in childhood. *Cancer* **32**:973–984, 1973.

150. LiVolsi VA, Perzin KH, Badder EM, et al: Granular cell tumors of the biliary tract. *Arch Pathol* **95**:13–17, 1973.

151. Whisnant JD, Bennett SE, Huffman SR, et al: Common bile duct obstruction by granular cell tumor (Schwannoma). *Am J Dig Dis* **19**:471–476, 1974.

152. Evans N, Hoxie HJ: Primary myxosarcoma of liver. *Am J Med* **91**:290–294, 1937.

CHAPTER 13 BENIGN EPITHELIAL TUMORS AND TUMORLIKE LESIONS OF THE LIVER

HUGH A. EDMONDSON, M.D.

Benign epithelial tumors and tumorlike lesions usually become manifest *(a)* in infancy before the age of two years, *(b)* in childhood, or *(c)* in adults before the age of 50. Most commonly an enlarged abdomen is noted by the patient or by the parents in the case of infants or children (1). Some tumors are unsuspected, and the diagnosis is made by the physician when the abdomen is examined. Older children often complain of pain (1). Other symptoms include a sense of fullness or indigestion. Jaundice is rare (2). Adenomas in women may produce pain by hemorrhage into their substance or they may rupture into the abdominal cavity with consequent shock. Roentgenograms often disclose that the colon and stomach are displaced downward and to the left. Arteriograms and radionuclide imaging have proved to be of great help in the differential diagnosis of focal intrahepatic lesions (3). These indicate the degree of vascularity of the hepatic mass as compared with that in normal surrounding liver. The adenomas are "vascu-

lar"; cysts, infarcts, abscesses, and cirrhotic pseudomasses are "avascular" or "hypovascular."

CLASSIFICATION

The author's classification of tumors and tumorlike lesions for all age groups as well as for infants and children has been published (4, 5). The present classification (Table 1) is slightly modified but includes only the benign epithelial tumors and tumorlike lesions. For diagnostic purposes these may be divided into solid and cystic varieties. Most of the entities included in the classification have at one time or another been labeled "hamartomas." Albrecht's concept of a hamartoma (6) is that of a tumorous mass that is developmental in origin. It hardly seems likely that most of reported hamartomas, covering such a wide range of gross and microscopic change and occurring in nearly every decade of life, could truly be developmental

Table 1 Classification

Lesion	Solid	Cystic
Benign epithelial tumors		
Liver cell adenoma	X	
Bile duct adenoma	X	
Bile duct cystadenoma		X
Adrenal rest tumor	X	
Tumorlike lesions		
Adenomatous hyperplasia	X	
Focal nodular hyperplasia	X	
Mixed hamartoma (mixed adenoma)	X	
Solitary and multiple nonparasitic cysts	X	
Congenital hepatic fibrosis and polycystic disease		X
	X	X
Mesenchymal hamartoma		X
Anoxic necrosis	X	

in origin. It seems to the author far better to give a particular lesion a specific name that is not used for any other tumor or tumorlike lesion. This is not an easy task because such a plethora of terms have been used and so little is known of the etiology of the various entities. Three tumors derived from epithelial cells may occur in the liver. The liver cell adenoma arises from hepatocytes; the bile ducts give origin to small bile duct adenomas and rarely to large multiloculated cystadenomas.

LIVER CELL ADENOMAS

Adenomas of the liver were rarely reported previous to the use of oral contraceptives. However, in recent years an increasing number of liver cell adenomas have been noted (7–12). The author now has studied 29 reported cases. Clinically, they fall into four categories: (a) those who have a mass in the region of the liver; (b) those who have pain in the region of the liver; (c) those with symptoms of intraabdominal hemorrhage and shock; or (d) the rare instance of an incidental tumor noted during surgery. In 28 or 29 cases in the author's series, the entire tumor was removed and all the patients have remained well. In 9 of the patients the tumor had ruptured and intraabdominal bleeding had occurred so that emergency surgery had to be performed. Fortunately, all of these patients recovered. Liver scans and arteriograms are helpful in the diagnosis of tumors that have not ruptured.

The frequency of adenomas is doserelated as most patients had been on oral contraceptives for more than five years. Mestranol-containing compounds were the most commonly used oral contraceptives among the patients with tumors. It is of interest that several of the tumors became symptomatic at the time of menstruation, especially those that had ruptured. This raises the question of whether the blood vessels in the liver tumor may respond in a similar fashion to those in the endometrium at the time of menstruation.

The gross appearance of these adenomas in women on the "pill" varies considerably depending on the presence or absence of degenerative change and hemorrhage. Usually adenomas are sharply demarcated, encapsulated, and somewhat lighter in color than normal liver (Fig. 1). They may have a fairly homogeneous appearance, or blood vessels and a small amount of connective tissue may subdivide the tumor into segments of irregular size. Degenerative change may lead to necrosis, partial fibrosis, and hemorrhage. An occasional tumor may be light yellow due to fatty change or bile formation. Adenomas vary in size from about 2 to 20 or 30 cm in dimension. They are usually solitary, but multiple tumors have occurred.

On microscopic examination the neoplastic hepatocytes are larger than normal and form a cord pattern (Fig. 2) with visible canaliculi. In many tumors the hepatocytes have an acinar arrangement and may contain bile. The liver cords have the usual

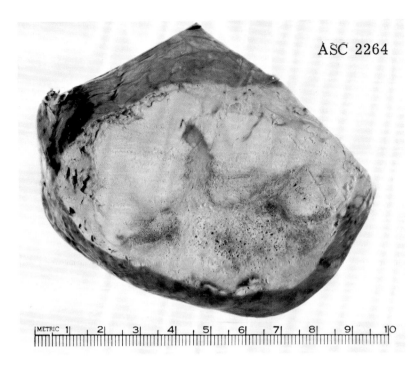

ASC 2264

Figure 1 Adenoma of the liver in a 26-year-old woman who complained only of a mass in the right upper quadrant. She has been taking oral contraceptives for 48 months. Patient has remained well since surgical removal of the tumor. (ASC 2264).

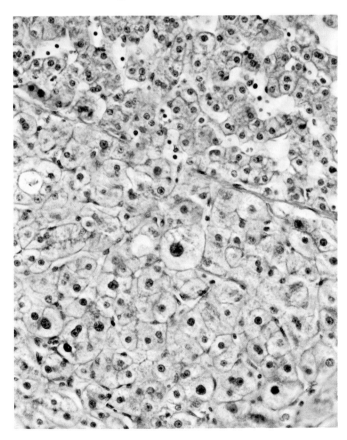

Figure 2 Margin of an adenoma with a thin capsule and large hyperplastic cells. The cords and sinusoids are more compressed than in the normal adjacent liver. (hematoxylin and eosin X250; ASC 2445).

311

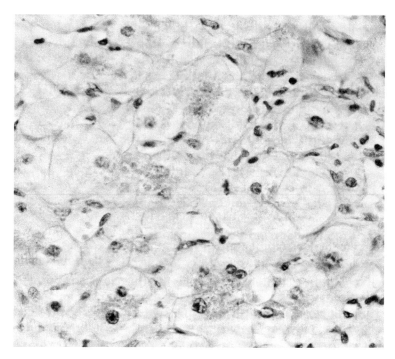

Figure 3 Lipochrome and a small amount of bile pigment are present around canaliculi in this liver cell adenoma (hematoxylin and eosin, X500).

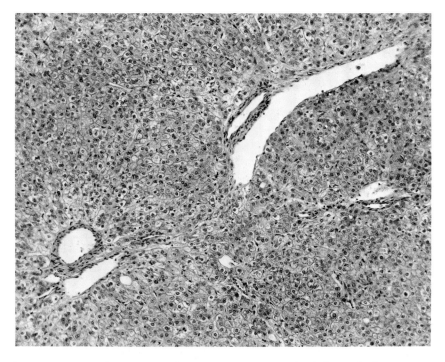

Figure 4 Arteries and veins commonly accompanying one another in liver cell adenomas (hematoxylin and eosin, X100; ASC 2141).

relationship to the sinusoids but often the latter appear compressed. The nuclei are usually of normal size, although occasional hyperchromatic nuclei with larger than normal nucleoli are observed. Binuclear forms are common. Except in a rare case, mitoses are absent. A few of the tumors show a variable amount of fatty change. The cytoplasm is acidophilic and similar to that of normal hepatocytes. In about one half of the adenomas studied there was lipochrome in the cytoplasm (Fig. 3). Occasionally this pigment is an outstanding feature. Adenomas have an abundant blood supply composed of both small arteries and accompanying veins (Fig. 4). Many large veins that are not accompanied by arteries are presumably outflow veins. Large vascular complexes are sometimes observed that give the tumor an angiomatous appearance. Infarcts and hemorrhage occurred in 20 of the 29 unreported cases studied by the author (13). The capsule is composed of a relatively acellular layer of collagenous connective tissue. In some instances the capsule was partially missing and the margin of the tumor was irregular.

The mechanism of formation of adenomas in women on oral contraceptives is not known. It is of interest that one of the women in the author's study had only a biopsy because the liver contained numerous nodules, some of which were approximately 10 cm in diameter. The biopsy taken from one of the small nodules showed transformation of cord cells to neoplastic type cells but no evidence of capsule formation. The appearance of the transformed cells was similar in all respects to the other adenomas that followed the use of oral contraceptives. This patient was taken off medication after surgery and the liver became much smaller. The patient died of carcinoma of the ovary many years later, at which time no evidence of adenomas was seen in the liver.

In addition to the tumors in women who use oral contraceptives, the author has had available for study four liver cell adenomas in infants and children, five in men, and seven in women on whom there was no history of use of oral contraceptives. All of these tumors have a histologic appearance similar to that of the adenomas described above. However, there was one major difference. Infarction and hemorrhage, with or without rupture, were seen only in the women taking oral contraceptives. The author knows of only one exception, that of a 40-year-old woman with rupture and fatal hemorrhage. This was noted at the time of autopsy at the Los Angeles County-University of Southern California Medical Center in 1955, before the era of oral contraceptives.

BILE DUCT ADENOMAS

Bile duct adenomas are small (usually less than 2 cm in diameter), firm, gray-white lesions that are located beneath Glisson's capsule. These symptomless tumors are sometimes observed and removed at surgery. Microscopically, they are composed of rather small ductular structures separated by a variable amount of connective tissue (Fig. 5). The epithelium is similar to that of bile ducts, but the acini do not contain bile as they sometimes do in polycystic disease. The etiology of bile duct adenomas is not known. There are no reports to indicate that they may become malignant.

The author has never seen an example of a papillary tumor of the *intrahepatic bile ducts*.

CYSTADENOMAS

Multilocular cystadenomas have been noted almost exclusively in women (14), usually in the middle age group. The symptoms are those of a growing abdominal mass. Right upper quadrant abdominal pain, occasionally radiating to the scapula, was the chief complaint in 60% of the cases. Biliary obstruction developed in some 35%. Roentgenograms, angiograms,

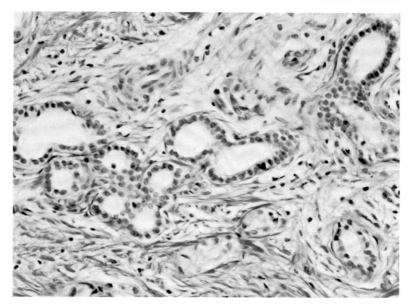

Figure 5 Bile duct adenoma composed of multiple glands of bile duct-type interspersed with a moderate amount of stroma (hematoxylin and eosin, X300; ASC 2261).

and radioisotopic scans outline the lesions. Ultrasonograms may be helpful in diagnosing their cystic nature. The majority of the reported tumors have been present in the right lobe. However, among 11 unreported cases that have been sent to the author, four arose in the left lobe and two in the right. The lobe of origin of the others was not mentioned.

Grossly, cystadenomas vary from a few centimeters in diagmeter to large multicystic structures 15 to 18 cm in greatest dimension. Most of the tumors are composed of cysts of variable size (Fig. 6), but occasionally there is one large cyst with many small locules around the periphery. Several examples of ductal cystadenomas have been reported (15). They may be polypoid and produce jaundice. The cysts contain a mucinous fluid that may be clear or colored by old hemorrhage.

Microscopically, cystadenomas differ from simple cysts in that they are multilocular and have mucoid material in their compartments; their columnar lining cells stain positively for mucin. The lining of the cysts may have a smooth contour but often contains folds (Fig. 7). Papillary processes of various size are noted in some of the cysts. Often these papillae are short and stubby. Hemosiderin and cholesterol clefts due to old hemorrhage are often present in the subepithelial tissue (Fig. 8). A characteristic feature of cystadenoma is the presence of densely cellular connective tissue just beneath the epithelial lining (Fig. 9). This tissue bears some resemblance to ovarian stroma. The connective tissue between the cysts contains many blood vessels. Small linear areas of calcification are frequent; these are probably not large enough to be visible on roentgenograms.

The treatment is complete surgical excision when possible. Many patients have had recurrences after surgery but, nevertheless, the prognosis seems to be good. Two instances of cystadenocarcinoma have been reported (14).

The origin of cystadenomas is unknown.

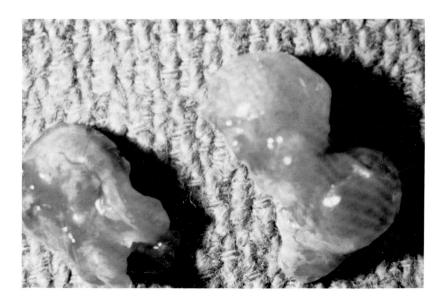

Figure 6 Multiple mucus-filled cysts in a cystadenoma. The tumor comprising the entire left lobe of the liver and weighing 4200 g was removed surgically from a 46-year-old white woman (ASC 2156).

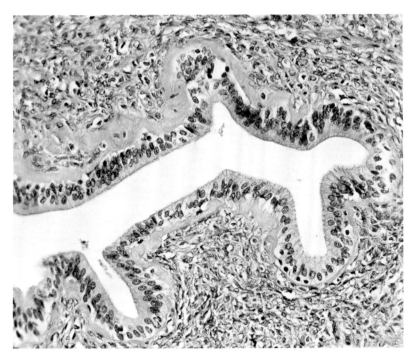

Figure 7 The lining cells of this small outpocket of a cystadenoma are tall columnar, and tend to have folds (hematoxylin and eosin, X250; ASC 2788).

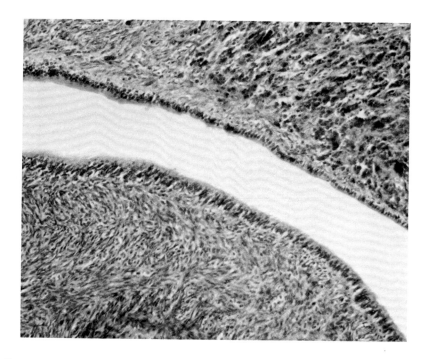

Figure 8   Subepithelial pigment and dense cellular stroma in a cystadenoma (hematoxylin and eosin, X150; ASC 1191).

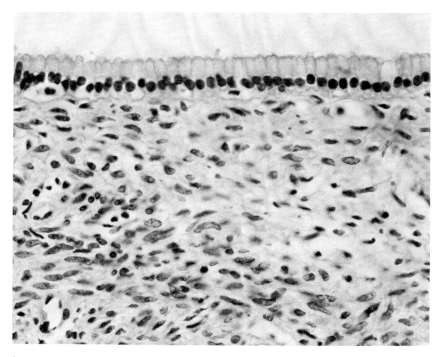

Figure 9   The lining cells of this cystadenoma are tall, columnar, and stain positively for mucin. The subepithelial stroma is densely cellular (hematoxylin and eosin, X500; ASC 2156). Figures 6 and 9 from the same case.

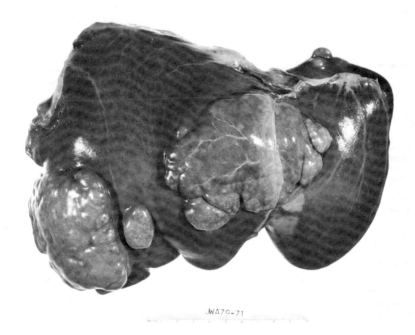

Figure 10   Large areas of adenomatous hyperplasia in a patient who died of submassive necrosis of the liver (JWA 79-71).

They are difficult to distinguish microscopically from cystadenomas of the pancreas. It is possible that both have a similar origin. The presence of a cystadenoma in both the liver and pancreas has been reported (16).

ADRENAL REST TUMORS

Adrenal rest tumors are extremely rare. Occasionally a portion or all of the right adrenal may be present beneath Glisson's capsule; thus the possibility of tumor formation exists.

ADENOMATOUS HYPERPLASIA

The formation of sizeable nodules following liver injury, either acute or chronic, has received many names but the choice of "adenomatous hyperplasia" seems appropriate. Large nodular areas of hyperplasia are a common finding in submassive necrosis of the liver; they are usually few in number and have an eccentric distribution (Fig. 10). Occasionally the nodules are more or less uniformly present in both lobes. They vary greatly in size, and sometimes they are palpable and are mistaken for neoplasms. Most often they are lighter in color, slightly bile-stained, and stand out strongly in contrast to the collapsed deep brown hepatic framework that remains after severe necrosis (Fig. 11).

In chronic liver disease, especially cirrhosis, adenomatous hyperplasia frequently develops. These nodules are usually discrete and rarely average more than 6 to 8 cm in diameter. Many such patients with known cirrhosis who develop a palpable mass have had unnecessary surgery. The nodules of adenomatous hyperplasia are of variable size and do not have a true capsule. Grossly, the surrounding septa pres-

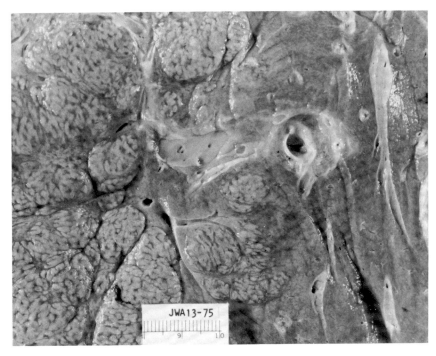

Figure 11   Large nodules of adenomatous hyperplasia stand out in sharp contrast to collapsed necrotic parenchyma in a patient with submassive necrosis (JWA 13-75).

ent in cirrhosis expand and thus form a pseudocapsule (Fig. 12) that microscopically contains many blood vessels and bile ducts. This differs markedly from the laminated layer of poorly cellular connective tissue in the capsule of an adenoma. The nodules do not have the homogeneous appearance of a true adenoma because small septa that carry blood vessels and even small bile ducts enter from the perimeter (Fig. 13). These usually subdivide the nodule. Rarely does a nodule arise in the cirrhotic liver that satisfies the criteria for a true adenoma. These seem to have limited growth potential and apparently are not complicated by hemorrhage and rupture. Larger lesions that have been called the macroregenerating lesion in cirrhosis may be correctly diagnosed by arteriograms and a liver scan (17). These are probably composed of several discrete areas of adenomatous hyperplasia.

The adenomatous foci in tyrosinemia are not encapsulated but apparently may become malignant. The author has seen one case of adenomatous hyperplasia in congenital hepatic fibrosis.

FOCAL NODULAR HYPERPLASIA

Nonencapsulated, nodular gray-white to tan tumors, usually solitary, composed of hepatocytic units with a distinct connective tissue pattern, are fairly common in women. The author's collection now consists of 50 cases, 35 of which are surgical specimens. Thirty-one of these were removed incidentally; only 4 patients had surgery for a palpable mass. Thirty-three were females aged 14 months to 74 years. The 2 males were 17 and 51 years old. All but 4 of the women were between 20 and 50 years old. The average age was 32 years.

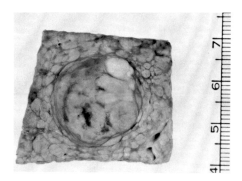

Figure 12 Area of adenomatous hyperplasia in a cirrhotic liver (LAC-USCMC 61070). Figures 12 and 13 are from the same patient).

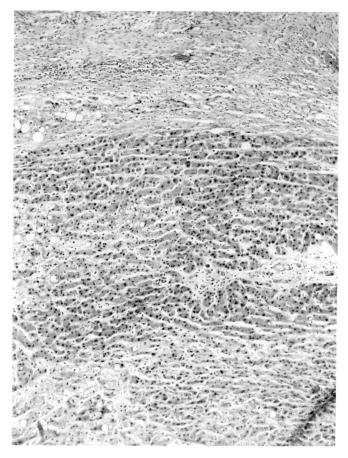

Figure 13 In this area of adenomatous hyperplasia the fibrous septa are pushed aside by the expansion of the nodule. Small bile ducts and blood vessels are noted in the lower right (hematoxylin and eosin, X75; LAC-USCMC 61070).

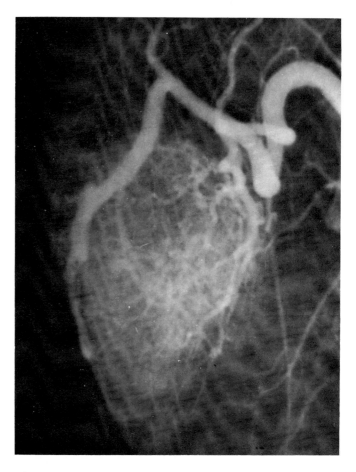

Figure 14   This angiogram shows the marked vascularity of focal nodular hyperplasia. The patient was a 29-year-old woman in whom a tumor of the liver was palpated at the time of pelvic surgery (ASC 2504).

The nodules are usually subcapsular but occasionally they are pedunculated or deep within the liver. A few have been too large to remove at surgery. Occasionally the gallbladder bed was involved so that this organ had to be removed. In autopsy material multiple nodules are occasionally observed that vary in size from 1 cm to 18 cm in greatest dimension. In some instances focal nodular hyperplasia is accompanied by one or more cavernous hemangiomas (18).

Angiograms have disclosed an abundant arterial supply in several cases (19). The angiograms on a large nodule in a 29-year-old white woman is shown in Fig. 14. This tumor was removed surgically in 1974. The patient has remained well.

Grossly, focal nodular hyperplasia usually has a central stellate mass of connective tissue with many fine septa radiating to the periphery (Fig. 15). The color of the tumor is lighter than that of the surrounding liver. In rare instances the nodules may be fatty or lightly bile-stained. Hemorrhage has been reported in patients with focal nodular hyperplasia who are taking oral contraceptives (20).

On microscopic examination the central area contains dense connective tissue in which there are many large blood vessels. The arteries often have thick myxomatous-like walls and constricted lumens. It may be assumed that the blood supply of the nodule is primarily derived from the hepa-

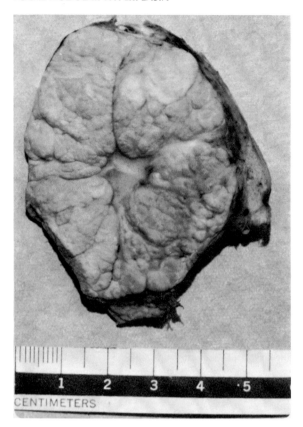

Figure 15 Focal nodular hyperplasia in a 21-year-old woman who was operated on for a mass in the mid-upper abdomen. The tumor was present in the left lobe of the liver (ASC 1427A).

tic artery and not from the portal vein. The hepatocytes are difficult to distinguish from adjacent liver cells. They are characteristically arranged in units around a tiny central core of connective tissue, blood vessels, and ductules. These units are best seen at the periphery of the lobules, next to surrounding liver (Fig. 16). A line of demarcation usually separates the hyperplastic units from adjacent liver but this may be indistinct because there is little difference between the hepatocytes of focal nodular hyperplasia and the normal liver. Connective tissue septa radiate from the central mass toward the periphery where they disappear; penetration into the adjacent liver was not observed in the author's material. A zone of widened sinusoids is frequently observed in the adjacent liver, possibly due to runoff from the heavy arterial blood supply in focal nodular hyperplasia.

The *prognosis* is good. There is no proof that focal nodular hyperplasia ever becomes malignant. A few have grown too large to remove but no complications have been reported in these patients.

Differential Diagnosis

Focal nodular hyperplasia is easily distinguished from liver cell adenoma by the presence of septa, ductules, and the individual hyperplastic units (Fig. 16). The so-

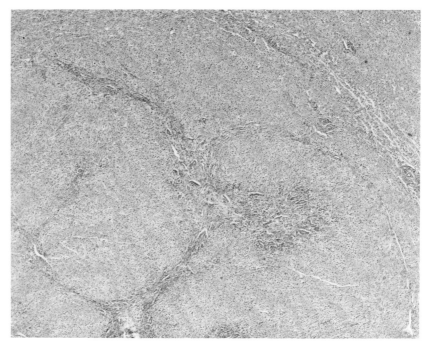

Figure 16   Margin of area of focal nodular hyperplasia showing multiple hyperplastic units with central connective tissue core and an ill-defined line of separation from adjacent liver (hematoxylin and eosin, X30); ASC 1708).

called mixed adenoma or hamartoma has wider septa, many small ducts, and much more of a pseudolobular pattern.

MIXED HAMARTOMA (MIXED ADENOMA)

Although described in the literature as a mixed adenoma, this lesion is not truly an adenoma. The fibrous tracts, bile ducts, and pseudolobules bear no resemblance to an adenoma. After perusing the literature, the author accepts only five instances of this disorder; four were in infants and one in an adult. The author has one unreported case (21). All presented with a palpable mass in the liver region and were removed surgically. They presented as localized nodular masses (8 to 10 cm in diameter). On gross examination all were multinodular, with tough fibrous bands separating the parenchyma (Fig. 17). Microscopic study disclosed a multitude of pseudolobules that varied greatly in size and that were composed of rather normal appearing hepatocytes that were separated by fibrous septa containing myriads of bile ductules (Fig. 18). Many of the latter seemed to arise from cord cells as fibrous tissue invaded the margins of the pseudolobules (Fig. 19). The connective tissue in the septa was often mature, compact, and arranged in thick bundles (Fig. 19), a type that the author has rarely observed in any other liver disease. Many large triads were present containing hepatic arterial branches with unusually thick walls. The outflow veins likewise were thick and their lumens small. Cholestasis has not been reported.

The nature of this lesion, its etiology, and the sequence of events that lead to the

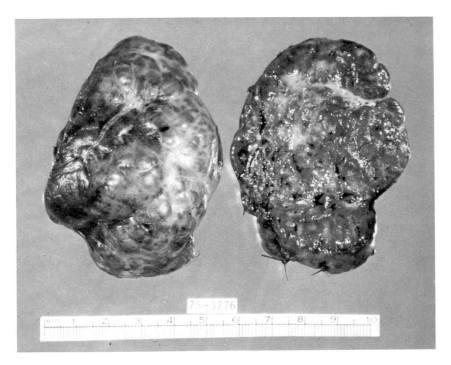

Figure 17 Mixed hamartoma of liver in a female aged 4 months (ASC 2710).

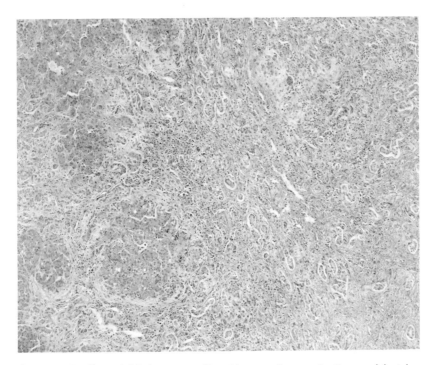

Figure 18 Small pseudolobules separated by wide areas of connective tissue and ductules. Tumor successfully removed from a 3-month-old baby boy (hematoxylin and eosin, X75; LAC-USCMC 53776). Figures 18 and 19 are from the same patient.

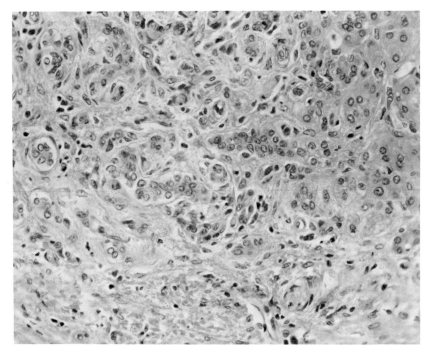

Figure 19 Margin of pseudolobule showing conversion of cord cells to ductular type (hematoxylin and eosin, X250; LAC-USCMC 5376).

unusual microscopic changes are not known. It appears to be a developmental anomaly that has many vascular peculiarities and progressive fibrosis.

NONPARASITIC CYSTS

Nonparasitic cysts of the liver are usually asymptomatic except for enlargement of the abdomen and a palpable mass (22–24). A few patients complain of pain which may become acute because of hemorrhage into the cyst or rupture. The disease is predominantly seen in females, the ratio being about 4 or 5 to 1. The cysts may occur at any age in life, but the majority have been noted in the middle age group (23, 24). Hepatic scans and arteriograms help to localize the lesions before surgery. Occasionally the wall of the cyst undergoes calcification and can be seen on x-ray. The

treatment is surgical, although some of the cysts are so deeply placed within the liver that removal is impossible. Under these circumstances marsupialization and other procedures are recommended (24).

Nonparasitic cysts of the liver are usually solitary but occasionally multiple. Grossly, they are round and vary from a few centimeters in diameter to some 15 to 20 cm (Fig. 20). They have a single layer of cuboidal to low columnar epithelium (Fig. 21) that secretes a serous type of clear fluid. This may become brown due to hemorrhage and undergo a degenerative change of the lining. Occasionally the cysts have a squamous epithelial lining. A thick fibrous capsule comprises the wall and outside of this is a heavily vascularized layer of connective tissue.

Multiple cysts may produce symptoms and necessitate surgery. Most often, however, a small group of simple cysts that had

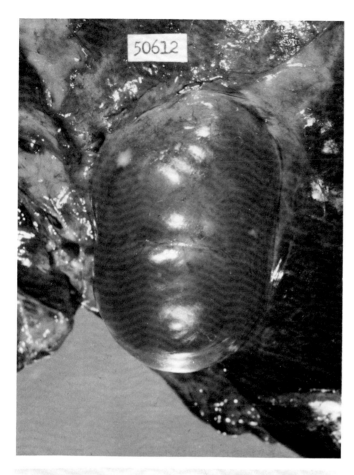

Figure 20 This large nonparasitic cyst was located adjacent to the porta hepatis in a 93-year-old woman (LAC-USCMC 50612).

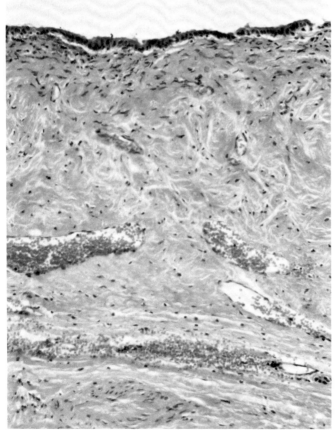

Figure 21 Low columnar epithelium lining this solitary cyst was removed surgically. Dense subepithelial connective tissue and marked vascularity of the capsular area is characteristic (hematoxylin and eosin, X150; LAC-USCMC 59-13514).

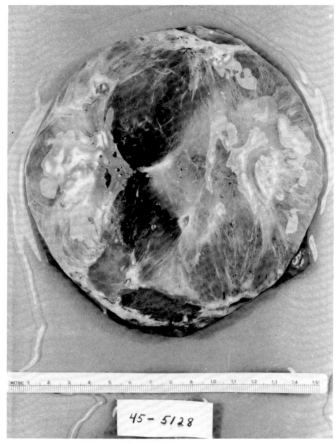

Figure 22 This markedly edematous mesenchymal hamartoma contains areas of necrosis. Serous fluid is seen alongside as it freely escapes from the hamartoma when incised. This hamartoma was removed from the right lobe of a 20-month-old girl (LAC-USCMC 45-5128). Figures 22 and 24 are from the same patient.

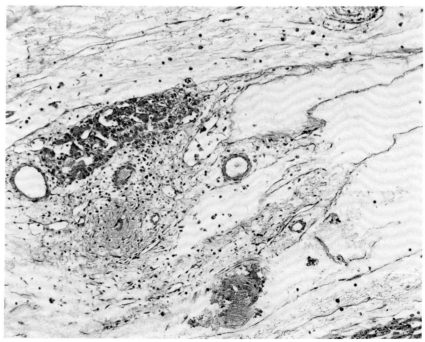

Figure 23 The tissue in this mesenchymal hamartoma is widely distended with fluid. A small island of hepatocytes remains. From a 10-month-old boy, the tumor measured 15 cm in greatest diameter. (hematoxylin and eosin, X125; ASC 2810).

not been clinically detectable may be noted at the time of autopsy.

CONGENITAL HEPATIC FIBROSIS AND POLYCYSTIC DISEASE

Polycystic disease of the liver, because of widespread involvement, offers no problem in differential diagnosis. Polycystic disease arises from Meyenberg complexes (25). Many of these small gray-white fibrous foci are often intermixed with the cysts in polycystic disease but they are also seen in variable number in patients either without cysts or in those patients who have only a few grossly visible minute cysts. In rare instances, much of the liver may be occupied by these complexes and metastatic carcinoma is suspected either at the time of surgery or autopsy.

In both infants and adults various forms of fibrosis may accompany the malformations of the bile ducts that form the basis for the Meyenburg complexes. In both children and adults fibrous septa may surround the lobules and the disease became known as congenital hepatic fibrosis (26). Patients may have symptoms of portal hypertension either during childhood or later in life.

MESENCHYMAL HAMARTOMAS

In infants with mesenchymal hamartomas there is increasing enlargement of the abdomen and a palpable mass. These watery oddities occur during the first one to two years of life; they may grow so rapidly that they are life-threatening because of difficulty in respiration (27). At the time of surgery the lesions are not encapsulated but merge gradually with the adjacent liver; occasionally they are pedunculated. On gross examination they are gray to gray-brown and edematous; ill-defined pseudo-

cysts and areas of necrosis are often present (Fig. 22). Occasionally areas of hemorrhage are seen. On microscopic examination the loose, relatively acellular connective tissue with marked edema is pathognomonic (Fig. 23). These may alternate with areas of dense, stringy connective tissue (Fig. 24). At least a few remnants of triads and periportal hepatocytes can be found. Many variations are observed as some lesions contain angiomatous areas and other lesions cause distortion of the portal areas for some distance from the primary area of involvement.

Electron microscopic studies have shown that the epithelial elements are well differentiated and that the bile ducts are typical of those in the normal liver. The myxomatous foci consist of fibroblasts, mature collagen, and only a few endothelial lined spaces (28).

Inflammatory lesions of the liver have been reported that may be confused with a neoplasm. The nature of these is unknown (29).

ANOXIC NECROSIS

In patients with cirrhosis who suffer from shock, especially in those with fatal hemorrhage, there may be extensive infarction of the centers of the pseudolobules. If hemorrhage also occurs within the infarcts or around their margins, the gross appearance may closely simulate primary carcinoma of the liver (Fig. 25). The correct diagnosis is easily made on microscopic examination (Fig. 26). In the cirrhotic liver a larger than normal proportion of oxygen is supplied by the hepatic artery. Thus, in shock with a fall in systolic blood pressure, infarcts may be widespread. Anoxic necrosis involving a variable amount of liver tissue may complicate hypotension due to any one of many conditions including myocardial infarction and exsanguinat-

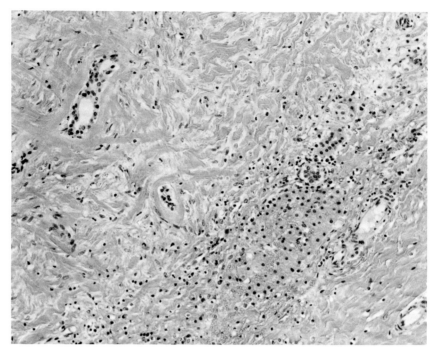

Figure 24 Dense connective tissue surrounding a distorted remnant of a triad (hematoxylin and eosin, X150; LAC-USCMC 45-5128).

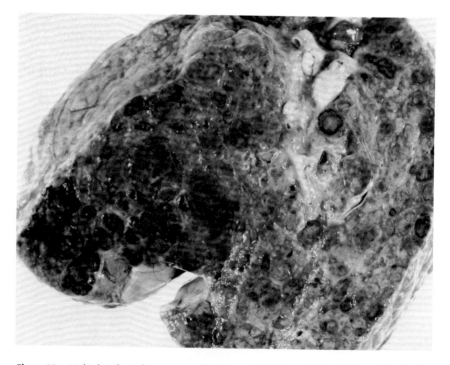

Figure 25 Multiple infarcts have occurred in the pseudolobules of cirrhosis. The patient had severe hemorrhage due to esophageal varices (JWA 80-74). Figures 25 and 26 are from the same patient.

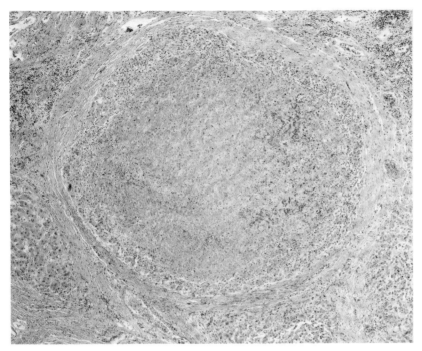

Figure 26 Infarction of central portion of small pseudolobules in cirrhosis (hematoxylin and eosin, X45; JWA 80-74).

ing hemorrhage. In these conditions the areas of infarction are often smaller than those in cirrhosis and frequently are located under Glisson's capsule. Little attention seems to have been given to anoxic necrosis in the literature.

REFERENCES

1. Ein, SH, Stephens CA: Benign liver tumors and cysts in childhood. *J Pediatr Surg* **9**:847–851, 1974.

2. Hepatic tumors in childhood. *Br Med J* **1**:394–395, 1972.

3. Muroff, LR, Johnson, PM: The use of multiple radionuclide imaging to differentiate the focal intrahepatic lesion. *Am J Roentgenol Radiat Ther Nucl Med* **121**:728–734, 1974.

4. Edmondson HA: *Tumors of the Liver and Intrahepatic Bile Ducts. Atlas of Tumor Pathology,* fascicle 25. Armed Forces Institute of Pathology, Washington, D.C., 1958.

5. Edmondson HA: Differential diagnosis of tumors and tumor-like lesions of the liver in infancy and childhood. *AMA J Dis Child* **91**:168–186, 1956.

6. Albrecht: Ueber Hamartome. *Verhandl Dtsch Pathol Gesellsch* **7**:153–157, 1904.

7. Baum JK, Bookstein JJ, Holtz, F, Klein EW: Possible association between benign hepatomas and oral contraceptives. *Lancet* **2**:926–929, 1973.

8. Knapp WC, Ruebner BH: Hepatomas and oral contraceptives. *Lancet* **1**:270, 1974.

9. Vosnides G, Brander W, O'Keefe B, et al: Oral contraceptives and the liver. *Br. Med J* **4**:430, 1974.

10. O'Sullivan JP, Wilding RP: Liver hamartomas in patients on oral contraceptives. *Br Med J* **3**:7–10, 1974.

11. Tountas C, Parskevas G, Deligeorgi H: Benign hepatoma and oral contraceptives. *Lancet* **1**:1351, 1974.

12. Vosnides G, O'Keeffe B, Brander W, Bewick M, Ogg C: Liver hamartomas in patients on oral contraceptives. *Br Med J* **3**:580, 1974.

13. Edmondson HA, Henderson BE, Benton B: Liver cell adenoma, in preparation.

14. Marsh JL, Dahms B, Longmire WP, Jr: Cysta-

denoma and cystadenocarcinoma of the biliary system *Arch Surg* **109**:41–43, 1974.

15. Short WF, Nedwich A, Levy HA, Howard JM: Biliary cystadenoma. Report of a case and review of the literature. *Arch Surg* **102**:78–80, 1975.

16. Keech MK: Cystadenoma of the pancreas and intrahepatic bile ducts. *Gastroenterology* **19**:568–574 1951.

17. Rabinowitz JG, Kinkabwala M, Ulreich S: Macroregenerating nodules in the cirrhotic liver. Radiologic features and differential diagnosis. *Am J Roentgenol Radiat Ther Nucl Med* **121**:401–411, 1974.

18. Benz EJ, Baggenstoss AH: Focal cirrhosis of the liver: its relation to the so-called hamartoma (adenoma, benign hepatoma). *Cancer* **6**:743–755, 1953.

19. Whelan TJ Jr, Baugh JH, Chandor, S: Focal nodular hyperplasia of the liver. *Ann Surg* **177**:150–158, 1973.

20. Mays ET, Christopherson WM, Barrows GH: Focal nodular hyperplasia of the liver: possible relationship to oral contraceptives. *Am J Clin Pathol* **61**:735–746, 1974.

21. Rhodes RH, Marchildon MB, Luebke DC, Edmondson HA, Mikity V: A mixed hamartoma of the liver: light and electron microscopy, in preparation.

22. Coutsoftides T, Hermann RE: Nonparasitic cysts of liver. *Surg Gynecol Obstet* **138**:906–910, 1974.

23. Longmire WP, Mandiola SA, Gordon HE: Congenital cystic disease of the liver and biliary system. *Ann Surg* **174**:711–726, 1971.

24. Jones WL, Mountain JC, Warren KW: Symptomatic non-parasitic cysts of the liver. *Br J Surg* **61**:118–123, 1974.

25. Melnick PJ: Polycystic liver: analysis of seventy cases. *AMA Arch Pathol* **59**:162–172, 1955.

26. Sherlock S: *Diseases of the Liver and Biliary System,* 4th ed. F. A. Davis Company, Philadelphia, 1968, pp 538–540.

27. Patil SD, Talib VH, Sultana Z, Talib NS, Bhagwat DS: Mesenchymal hamartoma of the liver. *Indian J Pediatr* **41**:283–286, 1974.

28. Dehner LP, Ewing SL, Sumner HW: Infantile mesenchymal hamartoma of the liver. Histologic and ultrastructural observations. *Arch Pathol* **99**:379–382, 1975.

29. Hertzer NR, Hawk WA, Hermann RE: Inflammatory lesions of the liver which simulate tumor: report of two cases in children. *Surgery* **69**:839–846, 1971.

Part Four PATHOPHYSIOLOGY

CHAPTER 14 HUMORAL EFFECTS OF HEPATOCELLULAR CARCINOMA

MALCOLM COCHRANE, M.D., M.B., M.R.C.P.
ROGER WILLIAMS, M.D., F.R.C.P.

As long ago as 1929 Nadler and Wolfer described the association of hypoglycemia with hepatocellular carcinoma (HCC) (1), and since that time a great many other systemic or humoral effects have been recognized, not directly related to dissemination of tumor tissue (2, 3) (Table 1). Some of these, such as hypoglycemia (4) and erythrocytosis (5) and alpha-fetoprotein synthesis (6) occur relatively frequently, often antedating local symptoms related to the primary growth, and secondly, in an established tumor they may be the cause of the most profound symptomatology requiring prompt and active treatment. The presence of an underlying cirrhosis—58% in our series of 85 cases of HCC—makes the interpretation of some of these manifestations, such as gynecomastia and protein abnormalities difficult, as they may be related to the underlying cirrhosis rather than to the neoplasm (7).

The pathophysiological mechanisms underlying these systemic manifestations fall into three major categories:

1. The synthesis by the tumor of proteins, hormones and hormonelike substances.

2. An alteration in the intracellular enzymes of the tumor cells and possibly the normal hepatocytes leading to deranged metabolism and loss of regulatory mechanisms.

3. Increased utilization of normal serum constituents by the massive tumor bulk and their decreased production due to insufficient remaining normal liver tissue.

The loss of enzymic pathways that serve to distinguish one cell from another and result in metabolic similarity between tumor cells arising from a variety of sites has been termed convergence by Greenstein (8).

The concept that the DNA of any nucleated cell retains the same genetic information to direct biochemical pathways for the synthesis of any protein or hormone, regardless of any subsequent specialization, would account for the occurrence of similar systemic manifestations with neoplasms derived from a wide variety of embryologically different cell lines.

333

Table 1 Systemic Manifestations of Primary Liver Cell Carcinomas

Endocrine Manifestations

  Hypercalcaemia
  Erythrocytosis
  Precocious puberty
  Gynaecomastia
  Raised levels of choronic gonadotrophin
  Raised levels of choronic somatotrophin

Metabolic Changes

Glucose	Hypoglycaemia
Lipids	Hypercholesterolaemia
	Hypertriglyceridaemia
Proteins	Increased foetoprotein
	Macroglobulinaemia
	Myelomatous-globulinaemia
	Increased haptoglobin
	Increased caeruloplasmin
Others	Porphyria
	Varient alkaline phosphatase
	Cystathioninuria
	Ethanolaminuria

Haematological Changes

  Hyperfibrinogenaemia
  Cryofibrinogenaemia
  Functional dysfibrinogenaemia
  Antifibrinolysis
  Plasmacytosis
  Haemolytic anaemia

In the process of malignant transformation, portions of nuclear DNA normally suppressed in that particular tissue, may escape from their inactivation and synthesize polypeptide hormones or proteins not normally produced, but coded for on the derepressed DNA. These new secretory products may be identical to the true hormones or proteins. However, if derepression is incomplete, then hormones with slightly different structures, and immunochemically distinct from the true hormone, may be produced.

An alternative hypothesis and one that does not involve dedifferentiation or convergence has recently been proposed by Warner (9). The production of hybrid cells by the fusion of a neoplastic with a nearby nonneoplastic cell may result in the expression of functions not present in the parent cells (10). Genes in the normal cells responsible for the suppression of malignancy may inhibit the tumorigenic potential of the hybrid cell, which only becomes overt after certain chromosomal alterations. This cell hybridization may be a relatively common phenomenon in tumors, although usually suppression of the malignant trait allows overgrowth by the original tumor cells. However, if the hybrid cells had a selective advantage over the malignant parent cells, such as the secretion of trophic or immunosuppressive hormones, their growth may be accentuated. The demonstration of the inhibitory effect of chorionic gonadotrophin, a commonly produced ectopic hormone (11), on phytohemagglutinin-induced lymphocyte blastogenesis (12) may be an example of such a selective advantage. This hypothesis of phenotypic mixing generated by cell hybridization would offer a reasonable alternative explanation for the association of polypeptide hormone secretion with a heterogenous group of tumor.

ERYTHROCYTOSIS

An association between erythrocytosis and hepatoma was first reported by McFadzean et al (13). He found an increased red cell mass and erythroid hyperplasia of the marrow in 10% of male Chinese patients with hepatoma developing on cirrhosis. The other types of neoplasm with which it is particularly associated are hypernephroma (14) and cerebellar hemangioblastoma (15).

At least 65 cases of erythrocytosis and HCC are now documented, and it is striking that more than 95% have developed on an underlying cirrhosis. Indeed, Brownstein and Billard have suggested that the finding of erythrocytosis in a cirrhotic patient is an indication of neoplastic transformation (16). Only one case has been reported in a woman (17), and it is of interest that a similar but less pronounced male dominance is found when erythrocytosis is associated with hypernephroma and cerebellar hemangioblastoma. In all cases, polycythemia rubra vera and arterial hypoxia were excluded as possible causes of the erythrocytosis. The diagnosis of erythrocytosis is made more difficult by the increase in plasma volume commonly found in cirrhosis—43 of 54 cases in one series in which it was measured (18). Thus if the hematocrit alone is used as an index of erythrocytosis, many cases will be missed. True increase in red cell mass have been found with hematocrits as low as 48% (19).

MECHANISMS UNDERLYING ERYTHROCYTOSIS

Three main theories have been proposed (Fig. 1).

Erythropoietin production by tumor.

The combined results of 11 publications show positive assays in 9 out of 17 sera from patients with erythrocytosis and HCC (18). In the three patients with neoplasms (including one HCC) and erythrocytosis, described by Adamson et al, urinary ery-

thropoitin was not increased after phlebotomy, whereas an increase was demonstrated in normal subjects and in patients with polycythemia rubra vera or secondary erythrocytosis from anoxia (20). These results indicate that the erythropoietin production is autonomous rather than part of a normal regulatory system. Assays on extracts of tumor tissue for erythropoietin have been less rewarding, with only two questionably positive results from the 10 extracts examined. In one of these, the slightly increased activity in the tumor extract could be completely neutralized by antiserum against erythropoietin (21). These mainly negative results may simply reflect inadequate tissue preparations, but erythropoietin production by the tumor is as yet unproven.

Tumor product as substrate for a renal erythropoietic factor.

Gordon and co-workers have postulated that the production of erythropoietin is a result of an enzymic interaction between a renal erythropoietic factor (REF), itself erythropoietically inactive and antigenically distinct from erythropoietin, and a globulin substrate secreted by the liver (22, 23, 24). In one patient with HCC neither the normal liver nor the hepatoma tissue possessed erythropoiesis stimulating activity or

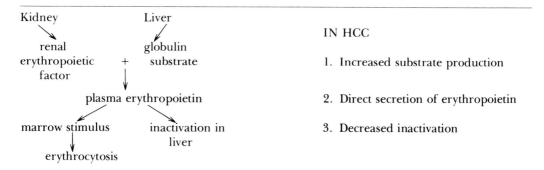

Figure 1 Postulated normal pathway for production of erythrocytosis with possible abnormalities in hepatocellular carcinoma.

the capacity to generate erythropoietin when incubated with normal human serum. However, homogenates of tumor tissue but not of normal liver were effective substrates for renal erythropoietic factor in the production of erythropoietin. Excess formation of substrate by the hepatoma for the renal erythropoietic factor could therefore explain the development of erythrocytosis. Several other workers support this mechanism of erythropoietin formation (25, 26), although some have been unable to reproduce Gordon's experimental results (27).

Failure to inactivate erythropoietin.

A third theory is based on evidence that the liver may be the normal site for inactivation of the erythropoietin (28, 29, 30). In the presence of extensive tumor masses there may be insufficient normal liver tissue remaining for effective inactivation. Some support for this is given by Gordon et al (24) who demonstrated marked reduction in erythropoietin activity by homogenates of the nontumorous portion of the liver, but not by the HCC tissue. The inactivation process correlates with the levels a lysosomal marker enzyme, B-glucuronidase (31), and it would be of considerable interest to assay for this enzyme both in the tumor and in the surrounding normal liver.

HYPERCALCEMIA

The hypercalcemia of patients with neoplastic disease is most frequently due to the presence of skeletal metastases, but it may also be found in the absence of metastases or parathyroid adenomata. This was first recognized by Gutman et al (36) and termed pseudohyperparathyroidism by Fry (33). Primary hyperparathyroidism coexisting with malignant tumors is another cause but is extremely rare (34).

To account for pseudohyperparathyroidism, Albright suggested that malignant tumors may be capable of producing a substance with actions similar to parathyroid hormone (35). A significant reduction of serum calcium following resection of the neoplasm, or a positive parathormone immunoassay of an extract for the neoplasm is required to provide conclusive evidence for the syndrome of pseudoparathyroidism, but for obvious reasons these are not always available. This condition is now recognized as the third commonest cause of hypercalcemia, accounting for 15% of the cases; metastatic bone disease and multiple myeloma together account for 55% and primary hyperparathyroidism accounts for 20%. Bronchogenic carcinoma and hypernephroma account for 60% of such cases (36), but there are many instances of its association with hepatoma (37–41).

We have had experience of three cases in the Liver Unit of King's College Hospital. One of these, a patient with an intrahepatic bile duct carcinoma, presented with an abdominal mass and during investigation was found to have a serum calcium of 17.6 mg/100 ml, serum inorganic phosphorus of 1.4 mg/100 ml and a urinary calcium excretion of up to 1000 mg per day (normal 300 mg). A decrease in serum calcium from 18 mg to 11 mg/100 ml followed corticosteroid therapy. Since no extension of the growth outside the liver could be demonstrated, orthotopic liver transplantation was carried out. Following this, the raised plasma parathormone and serum calcium levels rapidly returned to normal (Fig. 2). Significant arteriovenous and venovenous parathyroid hormone gradients (Table 2) were demonstrated across the liver at the time of operation, suggesting active secretion of the hormone into the hepatic vein. Assay of the tumor tissue, but not the surrounding normal liver, showed it to contain relatively high concentrations of parathyroid hormonelike material (42).

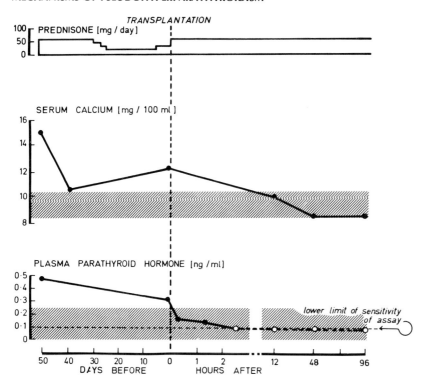

Figure 14.2 Plasma parathyroid hormone levels before and after hepatic transplantation.

Table 2   Postulated Mechanisms for the Production of Hypoglycemia in Hepatoma

Increased Rate of Glucose Utilization

a. In peripheral tissues by:
   i.   Insulin or insulin-like substances
   ii.   Potentiation of insulin activity
   iii. Stimulation of pancreatic insulin release
   iv.   Inhibition of counter-regulatory hormone opposing action of insulin
b. By the tumor

Decreased Rate of Glucose Production by Liver:

a. Massive replacement of normal liver by hepatoma
b. Alteration of hepatic enzymes of glucose metabolism
c. Failure of compensatory mechanisms

MECHANISMS OF PSEUDOHYPERPARATHYROIDISM

Production of Parathormone and Parathormonelike Substances

The first direct evidence that tumors were capable of secreting a parathyroid hormone-like substance came with the development in 1964 of a complement fixation technique by Tashjian et al (43). These authors demonstrated an immunological cross-reactivity but not identity between bovine parathyroid hormone and an antigenic extract from 6 out of 12 tumors. Riggs et al (44) measuring serum levels of immunoreactive parathyroid hormone (IPTH) in a series of 54 patients with primary hyperparathyroidism and 18 with pseudohyperparathyroidism (including 4 with HCC) found that although serum calcium levels were higher in the patients with pseudohyperparathyroidism, IPTH levels were in general lower. Different antisera could differentiate IPTH from the two groups with only minor overlap, thus confirming the findings of Berson and Yalow (45) who suggested that parathormone was immunoheterogenous. More recently, Root et al (46) have demonstrated several varieties of parathyroid hormonelike activity in association with malignant tumors—one being indistinguishable from the normal hormone, another immunologically distinct, and a third which was often associated with normal calcium levels. Thus in some cases the immunoreactive material in the serum of patients with pseudohyperparathyroidism is probably a precursor or intermediate form of parathormone, the tumor cells lacking the ability to synthesize the normally secreted hormone. Some support for this hypothesis is provided by the fact that the hormone within cultured tumor cells is a protein with an approximate molecular weight of 9000 which on secretion is degraded to a smaller peptide hormone (predicted MW 7000) which is immunologically distinct from hormone within the cells).

Alternative Humoral Substances

The inability to demonstrate parathormone or parathormonelike activity in the serum of almost 50% of patients with hypercalcemia associated with malignant tumors (47) suggests the possibility of a humoral substance not structurally related to parathyroid hormone, but capable of producing hypercalcemia. Tashijian et al has demonstrated a relationship between hypercalcemia and raised levels of prostaglandin E2 in a mouse fibrosarcoma (48). Organ culture of these tumors were shown to secrete prostaglandins, and supernatants from these cultures possess bone

reabsorbing activity. Administration of indomethacin, an antagonist of prostaglandins, decreases the hyperglycemia of the animals and its addition to the organ cultures also suggests the bone reabsorbing activity of the supernatants (49). Recently, additional evidence is that of Powell et al who failed to demonstrate parathormonelike activity using a variety of antisera, in 10 patients with pseudohyperparathyroidism, although resorption of Ca from bone by the tumor extracts was demonstrable (50). Certain sterols, chemically close to but not identical with 7-dehydrocholesterol (pro-VitD3) and which have osteolytic activity have also been found in patients with carcinoma of the breast (23). Humoral substances possibly related to abnormalities in vitamin D metabolism, may also be implicated (51).

HYPOGLYCEMIA

The association of hypoglycemia with HCC was first described by Nadler and Wolfer in 1929 (1). Since that time it has been recognized as a relatively common complication with a reported incidence of 24% (52) and 30% (53) in two small series. Many single case reports of hypoglycemia are quoted by the latter authors occurring alone or in association with erythrocytosis (54) or hypercalcemia (37), and the overall frequency in their own personal series of 142 cases (all Chinese) was 27%. In reviews of a large series of HCC from Africa, the United States, and England the frequency either of hypoglycemia or of erythrocytosis has not been as high. Why these occur more commonly in the Far East is not known.

Two clinically and histologically distinct groups have been identified by McFadzean (4) differing in the frequency and character of the hypoglycemia. Type A patients constituted 87% of cases. The tumors were rapidly growing and poorly differentiated; rapid wasting and profound muscle weakness were prominent features. Hypoglycemia which developed in 17% was usually preterminal and occurred within two weeks of death. Blood glucose decreased slowly on fasting and was relatively easily controled. Type B patients, on the other hand, had well-differentiated, slowly growing tumors with little weight loss or muscle weakness until late in the disease. The hypoglycemia developed in 100% of cases within 2 to 10 months of death and was characterized by a precipitous fall in glucose on fasting which was extremely difficult to control. The changes underlying the development of the hypoglycemia in the two groups is discussed later.

Table 3 Comparison of the Concentration of Parathyroid Hormone in the Arterial and Venous Supply to the Liver and the Venous Drainage from the Liver [a]

Concentration (Ng/ml) [b]				
In Hepatic Artery	In Portal Vein	In Hepatic Vein	Hepatic-Vein-Hepatic-Artery Gradient [c]	Hepatic-Vein-Portal-Vein Gradient [c]
0.39± 0.015	0.20± 0.015	0.54± 0.018	0.15	0.34

[a] Parathyroid hormone expressed in terms of its bovine equivalent.
[b] Mean ± SE of three dilutions in three separate assays.
[c] All gradients significant - p 0.0001 (Student's t test).

MECHANISMS OF HYPOGLYCEMIA

There are many possible explanations for the production of hypoglycemia (Table 3) related either to an increased rate of utilization or decreased rate of production of glucose (55). The diversity of the proposed mechanisms reflects not only our lack of understanding but also the probability of a multifactorial aetiology.

Production of Insulin or Insulinlike Substances by the Tumor

No convincing evidence for the secretion of insulin or insulinlike substances has been produced. Schonfeld et al demonstrated large amounts of a substance with an insulinlike activity (ILA) in one tumor although serum levels were normal (56). The possibility that tumors may act as sponges concentrating substance with insulinlike activity from the serum would account for the above findings and underlines the difficulty in attributing a true secretory function of tumors (57). Most authors have failed to show increases in insulin or insulinlike activity in the serum of patients during hypoglycemic episodes (5, 58). Immunoassays of the ILA found in a variety of other neoplasms failed to demonstrate cross reactivity with bovine insulin, suggesting, as for other hormones produced by tumors, antigenic heterogeneity (59, 60). High normal levels of free fatty acids and normal serum phosphorus levels (59) found in association with hypoglycemia would be unusual if insulin or substances with insulinlike activity were responsible. Further evidence against increased insulinlike activity with an increased peripheral utilization of glucose was also demonstrated by the normal disappearance rates of glucose after an intravenous lead (53). Indeed, in these studies the degree of peripheral assimilation, as assessed by the decrease in serum inorganic phosphate, was significantly lower than normal, suggesting diversion of glucose from the periphery to the tumor.

There is also no evidence for stimulation of pancreatic insulin release, as pancreatectomy has not influenced the course of tumor hypoglycemia (61, 62).

Increased Glucose Utilization by the Tumor

Some evidence for increased glucose utilization by the tumor is provided by the finding of high blood lactate levels that would be consistent with anaerobic glycolysis in the tumors (63). It has also been postulated that depletion of ATP levels, by the high energy requirements for protein synthesis of the tumor, removes its inhibiting influence on phosphofructokinase, a rate limiting glycolytic enzyme (64). It is also possible that glucose transport across tumor cells is independent of insulin (65). Both these factors could lead to uninhibited glycolysis in the tumor. However, until significant differences in arteriovenous glucose and lactic acid concentrations across the tumor have been demonstrated, this mechanism can only be considered as speculative.

Decreased Rate of Glucose Production by the Liver

The evidence here is more substantial. Kreisberg and Pennington, using isotope dilution techniques, demonstrated marked reduction in endogenous glucose production (66), although Chandalia and Boshell, using the more sensitive technique of glucose recycling, was unable to demonstrate inhibition of gluconeogenesis in the single case studied (63). Previously, McFadzean and Young (4) had found only a minimal response to glucagon in their type B patients (Fig. 3), which could be explained by a high glycogen content in the normal liver and tumor in type B patients but not in type A, and a markedly reduced phosphorylase activity required for the breakdown of glycogen in both types of tumor. Incubation at 37°C of residual liver tissue from type B patients resulted in little glycogenolysis, although glycogen breakdown was considerable in type A patients. Glucose-6 phosphatase, the final enzyme of the gluconeogenic pathway was completely absent from the tumors of both type A and type B tumors and also reduced in the residual tissue of both, whereas glucose-6-phosphate dehydrogenase activity was increased. These findings in conjunction with raised levels of lactic and pyruvic acid suggest a preferential increase in pentose production, which is required for nucleic acid synthesis in rapidly growing tumors at the expense of gluconeogenesis. Landau et al also found a decreased output of glucose by the liver but no detectable glucose-6-phosphatase activity in the tumor tissue (58).

In conclusion, hypoglycemia in the type A patient of MacFadzean is due to the glucose requirements of a massive tumor being greater than the gluconeogenic capability of the residual normal liver. That of the type B patient is secondary to abnormal enzyme patterns resulting in an acquired form of glycogen storage disease with defective glycogenolysis.

MANAGEMENT

If the mechanism of hypoglycemia proposed by McFadzean also applies to tumors from other races and countries, then adequate control of hypoglycemia in the type A patient should be obtained with an additional supply of glucose, either intravenously or orally of about 300 to 500 g per day. Control of type B hypoglycemia is much more difficult. Many forms of pharmacological therapy has been tried including glucagon (4), methyl prednisolone, 60 mg/day (56), diazoxide 400 mg/day, and trichloromethiazide, 4 mg/day (66) but without effect. The only satisfactory therapy has been the infusion of large quantities—2 to 3 L/day or more—of 10% dextrose. A carbohydrate intake—as high as 1500 g per day—may control symptoms in some of the cases, but others are dependent on continuous intravenous administration to sustain life.

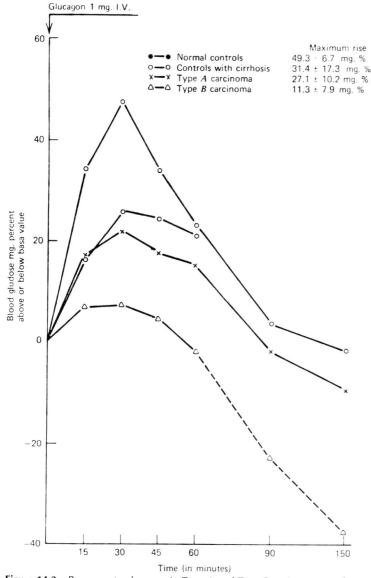

Glucagon 1 mg. I.V.

Maximum rise
●—● Normal controls   49.3 · 6.7 mg. %
○—○ Controls with cirrhosis   31.4 ± 17.3 mg. %
x—x Type *A* carcinoma   27.1 ± 10.2 mg. %
△—△ Type *B* carcinoma   11.3 ± 7.9 mg. %

Blood gludose mg. percent above or below basa value

Time (in minutes)

Figure 14.3   Response to glucagon in Type A and Type B patients, normal controls, and controls with cirrhosis.

SYNDROME OF SEXUAL PRECOCITY AND GONADOTROPHIN SECRETION

There are several reports of sexual precocity occurring in children with liver tumors. These tumors have usually been of the hepatocellular type that occur after five years of age rather than of the more primitive hepatoblastoma variety seen usually before the age of 40 months (67). A review of 10 cases of precocious puberty associated with HCC showed all patients to be male. Most

had gross hepatic enlargement, a deep voice, and pubic hair as well as enlargement of the penis, although testicular enlargement was rare. Growth was accelerated and bone age advanced. Urinary gonadotropin and testosterone excretion was increased whereas 17 ketosteroids were normal or only slightly increased (68).

Clinical gynecomastia is a rare finding in patients with hepatomas; however, histological changes showing increase in ducts, stroma, and apocrine glands in the breast were found in three of six cases examined by Williams (69). Regression of gynecomastia in a 58-year-old male with a hepatoma followed partial hepatectomy (70), as did the mammary hypertrophy amenorrhea and galactorrhea in a young woman reported by Couinaud et al (71). Chorionic gonadotropin or somatotropin levels were not estimated in any of these cases. The following is a discussion of mechanisms underlying precocious puberty.

The syndrome of sexual precocity is usually attributed to the secretion of ectopic gonadotropin by the tumor, as positive biological test for chorionic gonadotropin in serum (72) and tumor extracts (73) have been reported. This view has recently been confirmed by Braunstein et al with the demonstration that increased levels of immunoreactive human chorionic gonadotropin (and alpha fetoprotein) and signs of virilism decreased after resection of a hepatoblastoma in an 8-month-old boy (74). Development of pulmonary metastases was accompanied by a return of the signs of virilism and raised levels of human chorionic gonadotropin (and alpha-fetoprotein). Furthermore, cultures of tumor tissue were shown to secrete human chorionic gonadotropin and alpha-fetoprotein. The limitation of the syndrome to males is suggestive of the production of a secretion with mainly interstitial cell stimulating properties as this is the only stimulus required by the testis for sex hormone production; the ovary requires follicular stimulating as well as interstitial cell stimulating hormone to elaborate estrogen. The increased urinary levels of testosterone found in some cases were thought to be elaborated by the testis rather than the adrenals as the Leydig cells showed signs of stimulation whereas the adrenal cortex appeared atrophic (68). The following are descriptions of human chorionic gonadotropin and gonadotropin assays.

Braunstein et al (11), using a sensitive radioimmunoassay specific for human chorionic gonadotropin, found increased levels in the serum of 113 of 819 patients with various neoplasms including nongenital sites, that is, the breast and the gastrointestinal tract, as well as with primary growths of the testis (Table 4). It has been suggested that trophoblastic elements may be produced in primary or secondary tumors in other sites (i.e., nontrophoblastic) by morphologic retrodifferentiation of adenocarcinoma to choriocarcinoma (75, 76, 77). This finding could possibly account for the high proportion of positive results in some of the gastrointestinal tumors. Significant levels of gonadotropin were found in 14 (12%) of 81 patients with hepatomas. Unfortunately, few clinical details are given and there was no indication of associated symptoms or signs related to the hormone apart from gynecomastia, which was noted in four male patients with primaries in sites other than testes, but not in any of the 14 hepatomas.

More recently the ectopic production of a further placental protein, chorionic somatotropin, has been demonstrated using a sensitive radioimmunoassay (78). Significant levels were demonstrated in the serum of 11 of 128 nontrophoblastic neoplasms, 2 of 15 with hepatomas, 7 of 64 with bronchogenic carcinomas, 1 of 6 with malignant phaeochromocytomas, and 1 of 13 patients with lymphomas. The hormone was demonstrated in tissue extracts of one bronchogenic neoplasm, but no assays were available for the hepatoma cases.

HYPERLIPIDEMIA

Hyperlipidemia is an uncommon complication of hepatoma, but its mechanism has been extensively investigated in the chemically induced hepatoma of the rat, making it of considerable interest (79–82). Extremely high levels of cholesterol (1100 mg/100 ml) and fatty acids (2200

Table 4   Human Chorionic Gonadotrophin Assays in 819 Cases with Malignant Disease

Type of Tumor or Primary Situ	Patients	Positive Chorionic Gonadotrophin (%)
Testis	90	53 (59%)
Gastrointestinal tract	62	16 (26%)
Hepatoma/hepatoblastoma	81	14 (17%)
Hemopoietic	256	7 (3%)
Lymphoma	249	5 (2%)
Sarcoma	36	2 (5%)
Breast	33	4 (12%)
Melanoma	77	8 (10%)
Bronchogenic carcinoma	15	1 (7%)
Miscellaneous	20	3 (15%)

Source. G.D. Braunstein et al (11).

mg/100 ml) have been recorded in children with hepatoma (83). In an adult with a cholangiocarcinoma of the liver a cholesterol level of 700 mg/100 ml and total lipids of 3700 mg/100 ml have been recorded (84). There is also one adult case reported of HCC developing in a cirrhotic liver with both erythrocytosis and hypertriglyceridemia (190 to 338 mg/100 ml) and fluctuant hypercholesterolemia (536 to 895 mg/100 ml). β-Lipoprotein levels were normal but there was an abnormal pre-β band. At autopsy both the tumor and residual cirrhotic liver contained increased levels of cholesterol and triglycerides and it was assumed that the tumor had been responsible for the production of the abnormal lipoprotein.

Alpert et al demonstrated a significantly higher mean cholesterol in 15 of 46 patients from Uganda with HCC compared with controls (218 mg/100 ml and 130 mg/100 ml, respectively). In 38% of the patients, cholesterol levels were over 200 mg/100 ml, a most unusual level since the average Ugandan diet contains less than 20 mg of cholesterol daily. The synthesis of cholesterol from ^{14}C-glycine was demonstrated to be decreased in 7 of these patients as compared with a control group of patients with other types of liver disease,

but the cause of the hypercholesterolemia was not established (85). In no other series, however, has there been such a high frequency.

A possible explanation for hyperlipidemia has been developed by Siperstein et al (79–82) and Bricker (86). First, they have demonstrated in the normal rat that the regulation of cholesterol synthesis was through a sensitive negative feedback system in which dietary cholesterol specifically inhibited the reductase enzyme in the biosynthetic pathway responsible for the conversion of β-hydroxy β-methylglutarate to mevalonate. In rats with chemically induced hepatoma, such a feedback mechanism was not demonstrable, although the tumors possessed the enzymatic mechanisms required for cholesterogenesis. There appeared to be a similar defect in the two patients with HCC investigated. A high cholesterol diet failed to decrease cholesterol synthesis from ^{14}C-acetate as assessed in sequential biopsy specimens.

Study of the feedback mechanism in rats after partial hepatectomy, when hepatic regeneration is occurring with a rapid cellular turnover, shows it to be normal, whereas it is inoperative in the more slowly dividing and highly differentiated Morris hepatomas. This suggests the defect may be a property of malignancy per se rather than a nonspecific effect of dedifferentiation.

DYSFIBRINOGENEMIA

The increase in fibrinolytic activity often found in serum of a patient with cirrhosis has been shown to return to normal or even be depressed with the development of HCC (87). This could have been due to the release of an antifibrinolytic agent from the tumor, and an increase in antifibrinolytic activity may also account for raised fibrinogen levels sometimes encountered in patients with HCC. In the case reported by Bell (88), the raised fibrinogen level was associated with multiple dysproteinemias, including raised levels of cryofibrinogen, haptoglobin, and ceruloplasmin. Plasma fibrinogen concentration was 6 times normal and the circulating pool 14 times increased, a level that would have required a daily hepatic synthesis of 60 g/day as compared with the normal of 3.4 g/day. This, as well as the finding of electrophoretic and immunological identity of the cryofibrinogen with normal fibrinogen, and the failure to localize cryofibrinogen within the tumor by indirect immunofluorescent techniques, would again suggest an increase in antifibrinolytic activity rather than an increased synthesis by the tumor. Although cryofibrinogenemia is commonly encountered in a variety of malignant tumors—levels in excess of 100 mg/100 ml being found especially after metastatic spread (89)—there is one other single case report of its occurrence in a patient with HCC (90).

PORPHYRIA CUTANEA TARDA

The occurrence of cutaneous porphyria in cirrhosis is well known, as is its appearance in patients with cirrhosis at the time of developing a hepatoma (91). The only case

to our knowledge of porphyria cutanea tarda occurring in a patient with a hepatoma without an underlying cirrhosis has been reported from this unit (92). There is also one case in the literature of a benign hepatic tumor associated with photosensitivity and excess porphyrinuria. The patient was relieved of her symptoms by removal of the tumor which was shown to be rich in porhyrins (93).*

The patient we described was a 77-year-old lady who presented with a photosensitive painful hemorrhagic bullous eruption. The urine contained a great excess of uroporphyrin (355 μg/24 hr; normal range 5 to 30 μg/24 hr) (Fig. 4) and fecal coproporphyrin and protoporphyrin levels were also markedly raised (88 and 59 μg/g of dried stool μg/g, normal range of 3 to 11 μg/g and 8.39 respectively). Four months after presentation liver biopsy confirmed the presence of a hepatoma, and as in one of the patients with cutaneous porphyria, hepatoma and underlying cirrhosis reported by Braun and Berman (94), the tumor tissue but not surrounding normal liver fluoresced in ultraviolet light. After arterial perfusion of 5-fluorouracil there was a marked rise in porphyrin excretion in urine and feces (Fig. 4) probably due to necrosis or damage of the tumor cells. There was some relief of photosensitivity following this chemotherapy, and radiotherapy was also given. When she died four months later, autopsy revealed multiple tumor nodules in the liver, many with hemorrhagic centers, with normal intervening liver.

We suggested that the tumor cells themselves were the site of the excess porphyrin production and estimates of total content of coproporphyrin in the tumor at the time of autopsy was estimated to be at least 2

*Editor's note. Both Edmondson and Peters, who reviewed the histology of the reported adenoma in preparation of their respective chapters, consider the reported "adenoma" to be definitely malignant.

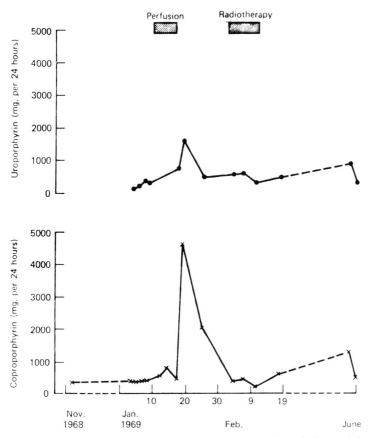

Figure 14.4 Levels of urinary coproporphyrin and uroporphyrin before and during treatment. Normal values coproporphyrin 134 ± 42; uroporphyrin 5 to 30 μg per 24 hours.

mg and that of uroporphyrin, 300 ug. The defect in the neoplastic cells responsible for these striking changes in porphyrin metabolism is unknown. It is unlikely to be related to increased activity of aminolevulinic acid (ALA) synthetase as urinary levels of ALA and prophobilinogen were normal. The predominant excretion of the normal type III porphyria isomers rather than the type I suggests that the activities of the cosynthetase and deaminase enzymes responsible for the conversion of porphobilinogen to coproporphyria III were normal. Abnormal metabolism of the porphyrinogens may have occurred within the tumor cells; the resulting prophyrin, being metabolically inert, could then only accumulate and be excreted.

HYPERTROPHIC PULMONARY OSTEOARTHROPATHY

The association of hypertrophic pulmonary osteoarthropathy (HPOA) with primary and secondary biliary cirrhosis is well recognized (95), as is its association with portal cirrhosis (96). There is also a report of two cases of HCC with hypertrophic pulmonary osteoarthropathy (97). One of the patients had been known to have cirrhosis for many years prior to the development of the hepatoma, but the HPOA seemingly developed at the same time as the malignancy. The second patient presented with a year's history of lassitude, and abdominal pains, HPOA, and multiple lung secondaries were also present at the time of diagnosis. It is of interest that extensive calcification was present in both these tumors. This is a rare finding in adult hepatoma, there being only six other recorded cases (97). It is more frequently seen in the hepatoblastoma of infancy (98) being caused by inclusion of bone as a mesenchymal component of an embryonic tumor (99).

Mechanism

Many hypotheses have been proposed to explain hypertrophic pulmonary osteoarthropathy including the escape of reduced ferritin into the systemic circulation (100), elevated estrogen levels (101), or a defect in the autonomic nervous system (102). The only consistent finding is an increased blood flow in the affected parts with vasodilatation (103).

OTHER RARE MANIFESTATIONS

Carcinoid Syndrome

It is well known that the carcinoid syndrome depends on the presence of hepatic secondaries, whatever the site of the primary tumor. Less well known is the fact that a primary carcinoid tumor may arise in the liver (104). There is also a very interesting case reported by Primack et al (105) who presented with an abdominal mass, bouts of explosive diarrhea, and fainting. 5-Hydroxyindole acetic acid, 5-hydroxtryptophan, and serotonin levels were increased in the urine. However, no evidence of a primary carcinoid tumor was found. Histology of the hepatic tumor was characteristic of an HCC. Synthesis of albumin and fibrinogen was demonstrated with cultures of tumor cells, again a characteristic of hepatic cells; indole derivatives were also detectable within the tumor. Increased tryptophan hydroxolase activity, reflecting raised levels of 5-hydroxytryptophan were also found in the liver tumor and in a single lung secondary.

An Isoenzyme of Alkaline Phosphatase

Tumor alkaline phosphatase differs from that normally present in the serum, by its faster electrophoretic mobility, increased resistance to heat denaturation, and increased inhibition by L-phenylalanine (106). It was first detected in 8 of 10 tumor homogenates from patients with HCC and in the serum of three others. It has been found in cholangiocarcinoma, fetal liver, or secondary hepatic tumors, but was detected in one case of postnecrotic cirrhosis and in another with a fatty liver. Portugal et al (107) found the isoenzyme in 28.6% of 37 patients with a hepatoma, and this was a close correlation between its presence in the serum and the appearance of alpha fetoprotein. This isoenzyme is probably different from the Regan isoenzyme (108, 109) which is biochemically and immunologically indistinguishable from placental alkaline phosphatase, which has also been found in many neoplasms but not so far in HCC.

Macroglobulinemia and Myelomatous Globulin

Macroglobulinemia has been reported in sera of two patients with HCC arising in cirrhotic livers (110, 111), but it may also appear in association with uncomplicated cirrhosis (112). This also applies to myelomatous globulin and plasmacytosis which have been reported in association with HCC with or without an underlying cirrhosis (2, 113).

Hyperaminoacidemia and Hyperaminoaciduria

These conditions are relatively common in cirrhosis (114) and have also rarely been reported in association with HCC. Dent and Walshe reported a case in which ethanolamine could be detected in the urine (115), and it is possible that this may be related to the accumulation of phosphoethanolamine that has been found in induced rat hepatomas (116).

Hemolytic Anemias

There is one case report of Coombs negative hemolytic anemia in association with HCC (117). Microangiopathic hemolytic anemias commonly complicate hemangioendotheliomas of the liver (118).

HEPATOBLASTOMAS AND CONGENITAL ANOMALIES

Representing a different type of systemic manifestation are the congenital anomalies described in association with the hepatoblastoma of infancy. This may be perhaps a reflection of the dysontogenetic origin of this tumor and of the possible relationship between teratogenesis and oncogenesis.

Geiser et al (119) have described the case of a 13-month-old child with a hepatoblastoma in whom both hemihypertrophy and cystathioninuria were present. The increase in size of organs on the left side was attributed to hyperplasia rather than hypertrophy of individual cells. Four other cases had been recorded; as well as that reported by Gieser et al there was one other in whom significantly raised levels of cystathionine were found in the tumor. However, cystathionine, a sulphur-containing amino acid and intermediate metabolite of methionine, has been demonstrated in the urine of many patients with hepatoblastoma without hemihypertrophy (120) as well as in 50% of cases with neuroblastoma (121).

A multiplicity of congenital abnormalities and other systemic manifestations have been reported in association with hepatoblastoma and to a lesser extent hepatocellular carcinoma in infants and children (67). Many of these such as macroglossia (122), Meckel's diverticulum and umbilical hernia (123), lipid storage disease (124) and glycogen storage disease (125) are sin-

gle instances and probably represent nothing more than chance association, whereas others which occur more frequently are more likely to be true associations. Osteoporosis has been the subject of many reports and might according to Teng et al (126) be the result of "active tumour metabolism" inducing a generalized catabolic state with an increased bone resorption. There is, however, little direct evidence to support this hypothesis.

CONCLUSIONS

Although the humoral syndromes associated with hepatoma are many and varied, it must be stressed that they are nevertheless extremely rare, many large series reporting only one or two such cases (7, 127, 128). Their incidence is obviously related to the availability of the various hormone assays and the extent of other investigations. Many syndromes will be grossly underestimated either because the clinical syndrome is poorly defined and has no direct short-term clinical effect, or because the ectopic hormones secreted are biologically inactive or secreted in amounts sufficient only to suppress the hormones but not to produce symptoms of hypersecretion.

The high incidence of erythrocytosis (10%) (13) and hypoglycemia (27%) reported in Chinese patients (53) and hypercholesterolemia (38%) in African patients (85) are unusual but of great interest. It may be that tumors from different parts of the world may behave in different ways either because of different etiological factors or possibly a different genetic composition which predisposes some races to metabolic derangements more readily than others.

What is the clinical significance of these syndromes? Their recognition in some instances may lead to an earlier diagnosis of the tumor; however, most occur late in the course of the disease when the diagnosis is only too obvious. Some of the manifestations, especially hypoglycemia and hypercalcemia, may provide profound management problems, and in these few cases are clearly of the utmost importance. However, most cases at the present time are unfortunately little more than medical curiosities worthy of case reports. At a more basic level these syndromes have provided a rich source of material, both human and animal, for the identification of the underlying mechanisms involved in cancer metabolism and evolution.

REFERENCES

1. Nadler WH, Wolfer JA: Hepatogenic hypoglycemia associated with primary liver cell carcinoma. *Arch Intern Med* **44**:700–710, 1929.

2. Viallet A, Benhamou JP, Fauvert R: Les manifestations paraneoplasiques des cancers primitifs du foie. *Rev Fr Etud Clin Biol* **6**:1087–1100, 1961.

3. Margolis S, Homcy C: Systemic manifestation of hepatoma. *Medicine* **51**:381–391, 1972.

4. McFadzean AJS, Young RTT: Further observations on hypoglycemia in hepatocellular carcinoma. *Am J Med* **47**:220–235, 1969.

5. McFadzean AJS, Todd D: Erythrocytosis associated with hepatocellular carcinoma. *Blood* **29**:808–811, 1967.

6. Abelev GI: Production of embryonal serum alpha globulin by hepatoma: review of experimental and clinical data. *Cancer Res* **28**:1344–1350, 1968.

7. Davidson AR, Tomlinson S, Calne RY, et al: The variable course of primary hepatocellular carcinoma. *Br J Surg* **61**:349–352, 1974.

8. Greenstein JP: *Biochemistry of Cancer.* Academic Press, New York, 1974.

9. Warner TFCS: Cell hybridization in the genesis of ectopic hormone secreting tumors. *Lancet* **1**:1259–1260, 1974.

10. Grzeschik KH: Utilization of somatic cell hybrids for genetic studies in man. *Humangenetik* **19**:1–40, 1973.

11. Braunstein GD, Vaitukaitis JL, Carbone PP, et al: Ectopic production of human chorionic gonadotrophin by neoplasms. *Ann Intern Med* **78**:39–45, 1973.

12. Contractor SR, Davies H: Effects of human chorionic gonadotrophin and chorionic gonadotrophin on phytohaemagglutinin-induced lymphocyte transformation. *Nat New Biol* **243**:284–286, 1973.

13. McFadzean AJS, Todd D, Tsang KC: Polycythemia in primary carcinoma of the liver. *Blood* **13**:427, 435, 1958.

14. Hewlett JS, Hoffman GC, Senhauser DA, et al: Hypernephroma with erythrocythemia. Report of a case and assay of the tumor for erythropoietic-stimulating substance. *New Engl J Med* **262**:1058–1062, 1960.

15. Waldmann TA, Levin EH, Baldwin M: The association of polycythemia with a cerebellar hemangioblastoma: The production of an erythropoiesis stimulating factor by the tumor. *Am J Med* **31**:318–324, 1961.

16. Brownstein MH, Ballard HS: Hepatoma associated with erythrocytosis. *Am J Med* **40**:204–210, 1966.

17. Fauvert R, Benhamson JP, Borvin P: Polyglobulia and primary cancer of the liver. *Bull Soc Med Hop Paris* **76**:757–767, 1960.

18. Thorling EB: In paraneoplastic erythrocytosis and inappropriate erythropoietin production–A review. *Scand J Haematol Suppl* **17**:1–166, 1972.

19. Kan YW, McFadzean AJS, Todd D, et al: Further observation on polycythemia in hepatocellular carcinoma. *Blood* **28**:592–598, 1961.

20. Adamson JW, Eschbach J. Finch CA: The kidney and erythropoiesis. *Am J Med* **44**:725–733, 1968.

21. Santer MA, Waldmann TA, Fallon HJ: Erythrocytosis and hyperlipemia as manifestations of hepatic carcinoma. *Arch Intern Med* **120**:735–739, 1967.

22. Gordon AS, Cooper GW, Zanjani ED: The kidney and erythropoiesis. *Semin Hematol* **4**:337–358, 1967.

23. Gordan GS, Cantino TJ, Erhardt L, et al: Osteolytic sterols in human breast cancer. *Science* **151**:1226–1228, 1966.

24. Gordon AS, Zanjani ED, Zalusky R: A possible mechanism for the erythrocytosis associated with hepatocellular carcinoma in man. *Blood* **35**:151–157, 1970.

25 Zanjani ED, Gordon AS, Wong KK, et al: The renal erythropoietic factor (REF). X. The question of species and class specificity. *Proc Soc Exp Biol Med* **131**:1095–1098, 1969.

26 Cantor LN, Zanjani ED, Wong KK, et al: The renal erythropoietic factor (REF). IX. Its subcellular distribution. *Proc Soc Exp Biol Med* **130**:950–952, 1969.

27. Erslev AJ, Kazal LA: Renal erythropoietic factor. Lack of effect on hypertransfused mice. *Blood* **34**:222–229, 1969.

28. Jacobsen EM, Davis AK, Alpen EL: Relative effectiveness of phenyl-hydrazine treatment and hemorrhage in the production of an erythropoietic factor. *Blood* **11**:937–945, 1956.

29. Prentice TC, Mirand, EA: Effect of acute liver damage plus hypoxia on plasma erythropoietin content. *Proc Soc Exp Biol Med* **95**:231–234, 1957.

30. Erslev AJ, Kazal LA: Inactivation of erythropoietin by tissue homogenates. *Proc Soc Exp Biol Med* **129**:845–849, 1968.

31. Briggs DW, George WJ, Fisher JW: Inactivation of erythropoietin by hepatic lysosomes. *Proc Soc Exp Biol Med* **144**:394–399, 1973.

32. Gutman AB, Tyson TL, Gutman EB: Serum calcium inorganic phosphorus and alkaline phosphatase activity in hyperparathyroidism, Paget's disease, multiple myeloma and neoplastic disease of bone. *Arch Intern Med* **57**:379–390, 1963.

33. Fry L: Pseudohyperparathyroidism with carcinoma of the bronchus. *Brit Med J* **1**:301–302, 1962.

34. Dent CE, Watson LCA: Hyperparathyroidism and cancer. *Brit Med J* **2**:218–221, 1964.

35. Mallory TB (Ed): Case records of the Massachusetts General Hospital. *New Engl J Med* **225**:789–794, 1941.

36. Lafferty FW: Pseudohyperparathyroidism. *Medicine* **45**:247–260, 1966.

37. Becker DJ, Sternberg MS, Kalser MH: Hepatoma associated with hypercalcemia. *JAMA* **186**:1018–1019, 1963.

38. Samuelson SM, Werner I: Hepatic carcinoma simulating hyperparathyroidism. *Acta Med Scand* **173**:539–547, 1963.

39. Keller RT, Goldschneider F, Lafferty FW: Hypercalcemia secondary to a primary hepatoma. *JAMA* **192**:782–784, 1965.

40. Naide W, Matz R, Spear PW: Cholangiocarcinoma causing hypercalcemia and hypophosphatemia without skeletal metastases (pseudohyperparathyroidism). *Am J Dig Dis* **13**:705–708, 1968.

41. Dunn RP, Nystrom JS: Association of ectopically produced hyperparathyroidism with hepatoma. *Calif Med* **118**:48–51, 1973.

42. Knill-Jones RP, Buckle RM, Parsons V, et al: Hypercalcemia and increased parathyroid hormone activity in primary hepatoma. Studies before and after hepatic transplantation. *New Engl J Med* **282**:704–708, 1970.

43. Tashjian AH Jr, Levine L, Munson PL: Immunochemical identification of parathyroid hormone in non-parathyroid neoplasms associated with hypercalcemia. *J Exp Med* **119**:467–484, 1964.

44. Riggs BL, Arnaud CD, Reynolds LC, et al: Immunologic differentiation of primary hyperparathyroidism from hyperparathyroidism due to non-parathyroid cancer. *J Clin Invest* **50**:2079–2083, 1971.

45. Berson SA, Yalow RS: Immunochemical heterogeneity of parathyroid hormone in plasma. *J Clin Endocr Biol Metab* **28**:1037–1047, 1968.

46. Roof BS, Carpenter B, Fink DJ, et al: Some thoughts on the nature of ectopic parathyroid hormones. *Am J Med* **50**:686–691, 1971.

47. Sherwood LM, O'Riordan JLH, Aurbach GD, et al: Preliminary communication. Production of parathyroid hormone by non parathyroid tissue. *J Clin Endocr Biol Metab* **27**:140–146, 1967.

48. Tashjian AH Jr, Voelkel EF, Levine L, et al: Evidence that the bone resorption-stimulating factor produced by mouse fibrosarcoma cells in prostoglandin E2. A new model for the hypercalcemia of cancer. *J Exp Med* **136**:1329–1343, 1972.

49. Tashjian AH Jr, Voelkel EF, Goldmaker P, et al: Successful treatment of hypercalcemia by indomethacin in mice bearing a prostaglandin producing fibrosarcoma. *Prostaglandins* **3**:515–524, 1973.

50. Powell D, Singer FR, Murray TM, et al: Non-parathyroid humoral hypercalcemia in patients with neoplastic disease. *New Engl J Med* **289**:176–181, 1973.

51. Raiszl LG: Prostaglandins and the hypercalcemia of cancer. *New Engl J Med* **289**:214–215, 1973.

52. Urteaga OB, Dieguez JN, Villanueva AY: Cancer primario del higado y de las vias biliares. *Arch Peru Patol Clin* **3**:3, 1949.

53. McFadzean AJS, Yeung TT: Hypoglycemia in primary carcinoma of the liver. *Arch Intern Med* **98**:720–736, 1956.

54. Bundith V, Chandraprasert S, Sriratanaban A: Hypoglycemia and erythrocytosis associated with hepatoma. *J Med Assoc Thailand* **55**:110–115, 1972.

55. Unger RH: Editorial: The riddle of tumor hypoglycemia. *Am J Med* **40**:325–330, 1966.

56. Schonfeld A, Babbott D, Gundersen K: Hypoglycemia and polycythemia associated with primary hepatoma. *New Engl J Med* **265**:231–235, 1961.

57. Unger RH, Lochner JD, Eisentraut AM: Identification of insulin and glucagon in a bronchogenic metastases. *J Clin Endocr* **24**:823–831, 1964.

58. Landau BR, Wills N, Craig JW, et al: The mechanism of hepatoma-induced hypoglycemia. *Cancer* **15**:1188–1196, 1962.

59. Field JB, Keen H, Johnson P, et al: Insulin-like activity of nonpancreatic tumors associated with hypoglycemia. *J Clin Endocr* **23**:1229–1236, 1963.

60. Tranquada RE, Bender AB, Beigelman PM: Hypoglycemia associated with carcinoma of the cecum and syndrome of testicular feminization. *New Engl J Med* **266**:1302–1306, 1962.

61. Miller DR, Bolinger RE, Janigan D, et al: Hypoglycemia due to nonpancreatic mesodermal tumors. *Ann Surg* **150**:684–696, 1956.

62. Silverstein MN, Wakim KG, Bahn RC, et al: A hypoglycemia factor in leukemic tumors. *Proc Soc Exp Biol Med* **103**:824–826, 1960.

63. Chandalia HB, Boshell BR: Hypoglycemia associated with extrapancreatic tumors. *Arch Intern Med* **129**:447–456, 1972.

64. Passoneau JV, Lowry OH: The role of phosphofructokinase in metabolic regulation. In *Advances in Enzyme Regulation*, Vol 2. McMillan, New York, 1964, pp 265–273.

65. Horecker BL, Hiatt HH: Pathways of carbohydrate metabolism in normal and neoplastic cells. *New Engl J Med* **258**:177–184, 1958.

66. Kreisberg RA, Pennington LF: Tumor hypoglycemia: A heterogenous disorder. *Metabolism*, **19**:445–452, 1970.

67. Ishak KG, Glunz PR: Hepatoblastoma and hepatocarcinoma in infants and children: Report of 47 cases. *Cancer* **20**:396–422, 1967.

68. McArthur JW, Toll GD, Russfield AB, et al: Sexual precocity attributable to ectopic gonadotrophin secretion by hepatoblastoma. *Am J Med* **54**:390–403, 1973.

69. Williams MJ: Gynecomastia. *Am J Med* **34**:103–112, 1963.

70. Summerskill WHS, Adson MA: Gynecomastia as a sign of hepatoma. *Am J Dig Dis* **7**:250–254, 1962.

71. Couinaud C, Schwarzmann V, Ceoara B, et al: Hepatome malin avec amenorrhee et galactorrhee. Disparition du syndrome endocrinien apres hepatectomie droite. *An Chir* **27**(2): C151–156, 1973.

72. Hung W, Blizzard RM, Migeon CJ, et al: Precocious puberty in a boy with hepatoma and circulating gonadotropin. *J Pediatr* **63**:895–903, 1963.

73. Reeves RL, Tesluk H, Harrison CE: Precocious puberty associated with hepatoma. *J Clin Endocr* **19**:1651–1660, 1959.

74. Braunstein GD, Bridson WE, Glass A, et al: *In vivo* and *in vitro* production of human chorionic gonadotrophin and alpha-fetoprotein by a virilising hepatoblastoma. *J Clin Endocr Metab* **35**:857–862, 1972.

75. Fine G, Smith RW Jr, Pachter MR: Primary extragenital choriocarcinoma in the male subject. Case report and review of the literature. *Am J Med* **32**:776–794, 1962.

76. McKenchnie JC, Fechner RE: Choriocarcinoma and adenocarcinoma of the esophagus with gonadotropin secretion. *Cancer* **27**:694–702, 1971.

77. Ozaki H, Ito I, Sano R, et al: A case of choriocarcinoma of the stomach. *Jap J Clin Oncol* **1**:83–94, 1971.

78. Weintraub BD, Rosen SW: Ectopic production of chorionic somatomammatropin by nontrophoblastic cancers. *J Clin Endocr Metab* **32**:94–101, 1971.

79. Siperstein MD, Fagan VM: Deletion of the cholesterol-negative feedback system in liver tumors. *Cancer Res* **24**:1108–1115, 1964.

80. Siperstein MD: In *Current Topics in Cellular Regulations*, Vol 2. Stadtman E, Horecker B (Eds). Academic Press, New York, 1970, p 65.

81. Siperstein MD, Fagan VM, Morris HP: Further studies on the deletion of the cholesterol feedback system in hepatomas. *Cancer Res* **26**:7–11, 1966.

82. Siperstein MD, Gyde AM, Morris HP: Loss of feedback control of hydroxymethylglutaryl coenzyme. A reductase in hepatomas. *Proc Natl Acad Sci USA* **68**:315–317, 1971.

83. Hansen AE, Ziegler MR, McQuarrie I: Disturbance of osseous and lipid metabolism in a child with primary carcinoma of the liver. *J Pediatr* **17**:9–30, 1940.

84. Viallett A, Benhamou JP, Fauvert RP: Primary carcinoma of the liver and hyperlipaemia. *Can Med Assoc J* **86**:1118–1121, 1962.

85. Alpert ME, Hutt MSR, Davidson CS: Primary hepatoma in Uganda. A prospective clinical and epidemiologic study of forty-six patients. *Am J Med* **46**:794–802, 1969.

86. Bricker LA, Morris HP, Siperstein MD: Loss of cholesterol feedback system in the intact hepatoma bearing rat. *J Clin Invest* **51**:206–215, 1972.

87. Kwaan HC, Lo R, McFadzean AJS: Antifibrinolytic activity in primary carcinoma of the liver. *Clin Sci* **18**:251–261, 1959.

88. Bell W, Bahr R, Waldmann TA, et al: Cryofi-brinogenemia, multiple dysproteinemias and hypervolemia in patient with primary hepatoma. *Ann Intern Med* **64**:658–664, 1966.

89. McKee PA, Kalbfleisch JM, Bird RM: Incidence and significance of cryofibrinogenemia. *J Lab Clin Med* **61**:203–210, 1963.

90. Levin WC, Long PA, Gregory R, et al: Secondary cryofibrinogenemia associated with cryopathy. *Proceedings of the Ninth Congress of the International Society of Hematology,* Vol 3. Universidad Nacional Autonoma de Mexico, Mexico, 1964, p 239.

91. Berman J, Braun A: Incidence of hepatoma in porphyria cutanea tarda. *Rev Czech Med* **8**:290–295, 1962.

92. Thompson RPH, Nicholson DC, Farnan T, et al: Cutaneous porphyria due to a malignant primary hepatoma. *Gastroenterology* **59**:779, 1970.

93. Tio TH, Leijnse B, Jarrett A, et al: Acquired porphyria from a liver tumor. *Clin Sci* **16**:517–527, 1957.

94. Braun A, Berman J: Patologicko-anatomicke nalezy pri porfyria cutanea tarda. *Acta Univ Carol (Med) (Praha)* **8**:597–605, 1959.

95. Leeson PM, Fourman P: A disorder of copper metabolism treated with penicillamine in a patient with primary biliary cirrhosis and renal tubular acidosis. *Am J Med* **43**:620–635, 1967.

96. Kieff ED, McCarty DJ Jr: Hypertrophic osteoarthropathy with arthritis and synovial calcification in a patient with alcoholic cirrhosis. *Arthritis Rheum* **12**:261–269, 1969.

97. Morgan AG, Walker WC, Mason MK, et al: A new syndrome associated with hepatocellular carcinoma. *Gastroenterology* **63**:340–345, 1972.

98. Margulis AR, Nice CM, Rigler LG: The roentgen findings in primary hepatoma in infants and children. *Radiology* **66**:809–816, 1956.

99. Kasai M, Watanabe I: Histological classification of liver cell carcinoma in infancy and childhood and its clinical evaluation. *Cancer* **25**:551–563, 1970.

100. Hall GH, Laidlaw CD: Further experimental evidence implicating reduced ferritin as a cause of digital clubbing. *Clin Sci* **24**:121–126, 1963.

101. Ginsburg J, Brown JB: Increased estrogen excretion in hypertrophic pulmonary osteoarthropathy. *Lancet* **2**:1274–1276, 1961.

102. Holling HE: Editorial notes. Pulmonary hypertrophic osteoarthropathy. *Ann Intern Med* **66**:232–234, 1967.

103. Holling HE, Brodey RS: Pulmonary hypertro-phic osteoarthropathy. *J Am Med Assoc* **178**:977–982, 1961.

104. Edmondson HA: *Tumors of the Liver and Intrahepatic Bile Ducts. Atlas of Tumor Pathology,* Section VII, fascicle 25. Armed Forces Institute of Pathology, Washington D.C., 1958.

105. Primack A, Wilson J, O'Conner GT, et al: Hepatocellular carcinoma with the carcinoid syndrome. *Cancer* **27**:1182–1189, 1971.

106. Warnock M, Reisman R: Variant alkaline phosphatase in human hepatocellular cancers. *Clin Chim Acta* **24**:5–11, 1969.

107. Portugal ML, Azevedo MS, Manso C: Serum alpha-fetoprotein and variant alkaline phosphatase in human hepatocellular carcinoma. *Int J Cancer* **6**:383–387, 1970.

108. Fishman W: Immunologic and biochemical approaches to alkaline phosphatase isoenzyme analysis. The Regan Isoenzyme. *Ann N Y Acad Sci* **166**:745–757, 1969.

109. Stolbach LL, Krant MJ, Fishman WH: Ectopic production of an alkaline phosphatase isoenzyme in patients with cancer. *New Engl J Med* **281**:757–762, 1969.

110. Olmer J, Mongin M, Muratore R: Le retentissement hepatique de la macroglobulinemie de Waldenstrom. *Presse Med* **65**:524–527, 1957.

111. Laurell CB, Laurell H, Waldenstrom J: Glycoproteins in serum from patients with myeloma, macroglobulinemia and related conditions. *Am J Med* **22**:24–36, 1957.

112. Waldenstrom J: Clinical diagnosis and biochemical findings in material of 296 sera with M-type narrow gamma-globulins. *Acta Med Scand Suppl* **367**:110–126, 1961.

113. Creyssel R, Fine JM, Morel P: Etude biochimique de quelques formes atypiques de dysproteinemies. *Rev Hematol* **14**:238–000, 1959.

114. Bigwood EJ, Crokaert R, Schram E, et al: Amino aciduria. *Adv Clin Chem* **2**:201–265, 1959.

115. Dent CE, Walshe JM: primary carcinoma of liver: description of case with ethanolaminuria, new and obscure metabolic defect. *Brit J Cancer* **7**:166–180, 1953.

116. Neish WJP, Rylett A: Accumulation of phosphoethanolamine in the livers of rats injected with hepatocarcinogens. *Brit J Cancer* **14**:737–745, 1960.

117. Prat JR, Obradors MS, Noguora RB, Sauras EC: Anaemia hemolitica asociada a hepatocarcinoma. *Revista espanala de las Enfermedades del aparato Digestivo* **39**:577–582, 1973.

118. Alpert LI, Benisch B: Hemangioendothelioma of the liver associated with microangiopathic hemolytic anemia. *Am J Med* **48**:624–628, 1970.

119. Geiser CF, Baez A, Schindler AM, et al: Epithelial hepatoblastoma associated with congenital hemihypertrophy and cystathioninuria. Presentation of a case. *Pediatrics* **46**:66–73, 1970.

120. Voute PA Jr, Wadman SK: Cystathioninuria in hepatoblastoma. *Clin Chim Acta* **22**:373–378, 1968.

121. Geiser CF, Efron ML: Cystathioneuria in patients with neuroblastoma and gamma glioneuroblastoma. Its correlation to vanilmandelic acid excretion and its value in diagnosis and therapy. *Cancer* **22**:856–860, 1968.

122. Leffers I: Uber eine seltern, maligne Mischgeschwulst der Leber bei einem 16 monate alten Knaben. *Beitr Pathol Anat* **105**:203–218, 1941.

123. MacNab GH, Moncrieff AA, Budian M: Primary malignant hepatic tumors in childhood. *British Empire Cancer Campaign, 13th Annual Report,* Vol 30. Sumfield and Day, Ltd., Eastbourne, Sussex, 1952, pp 168–176.

124. Cleland RS: Benign and malignant tumors of the liver. *Pediatr Clin North Am* **6**:427–447, 1959.

125. Mason HH, Andersen DH: Glycogen disease of the liver (von Gierke's disease) with hepatoma. *Pediatrics* **16**:785–799, 1955.

126. Teng CT, Daeschner CW, Singleton EB, et al: Liver disease and osteoporosis in children. Clinical Observations. *J Pedr* **59**:684–702, 1961.

127. El-Domeiri AA, Huvos AG, Goldsmith HS, et al: Primary malignant tumors of the liver. *Cancer* **27**:7–11, 1971.

128. Geddes EW, Falkson G: Malignant hepatoma in the Bantu. *Cancer* **25**:1271–1278, 1970.

CHAPTER 15 HUMAN ALPHA-1 FETOPROTEIN

ELLIOT ALPERT, M.D.

Alpha fetoprotein (AFP) is a serum alpha-1-globulin found normally in high concentrations in fetal sera, particularly in early gestation. In 1944, shortly after electrophoretic procedures became available, Pedersen discovered a protein band with alpha-1 mobility in fetal calf sera, not detectable in adult bovine sera, which he called fetuin (1). In 1956 Bergstrand and Czar discovered an apparently similar alpha-1 globulin in human fetal sera, which was not detectable in normal adult or maternal sera (2, 3). Similar alpha-1-globulins, apparently fetal specific, were found by Gitlin in the fetal sera of a wide variety of mammals (4), birds (5), and in sharks (6), indicating the early evolutionary appearance of this serum protein. All these fetal specific proteins are generally alpha globulins, but are electrophoretically and antigenically distinguishable, with little species cross-reactivity, except between closely related species (4). Fetuin, the initial fetal specific protein to be described and now one of the best chemically defined

Original work cited was supported by grants from the USPHS (CA 12389) and the American Cancer Society.

serum glycoproteins, does not really belong to the class of fetoproteins analogous to human AFP which is found in many species. Its time of appearance, chemical structure, and preponderance of carbohydrates make fetuin a distinctive bovine serum glycoprotein. In contrast, a different bovine alpha-1 globulin, found only in fetal calf sera, does seem to share many of the biochemical and biological features of other mammalian alpha-1 fetoproteins (7). The early evolutionary appearance of these fetal specific alpha-1-globulins and their high concentration early in gestation suggest an important normal biologic role which remains undefined.

In 1963 Abelev reported that a hepatoma specific antigen extracted from mouse hepatoma cells was immunologically identical to normal mouse AFP (8). The resynthesis of this fetal protein by the malignant cell represented a biochemical form of dedifferentiation and led to two major clinically important observations. First, it led to the detection of human fetoprotein in the serum of a hepatoma patient (9), suggesting that fetoprotein may be a helpful diagnostic test for human primary liver carcinoma. Its diagnostic usefulness was rapidly established in clinical studies in many parts of the world (10–16). Second, Abelev's discovery of AFP in hepatoma reemphasized earlier suggestions that some biochemical features of the malignant cell may resemble those found normally in the undifferentiated embryonic cell. Altered enzyme and isoenzyme patterns in cancer cells, thought to be tumor specific, were subsequently found to resemble frequently the activity and isoenzyme profile of the undifferentiated fetal cell (17). Some of the characteristics of the surface membrane of tumor cells also appear to be similar to normal fetal cells (18). A tumor specific surface membrane antigen in colon carcinoma described by Gold in 1965 (19) was subsequently found in fetal colon and renamed Carcino-Embryonic Antigen of the Digestive Tract (CEA) (20). The detection of CEA in the serum of colon cancer patients (21) led to extensive clinical trials establishing the diagnostic value of this fetal antigen. These findings have stimulated much recent work in experimental systems concerning the biology of AFP and the mechanism of its renewed synthesis in hepatoma, which have recently been reviewed (22–24). This chapter concerns itself largely with the chemical nature, biology, and clinical significance of *human* fetoprotein.*

CHEMICAL CHARACTERISTICS

AFP is antigenically distinct, and antisera against human AFP can be easily elicited in a number of heterologous species, including rabbit, guinea pig, sheep, goat, and horse. Since AFP is usually not identifiable by the routine electrophoretic techniques, the detection of AFP and its characterization rely completely on its unique antigenic determinants and the develop-

*The reader is referred to previous reviews of human AFP by GI Abelev, *Adv Cancer Res* **14**:295, 1971, and by R Massayeff, *Pathol Biol* **20**:703, 1972.

ment of a number of types of specific immunoassays. Antisera can be elicited by immunizing with purified AFP, fetal or hepatoma sera, and made specific by absorbing adequately with sera from normal adults. Antisera to AFP does not cross-react with any other known human serum protein.

The surface charge of AFP is actually very acidic and quite similar to that of albumin. Therefore, AFP migrates rapidly in the alpha region in most forms of electrophoresis at the usual alkaline pH. Human AFP migrates just posterior to albumin in alkaline pH on paper (2, 3), agar (3), cellulose acetate (25), starch gel (26), and starch or agarose (27, 28). After polyacrylamide gel electrophoresis, a high concentration of AFP is visible as a distinct band between albumin and alpha-1-antitrypsin (29). The molecular weight has been reported to be 64,600 by ultracentrifugation (30), between 70 and 75,000 by gel filtration (25, 27, 29–32) and between 72 and 74,000 by SDS polyacrylamide gel electrophoresis (27, 28, 31). It is commonly accepted to be about 72,000, only slightly larger than human serum albumin. AFP is a single polypeptide chain, with no detectable subunit structure (28, 31, 37). Aggregation of AFP may occur in highly purified form (31), but does not normally occur in whole sera (28). Human AFP has been purified biochemically (27, 28, 33–35) as well as by specific immunoprecipitation (30, 31, 37). The amino acid composition described by Nishi (30) and Ruoslahti (31) shows no unusual distribution. Approximately 3% of the molecule is composed of carbohydrate, including sialic acid (30, 31). Molecular heterogeneity has been described as with many other glycoproteins, and at least two forms can be demonstrated with slightly different net charges (27, 28, 36). The isoelectric point of these forms have been found to be 4.8 and 5.1 (27, 32, 35). Experiments with neuraminidase, which causes slight but definite alteration in electrophoretic mobility (28, 33, 37), suggest that the presence of 2 M of sialic acid per molecule probably accounts for the charge heterogeneity (27, 33). The sedimentation constant has been found to be between 4.5 and 5.0 (30–32). The solubility characteristics of AFP in rivanol and ammonium sulfate have been described by Masopust (32), and human AFP has been crystallized by Lehmann (34).

The AFP synthesized by hepatoma tissue and that synthesized by fetal liver have been shown to be biochemically as well as immunologically identical. The amino acid distribution, peptic tryptic digest patterns, and physical characteristics of fetal and hepatoma AFP are indistinguishable (30, 31, 38).

METHODS OF ASSAY

The early experimental (8) and clinical observations (10–16) were made with a relatively crude double agar gel-diffusion (AGD) technique that had a limited sensitivity of probably no more than 1 to 10 μg/ml. At this level of sensitivity, the detection of fetoprotein became widely used as a diagnostic test for hepatocellular carcinoma with few false-positive reactions (10–16). A number of other more sensitive techniques have been used in more recent studies (see Table 1). Counterimmunoelectrophoresis (CIEP) (39), electroimmunodiffusion (EID) (40), and latex fixation (41) can detect approximately 250 to 500 ng/ml of AFP. The use of prior rivanol precipitation can increase the sensitivity of these assays slightly (42). Hemagglutination (23), double antibody radio-labeled electroimmunodiffusion (REID) (23, 40, 43) and immunoenzymatic assays (44) can detect and quantitate as little as 50 ng/ml. Modifications of immunoenzymatic (45) and double antibody radio-labeled electroimmunodiffusion (radioelectro complexing) (46) have been reported to be able to detect 1 to 10 ng/ml. Radioimmunoassays

(RIA), measuring the competitive inhibition by human sera of radio-labeled purified AFP were first developed and used extensively by Purves (47) and Ruoslahti (48) and are able to detect a few nanograms per milliliter of fetoprotein. A variable low level of inhibitory activity in RIA has been found by different laboratories in the sera of many normal people, varying between 2.3 ng up to 30 ng/ml (48–53). Part of this wide variation in baseline represents differences between laboratory reagents and standards. In fact, the same reference preparation measured in different laboratories has given varying results. Another source of the variation in baseline levels may be due to nonspecific inhibition by serum factors (50, 52), antigen denaturation or oxidation, protein concentrations, etc. (54). Ruoslahti has recently provided direct evidence for the presence of AFP in some normal sera by extracting it from a large pool of sera by immunoabsorption (55). Nevertheless, there is still uncertainty as to the precise normal level (48–53) or whether the "normal" level is higher in populations with a high incidence of hepatoma (56). The use of a reference standard and comparative studies are needed to clarify this problem.

NORMAL BIOLOGY

Human AFP is synthesized normally in very large amounts early in fetal life (25). AFP is normally synthesized by fetal liver cells (57–59) and in trace amounts by the fetal GI tract (60). The AFP is secreted into serum, amniotic fluid, urine, CSF, and can be found in extracellular fluid. Since human fetal yolk sac cells also synthesize AFP (61), the synthesis of AFP in a few human placental tissues (58, 60) may be due to these yolk cell elements. The serum concentration in the first trimester can reach as high as 300 to 400 mg%, and represents the major serum globulin in

Table 1   Assays for AFP in Current Use

	Sensitivity ng/ml)	Positive Hepatomas (%)	Reference
Qualitative tests			
Double agar gel diffusion (AGD)	1000–10,000	28–95	10–16
Counter immunoelectrophoresis (CIEP)	250–500	50–95	39, 91
Latex fixation	250–500	50	41
Quantitative tests			
Electroimmunodiffusion (EID)	250–500	70	40
Radio-labeled electrodiffusion (REID)	50–100		23, 43, 111
Immunoenzymatic (ENZ)	50–100	78	89
Radioelectro complexing (REC)	1–10	—	46
Competitive inhibition radioimmuno assay (RIA)	0.5–20	78–95	51–53, 56, 91, 103

early gestation (25). Fetoprotein synthesis has been detected as early as 6 to 8 weeks of gestation (25) at the time of earliest liver cell differentiation. In isolated, perfused human fetal livers, as much as 19 to 26 μg of AFP can be synthesized per minute (62). The synthetic rate appears to stabilize with a rapidly enlarging fetal serum pool during mid-gestation, causing the serum concentrations to fall slightly (25). AFP is secreted into amniotic fluid, probably via fetal urine (25, 63). AFP can reach a concentration in amniotic fluid of up to 50 μg/ml (25), or 1 to 2% of the fetal serum concentration in early gestation and falls to below 10 to 15 μg/ml near term (64–66). After birth, the serum concentration of AFP rapidly falls with a half-life of 3.5 days (25). This half-life is very similar to the degradation and disappearance curve of fetoprotein infused into adult man (67), suggesting cessation of synthesis and subsequent metabolic degradation in the early postpartum period. The protein becomes undetectable except by radioimmunoassay after 3 to 4 months of life. Low levels of AFP, perhaps as high as 5 to 10 ng/ml, appear to persist in normal adults, but this is detectable only by RIA (49, 56).

The biologic function of AFP is un-known. Its early evolutionary appearance, its rapid synthetic rate, and high serum concentration in early fetal life, the period of most rapid differentiation and growth, suggest that the protein must have an important function. Its similarity to albumin in molecular weight and charge (28) must enable AFP to function as an osmotically active molecule protecting the intravascular volume. In fact, AFP biosynthesis diminishes during gestation as albumin synthesis and serum concentration rise, suggesting a homeostatic relationship (25, 62).

AFP certainly does not have the general binding characteristics of albumin. Experimentally, rat and human AFP bind estrogenic hormones selectively *in vitro* (68, 69). This has led Uriel to suggest that AFP may be involved in the regulation of protein synthesis and therefore differentiation, mediated by estrogen hormones (68). The estrogenic binding cells in fetal liver appear to be identical to the AFP-producing cells (70). However, the binding affinity of estrogen to *human* AFP appears to be much lower than for rat AFP (68, 69), and its role in man remains unclear.

There are many serum factors, including fetuin (71), that affect growth in tissue culture systems. Despite many experimental trials, AFP has shown no convincing effect on growth. Indeed, the factors in fetuin preparations thought to be growth promotors were later demonstrated to be insulin and other hormones contaminating the isolated fetuin (72). Similarly, although there are many factors in serum that affect lymphocyte responsiveness, including some in the alpha globulin fraction of serum, none have been identified as AFP. The alpha-1 globulin fraction of serum also contains alpha-1 antitrypsin and alpha-1 macroglobulins, which inhibit proteolytic enzymes. AFP does not appear to have any proteolytic enzyme activity or any inhibitory function on proteolytic enzyme systems (73), and is unrelated chemically and immunologically to alpha-1 antitrypsin. AFP does not appear to be an acute phase reactant, such as a number of other serum proteins. Human AFP elevations do not occur after trauma or infections (74). Experimentally, small elevations of AFP can be seen after 70% hepatectomy (75) or in carbon tetrachloride poisoning in neonatal rats (76), and is thought to be a product of regeneration (22–24). However, in man partial hepatectomy does not appear to result in significant AFP elevations (43).

During gestation, AFP is secreted into serum and into amniotic fluid. The amniotic fluid concentration reaches a peak concentration in the first trimester (25). During normal pregnancy, there is a small amount of fetal maternal transfusion, evidenced by the increase in detectable fetal red cells and other proteins which, in fact, may cause isoimmunization. There is a slight increase of AFP serum concentration in maternal sera during gestation, particularly near term (50, 77), presumably by means of fetal placental transfer. Maternal serum concentration of AFP can reach levels as high as 500 ng/ml transiently near term or during birth with placental disruption (50, 79). Normally, this increased AFP is transient and falls quickly.

There is an apparent life-long tolerance to AFP, since no homologous host immune response has been demonstrated. Animals immunized with homologous AFP show no immune response. Animals immunized with *human* fetoprotein produce antibodies to human fetoprotein, which may also cross-react with some determinants on its homologous AFP (78). However, no natural homologous antibody has been demonstrated.

AFP is present in normal adult sera, in trace amounts normally undetectable by any method other than competitive inhibition RIA (48, 56). The precise level is unclear because of the lack of a standard, but appears to be between 2 and 10 ng/ml. The source and function of this residual AFP is also unclear. However, the constant exposure of the immune system to low levels of AFP may be the mechanism by which life-long tolerance to AFP and subsequent lack of immune recognition is maintained.

AFP IN PATHOLOGIC CONDITIONS

Intrauterine Diseases

Abnormally high concentrations of AFP have been found in maternal sera associated with severe fetal distress and fetal death (79, 80), suggesting that AFP may be a useful marker of fetal placental dysfunction. However, there appears to be great variability in maternal levels that may limit its diagnostic usefulness (67). Amniotic fluid AFP concentrations are more consistently elevated (81). In fact, total protein concentration, as well as AFP concentration, rises with transudation of fetal serum through hypoxic or dead tissue (82). Large prospective clinical studies are still required to define the usefulness of amniotic and maternal AFP in predicting clinically significant and still treatable fetal distress.

Amniotic fluid AFP levels were first reported by Brock et al to be elevated in the presence of most cases of anencephaly (83). This observation was rapidly confirmed in a number of reports (84). Studies of amniotic fluid obtained by amniocentesis during pregnancy have indicated that elevated AFP levels in an apparently normal pregnancy may be an early diagnostic clue to the presence of anencephaly or certain other neural tube defects (84). There appears to be a selective increase in AFP, since total protein concentration in these amniotic fluids remains normal (82). Whether maternal AFP serum concentrations are elevated constantly enough in anencephaly to be useful is still not clear (84). Elevated amniotic fluid AFP levels have also been reported in a case of congenital esophageal atresia (85).

CHILDHOOD

Experimentally, increased serum AFP levels may also be induced after carbon tetrachloride poisoning in neonatal rats who may still have AFP secreting hepatocytes (76). In the human neonatal period, the serum concentration of AFP is increased in the presence of almost any kind of hepatic disease. Elevations have been reported in infants with viral hepatitis (86, 87), biliary atresia (87), neonatal hepatitis (87), and congestive hepatomegaly from cardiac defects (43). The degree of elevation seems to be a function of age, with the higher serum concentrations, up to several mg%, found in the early neonatal period (43). The serum AFP concentrations occurring with neonatal hepatitis appear to be significantly greater than that found in biliary atresia at an equivalent age in the neonatal period (88). If this observation is confirmed, AFP serum concentrations may be helpful in differentiating these conditions. These AFP elevations are transient and return to normal with resolution of the liver disease.

Fetoprotein reaches its normal level sometime during the first year of postnatal life. AFP elevations in children have been reported only in a few specific conditions. Significant AFP elevations occur in almost all reported cases of *hepatoblastoma*, reaching levels as high as several hundred mg% (89). Significant AFP elevations also occur in *teratoblastomas*, involving the ovaries and testes. Approximately one-third of such patients will have AFP elevations high enough to be detectable by gel diffusion (10, 90, 91). These AFP positive teratoblastomas may have elements of yolk cell, embyronal cell carcinomas, or chorionepithelioma. Although these are usually childhood gonadal tumors, they may occur in extragonadal sites and rarely in adults (43). Ovarian endodermal sinus tumors, which may be of yolk cell origin, may also be positive (92).

AFP serum concentrations have been helpful both in diagnosis and in evaluating the effect of chemotherapy or surgical excision (90). AFP has been localized by immunofluorescence in some of these tumors to cells of yolk sac origin (92, 93), which can synthesize AFP during fetal life (61).

Two genetically determined diseases have also been associated with significant elevations of AFP. Waldmann and McIntire have described elevated AFP in most children with *ataxia telangiactasia* but not in any other form of immune deficiency disease (94). The disease is thought to be a defect in maturation of the immune process and the authors hypothesize that AFP may be another manifestation of this defect in maturation (94).

Hereditary tyrosinosis is a second genetic defect associated with significantly elevated AFP levels (95). This elevation appears to be specific for congenital tyrosinosis, since a variety of other metabolic defects and glycogen storage diseases studied by the authors were not associated with AFP elevations. The levels of AFP in tyrosinosis had some rough relationship to the severity of the liver disease associated with this genetic defect (96). Although much is known about the metabolic pathways affected in tyrosinosis (97), the mechanism of AFP synthesis in this condition and its relationship to the metabolic defect in tyrosinosis are unknown.

A third benign disease associated with AFP elevations in childhood is *viral hepatitis* (86). As in the adult (discussed later), AFP serum concentrations are increased in a significant percentage of children with viral hepatitis. The levels fall with resolution of the disease. AFP elevations have been reported in Indian childhood cirrhosis, a unique chronic liver disease in Indian children (98). However this observation could not be confirmed by others (99).

Except for these few benign conditions, significant elevations of AFP occur only in primary liver cell carcinoma, hepatoblastoma, and teratoblastoma. Therefore, in the appropriate clinical setting, persistently elevated AFP concentrations can be quite helpful in the diagnosis of these tumors and serum concentrations may help in evaluating therapy.

AFP IN THE ADULT

Primary Liver Carcinoma

The reappearance of AFP in the sera of adult patients with hepatoma has been well documented since Tatarinov's observation in the Russian literature in 1964 (9). Elevations of AFP have been found in a high percentage of patients with hepatoma and have proven to be quite useful clinically in the diagnosis of this frequently occult malignancy (10–16).

The frequency of AFP elevations in liver cell carcinoma has varied widely in different series, between 23 and 95% (see Table 1). This variability has been due in large part to two main factors: sensitivity of the method used and a definite geographic variation (100). The serum concentration of AFP in patients with liver carcinoma varies widely from the several nanograms per milliliter found in normal individuals

to as high as 6 or 7 mg/ml, a range of 6 logs (16, 39, 40, 101, 102). The frequency of detectable AFP elevations, therefore, will depend on the sensitivity of the method used (see Table 1). Early clinical studies were routinely done with double gel diffusion with a sensitivity probably no greater than 1 to 10 μg/ml (10–16). In parts of Africa where the incidence of hepatoma is very high, fetoprotein elevations were reported in from 50% of hepatoma patients in Uganda (12) to as high as 80% in Senegal and South Africa (11, 13, 16). In the United States, using the same agar gel-diffusion method and antisera, only 28% of Caucasian hepatoma patients were positive (100). These early studies suggested a geographic variation in AFP levels independent of methodology.

As more sensitive and quantitative methods began to be employed for AFP detection and measurement, it became apparent that most of the variation in reported prevalence rates of AFP and liver carcinoma were quantitative differences (39) (see Table 1). Sensitive radioimmunoassays or immunoenzymatic assays can detect AFP elevations greater than 50 ng/ml in 78% of United States Caucasian hepatoma patients (89), 79% of European hepatoma patients (103), and 89% of Japanese patients (52). Purves has shown that there is a continuum of AFP serum concentrations in Bantu hepatoma patients merging with background levels (50, 56), but it seems clear that about 10 to 20% of hepatomas in various ethnic populations are not AFP producers. It is not yet clear whether these tumors are biologically different. The previously reported geographic variation probably was due to the higher AFP serum concentrations seen more frequently in some parts of the world where hepatoma incidence is high (56). The reason for the geographic variation in AFP serum concentrations is not clear but a number of factors have been thought to be important. A higher frequency of AFP-positive patients were noted among the younger age groups in a number of small studies, and age has been thought to be a significant factor by some authors (104, 105). A similar trend of male hepatoma patients having higher AFP levels more frequently than females has been suggested (14, 39). However, these differences are probably not statistically significant due to the wide variation in sera concentrations in all age groups.

AFP has been thought to reflect the degree of dedifferentiation and malignancy. Indeed, experimentally, AFP has been shown to be synthesized in a higher titer in the faster growing hepatoma cell lines (22, 23) and related to the degree of malignancy and aneuploidy (106, 107). One prospective and objective study in man has suggested a similar general correlation of AFP to the degree of histologic dedifferentiation, size of the tumor, and duration of survival (39). The few patients who survived longer than one year with liver cell carcinoma without treatment, having obviously very slowly growing tumors, had undetectable AFP by CIEP (39). Also, there was a general tendency for the larger tumors to have AFP elevations more frequently (39, 108). However, due to the large variation in both serum AFP concentration and pathologic and histologic appearance, no clinical significance should be inferred by the absolute serum concentration in any individual patient (15, 16, 39).

AFP has been localized by immunoflourescence in histologically malignant liver cells (109). There does not appear to be any reactive synthesis by surrounding normal cells. However, there is great variation in AFP synthesis in different parts of the same tumor in primates (110) and probably in man, similar to the morphologic variation that is characteristic of hepatoma. In addition, little is known of the factors that govern metabolic degradation and clearance of AFP. In view of all these variables, it is not surprising to see the serum concentration, which reflects net synthesis and degradation, to be so variable.

Serial clinical studies have shown that the serum concentration generally tends to stabilize or gradually increase with progression of disease (16, 39, 111). Rarely, dramatic falls in AFP serum concentration have occurred in the terminal period (16, 39), perhaps reflecting necrosis of AFP secreting tumor nodules or repression of synthesis. Despite this variability and the occasional fluctuations of AFP levels, surgical excision or chemotherapy has resulted in a marked drop in serum concentration (74, 111, 112). Persistently elevated levels or rising levels after presumed curative therapy have indicated growth of residual tumor (74). Therefore, measurement of serum concentration before and after presumably curative surgery of small hepatomas or hepatoblastomas can be quite helpful in the management of these patients.

Other Primary Liver Tumors

Although cholangiocarcinoma, a tumor arising from bile ductular epithelium, has been thought to be AFP-negative (8, 12, 15), mixed tumors with hepatocellular elements may be positive. One case of intrahepatic cholangiocarcinoma reported to be positive was diagnosed by percutaneous biopsy but postmortem confirmation could not be obtained (113). We have seen one AFP-positive patient with extrahepatic gall bladder carcinoma, and no hepatic pathology seen at postmorten, with significant AFP elevation of several hundred ng/ml (89). AFP does not appear to be elevated in other primary liver tumors. We have tested several patients with malignant hemangioblastomas and benign hepatic adenoma and lymphoma involving only the liver and found no detectable AFP (89).

Teratoblastoma

Gonadal teratoblastomas and embryonal

Table 2   AFP in Benign and Malignant Liver Disease

Reference	Method[b]	Secondary (Metastatic) Liver Cancer	Other Gastro-intestinal Cancer	Acute Viral Hepatitis	Chronic Active Hepatitis	"Cirrhosis"
		Number of AFP-Positive[a]/Total Patients				
Abelev (23)	REID	3/21	1/26	23/176		1/108
Alpert (43)	REID	2/28		2/56	1/6	0/30
Alpert (89)	ENZ	1/19	1/48	7/54	4/17	1/69
Ruoslahti (103)	RIA	7/79		5/25	2/21	9/61
Chayvialle (51)	RIA	0/13	0/23			
Hirai (52)	RIA	2/8	3/36	14/27	14/35	18/38
Silver (53, 132)	RIA	1/18		6/11	0/5	1/12
Total number		16/186	5/133	80/349	21/84	30/138
of positive[a]/total cases		8.6	3.8	22.9	25	9.4
		% Positive[a]				

[a] Positive = greater than ~ 50 ng/ml.
[b] See Table 1 for assay methods.

carcinomas are generally childhood tumors and about ⅓ have been reported to have significant AFP elevations (10, 90, 91). Rarely, these tumors may occur in adults and even in extragonadal sites and still be AFP-positive (43, 114).

The usefulness of serial serum AFP concentrations has also been demonstrated in evaluating the treatment of teratoblastomas in children (43, 90) and adults (43, 114). Changes in serum concentration have usually reflected the completeness of surgical reaction or chemotherapy. Recurrences have frequently but not invariably been associated with persistent or rising serum concentrations (43, 90, 115).

Liver Metastases

AFP elevations have also been reported in a number of isolated patients with gastrointestinal tract tumors and large liver metastases (15, 116–120). AFP elevations over 50 ng/ml were detected by immunoenzymatic assay (89) in only 2 of 67 patients with gastrointestinal cancer, including 1 of 19 with liver metastases. Only 5 to 10% of patients with metastic liver car-

cinoma have been positive by radioimmunoassay in various parts of the world (23, 52, 53, 103) (see Table 2). The primaries are generally of the stomach, pancreas, and gallbladder; all of embryonal foregut origin. Tumors of the hind gut (colon carcinoma) with liver metastases frequently secrete CEA (21) but only *rarely* AFP. It is interesting that, although the fetal gut can synthesize trace amounts of AFP (60), the distribution of these AFP-secreting cells in the GI tract is not known.

Individual case reports have described patients with carcinoma of the gallbladder (89), bronchogenic carcinoma of the lung with hepatic metastases (53), and without liver metastases (121), to be AFP-positive, but these must be very rare. AFP elevations in these metastatic tumors are uniformly low and only rarely exceed 1000 ng/ml which may be detectable by gel diffusion (15, 52, 53, 89, 103).

AFP and Benign Disease

Serum AFP levels are elevated in a small but significant number of patients with acute and chronic viral hepatitis (see Table

2). In 1967 we noted a patient with viral hepatitis to be AFP-positive but thought it might have been due to an unrecognized coding error in what was a double blind prospective study (12). Subsequently, AFP was reported to be elevated in children with hepatitis (14) and several reports appeared documenting the presence of elevated AFP levels in adults with acute viral hepatitis (122, 123). Approximately 23% of patients with acute viral hepatitis were found to have elevations of AFP detectable in several series by double antibody radioautography (23, 43), radioimmunoassay (52, 124), or immunoenzymatic assay (89) (see Table 2). These elevations were uniformly low, usually less than 500 ng/ml, and were not appreciated in initial studies when the relatively crude technique of gel diffusion was being employed for AFP detection. The elevations in fetoprotein are transient and tend to disappear with resolution of the disease. Several reports have suggested a correlation of AFP with hepatitis B surface antigen (HBsAg) (125–129). Other reports have found no relationship to the presence (130) or titer of HBsAg (124) in other populations. The AFP found in viral hepatitis is immunologically identical to that found in liver carcinoma and fetal sera (43). Quantitively, the AFP titer appears to be highest shortly after the peak of serum glutamic oxalacetic transaminase (SGOT) and clinical jaundice (131, 132). The levels do not seem to have a clear-cut relationship to clinical severity and prognosis in benign viral hepatitis, despite a general correlation to SGOT levels (132). The presence of a high concentration (detectable by agar gel diffusion) of AFP in some patients with massive hepatic necrosis has been reported to be associated with a good prognosis (133). However, elevated AFP serum concentrations occur more frequently in patients with massive hepatic necrosis that is fatal, than in the benign self-limited disease, suggesting a poorer prognosis (43).

Because of the temporal appearance during the course of viral hepatitis, AFP has been thought to be the product of liver regeneration (23, 131, 132). However, it should be noted that similar AFP elevations are not usually found in nonviral hepatitis, despite the similar degree of clinical jaundice and acute hepatic necrosis (43). Patients with massive hepatic necrosis due to *nonviral* toxic agents, drugs, or alcoholic hepatitis only rarely have significant AFP elevations (43, 53, 134). AFP also does not increase with hepatic trauma or infection (74). Therefore, it is unlikely that hepatic necrosis is responsible for significant AFP synthesis. Although, experimentally, rat AFP levels can rise slightly after 70% hepatectomy (23, 75), no such increase has been seen in humans subjected to smaller but significant partial hepatectomies (43). AFP elevations have not been detected during the early postoperative period following partial hepatectomy, when hepatic regeneration is presumably most active. Therefore, it appears unlikely that AFP elevations in hepatitis are simply due to hepatic regeneration; the presence of an additional factor, such as the hepatitis virus is probably required (43). The significance of this association to viral infection is unclear, but may indicate the oncogenic potential of the hepatitis virus, particularly if superimposed on an already compromised liver.

AFP elevations also occur in some patients with *chronic* active hepatitis (see Table 2). Approximately 25% of patients with chronic active hepatitis and less than 10% of patients with established cirrhosis (23, 43, 52, 103, 132) have small but significant AFP elevations, usually less than 500 ng/ml (See Table 2). These levels generally are detectable only by CIEP (43), radioimmunoassay (23, 52), or radioimmunoenzymatic assay (89), and only rarely reach the levels detectable by gel diffusion. Whether these small elevations in chronic hepatitis and cirrhosis represent the effects of occult viral infection or coexistent viral hepatitis is unknown.

It appears that the reappearance of AFP in the serum of patients with benign liver diseases is largely restricted to patients having acute viral or chronic active hepatitis. The serum AFP concentrations in chronic hepatitis and cirrhosis are usually low. Therefore, although there may be overlap of low fetoprotein levels in some patients with benign liver disease, using sensitive techniques, quantitatively significant elevations of over 500 ng/ml are still highly suggestive of malignancy. The significance and relationship of the elevations of AFP to the long-term prognosis in acute and chronic hepatitis is unknown. Recent experimental work indicates that transient AFP synthesis can be induced in rats by carcinogens after a small subcarcinogenic dose (135). Small amounts of naturally occurring carcinogens and hepatotoxins are ingested by man, particularly in some parts of the world. The transient induction of AFP synthesis by the hepatitis virus in man may indicate an additional, perhaps additive, type of potentially premalignant hepatotoxicity.

REFERENCES

1. Pedersen K: Fetuin, a new globulin isolated from serum. *Nature (London)* **154**:575, 1944.
2. Bergstrand CG, Czar B: Demonstration of a new protein fraction in serum from the human fetus. *Scand J Clin Lab Invest* **8**:174, 1956.
3. Bergstrand CG, Czar B: Paper electrophoretic study of human fetal serum proteins with demonstration of a new protein fraction. *Scand J Clin Lab Invest* **9**:277–286, 1957.
4. Gitlin D, Boesman M: Fetus specific serum proteins in several mammals and their relation to human alpha-fetoprotein. *Comp Biochem Physiol* **21**:327–336, 1967.
5. Gitlin D, Kitzes J: Synthesis of serum albumin, embryo-specific α-globulin and conalbumin by chick yolk sac. *Biochem Biophys Acta* **147**:234, 1967.
6. Gitlin D: Personal communication.
7. Kithier D, Masopust J, Radl J: Fetal alpha-globulin of bovine serum differing from fetuin. *Biochim Biophys Acta (Amsterdam)* **160**:135–137, 1968.
8. Abelev GI, Perova S, Khramkova NI, et al: Production of embryonal alpha-globulin by the transplantable mouse hepatomas. *Transplant Bull* **1**:174–180, 1963.
9. Tatarinov YS: Detection of embryospecific alpha-globulin in the blood sera of patients with primary liver tumour. *Vopr Med Khim* **10**:90–91, 1964.
10. Abelev GL, Assecritova IV, Kraevsky NA, et al: Embryonal serum alpha-globulin in cancer patients: diagnostic value. *Int J Cancer* **2**:551–558, 1967.
11. Uriel J, de Nechaud B, Stanislawski-Birencwajg M, et al: Le diagnostic du cancer primaire de foie par des me(thodes immunologiques. *Presse Me+d* **76**:1415–1416, 1968.
12. Alpert E, Uriel J, de Nechaud B: Alpha-1-fetoprotein in the diagnosis of human hepatoma. *New Engl J Med* **278**:984–986, 1968.
13. Masseyeff R, Sankale M, Onde M, et al: Valeur de la recherche de l'alpha-l-foetoproteine serique pour lediagnostic du cancer primitif du foie. *Bull Soc Me(d Afr Noire Langue Fr* **13**:537–548, 1968.
14. Masopust J, Kithier R, Radl J, et al: Occurrence of fetoprotein in patients with neoplasms and non-neoplastic diseases. *Int J Cancer* **3**:364–373, 1968.
15. O'Conor GT, Tatarinov YS, Abelev GI, et al: A collaborative study for the evaluation of a serologic test for primary liver cancer. *Cancer (Philadelphia)* **25**:1091–1098, 1970.
16. Purves LR, Bersohn I, Geddes EW: Serum alpha-fetoprotein and primary cancer of the liver in man. *Cancer (Philadelphia)* **25**:1261–1270, 1970.
17. Criss WE: A review of isozymes in cancer. *Cancer Res* **31**:1523–1542, 1971.
18. Moscona AA: Embryonic and neoplastic cell surfaces: availability of receptors for concanavalin A and wheat germ agglutinin. *Science* **171**:905–907, 1971.
19. Gold P, Freedman SO: Demonstration of tumor-specific antigens in human colonic carcinomata by immunological tolerance and absorption techniques. *J Exp Med* **121**:439–459, 1965.
20. Gold P, Freedman SO: Specific carcino embryonic antigens of the human digestive system. *J Exp Med* **122**:467–481, 1965.
21. Thomson DMP, Krupey J, Freedman SO, et al: The radioimmunoassay of circulating carcin-

oembryonic antigen of the human digestive system. *Proc Natl Acad Sci USA* **64**:161–167, 1969.

22. Abelev GI: Production of embryonal serum alpha-globulin by hepatomas: review of experimental and clinical data. *Cancer Res* **28**:1344–1350, 1968.

23. Abelev GI: Alpha-fetoprotein in ontogenesis and its association with malignant tumors. *Adv Cancer Res* **14**:295–357, 1971.

24. Sell S, Wepsic HT: Alpha fetoprotein. In *The Liver—The Molecular Biology of Its Diseases*. Becker F (Ed). Marcel Dekker Inc., New York, 1974.

25. Gitlin D, Boesman M: Serum alpha-fetoprotein albumin and globulin in the human conceptus. *J Clin Invest* **45**:1826–1838, 1966.

26. Purves LR, Rolle M, Bersohn I: Serum alpha-fetoprotein. III. Electrophoresis of sera from cases of primary cancer of the liver. An electrophoretic variant. *S Afr Med J* **43**:1194–1196, 1969.

27. Alpert E, Schur P, Drysdale J, et al: Human alpha-1-fetoprotein: purification and physical properties. *Fed Proc* **30**:246, 1971.

28. Alpert E, Drysdale JW, Isselbacher KJ, et al: Human α-fetoprotein: Isolation, characterization, and demonstration of microheterogeneity. *J Biol Chem* **247**:3792–3798, 1972.

29. Goussev A, Jasova AK: Isolation and purification of embryo specific alpha globulins of the human animals employing preparative disc electrophoresis in polyacrylamide gels. *Biochim USSR* **35**:172–181, 1970.

30. Nishi S: Isolation and characterization of a human fetal alpha-1-globulin from the sera of fetuses and a hepatoma patient. *Cancer Res* **30**:2507–2513, 1970.

31. Ruoslahti E, Seppala M: Studies of carcino-fetal proteins. Physical and chemical properties of human alpha-fetoprotein. *Int J Cancer* **7**:218–225, 1971.

32. Masopust J, Tomasova H, Kotal L: Some physicochemical characteristics of human alpha-1-fetoprotein. *Protides Biol Fluids* **18**:37–42, 1970.

33. Purves LR, Van der Merwe E, Bersohn I: Serum alpha-fetoprotein. V. The bulk preparation and some properties of alpha-fetoprotein obtained from patients with primary cancer of the liver. *S Afr Med J* **44**:1264–1268, 1970.

34. Lehmann FG, Lehmann D, Martini GA: Alpha-1-Fetoprotein Isolierung und Kristallisation aus menschlichen Plasma. *Clin Chim Acta* **33**:197–206, 1971.

35. Alpert E, Drysdale JW, Isselbacher KH: Isoelectric focusing of human α-fetoprotein: an aid in purification and characterization of microheter-

ogeneity. *Ann N Y Acad Sci* **209**:387–396, 1973.

36. Purves LR, Van der Merwe E, Bersohn I: Variants of alpha-fetoprotein. *Lancet* **2**:464–465, 1970.

37. Adinolfi fi, Adinolfi fi, Cohen S: Isolation and characterization of human foetal α-globulin (α₁F) from foetal and hepatoma sera. *Biochim Biophys Acta* **251**:197–207, 1971.

38. Ruoslahti E, Seppala M, Pihko H, et al: Studies of carcino-fetal proteins. II. Biochemical comparisons of alpha-fetoprotein from human fetuses and patients with hepato-cellular cancer. *Int J Cancer* **8**:283–288, 1971.

39. Alpert E, Hershberg R, Schur PH, et al: Alpha fetoprotein in human hepatoma: improved detection in serum and quantitative studies using a new sensitive technique. *Gastroenterology* **61**:137–143, 1971.

40. Sizaret PP, McIntire R, Princler GL: Quantitation of human α-fetoprotein by electroimmunodiffusion. *Cancer Res* **31**:1899–1902, 1971.

41. Alpert E, Coston RL: Evaluation of a rapid latex-agglutination test for detection of α₁-fetoprotein. *Clin Chem* **19**:1069–1070, 1973.

42. Mody NJ, Vogel CL, Patel IR, et al: Rivanol precipitation technique for the detection of α-fetoprotein. *J Lab Clin Med* **80**:125–133, 1972.

43. Alpert E: Alpha-1-fetoprotein: serologic marker of human hepatoma and embryonal carcinoma. *Natl Cancer Inst Monogr* **35**:415–420, 1972.

44. Alpert E, Coston R, Perrotto J: Immunoenzymatic assay for alpha-fetoprotein. *Lancet* **1**:626, 1974.

45. Belanger L, Sylvestre C, Dufour D: Enzyme-linked immunoassay for alpha-fetoprotein by competitive and sandwich procedures. *Clin Chim Acta* **48**:15–18, 1973.

46. Simons MJ: Australia antigen detection by radio electrocomplexing. *Bull WHO* (in press).

47. Purves LR, Geddes EW: A more sensitive test for alpha-fetoprotein. *Lancet* **1**:47–48, 1972.

48. Ruoslahti E, Seppala M: Studies of Carcino-fetal proteins. III. Development of a radioimmunoassay for α-fetoprotein. Demonstration of α-fetoprotein in serum of healthy human adults. *Int J Cancer* **8**:374–383, 1971.

49. Rouslahti E, Seppala M: α-foetoprotein in normal human serum. *Nature* **235**:461–462, 1972.

50. Purves LR, Purves M: Serum alpha-fetoprotein. VI. The radio-immunoassay evidence for the presence of AFP in the serum of normal people during pregnancy. *S Afr Med J* **46**:1290–1297, 1972.

51. Chayvialle JAP, Ganguli PC: Radioimmunoassay of alpha-fetoprotein in human plasma. *Lancet* **1**:1355–1357, 1973.

52. Hirai H, Nishi S, Watabe H: Radioimmunoassay of α-fetoprotein. *Protides Biol Fluida* **20**:579–587, 1973.

53. Silver HKB, Gold P, Feder S, et al: Radioimmunoassay for human alpha-1 fetoprotein. *Proc Nat Acad Sci USA* **70**:526–530, 1973.

54. Berson SA, Yalow RS: Principles of immunoassay of peptide hormones. In *Plasma. Clin End*, Vol 2. Astwood EB, et al (Eds). Grune & Stratton, New York, 1968.

55. Ruoslahti E, Pihko H, Vaheri A, et al: α-Fetoprotein, structure and expression in man and in inbred mouse strains under normal conditions and liver injury. In *Proceedings of the Seventh Miles Symposium*. The Johns Hopkins Institute, Baltimore, Md., (in press).

56. Purves LR, Branch WR, Geddes EW, et al: Serum alpha-feto-protein VII. The range of apparent serum values in normal people, pregnant women, and primary liver cancer high risk populations. *Cancer* **31**:578–587, 1973.

57. Gitlin D, Boesman M: Sites of serum alpha-fetoprotein synthesis in the human and in the rat. *J Clin Invest* **46**:1010–1016, 1967.

58. Linder E, Seppala M: Localization of the alpha-fetoprotein in the human fetus and placenta. *Acta Pathol Microbiol Scand* **73**:565–571, 1968.

59. Englehardt NV, Shipova LV, Goussev AI, et al: Immunohistochemical detection of alpha-fetoglobulin on sections of the liver of human embryo and newborn mice. *Bull Exp Biol Med* **12**:62–66, 1969.

60. Gitlin D, Perricelli A, Gitlin GM: Synthesis of alpha-fetoprotein by liver, yolk sac, and gastrointestinal tract of the human conceptus. *Cancer Res* **32**:979–982, 1972.

61. Gitlin D, Perricelli A: Synthesis of serum albumin, prealbumin, foetoprotein, α_1-antitrypsin and transferrin by the human yolk sac. *Nature* **228**:995–997, 1970.

62. Kekomaki M, Seppala M, Ehnholm C, et al: Perfusion of isolated human fetal liver: Synthesis and release of alpha-fetoprotein and albumin. *Int J Cancer* **8**:250–258, 1971.

63. Gitlin D, Kumate J, Morales C, et al: The turnover of amniotic fluid protein in the human conceptus. *Am J Obstet Gynecol* **113**:632–645, 1972.

64. Seppala M, Ruoslahti E: Alpha-fetoprotein in amniotic fluid: An index of gestational age. *Am J Obstet Gynecol* **114**:595–598, 1972.

65. Brock DJH, Sutcliffe RG: Alpha-fetoprotein in the antenatal diagnosis of anencephaly and spina bifida. *Lancet* **2**:197–199, 1972.

66. Milunsky A, Alpert E: The value of alpha-fetoprotein in the prenatal diagnosis of neural tube defects. *J Pediatr* **84**:889–893, 1974.

67. Purves LR, Branch WR, Boes WGM: Alpha-fetoprotein as a diagnostic aid. *Lancet* **1**:1007, 1973.

68. Uriel J, deNechaud B, Dupiers M: Estrogen-binding properties of rat, mouse and man fetospecific serum proteins. Demonstration by immunoautoradiographic methods. *Biochem Biophys Res Com* **46**:1175–1180, 1972.

69. Nunez E, Vallette G, Benassayag C, et al: Comparative study on the binding of estrogens by human and rat serum proteins in development. *Biochem Biophys Res Com* **57**:126–133, 1974.

70. Uriel J, Aussel C, Bouillon D, et al: Localization of rat liver alpha-fetoprotein by cell affinity labelling with tritiated oestrogens. *Nature* **244**:190–192, 1973.

71. Puck TT, Waldren CA, Jones C: Mammalian cell growth proteins. I. Growth stimulation by fetuin. *Proc Natl Acad Sci USA* **59**:192, 1968.

72. Jones C, Puck TT, Waldren C, et al: Mammalian cell growth proteins. *J Cell Biol* **39**:69A, 1968.

73. Alpert E, Talamo RC: Unpublished data.

74. Alpert E, Starzl TE, Schur PH, et al: Serum alpha-fetoprotein in hepatoma patients after liver transplantation. *Gastroenterology* **61**:144–148, 1971.

75. Perova SD, Elgort DA, Abelev GI: Alpha-fetoprotein in the sera of rats after partial hepatectomy. *Bull Eksp Biol Med* **71(3)**:45–47, 1971.

76. de Nechaud B, Uriel J: Antigenes allulaires transitoires du foie de rat. I. Secretions et synthese des proteines seriques foeto-specifiques au cours du developpement et de la regeneration hepatique. *Int J Cancer* **8**:71–80, 1971.

77. Seppala M, Ruoslahti E: Radioimmunoassay of maternal serum alphafetoprotein during pregnancy and delivery. *Am J Obstet Bynecol* **112**:208–212, 1972.

78. Nishi S, Watabe H, Hirai H: Production of antibody to homologous alpha-fetoprotein in rabbits, rats and horses by immunization with human alpha-fetoprotein. *J Immunol* **109**:957–960, 1972.

79. Seppala M, Ruoslahti E: Alpha-fetoprotein in maternal serum: A new marker for detection of fetal distress and intrauterine death. *Am J Obstet Gynecol* **115**:48–52, 1973.

80. Cohen H, Graham H, Lau HL: Alpha-1-

fetoprotein in pregnancy. *Am J Obstet Gynecol* **115**:881–883, 1973.

81. Seppala M, Ruoslahti E: Alpha-fetoprotein in abortion. *Brit Med J* **2**:769–770, 1972.

82. Milunsky A, Alpert E, Charles D: Amniotic fluid alpha-fetoprotein in anencephaly. *Obstet Gynecol* **43**:592–594, 1974.

83. Brock DJH, Sutcliffe RG: Alpha-fetoprotein in the antenatal diagnosis of anencephaly and spina bifida. *Lancet* **2**:197–199, 1972.

84. Editorial: Towards the prevention of spina bifida. *Lancet* **1**:907, 1974.

85. Seppala M: Increased alpha-fetoprotein in amniotic fluid associated with a congenital esophageal atresia of the fetus. *Obstet Gynecol* **42**:613–614, 1973.

86. Masopust J, Kithier K, Radl J, et al: Occurrence of fetoprotein in patients with neoplasms and non-neoplastic diseases. *Int J Cancer* **3**:364–373, 1968.

87. Kang K-Y, Higashino K, Takahashi Y, et al: Alpha-fetoprotein in infantile diseases. *Clin Chim Acta* **42**:175–180, 1972.

88. Zeltzer PM, Neerhout RC, Fonkalsrud EW, et al: Differentiation between neonatal hepatitis and biliary atresia by measuring serum alpha-fetoprotein. *Lancet* **1**:373–375, 1974.

89. Alpert E: Serum alpha-fetoprotein (AFP) in benign and malignant gastrointestinal diseases: Evaluation of an immuno-enzymatic assay. *Clin Chim Acta,* (in press).

90. Mawas C, Kohen M, Lemerle J, et al: Serum alpha-1-fetoprotein in children with malignant ovarian or testicular teratomas. Preliminary results. *Int J Cancer* **4**:76–79, 1969.

91. Kohn J, Weaver PC: Serum alpha-fetoprotein in hepatocellular carcinoma. *Lancet* **2**:334–337, 1974.

92. Wilkinson EJ, Friedrich EG, Hosty TA: Alpha-fetoprotein and endodermal sinus tumor of the ovary. *Am J Obstet Gynecol* **116**:711–714, 1973.

93. Teilum G, Albrechtsen R, Norgaard-Pedersen B: Immunofluorescent localization of alpha-fetoprotein synthesis in endodermal sinus tumor (yolk sac tumor). *Acta Pathol Microbiol Scand* **82**:586–588, 1974.

94. Waldmann TA, McIntire KR: Serum-alpha-fetoprotein levels in patients with ataxia-telangiectasia. *Lancet* **2**:1112–1115, 1972.

95. Belanger L, Belanger M, Larochelle J: Existence d'α-foeto-proteine circulate chez 8 patients souffrant de tyrosinenie hereditaire. *Union Med.* **101**:877–878, 1972.

96. Belanger, L: personal communication.

97. Scriver CR, Rosenberg LE, "Tyrosine." In *Amino Acid Metabolism and Its Disorders.* Scriver, Rosenberg (Eds). W. B. Saunders Co., 1973.

98. Nayak NC, Malaviya AN, Chawla V, et al: Alpha-fetoprotein in Indian childhood cirrhosis. *Lancet* **1**:68–69, 1972.

99. Agarwal SS, Mehta SK, Bajpai PC: Alpha-fetoprotein in Indian childhood cirrhosis. *Lancet* **2**:175–176, 1974.

100. Alpert ME: Alpha-1-fetoprotein in hepatoma. *Clin Res* **17**:461, 1969.

101. Purves LR, Macnab M, Bersohn I: Foetoglobin and primary liver cancer. *Lancet* **2**:634, 1968.

102. Purves LR, Bersohn I, Geddes EW, et al: Serum alpha-fetoprotein. IV. Effects of chemotherapy and radiotherapy on serum alpha-fetoprotein levels in cases of primary liver cancer. *S Afr J Med Sci* **44**:590–594, 1970.

103. Ruoslahti E, Salaspuro M, Pihko H, et al: Serum alpha-fetoprotein: Diagnostic significance in liver disease. *Brit Med J* **2**:527–529, 1974.

104. Mawas C, Buffe D, Burtin P: Influence of age on alpha-fetoprotein incidence. *Lancet* **1**:1292, 1970.

105. Baghshawe A, Parker AM: Age distribution of alpha-fetoprotein in hepato-cellular carcinoma. *Lancet* **2**:268, 1970.

106. Becker FF, Klein KM, Wolman SR, et al: Characterization of primary hepatocellular carcinomas and initial transplant generations. *Cancer Res* **33**:3330–3338, 1973.

107. Sell S, Morris HP: Relationship of rat alpha-1-fetoprotein to growth rate and chromosome composition of Morris hepatomas. *Cancer Res* **34**:1413–1417, 1984.

108. Masseyeff R, Basteris B, Leblanc L: Use of the alpha-fetoprotein test for the diagnosis of primary liver cancer. *Protides Biol Fluids* **18**:217–220, 1970.

109. Engelhardt NV, Goussev AI, Shipove J Jr, et al: Immunofluorescent study of alpha-fetoprotein in liver and liver tumours. I. Technique of localization in tissue sections. *Int J Cancer* **7**:198–206, 1971.

110. Hull E, Carbone P, Gitlin D, et al: Alpha-fetoprotein in monkeys with hepatoma. *J Natl Cancer Inst* **42**:1035–1044, 1969.

111. McIntire RK, Vogel CL, Princler GL, et al: Serum alpha-fetoprotein, a biochemical marker for hepatocellular carcinoma. *Cancer Res* **32**:1941–1946, 1972.

112. Purves LR, Bersohn I, Geddes EW, et al: Serum alpha-fetoprotein. IV. Effects of chemotherapy and radiotherapy on serum alpha-fetoprotein

levels in cases of primary liver cancer. *S Afr Med Sci* **44**:590–594, 1970.

113. Villeneuve JP, Richer G, Cote J, et al: Alpha fetoprotein and cholangiocellular carcinoma. *New Engl J Med* **290**:1260, 1974.

114. Mawas C, Buffe D, Schiversynth P, et al: Alpha-1-fetoprotein and children's cancer. *Rev Eur Clin Biol* **16**:430–435, 1971.

115. Esterhay RJ Jr, Shapiro HM, Sutherland JC, et al: Serum alpha-fetoprotein concentration and tumor growth dissociation in a patient with ovarian teratocarcinoma. *Cancer* **31**:835–839, 1973.

116. Bourreille J, Metager P, Sanger F, et al: Existence d'α-foeto-proteine au cones d'un canccer secondaire du foie d'origine gastrique. *Presse Med* **78**:1277–1278, 1970.

117. Alpert E, Pinn VW, Isselbacher KJ: Alpha-fetoprotein in a patient with gastric carcinoma metastatic to the liver. *New Engl J Med* **285**:1058–1059, 1971.

118. Mehlman DJ, Bulkley BH, Wiernik PH: Serum alpha-fetoglobulin with gastric and prostatic carcinoma. *New Engl J Med* **285**:1059–1060, 1971.

119. Kozower M, Fawaz KA, Miller HM, et al: Positive alpha-fetoprotein in a case of gastric carcinoma. *New Engl J Med* **285**:1060–1061, 1971.

120. Geoffrey Y, Melazer P, Dennis P: α-foeto-proteine et cancer secondaire du foie. *Presse Med* **78**:1896, 1970.

121. Corlin RF, Tompkins RK: Serum alpha-1-fetoglobulin in a patient with hepatic metastases from bronchogenic carcinoma. *Dig Dis* **17**:553–555, 1972.

122. Goeffrey Y, Dennis P, Colon R, et al: Presence d'α-1-foeto-proteine chez l'adulte au cours d'une hepatite virale traitee par cortitherapie. *Presse Med* **78**:1107–1108, 1970.

123. Smith JH: Occurrence of alpha-fetoprotein in acute viral hepatitis. *J Cancer* **8**:421–424, 1971.

124. Ruoslahti E, Seppala M, Rasanen JA, et al: Alpha-fetoprotein and hepatitis B. Antigens in acute hepatitis and primary cancer of the liver. *Scand J Gastroenterol* **8**:1–6, 1973.

125. Smith JB, Blumberg BS: Viral hepatitis postnecrotic cirrhosis and hepatocellular carcinoma. *Lancet* **2**:953, 1969.

126. Vogel GL, Mody N, Anthony PP, ET AL: Hepatitis-associated antigen in Ugandan patients with hepatocellular carcinoma. *Lancet* **2**:621–624, 1970.

127. Hersh T, Hollinger FB, Goyal RK, et al: Australian antigen and antibody and alpha-fetoglobulin in hepatoma patients. *Int J Cancer* **8**:259–263, 1971.

128. Denison EK, Peters RL, Reynolds TB: Familial hepatoma with hepatitis-associated antigen. *Ann Intern Med* **74**:391–394, 1970.

129. Smith JB: Occurrence of alpha-fetoprotein in acute viral hepatitis. *Int J Cancer* **8**:421–424, 1971.

130. Alpert E, Isselbacher KJ: Hepatitis-associated antigen and hepatoma in the U.S. *Lancet* **2**:1087, 1971.

131. Smith JB, Barker LF: Alpha-1-fetoprotein and liver-specific antigen in viral hepatitis type B. *Arch Intern Med* **133**:437–439, 1974.

132. Silver KHB, Deneault J, Gold P, et al: The detection of alpha-1-fetoprotein in patients with viral hepatitis. *Cancer Res* **34**:244–247, 1974.

133. Karvountzis GG, Redeker AG: Relation of alpha-fetoprotein in acute hepatitis to severity and prognosis. *Ann Intern Med* **80**: 156–160, 1974.

134. Meshkinpour H, Wepsic HT, Schmalhorst WR: Alpha-1-fetoprotein and alcoholic hepatitis. *Dig Dis* **19**:709–713, 1974.

135. Becker FF, Sell S: Early elevation of alpha-1-fetoprotein in *N*-2-fluorenylacetamide hepatocarcinogenesis. *Cancer Res*, (in press).

CHAPTER 16 LIPID METABOLISM IN PATIENTS WITH HEPATOCELLULAR CARCINOMA

EIJI ARAKI, M.D.
NOBUO OKAZAKI, M.D.

Considerable evidence has accumulated for certain metabolic abnormalities related to the so-called paraneoplastic syndrome (1) in human hepatocellular carcinoma (HCC). However, abnormalities of lipid metabolism in HCC have received very little attention in the past, perhaps because of the difficulty in providing clear evidence for or against its existence. With the advent of techniques for separating and quantitating various lipids, studies of the character of lipid metabolism in patients with HCC have become feasible (2). This review characterizes several types of disturbance in lipid metabolism that may develop as systemic manifestations of HCC beyond the abnormalities that may be associated with cancer in general or with underlying cirrhosis.

ABNORMALITIES IN SERUM LIPIDS OF PATIENTS WITH HCC

Serum lipids of tumor-bearing animals or of cancer patients have been studied extensively (3–7) because of ready availability of material, but only few relationships of malignancy to lipids have been characterized.

Hyperlipidemia

Varying degrees of hyperlipidemia associated with cancer are a rather constant finding, as shown not only in humans with cancer (8, 9), but also in animals with Jensen sarcoma (3) or Walker carcinosarcoma 256 (4, 10–13). Viallet et al (14) noted a serum total lipid of 3720 mg/100 ml in a patient with HCC, of which cholesterol comprised approximately 19%. Santer et al (15) described a patient with HCC who also had underlying cirrhosis and who presented with erythrocytosis and hyperlipidemia. The latter authors proposed that the elevated total lipid levels resulted from the presence of an abnormal lipoprotein with a "pre-β" mobility. Their study has been the only one on lipoprotein profile

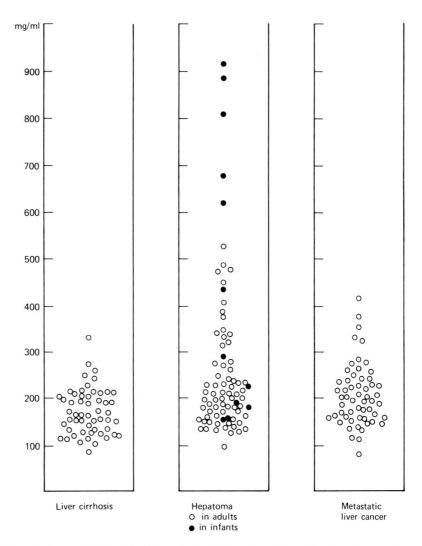

Figure 1 Serum cholesterol levels in patients with hepatoma, liver cirrhosis, and metastatic liver cancer. The solid circles represent cases of infant hepatoma.

in humans with HCC and hyperlipidemia. Although in earlier studies lipidemia had been attributed either to increased mobilization of free fatty acids for energy production (16–18) or to impaired clearing activity (19, 20), in patients with HCC, hyperlipidemias may also be produced by a different mechanisms. There is good evidence that some lipoproteins are produced by hepatoma tissue as discussed below.

Hypercholesterolemia

Elevation of serum cholesterol levels during tumor growth has been reported to occur in animals with Ehrlich ascites tumor

and other animal tumors (4, 8, 21). Human HCC is also often associated with an increased concentration of cholesterol in serum. Alpert et al (22) noted a significant elevation of serum cholesterol levels in one-third of 46 patients with HCC in Uganda. Okazaki and co-workers (23) at National Cancer Center Hospital, Tokyo, examined the association between hepatoma and hypercholesterolemia and found serum cholesterol levels in excess of 350 mg/100 ml in 14% and between 349 and 250 mg/100 ml in 32% of 50 cases of HCC (Fig. 1).

Hypercholesterolemia was also a dominant feature in 5 out of 10 infants with

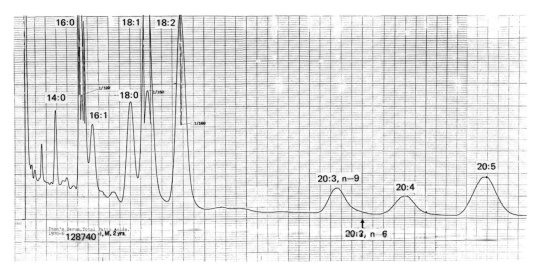

Figure 2 Gas-liquid chromatogram of serum fatty acids obtained from an infant with hepatocellular carcinoma (1 year-old male, #128740, National Cancer Center Hospital, Tokyo). Increased percentage composition of 5,8,11-eicosatrienoic acid is observed (the peak marked with an arrow).

hepatoblastoma from the same hospital (24). Tumor tissue resected during surgery from one infant with hypercholesterolemia (cholesterol 618 mg/100 ml) was analyzed for lipids, and a high concentration of cholesterol was found by silicic acid column chromatography (25). According to Hanawa (24), serum cholesterol level is of considerable diagnostic significance in the follow-up of hepatoma cases because the levels in serum fluctuate in parallel with the tumor size, decreasing after resection and increasing again with recurrence of the hepatoma. Simultaneous development of hypercholesterolemia and osteoporosis has been described in a 10-year-old boy with hepatoma (26). Viallet et al (14) reported hypercholesterolemia (approximately 700 mg/100 ml) in a patient with cholangiocarcinoma without underlying cirrhosis.

Phospholipids in Serum

Phospholipid levels of the serum have been reported to increase by a maximum of 30% in chickens with Rous sarcoma (27). Lee (28), in studying the serum lipids of patients with malignancy in Hong Kong, found high concentrations of choline-containing phospholipids, particularly in the serum of patients with carcinomas of the liver and of the head of the pancreas. We have no such experience of hyperphospholipidemia in HCC as yet.

Fatty Acid Composition of Serum

Accumulated evidence indicates that changes in fatty acid composition of serum in various diseases are generally only quantitative. An exception includes Refsum's disease in which unusual fatty acid, 3, 7, 11-tetramethyl hexadecanoic acid is detected in serum. However, in 1965 Collins and Connelly (29) found an unusual fatty acid in blood plasma, liver, and in HCC tissue of an 8-year-old girl with hypercholesterolemia. They identified this acid as 5,8,11-eicosatrienoic acid by gas-liquid chromatography from the relative retention time of its methyl ester in comparison with those obtained from various tissues. Independent of their investigation, we found an unphysiological isomer of eicosatrienoic acid in serum of an infant with hepatoblastoma during our survey analyses of serum fatty acids in malignancy (Fig. 2). This prompted us to study the serum fatty acids obtained from subjects under various nutritional and pathological conditions. This fatty acid was later fully identified as

Table 1   Serum Fatty Acid Composition in Patients with Hepatocellular Carcinoma, Metastatic Carcinoma, and Liver Cirrhosis

	Fatty Acids (%)										
	14:0	16:0	16:1	18:0	18:1	18:2	18:3	20:2	20:3ω9	20:3ω6	20:4
HCC 20:3, n-9 + (9)	1.2 ±0.8	28.6 ±3.9	6.4 ±0.3	7.0 ±1.6	27.1 ±3.9	21.6 ±4.1	0.9 ±0.3	0.6 ±0.4	0.4 ±0.3	1.0 ±1.0	5.0
HCC 20:3, n-9 − (15)	1.7 ±1.1	30.9 ±3.6	6.8 ±2.0	8.1 ±2.0	28.1 ±3.4	18.9 ±3.8	1.0 ±0.7	0.2^b ±0.1		0.6^a ±0.3	3.7^b ±1.4
Metastatic (14)	1.2 ±0.7	28.3 ±4.7	5.0^a ±1.8	7.6 ±1.0	27.2 ±4.2	24.6 ±4.0	0.7 ±0.1	0.2^b ±0.3		1.0 ±0.4	4.2 ±1.6
Cirrhosis (10)	1.8^a ±0.3	28.1 ±4.4	8.3^b ±1.5	7.7 ±1.6	26.4 ±4.1	22.0 ±3.0	0.5^a ±0.4	0.3 ±0.3		1.0 ±0.5	4.1 ±0.4

$^a p < 0.01.$
$^b p < 0.05.$

5,8,11-eicosatrienoic acid (20:3, n-9) by mass spectrometry of its trimethylsilyloxy derivative (30). The abnormal fatty acid was found in sera of 9 of 24 (37.5%) patients with HCC. None of 14 patients with metastatic carcinoma had detectable levels of the abnormal fatty acid and similarly none of 10 patients with cirrhosis. Of 105 normal individuals, none had the abnormal isomer. In our material, this fatty acid was only detected in patients with HCC who had alpha fetoprotein (AFP) in their sera (9 out of 19 cases or 47.4%) and was not detectable in the patients who had no detectable AFP (0 in 5 cases). The mean value of 20:3, n-9 in the positive group was 0.4% (Table 1).

This fatty acid, 20:3, n-9, has been known to occur, however, in the serum lipids of patients being maintained by prolonged intravenous hyperalimentation with a fat free preparation (31). There was no indication of systemic deficiency of essential fatty acids in the patients in whom this unphysiological fatty acid was detected. In the group positive for this fatty acid, the percentages of fatty acids of the linoleate family (18:2, 20:3, n-6, and 20:4) were somewhat higher than in the patients with HCC who lacked the abnormal fatty acid. No differences in the levels of essential fatty acids were observed between the fatty acid composition of serum of 20:3, n-9 positive hepatoma cases and those of metastatic liver carcinoma or of liver cirrhosis. In Table 2 the analytical results of several tissues of an autopsy case of hepatoma are summarized. Eicosatrienoic acid, n-9, was observed in the primary tumor, metastatic tumors and also in the serum. The fatty acid compositions of the primary liver cell carcinoma and of its metastatic tumor to the lung showed an almost identical composition. Furthermore, we found the presence of this fatty acid, 20:3, n-9, in the fetal liver before the middle of three months of gestation (32) and a close resemblance of fatty acid components in fetal liv-

Table 2 Composition of Total Fatty Acids from Tissues of a Patient with Hepatocellular Carcinoma

Organs	Fatty Acids (%)									
	14:0	16:0	16:1	18:0	18:1	18:2	20:3ω9	20:3ω6	20:4	Others
Primary tumor	1.2	22.6	8.1	9.2	38.3	11.3	0.3	0.9	6.0	2.1
Metastatic tumor	1.5	22.8	9.1	7.8	40.3	10.5	0.3	0.7	4.6	2.4
Serum	2.0	26.6	6.1	9.1	31.1	17.0	0.4	0.7	5.5	1.5
Cirrhotic liver	1.0	26.4	4.3	15.9	24.4	18.9	–	0.8	7.3	1.0
Lung	1.4	33.5	6.7	12.5	28.4	8.0	–	1.0	6.4	2.1
Spleen	0.6	25.0	4.8	15.5	25.3	10.3	–	2.0	14.0	2.5
Kidney	0.3	21.7	3.9	13.4	31.8	15.0	–	1.3	11.5	1.1
Heart muscle	2.3	17.3	4.3	10.8	31.2	21.5		0.8	10.3	1.0
Skeletal muscle	1.7	21.1	5.8	7.3	43.2	13.0	–	0.8	4.8	2.3
Adipose tissue	2.5	18.2	8.1	4.3	42.8	18.5	–	0.2	1.6	3.8
Pancreas	2.5	22.7	7.4	7.8	40.4	13.0	–	0.4	3.3	2.5
Intestine	1.6	18.2	6.3	7.8	43.3	15.7	–	0.5	3.9	2.7

er to those of infant hepatoblastoma (33). Although there has been no direct evidence to show the synthesis of this fatty acid by hepatoma tissue, the peculiar distribution pattern in the organs and serum and the fatty acid composition of fetal type strongly suggest an altered metabolism of fatty acids in hepatoma tissue.

Serum Lipoproteins

Early investigations in the field of serum lipoproteins (34) have demonstrated that in sera of patients with cancer, low-density lipoproteins increased and high-density lipoproteins decreased. A significant decrease in serum high-density lipoproteins (HDL2) has also been demonstrated in rats bearing a mammary tumor induced by 9,10-dimethyl-1,2-benzanthracene (35), in rats with Walker carcinosarcoma 256 (35), and in mice with Ehrlich ascites tumor (36). However, a striking increase in serum lipoproteins, particularly in high-density lipoproteins during N-2-fluorenylacetamide-induced hepatic carcinogenesis, has been found (37). From these results it might be speculated that the differences in serum lipoprotein profile in those malignancies depend on whether the carcinomas are hepatocellular; some hepatocellular carcinomas seem to have a capacity to synthesize high-density lipoproteins, while other tumors such as Ehrlich ascites tumor and Walker carcinosarcoma 256 do not. Abnormalities of individual serum lipid classes in patients with HCC suggest qualitative alterations in lipoproteins. In fact, marked deviations from normal have been observed in some lipoprotein fractions of the blood of hepatocellular tumor-bearing animals. Narayan and co-workers (36) found that some unusual high-density lipoprotein fractions, which had been detected in rats during chemical carcinogenesis with N-2-fluorenylacetamide (38), were also significantly elevated in the rats transplanted with Morris hepatoma 7777. In addition, analysis of the composition of lipid moiety of lipoproteins has demonstrated that the very low-density lipoprotein fraction of rats with Walker carcinosarcoma contained greater amounts of phosphatidylcholine, sphingomyelin, and triglyceride than found in sera of normal rats (35). Of particular interest in this regard are the analyses of the serum lipoproteins in patients with HCC.

LIPID COMPOSITION OF HEPATOCELLULAR CARCINOMA TISSUE

Many investigations on tumor lipids have

followed the first contribution of Bullock and Cramer (39); moreover, the work in this field up to 1956 was thoroughly reviewed by Haven and Bloor (18). Much interest has since been aroused in the possible role of lipids in the abnormal surface properties exhibited by malignant cells as well as in the alteration in enzymatic activities in which specific lipids act as co-factors.

The authors initiated a study of lipids in human hepatoma tissue in 1964 in order to determine the quantitative and qualitative differences between the lipids of hepatoma and liver tissue (40).

The general lipid composition in a whole homogenate from human HCC was studied with silicic acid column chromatography in comparison with that of normal liver (41, 42). The total lipids of each tissue was separated quantitatively into neutral lipid, glycolipid, and phospholipid fractions. These fractions were analyzed by thin-layer chromatography and their fatty acid moieties were converted to methyl esters for gas-liquid chromatographic analyses. When compared with normal liver tissue, the total amount of lipid in HCC tissue was generally higher; the lipid of one consisted of approximately 92% of dry weight of the tissue. The greater lipid content of the HCC tissue was due to the high percentage of neutral lipid. The phospholipid fraction of lipid from HCC tissue was much lower than that of liver (40).

Cholesterol in HCC Tissue

Neoplastic tissues generally contain large quantities of cholesterol, especially of esterified cholesterol (40, 43). An increase of the total cholesterol concentration in the Walker carcinosarcoma was demonstrated to be associated with the growth of malignant tissue (44). In our study, too, the concentration of cholesterol in human HCC tissue was found to be high by the colorimetric assay of the fraction separated by silicic acid column chromatography, as

shown in Figs. 3 and 4. Cholesterol ester comprised 60.2% of total cholesterol in one specimen of HCC, whereas in liver tissue it comprised only 11.8% (33). Cholesterol oleate was the molecular species most increased in HCC (32). The concentration of cholesterol esters is reported to be increased as HCC becomes more deviated (43). It is interesting to note that cholesterol content of the microsomal fraction is higher in HCC tissue than in the corresponding fractions of normal liver tissue (45), suggesting possible compositional alteration of its membrane. In animals synthesis of cholesterol is markedly suppressed by feeding of cholesterol-rich diets (46) or by fasting (47) and is increased by feeding cholestyramine (48). While indirect evidence suggested the site of this suppression to be before the step of mevalonate synthesis (9), measurement of the synthesis of mevalonate and 3-hydroxy-3-methylglutarate with gas-liquid chromatography (50) confirmed more specifically the biochemical site of feedback control of cholesterol synthesis to be the reaction involving mevalonate: NADP oxidoreductase (acylating CoA); EC1.1.34 (HMGCoA reductase). Direct evidence for decreased HMGCoA reductase activity following cholesterol feeding has been provided by Linn (51), who assayed ^{14}C-mevalonate derived from [3-^{14}C]-3-hydroxy-3-methylglutaryl coenzyme A and concluded that the primary site of cholesterol feedback control is the reaction responsible for mevalonate synthesis. The intracellular localization of this enzyme activity has been shown to be in the microsomes (52).

This enzyme in liver is known to be controlled physiologically by three independent mechanisms: endogeneous feedback (53), diurnal rhythm (54), and intermittent feeding and food deprivation (51). There is a considerable debate about how this control is mediated to the enzyme, however.

Cholesterogenesis has been shown to

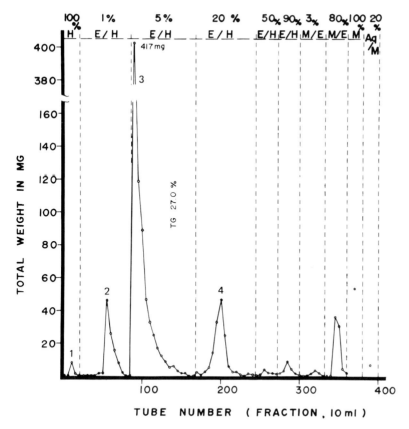

Figure 3 Silicic acid column chromatography of the simple lipid fraction of human hepatoma. Stepwise elution of lipids from silicic acid was performed on a column (3 x 60 cm) containing 60 g of adsorbent. Composition of the eluting solvents is given at the top. *H:* hexane; *E:* diethyl ether; *M:* methanol; *Aq:* water. Peaks: 1, carbohydrate; 2, cholesterol ester; 3, triglyceride and free fatty acid; 4, free cholesterol.

proceed not only in transplantable tumors, such as mouse hepatoma BW 7756 (55), Morris hepatoma 5123–t.c. (55), and others (56), but also in human hepatoma (55, 57).

The cholesterol feedback mechanism, present in normal liver of all species so far examined, has been found to be totally absent in every hepatoma that has been studied, whether in man (two hepatoma) (55, 57), the mouse (two transplantable and a spontaneous hepatomas) (55, 58, 60), the rat (19 minimal-deviation hepatomas) (52, 55, 57, 60, 64, 65), or rainbow trout (66). Thus, cholesterol synthesis in hepatoma is unrefractory to a variety of dietary manipulations known to alter synthesis in the liver, for example, fasting, cholesterol feeding, refeeding after fasting, and cholestyramine feeding (58, 62, 63). Regenerating liver possesses a normal feedback system and therefore the lack of feedback control may be a unique characteristic of malignancy per se rather than of rapid cellular proliferation (52). Furthermore, feedback control of cholesterol synthesis has been found to be absent also from precancerous liver, that is, liver of animals treated for only short periods of time with hepatocar-

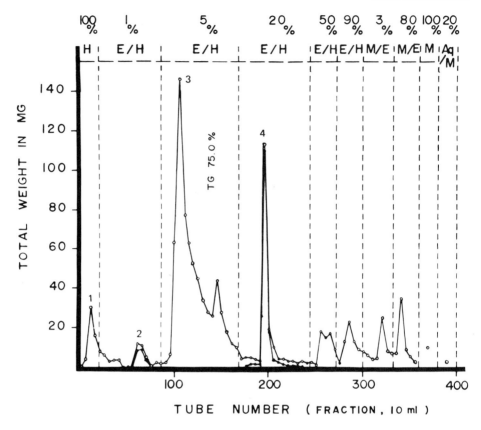

Figure 4 Silicic acid column chromatography of the simple lipid fraction of human liver. *H:* hexane, *E:* diethyl ether, *M:* methanol, *Aq:* water. For peaks 1 to 4, see legend for Fig. 3.

cinogens such as aflatoxin (68, 69), *N*-2-fluorenylacetamide (68, 70, 71), 3-methyl-4-dimethylaminoazobenzene (72), and ethionine (73). In those cases, disappearance of the cholesterol feedback system occurred at an early stage of carcinogenesis, many months before malignant transformation of the liver cell (66, 69); the degree of loss of control was variable, from complete to partial. The severity of early loss of control following carcinogen treatment correlated well with the subsequent development of hepatoma (68). In the early stage of hepatocarcinogen treatment, when feedback control of cholesterol synthesis is lost, most of the other controls of lipid synthesis are retained, and even normal

feedback control may be regained later (68, 70). Although in hepatomas abnormalities have been found in all three kinds of control, some hepatomas retain a diurnal rhythm while some lose it (63). During the latent period after *N*-2-fluorenylacetamide treatment, a normal response of cholesterol synthesis to fasting can be retained in liver, even at a time when feedback control is lost (63). Cholesterol synthesis is apparently unaffected by dietary cholesterol levels in the livers of normal mice who come from strains of mice in which there is a high incidence of spontaneous HCC. Bissel and Alpert (74) studied the feedback control of hepatic cholesterol synthesis in a group of male patients with liver disease in Uganda, where hepatoma is 20-fold more common than in North America, using another group of patients in Boston as a control. Cholesterol synthesis as measured in pieces of HCC obtained by needle biopsy was significantly lower as compared with similar nontumor liver tissue obtained from normal Ugandan control subjects, and even compared with synthesis by tissue obtained from patients in the United States (55, 57). It was confirmed that feedback mechanism remains quite normal in the presence of various liver diseases, for example, cirrhosis or fatty liver (75). However, the feedback mechanism was absent in several cases of nonmalignant liver disease in this country (74).

To account for the failure of dietary cholesterol to inhibit sterol synthesis from acetate in patients with HCC, Siperstein and Fagan (55) proposed an intracellular disturbance of the mechanism regulating cholesterol synthesis, that is, alteration in the structure of the HMG-CoA reductase, so that allosteric inhibition of enzyme activity by cholesterol is ineffective. However, Sabine and Chaikoff (59) postulated that the intact tumor failed to respond because the special metabolic regulators, active in a cell-free system, hardly penetrate the malignant cells in amounts resulting in sufficient intracellular concentrations to be effective. They suggested that a similar explanation would hold for the failure of feedback inhibition of fatty acid synthesis. However, attempts to demonstrate inhibition of the liver enzyme *in vitro* by cholesterol, by other steroids, or by microsomal preparations from cholesterol-fed animals have failed (58, 76). Analyses of Km values and heat stability for HMG-CoA reductase from liver and hepatomas did not show any difference in these properties (58). Harry and his co-workers (65) obtained results with rat hepatoma, which suggested that the capacity of hepatoma to take up dietary cholesterol from plasma is markedly impaired and that it cannot accumulate cholesterol or cholesterol esters even when high cholesterol diets are fed. These data may support the hypothesis of Sabine and Chaikoff (56). From these reports it seems that loss of regulation of cholesterol synthesis is innate in the process of hepatocarcinogenesis.

Hypercholesterolemia frequently associated with HCC can be explained by the recent investigation of Bricker et al (61). Using the desmosterol suppression technique, they demonstrated that HCC releases over 90% of synthesized cholesterol into circulation of the host; it may contribute significantly to the total serum cholesterol, even though the capacity of cholesterogenesis is relatively small.

Bile Acids in Hepatoma Tissue

Bricker et al (77) have demonstrated the capacity of hepatoma (Morris hepatoma 3924A) to synthesize bile acid from both acetate and mevalonate. Feeding of cholesterol to animals promptly suppresses the *de novo* synthesis of sterols by the normal liver and increases its capacity to convert cholesterol to bile acids (77). However, sterol syntheses in hepatoma tissue are unaffected by exogenous cholesterol and, unlike normal liver, exogenous cholesterol cannot be utilized by hepatoma tissue for bile acid synthesis (77). Feeding of cholestyramine to absorb bile salts causes an increase in cholesterol in normal liver but not in animal hepatomas (Morris hepatoma 5123C, mouse hepatoma BW7756) (76). In experiments with tissue slices, addition of sodium deoxycholate to an incubation medium inhibited cholesterol synthesis by liver tissue, but not with hepatoma (76), whereas direct addition of sodium deoxycholate *in vitro* to a cell-free system inhibited cholesterol synthesis both in liver and in hepatoma (76).

Phospholipids in Hepatoma Tissue

Extensive studies have been made of phospholipid content and intracellular distribution of lipid phosphorus in hepatomas and other tumors (78, 79). It has been shown with Novikoff hepatoma and human hepatomas that the total phospholipid content of hepatoma tissue is much smaller than normal liver (42, 78, 79).

Williams et al (80) reported that in hepatoma the percentage of phosphatidylcholine was lower than that of nontumor liver. Veerkamp et al (78), on the other hand, found the proportion of the major components of phospholipid to be nearly equal in both tissues. In Reuber H-35-hepatoma plasma membrane, the same percentage of individual phospholipids was found as in nontumor liver (81). In our study on human hepatoma, the proportions of the major phospholipid classes were not greatly altered, exhibiting only quantitative differences in composition (42). Using the partial hydrolysis technique of Dawson, we confirmed the relatively high contents of plasmalogen and sphingomyelin in human hepatoma, just as have been reported in several animal hepatomas (33). Veerkamp et al (78) have found high levels of plasmalogen in tumors induced with p-dimethylaminoazobenzene. The Morris hepatoma 3924A cell membrane exhibited a fourfold increase in sphingomyelin and also a significant increase in choline plasmalogen (81). In a case of human hepatoma, plasmalogen and sphingomyelin comprised 7.1% and 13.3%, respectively, of the total phospholipid of the liver compared to 4.1% and 3.1% in normal liver (33). Substantial amounts of plasmalogen found in hepatoma tissues are worthy of note, since liver contains the lowest plasmalogen content of all tissues (82). However, the tissues from 3-week-old rats were reported to contain more plasmalogen than the adult tissue, suggesting the possibility that increase of this substance may be a characteristic of rapid cellular proliferation.

Early investigators reported alterations in the proportion of phosphatidylethanol-amines to phosphatidylcholine in tumors (80, 84). Later, Figard and Greenberg (79) demonstrated that the enzyme which methylates phosphatidylethanolamine to phosphatidylcholine was definitely absent in such hepatomas as the Novikoff's and Dunning's type, whereas the activity found in Morris hepatoma was only 20% of the activity found in nontumor liver.

It is by no means clear whether the differences in phospholipid found between liver and hepatomas are due to malignancy per se, since phospholipids have been noted to differ with the stage of development, the portion of tissue, and also with individuals. A recent report (85) illustrates that the phospholipid patterns of normal cell (3T3) and potentially malignant cell (PY3T3) are the same, whereas another report (86) points out that in malignant transformed cell (W1-38VA13) phospholipid decreases compared with the normal cell.

The fatty acid composition of phosphatides of human hepatoma is characterized by its high content of monoenoic acids as compared with normal liver (42). Veerkamp et al (78) reported that the major difference between fatty acids extracted from hepatoma and those from nontumor liver was a shift in the ratio of stearic acid and oleic acid of phospholipid. Furthermore, a disturbance in the fatty acid positioning and pairing in phosphatidylcholine was found in hepatoma; the molecular composition of the hepatoma phosphatidylcholine was quite different from that found in the normal liver, and unusual molecular species of phosphatidylcholine, such as 18:2/20:4 and unsaturated/saturated, were found in hepatoma (87, 88). Those changes in phosphatidylcholine may suggest a severe derangement in the membrane properties of these hepatomas.

The turnover rate of phospholipid is generally increased in hepatoma (89), and the virus-transformed, potentially malignant cells have higher rate of phospholipid turnover than their counterparts (90). It has been proposed that this increased turnover rate is due primarily to phospholipid changes at the cell surface.

Fatty Acids in Hepatoma Tissue

We have determined the fatty acid compositions of lipids of human hepatoma and liver tissue (32). Thirty-five fatty acids were identified in hepatoma tissue, most of them corresponding to the counterpart in normal liver tissue. The levels of monoenoic acids were higher in total as well as in each lipid class, and those of linoleic and polyunsaturated fatty acids were lower in the hepatoma lipids. In some specimens of hepatoma, an unphysiological isomer of eicosatrienoic acid was detected and identified as 5,8, 11-eicosatrienoic acid. A detailed study of this compound demonstrated that it is distributed mainly in the central portion of the hepatoma mass and detected only in traces in the surrounding liver tissue. This piece of evidence suggests that the occurrence of this fatty acid is not secondary to a systemic essential fatty acid deficiency of the patient but is rather due to a localized disturbance in fatty acid metabolism. In order to elucidate the mechanism, positional isomers of the unsaturated fatty acids were analyzed in two hepatoma and two control liver tissues. The results indicated that every isomer of each family of fatty acids increased without any evidence of the competitive inhibition which is generally observed in mammalian cells.

Studies have demonstrated that tumor cells have the ability not only to oxidize fatty acids as a metabolic fuel (91) but also the capacity to synthesize long chain fatty acids from glucose or acetate (92). However, the data indicate that this synthetic process is too slow to provide lipids in sufficient amounts to meet requirements for the growth and that the tumor must obtain its lipids preformed from the host

(92). Investigations on Ehrlich ascites tumor indicated that the tumor cells are capable of synthesizing only 3% of the calculated requirement of fatty acid (93). In contrast, Morris hepatoma 9121 was shown to biosynthesize fatty acids as readily as normal liver tissue does, and even faster than the host liver (94). Furthermore, while dietary changes such as feeding of a fat-deficient diet or of a high-fat diet, lead to either elevated or decreased fatty acid synthesis in liver, such dietary regimens fail to influence fatty acid synthesis in hepatoma tissue (95). It has been shown that feedback inhibition of fatty acid synthesis in liver caused by dietary changes is localized at the acetyl-CoA carboxylase step (96). The defective feedback control of fatty acid synthesis, characteristic of hepatoma, is not always observed in the precancerous state, even when feedback control of cholesterol synthesis has been lost. Whereas the slow-growing, highly differentiated HCC, which resembles differentiated adult liver cells, has the capacity of oxidizing fatty acid and utilizes little, if any, glucose, rapid-growing, poorly differentiated hepatomas have largely lost the capacity for fatty acid oxidation, but have acquired the ability to utilize glucose (97). Such loss of oxidative capability is paralleled by decreased activities of β-hydroxybutyrate dehydrogenase, the enzyme localized to the inner compartment of mitochondria of the liver (96). There is a regular decrease of this enzyme activity with low degree of differentiation (96). Even minimally deviated HCC have lost most of their acyl-CoA synthetase activity, and in the poorly differentiated HCC, the activities ranged from 5% of the normal liver activity for butyrate to about 1% for palmitate (96).

Snyder et al reported the occurrence of relatively high quantities of glyceryl ether diesters in various tumor tissues from animals and man, but we failed to detect this substance in the neutral lipid fraction of

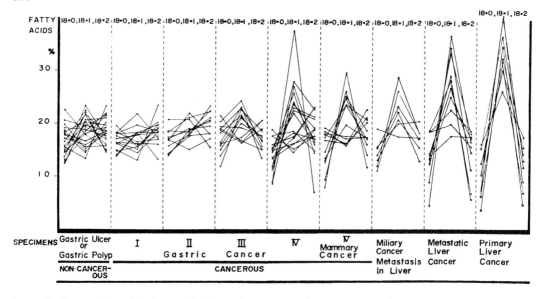

Figure 5 Compositions of C₁₈ fatty acid in livers of cancerous and noncancerous subjects and in liver carcinomas. The advances of cancer invasion are classified according to the *General Rules for the Gastric Cancer Study in Surgery and Pathology* (Japanese Research Society for Gastric Cancer, Kanehara Press, Tokyo, 8th ed, 1971).

human HCC (42).

Lipid Peroxides in Hepatoma Tissue

It has been reported that the serum levels of lipid peroxides increase (98) and those of vitamin E decrease (99) in the patients with liver disease. However, thiobarbituric acid (TBA) reaction has been found to be absent from the tissues in which cell proliferation is actively taking place, especially in tumors (100). Donnan (101) found that HCC induced by 3-methyl-4-dimethylaminoazobenzene had low TBA values as compared with nontumor liver tissue. Shuster (102) showed that the homogenate of Ehrlich ascites tumor produced no TBA-reacting substance on incubation or on irradiation of ultraviolet light, although this tumor contained more linoleic acid than normal liver. Ohnishi (103) observed that hepatoma and fibrosarcoma have minimal peroxide levels. Furthermore, he (103) demonstrated that the degree of unsaturation of choline-containing acetal phosphatide of tumor tissue was very low as compared with that of the lipid of homologous normal tissue, and that for this reason the neoplastic tissue was no longer capable of showing TBA-reaction. Recently, we also found that the purified lipids obtained from human hepatoma exhibited low TBA values as compared with hepatic lipids (42). Although there has been no direct evidence, the high levels of serum vitamin E, observed by Baumer and Beckmann (104) in HCC patients, may be induced by this lowered level of lipid peroxide in hepatoma.

EFFECTS OF MALIGNANCY ON THE COMPOSITION OF HEPATIC LIPID

To study the systemic effects of malignancy, such as on the composition of the hepatic lipid, chemical analyses have been made of biopsy specimens of the liver obtained for histological diagnosis in the patients with gastric carcinoma and noncancerous gastroduodenal diseases (105). In such liver tissue, proportion of neutral lipids to phospholipids remained essentially unchanged, but an increase of lysophosphatidylcholine was observed in the livers in which there were cancer metastases. A significant increase of monoenoic acid was also observed in the stage when there was cancer involvement (Fig. 5). As the tumor grows, the composition of fatty acid in the unaffected liver of the tumor-bearing patient approaches the composition of this particular fatty acid found in the tumor.

CONCLUSION

Evidence presented here indicates that many abnormalities of lipid metabolism occur in hepatoma, of which a defective feedback control of cholesterogenesis, occurrence of 5,8,11-eicosatrienoic acid, altered profiles of tissue phosphatides, and serum lipoproteins are the major ones observed both in animals and in man. However, more information of the structural and functional role of lipids is necessary for complete understanding of the correlation between lipid abnormalities and malignancy.

REFERENCES

1. Viallet A, Benhamou JP, Fauvert R: Les manifestations paraneoplasiques des cancers primitifs du foie. *Rev Fr Etudes Clin Biol* **6**:1087–1097, 1961.

2. Araki E, Okazaki N, Hattori N: Abnormalities in lipid and fatty acid composition in the patients of hepatocellular carcinoma. *Igaku-no Ayumi (Tokyo)* **80**:493–498, 1972.

3. Green HN: Changes in the esterase and fat content of the serum induced by cancer and cancer producing agents. *Brit J Exp Pathol* **15**:1–14, 1934.

4. Haven FL, Bloor WR, Randall C: Lipids of the carcass, blood plasma and adrenals of the rat in cancer. *Cancer Res* **9**:511–514, 1949.

5. Kaufmann HP, Schwarz HG: Zur Biologie der Fette VII: Die quantitative Bestimmung der Blutlipoide und ihre Menge im Blut gesunder und Krebskranken. *Fette Seifen Anstrichm* **56**:17–20, 1954.

6. Elmendorff HV: Serum lipide und Carcinom. *Fette Seifen Anstrichm* **67**:557–562, 1965.

7. Elmendorff HV, Rumpf D: Uber die Serumlipids von Gesunden und Krebskranken. *Fette Seifen Anstrichm* **68**:102–107, 1966.

8. Mattick WL, Buchwald KW: Blood cholesterol studies in cancer. IV. With special reference to other lipid partitions. *J Cancer Res* **13**:157–166, 1929.

9. Mueller PS, Watkin DM: Plasma unesterified fatty acid concentrations in neoplastic disease. *J Lab Clin Med* **57**:95–108, 1961.

10. Haven FL, Bloor WR, Randall C: The nature of the fatty acids of rats growing Walker carcinoma 256. *Cancer Res* **11**:619–623, 1951.

11. Stewart AG, Begg RW: Systemic effects of tumors in force-fed rats. III. Effect on the composition of the carcass and liver and on the plasma lipids. *Cancer Res* **13**:560–565, 1953.

12. Begg RW: Studies on hyperlipidemia in tumor-bearing rats. *Proc Am Assoc Cancer Res* **2**:4, 1955.

13. Frederick GL, Begg RW: A study of hyperlipemia in the tumor-bearing rat. *Cancer Res* **16**:548–552, 1956.

14. Viallet A, Benhamou JP, Fauvert R: Primary carcinoma of the liver and hyperlipemia, case report. *Can Med Assoc J* **86**:1118–1121, 1962.

15. Santer MA, Waldmann TA, Fallon HJ: Erythrocytosis and hyperlipemia as manifestations of hepatic carcinoma. *Arch Intern Med* **120**:735–739, 1967.

16. Mider GB, Sherman CD Jr, Morton JJ: The effect of Walker carcinoma 256 on the total lipid content of rats. *Cancer Res* **9**:222–224, 1949.

17. Mider GB, Fenninger LD Jr, Haven FL, et al:

The energy expenditure of rats bearing Walker carcinoma 256. *Cancer Res* **11**:731–736, 1951.

18. Haven FL, Bloor WR: Lipids in cancer. *Adv Cancer Res* **4**:237–314, 1956.

19. Begg RW, Lotz F: Clearing factor and hyperlipemia in tumor-bearing rats. *Proc Am Assoc Cancer Res* **2**:93–94, 1956.

20. Begg RW: Further studies on clearing activity in tumor-bearing rats. *Proc Am Assoc Cancer Res* **2**:187, 1956.

21a. Kabara JJ, Okita GT, LeRoy GV: The simultaneous use of H^3 and C^{14} to study cholesterol metabolism in normal and tumor mice. *Proc Am Assoc Cancer Res* **2**:219–220, 1957.

21b. Kabara JJ, Okita GT: Incorporation of H^3 and C^{14} cholesterol precursors in normal and tumorous mice. *Proc Am Assoc Cancer Res* **3**:31, 1959.

22. Alpert ME, Hutt MS, Davidson CS: Primary hepatoma in Uganda. A prospective clinical and epidemiologic study of forty-six patients. *Am J Med* **46**:794–802, 1969.

23. Okazaki N, Hattori N, Araki E: Primary carcinoma of the liver associated with erythrocytosis and hyperlipemia. *Jap J Gastroenterol* **69**:775, 1972.

24. Hanawa Y, Ise T, Hasegawa H, Sano R: Serum cholesterol in children with hepatoma. *Jap J Clin Oncol* **1**:129–136, 1971.

25. Araki E, Hanawa Y: Lipid analysis of hepatoma tissue obtained from a case of infant. *Acta Hepatol* **8**:251, 1967.

26. Hansen AE, Ziegler MR, McQuarrie I: Disturbance of osseous and lipid metabolism in a child with primary carcinoma of the liver. *J Pediatr* **17**:9–30, 1940.

27. Pentimalli F, Schmidt G: Über das Verhalten der Phosphorfraction im Blutplasma sarcomkranker Hühner. *Biochem Z* **282**:62–73, 1935.

28. Lee LMY: Serum phospholipids in neoplastic disorders. *Clin Chim Acta* **32**:25–32, 1971.

29. Collins FD, Connelly JF: A fatty acid characteristic of a deficiency of linoleic acid in a case of hepatoma. *Lancet* **2**:883–885, 1965.

30. Okazaki N, Araki E: Eicosatrienoic acid ω9 in serum lipids of patients with hepatocellular carcinoma. *Clin Chim Acta* **53**:11–21, 1974.

31. Paulsrud JR, Pensler L, Whitten CF, et al: Essential fatty acid deficiency in infants induced by fat-free intravenous feeding. *Am J Clin Nutr* **25**:897–904, 1972.

32. Araki E, Okazaki N: Fatty acids of human hepatoma. *Proc Jap Cancer Assoc* **27**:16, 1968.

33. Araki E, Okazaki N: Lipids of infant hepatoma.

Proc Jap Cancer Assoc **30**:85, 1971.

34. Barclay M, Cogin GE, Escher GC, et al: Human plasma lipoproteins. I. In normal women and in women with advanced carcinoma of the breast. *Cancer* **8**:253–260, 1955.

35. Barclay M, Skipski VP, Terebus-Kekisho, et al: Serum lipoproteins in rats with tumors induced by 9,10-dimethyl-1,2-benzanthracene and with transplanted Walker carcinosarcoma 256. *Cancer Res* **27**:1158–1167, 1967.

36 Narayan KA, Morris HP: Serum lipoproteins of rats bearing transplanted Morris hepatoma 7777. *Int J Cancer* **5**:410–414, 1970.

37. Narayan KA: Rat serum lipoproteins during carcinogenesis of the liver in the preneoplastic and the neoplastic state. *Int J Cancer* **8**:61–70, 1971.

38. Narayan KA: Serum lipoproteins during chemical carcinogenesis. *Biochem J* **103**:672–676, 1967.

39. Bullock WE, Cramer W: Contributions to the biochemistry of growth on the lipoid of transplantable tumors of the mice and rats. *Proc Soc Br* **87**:236–239, 1914.

40. Araki E, Okazaki N: Lipids in cancer tissues of human livers and in livers of patients with extrahepatic malignant lesion. *Proc Jap Cancer Assoc* **24**:143–144, 1965.

41. Araki E, Okazaki N, Ariga T: Lipids of human liver carcinoma. *Proc Jap Conf Lipid Biochem* 105–108, 1966.

42. Araki E, Phillips F, Privett OS: Studies on the lipid and fatty acid composition of human hepatoma tissue. *Lipids*, **9**:707–712, 1976.

43. Snyder F, Blank ML, Morris HP: Occurrence and nature of *o*-alkyl and *o*-alk-1-enyl moieties of glycerol in lipids of Morris transplantable hepatomas and normal rat liver. *Biochem Biophys Acta* **176**:502–510, 1969.

44. Boyd EM, McEwen HD: The concentration and accumulation of lipids in the tumor component of a tumor-host organism, Walker carcinoma 256 in albino rats. *Can J Med Sci* **30**:163–172, 1952.

45. Theise H, Bielka H: Die Lipidzusammensetzung der Mikrosomenfraktion von Leber und Hepatom. *Arch Geschwulstforsch* **32**:11–19, 1968.

46. Gould RG: Lipid metabolism and atherosclerosis. *Am J Med* **11**:209–227, 1951.

47. Tomkins GM, Chaikoff IL: Cholesterol synthesis by liver I. Influence of fasting and of diet. *J Biol Chem* **196**:569–573, 1952.

48. Huff JW, Gilfillan JL, Hunt VW: Effect of cholestyramine, a bile acid binding polymer on plasma cholesterol and fecal bile acid excretion in

the rat. *Proc Soc Exp Biol Med* **114**:352–355, 1963.

49. Siperstein MD, Gust MJ: Studies on the site of the feedback control of cholesterol synthesis. *J Clin Invest* **39**:642–652, 1960.

50. Siperstein MD, Fagan VM: Inhibition of mevalonate synthesis by dietary cholesterol. *Fed Proc* **21**:300, 1962.

51. Linn TC: The effect of cholesterol feeding and fasting upon β-hydroxy-β-methylglutaryl coenzyme A reductase. *J Biol Chem* **242**:990–993, 1967.

52. Siperstein MD, Fagan VM: Studies on the feedback regulation of cholesterol synthesis. *Avd. Enz Regulation,* Vol 2. Pergamon Press, New York, 1964, pp 249–264.

53. Weis HJ, Dietschy JM: Failure of bile acids to control hepatic cholesterogenesis: evidence for endogenous cholesterol feedback. *J Clin Invest* **48**:2398–2408, 1969.

54. Back P, Hamprecht B, Lynen F: Regulation of cholesterol biosynthesis in rat liver: diurnal changes of activity and influence of bile acids. *Arch Biochem Biophys* **133**:11–21, 1969.

55. Siperstein MD, Fagan VM: Deletion of the cholesterol-negative feedback system in liver tumors. *Cancer Res* **24**:1108–1115, 1964.

56. Sabine JR: Defective control of cholesterol synthesis and the development of liver cancer: A review. In *Tumor Lipids.* Wood R (Ed). American Oil Chemists' Society Press, 1973, pp 21–33.

57. Siperstein MD, Fagan VM, Morris HP: Further studies on the deletion of the cholesterol feedback system in hepatomas. *Cancer Res* **26**:7–11, 1966.

58. Kandutsch AA, Hancock RL: Regulation of the rate of sterol synthesis and the level of β-hydroxy-β-methylglutaryl coenzyme A reductase activity in mouse liver and hepatomas. *Cancer Res* **31**:1396–1401, 1971.

59. Sabine JR, Abraham S, Chaikoff IL: Control of lipid metabolism in hepatoma: Insensitivity of rate of fatty acid and cholesterol synthesis by mouse hepatoma BW-7756 to fasting and feedback control. *Cancer Res* **27**:793–799, 1967.

60. Siperstein MD: Regulation of cholesterol biosynthesis in normal and malignant tissues. *Curr Top Cell Reg* **2**:65–100, 1970.

61. Bricker LA, Morris HP, Siperstein MD: Loss of the cholesterol feedback system in the intact hepatoma-bearing rat. *J Clin Invest* **51**:206–215, 1972.

62. Siperstein MD, Gyde AM, Morris HP: Loss of feedback control of hydroxymethyl coenzyme A

reductase in hepatomas. *Proc Natl Acad Sci* **68**:315–317, 1971.

63. Goldfarb S, Pitot HC: The regulation of β-hydroxy-β-methylglutaryl coenzyme A reductase in Morris hepatoma 5123C, 7800, and 9618A. *Cancer Res* **31**:1879–1882, 1971.

64. Bricker LA, Siperstein MD: Demonstration of cholesterol feedback deletion in intact hepatoma-bearing rats. *J Clin Invest* **48**:11a, 1969.

65. Harry DS, Morris HP, McIntyre N: Cholesterol biosynthesis in transplantable hepatomas: evidence for impairment of uptake and storage of dietary cholesterol. *J Lipid Res* **12**:313–317, 1971.

66. Siperstein MD: Feedback control of cholesterol synthesis in normal, malignant and premalignant tissues. *Proc Can Cancer Res Conf* **7**:152, 1966.

67. Sabine JR, Horton BJ, Hickman PE: Control of cholesterol synthesis in hepatomas: absence of diurnal rhythm in hepatomas 7794 A and 9618A. *Eur J Cancer* **8**:29–32, 1972.

68. Horton BJ, Horton JD, Sabine JR: Metabolic controls in precancerous liver. II. Loss of feedback control of cholesterol synthesis, measured repeatedly *in vivo,* during treatment with the carcinogens N-2-fluorenylacetamide and aflatoxin. *Eur J Cancer* **8**:437–443, 1972.

69. Siperstein MD: Deletion of the cholesterol negative feedback system in precancerous liver. *J Clin Invest* **45**:1073, 1966.

70. Horton BJ, Sabine JR: Metabolic controls in precancerous liver. Defective control of cholesterol synthesis in rats fed N-2-fluorenyl-acetamide. *Eur J Cancer* **7**:459–465, 1971.

71. Horton BJ, Sabine JR: Metabolic controls in precancerous liver. III. Further studies on the control of lipid synthesis during N-2-fluorenylacetamide feeding. *Eur J Cancer* **9**:1–9, 1973.

72. Horton BJ: Ph.D. Thesis, University of Adelaide, 1972, cited from Reference 56.

73. Horton BJ, Sabine JR: Metabolic controls in precancerous liver. IV. Loss of feedback control of cholesterol synthesis and impaired cholesterol uptake in ethionine-fed rats. *Eur J Cancer* **9**:11–17, 1973.

74. Bissel M, Alpert E: The feedback control of hepatic cholesterol synthesis in Ugandan patients with liver disease. *Cancer Res* **32**:149–152, 1972.

75. Bhattathiry EP, Siperstein MD: Feedback control of cholesterol synthesis in man. *J Clin Invest* **42**:1613–1618, 1963.

76. Sabine JR: Control of cholesterol synthesis in

hepatomas: the effect of bile salts. *Biochim Biophys Acta* **176**:600–604, 1969.

77. Bricker LA, Marraccini JV, Rosenblatt S, et al: Effects of dietary cholesterol on bile acid synthesis in liver and hepatomas. *Cancer Res* **34**:449–453, 1974.

78. Veerkamp JH, Mulder I, vanDeenen LLM: Comparative studies on the phosphatides of normal rat liver and primary hepatoma. *Z Krebsforsch* **64**: 137–148, 1961.

79. Figard PH, Greenberg DM: The phosphatides of some mouse ascites tumors and rat hepatomas. *Cancer Res* **22**:361–367, 1962.

80. Williams HH, Kaucher M, Richards AJ, Moyer EZ: The lipid partition of isolated cell nuclei of dog and rat livers. *J Biol Chem* **160**:227–232, 1945.

81. Selkirk JK, Elwood JC, Morris HP: Study on the proposed role of phospholipid in tumor cell membrane. *Cancer Res* **31**:27–31, 1971.

82. Rapport MM, Norton WT: Chemistry of lipids. *Ann Rev Biochem* **31**:103–138, 1962.

83. Minder WH, Abelin I: Über die hormonale und nichthormonale Beeinflussung der Acetalphosphatide (plasmalogen). Hoppe-Seyler's *Z Physiol Chem* **298**:121–131, 1954.

84. Haven FL: The rate of turnover of the lecithins and cephalins of carcinosarcoma 256 as measured by radioactive phosphorus. *J Natl Cancer Inst* **1**:205–209, 1940.

85. Kulas HP, Marggraf WD, Koch MA, et al: Comparative studies of lipid content and lipid metabolism of normal and transformed mouse cells. *Hoppe-Seyler's Z Physiol Chem* **353**:1755–1760, 1972.

86. Haward BV, Kritchevsky D: The lipids of normal diploid (W1-38) and SV 40-transformed human cells. *Int J Cancer* **4**:393–402, 1969.

87. Bergelson LD: Dyatlovitskaya EV: Molecular structure of tumor lecithins and their relevance to some properties of tumor cell membranes. In *Tumor Lipids.* Wood R (Ed). American Oil Chemists' Press, 1973, pp 111–125.

88. Ruggieri S, Fallani A: A comparative study of lecithins from Yoshida hepatoma AH130, Morris hepatoma 5123 and host rat livers. In *Tumor Lipids.* Wood R (Ed). American Oil Chemists' Society Press, 1973, pp 89–110.

89. Pasternak CA: Phospholipid turnover in normal and cancer cells. In *Tumor Lipids.* Wood R (Ed). American Oil Chemists' Society Press, 1973, pp 66–74.

90. Cunningham DD: Changes in phospholipid turnover following growth of 3T3 mouse cells to confluency. *J Biol Chem* **247**:2464–2470, 1972.

91. Weinhouse S: Studies on the fate of isotopically labeled metabolites in the oxidative metabolism of tumors. *Cancer Res* **11**:585–591, 1951.

92. Medes G, Thomas A, Weinhouse S: Metabolism of neoplastic tissue. IV. A study of lipid synthesis in neoplastic tissue slices *in vitro*. *Cancer Res* **13**:27–29, 1953.

93. Spector AA, Steinberg D, Tanaka A: Uptake of free fatty acids by Ehrlich ascites tumor cells. *J Biol Chem* **240**:1032–1041, 1965.

94. Elwood JC, Morris HP: Lack of adaptation in lipogenesis by hepatoma 9121. *J Lipid Res* **9**:337–341, 1968.

95. Sabine JR, Abraham S, Chaikoff IL: Lack of feedback control of fatty acid synthesis in a transplantable hepatoma. *Biochim Biophys Acta* **116**:407–409, 1966.

96. Weinhouse S: Fatty acids as metabolic fuels of cancer cells. In *Tumor Lipids Wood R (Ed)*. American Oil Chemists' Society Press, 1973, pp 14–20.

97. Ohe K, Morris HP, Weinhouse S: β-hydroxybutyrate dehydrogenase activity in liver and liver tumors. *Cancer Res* **27**:1360–1371, 1967.

98. Schauenstein E, Burgermeister E, Heinzel H: Über den Serum-Lipoxyd-gehalt alter Menschen und seine Beeinflussung durch Gerusan. *Wien Med Wochenschr* **44**:758–762, 1961.

99. Kater RMH, Unterecker WJ, Kim CY, Davidson DS: Relationship of serum tocopherol to beta-lipoprotein concentrations in liver diseases. *Am J Clin Nutr* **23**:913–918, 1970.

100. Ohnishi T: Lipid-peroxide formation and phospholipid in normal and tumor tissues. *Gann* **49**:233–248, 1958.

101. Donnan SK: The thiobarbituric acid test applied to tissues from rats treated in various ways. *J Biol Chem* **182**:415–419, 1950.

102. Shuster CW: Effects of oxidized fatty acids on ascites tumor metabolism. *Proc Soc Exp Biol Med* **90**:423–426, 1955.

103. Ohnishi T: Choline-containing acetal phosphatide and thiobarbituric acid reaction in the rat liver. *Gann* **51**:1–10, 1960.

104. Bäumer A, Beckmann R: Zur Bedeutung einer Vitamin E-Erniedigung im Serum bei Leberkrankheiten. *Klin Wochenschr* **33**:431–434, 1955.

105. Araki E, Okazaki N, Nawa H: Hepatic lipids in cancer patients and in tumor-bearing rats. *Seikagaku* **39**:622, 1967.

Part Five *CLINICAL FEATURES*

CHAPTER 17 CLINICAL ASPECTS OF HEPATOCELLULAR CARCINOMA—ANALYSIS OF 134 CASES

KUNIO OKUDA, M.D.

INCIDENCE AND MATERIAL FOR STUDY

The incidence of hepatocellular carcinoma (HCC, synonymous with liver cell carcinoma or hepatoma) in Japan is 5 to 10 times that in Europe and the United States (1–4). The frequency varies from area to area even in a small country like Japan. Northern Kyushu, about 600 miles southwest of Tokyo and where a large part of the clinical observations have been made by the author, seems to have a higher incidence of HCC compared with Tokyo. The necropsies of patients with liver cirrhosis and HCC performed at Kurume University Hospital (northern Kyushu) and at Chiba University Hospital (near Tokyo) in the period from 1958 to 1972 were reviewed and compared. The frequency of HCC relative to cirrhosis was 110:70 in the former and 89:97 in the latter, with a peak incidence in the fifth and sixth decade, respectively, and the difference was significant ($p < .05$). Of 4611 necropsies made at Kurume University, HCC constituted 3.17%, whereas at Tokyo Medi-

cal and Dental College the comparable figures were 3232 and 1.36%(3). There were 2817 cases of HCC in 136,478 necropsies throughout Japan from 1958 to 1967 with an incidence of 2.06%(4).

The clinical statistics given in this chapter have mainly been derived from 134 patients with unequivocal HCC who had been admitted to the second Department of Medicine, Kurume University Hospital during the last 10 years. Pathological data have been drawn from 153 necropsies of HCC made at the author's disposal through the courtesy of Professor T. Nakashima, Pathology Department. Some of the illustrative cases have also been selected from the patients seen at Chiba University and affiliated hospitals.

Of the 134 clinical cases, autopsies were performed in 76, the diagnosis was made by needle or surgical biopsy in 34 cases, and in the remainder the diagnosis was based on clinical data, including positive alpha-fetoprotein (AFP), by exclusion of extrahepatic primary neoplasm as deter-

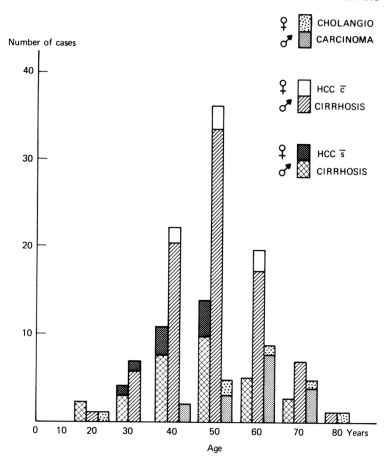

Figure 1 Age distribution of 134 cases of hepatocellular carcinoma (HCC) and 23 cases of cholangiocarcinoma. HCC was further divided clinically into two groups with (95) and without (39) associated cirrhosis. Note the age peak in the fifth decade for HCC compared with that in the sixth for cholangiocarcinoma.

mined by scanning, laparoscopy, celiac an-giography, complete radiographic study of the digestive tract, etc. Because of the importance of associated cirrhosis, patients have been clinically divided into those with and without cirrhosis. The diagnosis of cirrhosis was made by similar diagnostic procedures and from clinical signs of portal hypertension and biochemical changes. There were 95 cases of HCC with cirrhosis and 39 cases without; the age and sex are shown in Fig. 1. Antemortem distinction of the two groups is not absolute, but has been

fairly accurate as checked by autopsy. Some of the latter group were found to have fibrosis or very mild cirrhosis, but none had evidence of fully developed cirrhosis. The overall male to female ratio was 118:16, or 7.4:1. For comparison, 23 autopsy cases of cholangiocarcinoma are shown in the same diagram, demonstrating a less predominance of males (2.8:1) and a peak incidence of one decade later. (5).

NATURAL HISTORY AND ETIOLOGIC FACTORS

Personal history, past history, and other

Table 1 Natural History of Etiologic Importance (134 Cases)

History	Number of Patients (39 s̄ cirrhosis: 95 c̄ cirrhosis)	Percentage
Surgery, minor or major	47	35.1
Jaundice	34 (3:31)	25.4
Alcohol, habitual intake		
Moderate (50 to 125 ml EtOH)	33	24.6
Heavy (> 125 ml EtOH)	6	4.5
Liver disease [a]	32 (3:29)	23.9
Blood transfusion	13 (1:12)	9.7
Syphilis	11 (0:11)	8.2
Schistosomiasis	11 (7, unaware)	8.2
Malaria	8	6.0
Biliary tract disease	6	4.5
Other parasitic disease	3	2.2

[a] 18 undefined, 5 acute hepatitis, 4 chronic hepatitis, 4 cirrhosis, 1 liver abscess.

factors in the record have been analyzed from an etiologic point of view. Regarding occupation, 23.1% of the patients were office workers, 17.2% farmers, 17.2% other type of laborers, 12.7% merchants, 9.0% intellectuals such as teachers, doctors, pharmacists, and priests, and 6.0% housewives, etc. No predilection of the disease for a particular socioeconomic class has been implicated. Although the climate in Kyushu is more favorable for fungus growth than around Tokyo, evidence of food contamination by potential carcinogens has not yet been demonstrated.

In the personal and past histories, prior surgical operation of some sort was elicited in 35.1% of the patients, jaundice in 25.4%, habitual alcholic intake of more than 50 ml of ethanol in 29.1%, liver disease in 23.5%, and blood transfusion in 9.7% (Table 1). There was a significant difference between the groups with and without cirrhosis in the frequency of history of liver disease, including or not including jaundice and biliary tract disease—44 out of 95 cases with cirrhosis had a history of hepatobiliary disease, whereas only 5 of 39 without cirrhosis (p < .01) had the same history.

Hepatitis B antigen, recently linked etiologically to HCC (6, 7), was positive in

sera of 41 of 81 patients' when analysis was by radioimmunoassay. Counterelectrophoresis or single radial immunodiffusion testing was also undertaken, and it is significant that sera of more than half of the patients were positive by radioassay but only 8.6% were positive by less sensitive methods. The difference suggests low antigen concentrations in sera of patients with HCC in contrast to higher antigen concentration in patients with acute hepatitis and even chronic active hepatitis (Fig. 2). It is tempting to postulate that low antigenemia in HCC is the reflection of an altered immune response of the host which somehow conditions itself to carcinogenesis.

Schistosomiasis as diagnosed by clinical data, the demonstration of ova in liver or rectal mucosa or positive skin test, was present in 11 patients (8.2%). A recent study in another endemic area in Japan has suggested an etiologic role of this disease (9). A statistical analysis of necropsies done at Kurume University has indicated an incidence of HCC of 10.6% among those with schistosomiasis japonica compared with 2.78% among those without this disease (p < .01). Kurume is located along the Chikugo River where schistosomiasis japonica was endemic until 10 years ago.

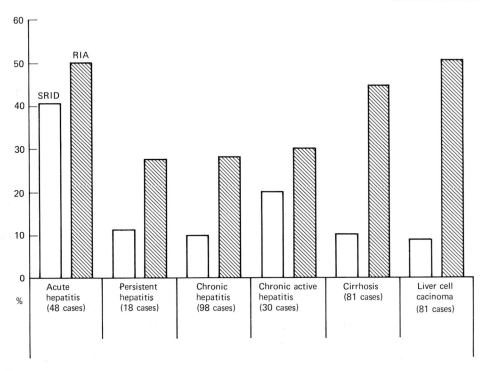

Figure 2 Detection rate of HBsAg in various liver diseases. It was positive in sera from 41 of 81 patients with HCC by radioimmunoassay (RIA), but in only 7 by the immunodiffusion method (SRID). The difference between the two methods was less in acute and chronic active hepatitis.

No fresh cases of schistosomiasis have been seen in recent years following the employment of vigorous control measures. Although the statistics suggest a possible etiologic role of chronic schistosomiasis, a careful study of the livers bearing both schistosome ova and HCC revealed that the majority had, in addition, the histopathological characteristics of posthepatitic cirrhosis with superimposed schistosomiasis. HBsAg was also positive in 27%. Thus, it is more likely that HBsAg and schistosomiasis rather than the latter alone predisposed the liver to this type carcinoma.

Clonorchiasis was found in only two cases in our series, each having a minute tumor nodule (minimal HCC) as revealed by autopsy. Clonorchiasis in Hong Kong was more often associated with cholangiocarcinoma (11).

A history of syphilis has occasionally been linked to HCC (12, 13) and was elicited from 11 patients with HCC and cirrhosis (11.6%), but in none with HCC without cirrhosis. Other factors that have allegedly been associated with HCC include thorotrast (14), hemochromatosis (15), androgen (16), etc. Chronic congestion of the liver as a result of idiopathic stenosis of the vena cava at the hepatic portion (Budd-Chiari disease) is often complicated by hepatic carcinoma—29 cases out of 71 in the Japanese literature up to 1967 according to Nakamura et al (17). Thus it seems that any chronic liver disease predisposes this organ to primary carcinoma, but the possible role of HBsAg acting directly as a carcinogen or indirectly via chronic parenchymal liver disease has not yet been fully elucidated.

SYMPTOMATOLOGY

The onset of symptoms is usually insidious unless ushered in by an acute abdominal event or hematemesis. Without clear definition of "onset," it is difficult to decide what was the first subjective complaint. The disease is more often a continuation of chronic hepatitis or cirrhosis in this country. The symptoms that are attributed to an enlarging tumor are pain in the upper abdomen (mostly right hypochondrium), malaise, a sense of epigastric fullness after meals, persistent oppression and discomfort in the upper abdomen, general abdominal distension, self-palpated mass, anorexia, nausea and vomiting, jaundice, and weight loss. Lumbago or other symptoms may be produced by metastases (Table 2).

The pain, which bears no direct relationship to liver size, is usually not severe but often annoying. It may be the first and most important sign among patients with cirrhosis, suggesting complication by HCC. Abdominal fullness and distension were common in patients with a huge liver or ascites. Comparing our data with those tabulated by Berman in Bantu patients (18), it is immediately apparent that in South Africa weight loss is a most common early sign and pain and fever are more frequent. We feel that the difference is due mainly to the fact that the frequency of associated cirrhosis was lower and the extent of hepatic involvement with cirrhosis was much less in South Africa as evidenced by large liver weights—the average weight of our HCC livers was 2036 g, the smallest being 520 g, as compared to an average of 3960 g with the smallest weighing 1900 g in Berman's material. In the former, weight of the liver with advanced cirrhosis and

Table 2   Early Symptoms in 134 Cases of Hepatocellular Carcinoma

Complaint	Percentage
Abdominal discomfort	
Fullness	32.0
Swelling, distension	11.9
Total	43.9
Pain	
Right upper abdomen	21.6
Epigastrium	12.7
Lumbago	4.5
Other area	3.0
Total	41.8
Malaise	30.6
Anorexia	10.4
Tumor felt	10.4
Jaundice, itch	8.3
Weight loss	4.5
Nausea, vomit	4.5
Diarrhea or constipation	3.7
Fever	3.0
Hematemesis, tarry stool	1.5
Change in psyche	0.7

HCC was less than 1200 g and livers weighing more than 4.5 kg had minimal or no cirrhosis (19). Patients with cirrhosis do not develop *acute* weight loss because of chronicity of the disease.

In a small number of patients, signs of acute blood loss into the abdominal cavity, fever, and symptoms related to hypoglycemia, hypercalcemia, and plethora may be the early manifestations. These latter signs are believed to be caused by humoral factors secreted by tumor cells as discussed in Chapter 14.

ONSET OR DEVELOPMENTAL STAGE

Recently, we are detecting relatively small HCC among the patients under long clinical observation by doing repeated blood tests and biopsies. The patient is first found to have some biochemical abnormalities, often by chance, and then a diagnosis of chronic hepatitis with minimal or moderate histological activities may be made by biopsy. Typically, the patients are seen by their physician over a number of years, the disease progressing very slowly. Suddenly, the physician is alarmed by increasing AFP or by seeing localized decrease in radioactivity on the scan. He is then surprised to realize that the tumor is already unmistakably large as studied by angiography or laparoscopy. We have experienced at least 16 such cases, and similar reports are rapidly increasing in Japan and probably in other countries as well. Based on our own cases and judging from these reports, we now believe that HCC develops not only in established cirrhosis but also in certain stages of chronic hepatitis. When it arises in advanced cirrhosis, the patient dies from hepatic failure before the carcinoma attains a large mass. Contrary to the generally held expectation, detection of early HCC by serum AFP measurement seems still difficult, if not impossible. In the following patients with 5 to 13 years of follow-up for chronic hepatitis, HCC was already peachsized when it was detected by scanning or AFP determinations.

CASE 1. K. M., a 68-year-old male, had the first episode of mild jaundice 31 years previously, a second episode 12 years later, and a diagnosis of chronic hepatitis was made 13 years prior to death. He had since been under medical care at another hospital. Because of increasing malaise and anorexia, he was admitted from March to June 1971; needle biopsy disclosed changes compatible with chronic active hepatitis with moderate activities (Fig. 3a). Blood chemistry included: SGOT 52 u (Karmen); SGPT 31 u (K); alkaline phosphatase (AL-P) 8 u (K.A.); total pro-

tein 7.5 g γ-globulin 2.2 g/100 ml; and BSP test 21% retention at 30 min. Liver scan was unremarkable. He was followed at two-month intervals after discharge for two years and during this time blood chemistry remained almost unchanged. AFP, which had remained less than 38 ng/ml but above 10 ng/ml (our absolute normal limit) in this follow-up period, started to rise sharply in March 1973, and was 1670 ng in April with concomitant positive turn for HBsAg (Fig. 3b). He was readmitted for evaluation. Celiac angiography disclosed an apple-shaped area with tumor vessels in the right lower liver. Laparoscopy also demonstrated a bulge in the same location of a mildly cirrhotic liver. Operation was carried out in June to resect the right half of the liver (Fig. 3c). Although it was a success technically there were several small metastases already outside the major mass that represented the typical "solitary form" by our nomenclature (19). The liver parenchyma revealed very mild or early cirrhosis with thin septa and macronodules. The liver functions gradually deteriorated after the operation, tumor recurred and he died four months postoperatively.

Note in this case that AFP dropped precipitously following resection and rose again sharply with increasing SGOT. The HBsAg became undetectable (by counterelectrophoresis) with decreasing AFP and detectable again with the rise of AFP. Destruction of HBsAg-containing liver cells by the rapidly expanding tumor, and the release of HBsAg into blood may explain the observed phenomenon.

CASE 2.2 K. K., a 55-year-old high official, was found to have abnormal liver tests (SGOT 85 Karmen u, AL-P 8.3 Bod. u, bilirubin 1.7 mg) in October 1968. In January 1969 he entered the hospital for complete liver study which disclosed chronic active hepatitis by biopsy (Fig. 4a) and an enlarged left lobe with some splenic activity on the scan (Fig. 4b). He was readmitted in April 1970 when laparoscopy disclosed a cirrhotic liver with no visible tumor, and biopsy histology was

Figure 3 Case 1. (a) Liver biopsy in March 1971, showing chronic hepatitis with some fibrosis and mild inflammation (Okuda, K. et al: Gastroenterology **69**:226, 1975). (b) Clinical course of Case 1 with respect to AFP levels and HBAg. Note the sudden rise in AFP with positive turn for HBAg. After removal of the tumor, AFP dropped precipitously, and recurrence of tumor was accompanied by a sharp rise of AFP and positive HBAg again. (c) Resected right lobe. The tumor was 5 x 5 cm and was of the solitary type with several small metastases already seen in a thin septal cirrhotic liver.

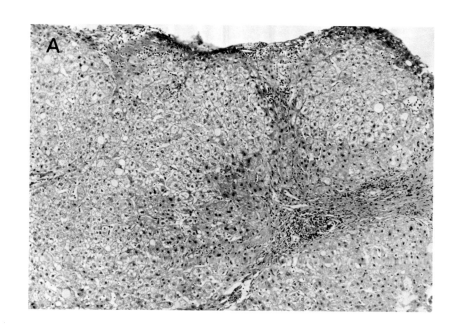

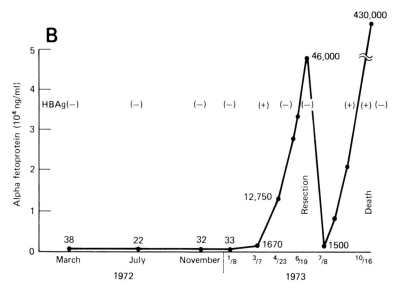

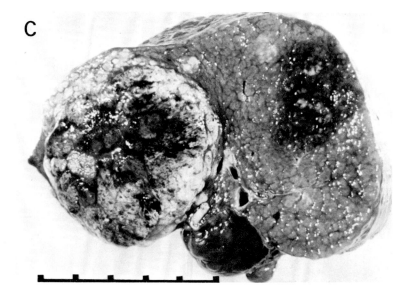

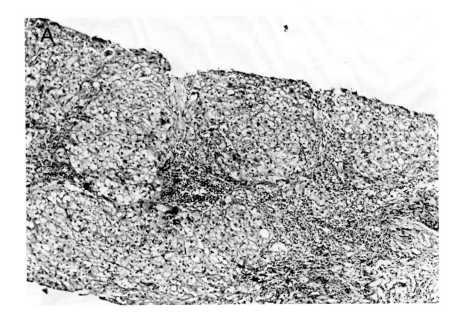

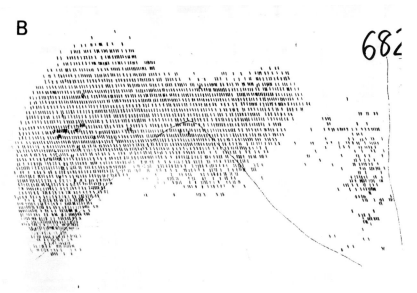

Figure 4 Case 2. *(a)* First liver biopsy in January 1969, demonstrating chronic active hepatitis with severe inflammation and disorganized lobules (Okuda, K. et al: *Gastroenterology* **69**:226, 1975). *(b)* Liver scan made at the same time as *(a)*, showing an enlarged left lobe and some splenic activity. *(c)* Scan 15 months after *(b)*. *(d)* Scan 3 years after *(c)*, revealing a clearly demarcated lesion in the left lobe inferiorly. The advancing cirrhotic changes are apparent compared with the previous scans. *(e)* The third biopsy made 4 years and 9 months after the first, showing persistent inflammation and formation of a regenerative nodule.

C

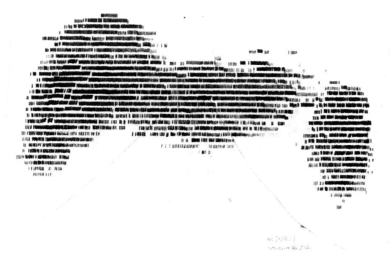

D

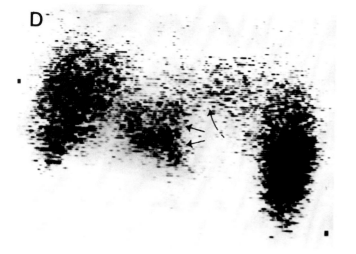

E

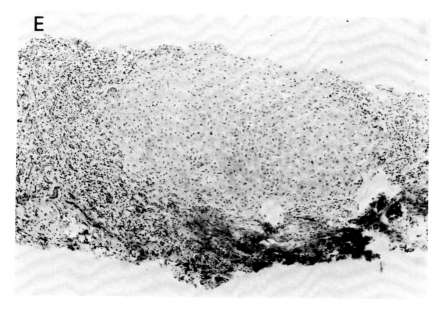

Table 3 Objective Signs on Admission (134 Cases)

Finding	Number of Patients	Percentage
Hepatomegaly		
2 to 3 fingerbreadths [a]	52	38.8
> 4 fingerbreadths	48	35.9
Undetermined	18	13.4
Ascites	66	49.3
Tenderness in upper abdomen	65	48.6
Vascular spider	53	39.6
Palpable mass	51	38.2
Jaundice	40	29.9
Dilated abdominal veins	39	29.1
Splenomegaly	22	16.4
Palmar erythema	21	15.7
Pigmentation	7	5.3
Gynecomastia	5	3.7

[a] Below the right costal margin in the mammillary line.

almost unchanged from the previous one. A liver scan made two years after the first showed slightly advanced atrophy of the right lobe of the liver and more activity in the spleen (Fig. 4c). He was almost without symptoms and blood chemistry was consistently but only mildly abnormal during this period. He developed abdominal pain and was admitted for the third time in October 1973. The scan this time revealed a clearly demarcated cold lesion in the left lobe (Fig. 4d) and liver histology showed cirrhosis with inflammation (Fig. 4e). His plasma AFP levels were 70 ng/ml in May 1972, 100 ng in November 1973, 620 ng in January 1974 and 1500 ng at the time of death in February. Evidently, AFP was abnormal but not high when the mass was already peach-sized.

In these two cases, the tumor was already of a considerable size at the time AFP was found rising from the previous unfluctuating subnormal levels. Taking into account the long latent period of cancer growth, the carcinoma must have evolved in these cases sometime during the precirrhotic phase of chronic hepatitis.

OBJECTIVE SIGNS

The physical signs differ considerably from patient to patient because of the variation in pathology. Those patients with advanced cirrhosis have clinical features very much like those of patients with hepatic cirrhosis and, in the terminal stage, of patients with cirrhosis in hepatic failure. When patients have little or no fibrosis in their liver, the tumor may develop to an extreme size with compensatory hypertrophy of the remaining liver parenchyma, turning the entire liver into a huge mass. In such cases, hepatomegaly is the most prominent objective finding with abdominal fullness as the chief complaint. There may be some tenderness on palpation of the liver, and bruit may be heard over the mass because of the increased arterial vessels (20). The right anterior chest may be pushed forward from within by the mass, making the costal margin almost continuous with the underlying liver on palpation. Asymmetry of the right and left costal margins is evident on inspection. The surface of the mass may be felt as coarse irregularities with increased consistency. In the Bantu, as described by Berman (18), this type of HCC seems to be predominant, making the average liver weight at the time of autopsy almost twice that in our series (19). Hepatomegaly is usually more prominent in metastatic liver carcinoma than HCC in Japan. The size of the liver in our series of cases is given in Table 3 in terms of the number of fingerbreadths that the liver was palpated below the right costal margin. In the patients without cirrhosis, the livers extended more than two fingerbreadths below the costal margin in 98% and greater than four fingerbreadths in 57%, while in those with cirrhosis the comparable figures were 63% and 17%, respectively. The spleen is palpable in patients with cirrhosis and portal hypertension. If the spleen becomes enlarged within a short period of time along with other manifestations of portal hypertension, then portal vein occlusion by the tumor should be suspected. Sometimes, an enlarged left lobe makes the palpation of the spleen difficult, or is mistaken for it (Fig. 5).

Skin manifestations include those seen in hepatic cirrhosis, such as vascular spiders, palmar erythema, and pigmentation. A somewhat localized area of vascular dilatation may be seen in the skin over the liver posteriorly, but very rarely. It is presumably caused by tumor compression of the right subcostal veins. Distended veins on the abdominal wall may be just as prominent as in cirrhosis.

Ascites sometimes form during progression of the disease but may be present at the first examination. When it appears suddenly and the patient goes into shock, paracentesis invariably yields bloody fluid, a grave prognostic sign that requires resuscitation followed by urgent laparotomy to stop the bleeding from rupture of a tumor nodule. In northern Kyusu, aspiration of hemorrhagic ascites is due to HCC in more than 50% of the patients in the author's experience. Edema of the lower extremities is usually less marked compared with edema in cases of cirrhosis. When leg edema and ascites are very marked but without severe hypoalbuminemia, the Budd-Chiari syndrome, resulting from tumor growth in the inferior vena cava, should be suspected. Hydrothorax is not an infrequent complication of massive ascites in cirrhosis and may also occur in patients with HCC.

Jaundice was seen on admission in approximately one out of three patients and in about 70% at the time of death. Once jaundice has become overt, it seldom regresses and, excepting rare cases of the "cholestatic form" as described below, overt jaundice more often indicates parenchymal damage.

The so-called paraneoplastic syndrome related to HCC includes polycythemia (21, 22), hypoglycemia (23), hypercalcemia (24), dysfibrinogenemia (25, 26), hyperlipemia (27), carconoid syndrome (28), pulmonary osteoarthropathy (29), etc.

CLINICAL TYPES

In view of the protean manifestations, several clinical forms have been separated according to the symptoms, signs, and courses. Such classification has certain merit in predicting the subsequent course and understanding the pathophysiology.

Ewing (3) suggested four well-defined clinical types: (1) those in which no symptoms are detected and the patient dies suddenly from hemorrhage or after an illness of a few days; (2) those in which latent carcinoma is found among patients who succumb to cirrhosis or other diseases; (3) those in which the usual history of cirrhosis terminates rapidly with hepatic tumor, jaundice, ascites, and cachexia, and (4) those in which the usual history of a malignant tumor from the first liver involvement develops among previously healthy patients. Berman (19) divided liver carcinomas into typical or frank cancer (group I) and atypical carcinomas which are further divided into acute abdominal cancer (group II), febrile cancer (group III), occult cancer (group IV), and metastatic cancer (group V). Both classifications are similar in that occult HCC found at autopsy and acute intraabdominal hemorrhage terminating rapidly are separated from the

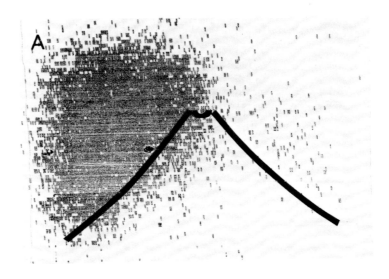

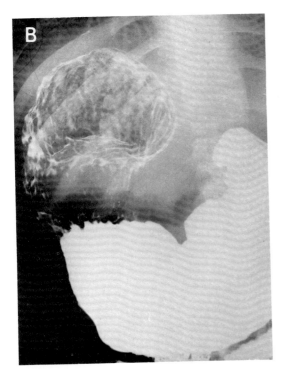

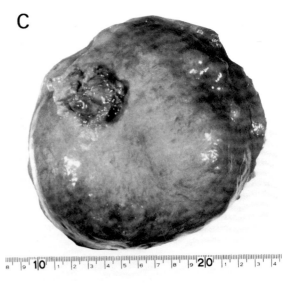

Figure 5 *(a)* This 51-year-old male had a left hypochondriac mass indistinguishable from the spleen by palpation. Because of polycythemia, a blood disease had been suspected. Liver scan obtained with ^{51}Cr-labeled denatured red cell disclosed very little activity in the spleen, and absence of the left liver. *(b)* Barium examination of the stomach (prone film) revealed an extragastric mass compressing the stomach from the front. *(c)* The resected left lobe containing HCC of the solitary (massive) type.

more common groups. However, it is difficult to decide what is the most typical clinical form for lack of pathognomonic clinical feature for HCC, and there is a geographical difference in frequency of the prominent anatomical type. For instance, in 108 cases of MacDonald's series (31), the nodular type accounted for 85.2%, while in our series of 112 cases (19) the corresponding figure was only 47.4%, and just as many cases were of the massive type. Group III in Berman's classification, which constituted 8% and in which fever was the presenting symptom and suggestive of liver abscess, is extremely rare in Japan.

In our patients the most common clinical features are general malaise, upper abdominal pain, abdominal fullness, and a palpable hepatic mass. The size of the liver bears little relation to the general condition of the patient. Rather, it is not uncommon to see a patient walking around with a huge liver and minimal complaints, and a very ill patient having a relatively small and nodular liver with ascites and other severe manifestations of cirrhosis. The nontumorous liver parenchyma in the former is not cirrhotic and is functioning well. In the latter, the diagnosis of carcinoma is barely possible by physical examination alone unless it is distinctly large.

Thus in a number of patients, the clinical feature is that of hepatic cirrhosis and the presence of carcinoma is demonstrated antemortem either by scintiscan, AFP, laparoscopy, or angiography. We call such patients the "cirrhotic type" and distinguish it from the Berman's occult type, which he defined as those latent cases that are discovered either during examination for complaints other than those attributable to liver disease or are accidentally found at autopsy. Discovery of small HCC in a cirrhotic liver at autopsy is seldom a surprise in this country because of its high incidence in nonalcoholic cirrhosis. In our classification, the occult type is defined as HCC not diagnosed with certainty antemortem. Occult

HCC would be discovered more frequently if the liver were subjected to more careful examination; we have found four cases of minimal HCC either by slicing the liver or by roentgenologic examination after injection of contrast medium into the hepatic artery during autopsy.

In a small proportion of patients, the clinical characteristics are those of acute or subacute hepatitis, and liver carcinoma is found as a surprise. We call such cases the "hepatitis type." In some cases, features of obstructive jaundice are predominant from the onset, and bile duct exploration reveals intraductal growth of HCC or compression of a large bile duct by the tumor—the "cholestatic type." Thus patients with HCC may be clinically divided into the following: (1) frank type, (2) cirrhotic type, (3) occult type, (4) febrile type, (5) acute abdominal type, (6) metastatic type, (7) hepatitis type, (8) cholestatic type, and (9) others. In this classification, the cirrhotic, hepatitis, and cholestatic types are additional to those described by Berman.

The following case descriptions illustrate some of these types.

Occult Type

A patient with typical features of cirrhosis dies from hepatic failure or rupture of a varix, and at the time of autopsy one to several, at most, nodules of carcinoma may be found in a highly atrophic liver. Unless AFP has been elevated, antemortem diagnosis of the complicating carcinoma is extremely difficult, and it may even escape the pathologist's eye.

CASE 3. K. G., a 54-year-old male, developed malaise and jaundice and was admitted to a hospital in September 1971, where a diagnosis of chronic hepatitis complicating chronic schistosomiasis japonica was made based on liver biopsy. Calcified schistosome ova and mononuclear cell infiltration were seen in the portal tract. In June 1973, he had hematemesis and was rushed to our hospital. He was emaciated but there was no evidence of ascites. Laboratory studies included: red cell count 3,100,000, serum total albumin 2.7 g, γ-globulin 2.9 g, total bilirubin 2.8 mg, direct bilirubin 1.3 mg/100 ml, SGOT 98 u (Karmen), SGPT 42 u (K.), AL-P 11.5 u (K.A.), HBsAg positive and AFP 463 ng/ml. BSP test showed 32.5% retention at 45 min. Liver scan disclosed an atypical inverted triangular pattern often seen in chronic schistosomiasis (32). Celiac angiography demonstrated a markedly shrunk right lobe. In the periphery of a superioposterior branch of the right hepatic artery, there was a change suggestive of a round lesion with displacement of the fourth order branches (Fig. 6a). Autopsy disclosed advanced cirrhosis with features of both posthepatitic cirrhosis and chronic schistosomiasis (Fig. 6b). A 1.5 × 1.5 cm lesion was found at the location corresponding to the angiographic changes. In Nakashima–Okuda's classification (19), this belongs to the "cirrhotic oligonodular" form of HCC which is usually well differentiated histologically.

Febrile Type

Although an occasional rise in temperature is not uncommon during the course of disease, the febrile type as designated by Berman (19), which is hardly distinguishable from liver abscess, is very seldom encountered in Japan. The course is usually rapidly downhill, the liver speedily enlarging while the general condition of the patient visibly deteriorates.

CASE 4. I. K., a 53-year-old farmer, began having a dull pain in the right upper quadrant in September 1973 and was admitted on November 2, 1973 because of malaise and fever. He seemed acutely ill, and there was much perspiration. A firm liver was felt two fingerbreadths below the right costal margin. Chest X-ray disclosed a scallop-shaped protrusion in the right diaphragm medially (Fig. 7a). Laboratory studies included: leukocyte count 14,000/mm³ with 23% stabs, 62% segs, 7% lymphocytes, 5% monocytes, and 3% eosinophils; erythrocyte sedimentation rate 118 mm/hr, CRP (+++), serum albumin 3.1 g, γ-globulin 0.92 g/100 ml, SGPT 44 IU, AL-P 272 IU, and AFP negative.

Liver scan disclosed two large space-occupying lesions in the right lobe of the liver, one located superiorly and the other inferiorly. ⁶⁷Ga-citrate scan showed activity only in the inferior lesion (Fig. 7b), and celiac angiography demonstrated the upper lesion to be hypovascular. Laparoscopy was not diagnostic.

Despite intensive treatment with antibiotics, the patient continued to have fever and prostration (Fig. 7c). The leukocyte count increased and the right diaphragm rose rapidly (Fig. 7d). He was subsequently operated on for suspected liver abscesses. A tumor was seen infiltrating from the liver to the right kidney. Autopsy two months later disclosed a main tumor with a necrotic interior in the right lobe of the liver, and a smaller tumor in the inferior portion. Metastases were seen in the right diaphragm, both lungs, kidneys, and over the peritoneum with some dissemination. Histology was very similar to the case described by Edmondson and Steiner (33) for which they used the term "carcinosarcoma." The cells consisted in the main of spindle cells (Fig. 7e), but there were also epithelial cell components, giant cells, and cells in transition from epithelial to spindle cells (Fig. 7f). In the areas with epithelial cell arrangements, the tumor cells contained AFP as demonstrated by the immunofluorescent antibody technique. It is of interest that serum AFP became detectable by the immunodiffusion method terminally.

The author has seen a case of hepatocholangioma in which serum AFP decreased progressively without treatment, and it was found at autopsy that cholangiocellular component was predominant. Serum AFP level is related to the relative proportion of AFP-producing cells and, in these cases, there was probably some change in the population of such cells.

Acute Abdominal Type

CASE 5. K. O., a 73-year-old man, began having anorexia and pain in the right upper abdomen in July 1965. When he consulted a physician because of increasing malaise, the liver was already palpable three fingerbreadths and ascites apparent. He was admitted on December 16, 1965. Major tests included; red cell count 2,910,000/mm³, SGOT 36 u (Frankel), SGPT 23 u (F.), SLDH 890 u, serum bilirubin 4.6 mg, albumin 3.2g and γ-globulin 1.7 g/100 ml.

On December 21, shortly after splenoportography, he started having severe abdominal pain to the right of the umbilicus. Blood pressure dropped, aspirated ascites was grossly bloody, and he died the following day. Autopsy disclosed a small bleeding lesion, protruding on the right posterolateral surface of the liver (Fig. 8).

CASE 6. H. H., a 60-year-old male, entered the hospital on July 7, 1969 with chief complaints of malaise, abdominal distention, and leg edema. The massive ascites seen on admission was temporarily decreased with diuretics. The liver was then palpated 2.5 fingerbreadths below the right costal margin. The red cell count was 2,300,000/mm³, SGOT 57 u (Karmen), SGPT 40 u (K.), AL-P 18 u (K.A.), total protein 5.4 g,

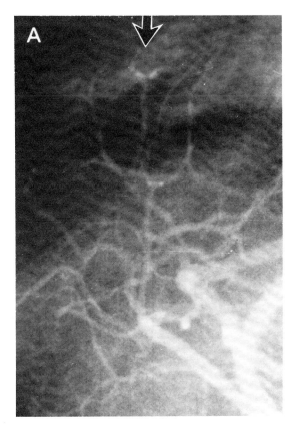

Figure 6   Case 3. *(a)* Celiac angiogram demonstrating a markedly shrunk right liver and a small lesion with displaced fourth order arterial branches (at arrows). *(b)* Mixed macronodular and micronodular cirrhosis superimposed on chronic schistosomiasis. Several small tumor lesions indistinguishable from cirrhotic nodules are seen. The 1.5 x 1.5 cm tumor located subcapsularly in the right superior area (arrow) corresponds to the angiographic change in *(a)*.

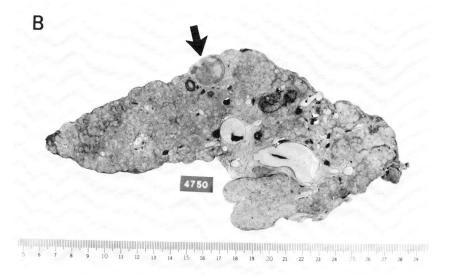

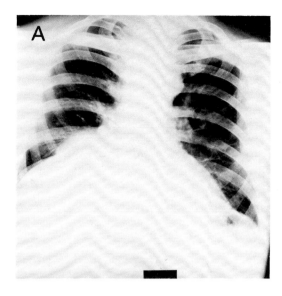

Figure 7   Case 4. (a) Chest film showing a scallop-shaped protrusion of the right diaphragm medially. *(b)* ⁶⁷Ga-citrate scan demonstrating the superior defect to be cold, and the inferior defect to be hot. *(c)* Clinical course of the patient with continuous fever and leukocytosis. *(d)* Chest film taken three weeks after the first film. Marked elevation of the diaphragm and reaction in the thorax are evident. *(e)* A large portion of the tumor showed this type of histology which resembled spindle-cell sarcoma. *(f)* An area where epithelial cells and spindle cells are mixed, suggesting transition between them. There were other areas where cells were in a typical epithelial cell arrangement, and AFP was positive by the immunofluorescent technique.

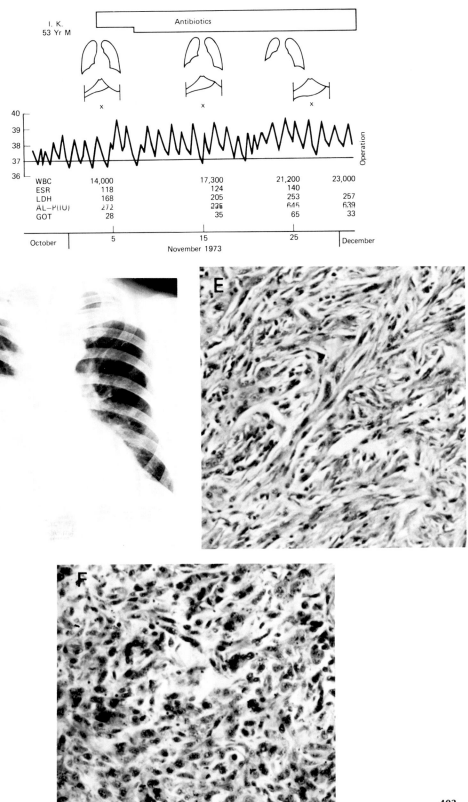

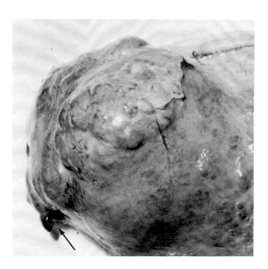

Figure 8 Case 5. A small bleeding lesion seen at autopsy. Although the lesion was small, bleeding was profuse and the patient died within 24 hours.

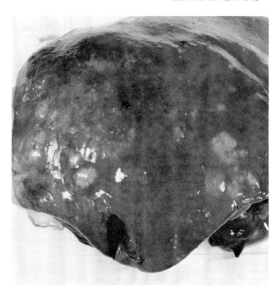

Figure 9 Case 6. A large hole was seen on the surface of a noncirrhotic liver at the time of autopsy. Apparently, a tumor nodule had sloughed off. This 60-year-old male had hemorrhagic ascites and was kept alive for about a month with 32 units of blood transfused.

albumin 2.9 g, γ-globulin 0.97 g/100 ml, and liver scan revealed a large defect in the right lobe of the liver. Ascites was grossly bloody with a hematocrit value of 6%. The red cell count dropped to 1,860,000/mm³ on August 4, which was restored to 4,600,000/mm³ on August 19 after 15 units of blood were transfused. He continued to have hemorrhagic ascites which had to be removed at weekly intervals. Starting August 28, 18 units of blood were transfused to keep the red cell count above 3 million but he succumbed on September 10.

Autopsy disclosed a noncirrhotic liver containing a main tumor in the center of the right lobe together with many small metastases, and a large hole on the right lower anterior edge (Fig. 9). This large defect had been produced by shedding of a tumor nodule. Also noted was a tumor thrombus growing in the hepatic vein and into the inferior veva. It explains the early appearance of leg edema, one of the presenting symptoms of the Budd-Chiari syndrome.

The latter case is rather unusual in the size of perforation. As evident from the photographs, forceful palpation or any self-inflicted physical force on the liver can break a fragile surface of a protruding carcinoma nodule. Once the bleeding has started, spontaneous hemostasis is very unlikely.

Ong and Taw recorded an incidence of tumor rupture in 14.5% of their patients in Hong Kong (34), and in Berman's series (18) the acute abdominal type constituted 8% of the total. Although ascites was bloody in 64 cases or 41.9% of our 153 cases at the time of autopsy, very few had presented with acute abdominal signs clinically. The difference from these reports may be because more of our patients had advanced cirrhosis with ascites, and gradual bleeding did not produce alarming clinical signs.

Metastatic Type

Extrahepatic metastases such as lung and bone lesions may be the first clinical sign to arouse suspicion of primary liver cancer. Metastases to other organs seldom become manifest before the liver tumor is found.

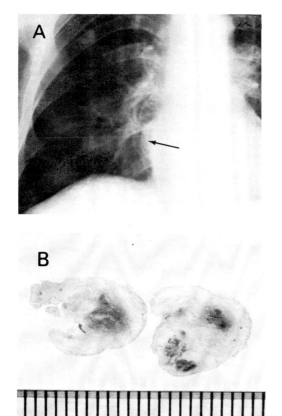

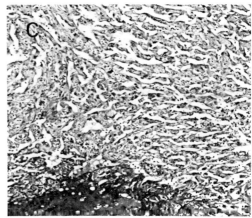

Figure 10 Case 7. *(a)* A small lesion is seen in the right lung along the mediastinum (arrow). This 57-year-old man had been given thorotrast for angiography years ago, and thorium densities are seen below the diaphragm. *(b)* Pieces of expectorate coughed up by the patient. *(c)* hepatocellular carcinoma with blood sinuses. (Courtesy of Dr. M. Igarashi)

CASE 7. C. M., a 57-year-old male, was admitted because of increasing fatigability and weight loss. During World War II, he had sustained a leg wound and malaria. An abdominal radiograph disclosed a typical thorotrast deposit in the liver and spleen. Obviously, thorotrast angiography had been carried out at the time of treatment for gunshot wound. Blood chemistry was not remarkable except for an elevated SLDH (685 u) and AL-P (4.6 Bessey u). Alpha fetoprotein and HBsAg were negative.

Two months after discharge, he started having chest pain and hemoptysis. A chest film demonstrated a round density in the right lower lung along the mediastinum (Fig. 10a). Shortly after readmission, he coughed up two small fragments with sputum (Fig. 10b). Histological study of the expectorated tissue disclosed typical HCC (Fig. 10c). Although the thorotrast densities spread throughout the liver had failed to indicate any cold area on the first admission, liver scan later demonstrated an area of decreased activity in the right lobe of the liver laterally and posteriorly.

Although lung lesions develop early in some patients and may be detected radiographically by chance before liver disease becomes apparent, it occurred in only two in our series. Berman (18) described Negro men with bone metastases producing prominent lumps, and pathologic fracture may be the first presenting symptoms (35). In our series, however, there were only two who first presented with pain due to bone destruction. According to Ohlsen and Norden (36), extrahepatic metastases are more frequent in patients without cirrhosis.

Hepatitis Type

The author has so far experienced five cases of HCC with a clinical course very similar to that of severe hepatitis or progressive hepatic failure. Two of them were diagnosed as acute severe hepatitis at onset, their course was exactly one of subacute hepatitis (submassive necrosis), and a small HCC was found in a cirrhotic liver at autopsy.

CASE 8. T. T. This otherwise healthy 74-year-old male had developed a small sarcoma in the upper pharynx for which ^{60}Co therapy was given. The lesion disappeared completely. Toward the end of the therapy, he developed anorexia and malaise and 4 days after the last dose he noticed pruritus and jaundice. On admission a week later, SGPT was 1270 u (K.) SGOT 880 u (K.), total bilirubin 8.2 mg/100 ml, AL-P 3.4 u (Bessey), and HBsAg was positive. Jaundice was deepening with a peak bilirubin level of 25 mg/100 ml after 3 weeks. At this point, corticosteroid was started with an initial dose of 60 mg prednisolone. The response seemed satisfactory, reducing the total bilirubin to 10 mg/100 ml in 12 days. Subsequent response was slow as shown in Fig. 11a; transaminase activities remained low during the cortisosteroid therapy and BSP retention improved from 29.2% retention to 18.2% at 45 min. HBsAg became negative after two months from the onset, and AFP was negative throughout. Despite improvements in all other liver test results, serum albumin remained in the range of 2.5 to 2.9g/100 ml, and he started having ascites after one month of treatment. Liver scan made two months before death disclosed relatively small but discrete space occupying lesions in the right lobe of the liver superiorly (Fig. 11b). The shape of the liver was compatible with chronic hepatitis, the spleen being small with low radioactivity, and the bone marrow not visualized. Thus the scan was not compatible with long standing cirrhosis or portal hypertension. Autopsy revealed a 5 × 5 × 6 cm tumor, and a small metastasis in the right lobe of a cirrhotic liver; histologically it was a well-differentiated HCC producing bilirubin. The liver cirrhosis was of the thin stromal multilobular type, with severe inflammatory reactions (Fig. 11c).

Another case happened to be the dean of our medical school. He developed jaundice and high serum transaminase levels while traveling. Because of the high γ-globulin and rapidly increasing serum bilirubin levels, a clinical diagnosis of severe hepatitis was made. Despite intensive corticosteroid treatment, his condition gradually deteriorated with continuous mild jaundice. Ascites developed after four months, and he died from massive intraabdominal hemorrhage two months later. A bleeding tumor 5 cm in diameter was found in the right inferoposterior surface of a cirrhotic liver. Cirrhosis was also of the thin stromal type with inflammatory cell infiltrations. Clinically, both cases resembled at the outset severe hepatitis which usually terminates within several months. However, histology of the liver at autopsy was quite different, lacking the features of postnecrotic cirrhosis or submassive necrosis with portal-central bridging.

There was no evidence of preexisting cirrhosis in these cases, but they apparently had had a small HCC at the time of the clinical onset that mimicked acute hepatitis. It is a reasonable postulate that they had unnoticed chronic hepatitis complicated by a small HCC, and hepatitis was exacerbated to progress rapidly to cirrhosis, with simultaneous accelerated growth of the tumor. Such an acutely downhill course is very unusual with chronic hepatitis that was not noticed before exacerbation.

Cholestatic Type

The patient may develop deep jaundice before the tumor becomes large, exhibiting features of surgical jaundice or cholestasis without evidence of severe parenchymal damage. The subsequent clinical course will be that of obstructive jaundice combined with liver carcinoma.

CASE 9.   T. O., a 56-year-old male, entered the hospital on March 17, 1973 because of abnormal blood chemistry. He had had easy fatigability for two years after gastrectomy for an ulcer. Physical examination was not remarkable, and slightly elevated serum bilirubin and alkaline phosphatase were the only abnormal tests. AFP was positive by radial immunodiffusion on admission. Liver scan disclosed a small cold area near the porta hepatis (Fig. 12a) and moderate activities in the spleen and spine. He became increasingly jaundiced, and started having colicky pains in the right upper quadrant suggestive of gallstones. Percutaneous transhepatic cholangiography (37) demonstrated dilated major bile ducts with filling defects both in the right and left hepatic ducts (Fig. 12b). SGOT was elevated mildly, alkaline phosphatase slowly rising, and serum bilirubin soon reached a level of 26 mg/100 ml. Bile duct carcinoma producing AFP was one possibility, and surgical exploration was carried out. No tumor growth was found at the porta hepatis, and he died two weeks later. Autopsy disclosed a cirrhotic liver with diffuse type HCC; the tumor had grown into the large intrahepatic bile ducts proximal to the common hepatic duct (Fig. 12c).

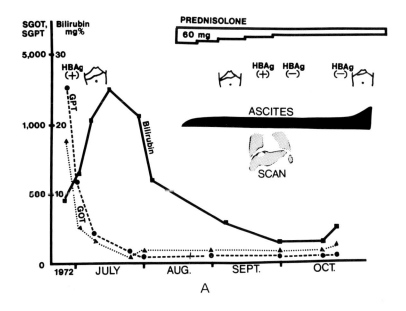

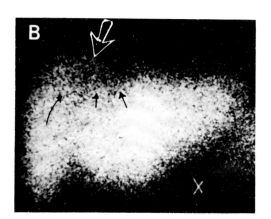

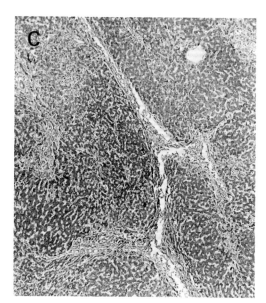

Figure 11 Case 8. *(a)* Chart depicting liver size, ascites, SGOT, SGPT, bilirubin, HBAg, and treatment in relation to the clinical course which was very similar to that of acute severe hepatitis. *(b)* Scintiscan made two months after the onset already showed a space-occupying lesion. There was no indication of fully developed cirrhosis. *(c)* Thin stromal multilobular cirrhosis with severe inflammatory reaction.

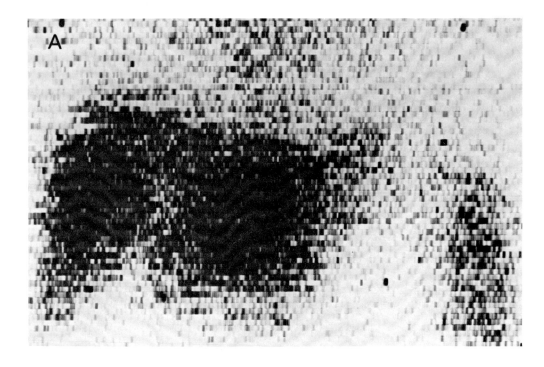

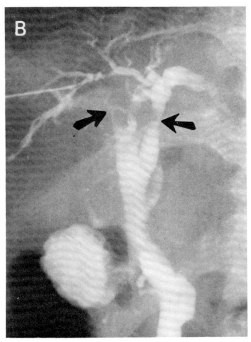

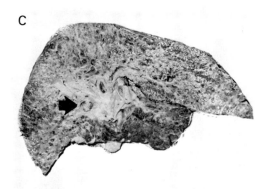

Figure 12 Case 9. *(a)* Liver scan was compatible with cirrhosis and showed a cold area in the center. *(b)* Percutaneous transhepatic cholangiography demonstrated dilated large bile ducts, filling defects in the right and left hepatic ducts (arrows), and irregularities of the intrahepatic ducts. *(c)* Beside small tumor nodules scattered in the cirrhotic liver, tumor growth is seen in the right hepatic duct (at arrow). (Courtesy of Dr. T. Kumagai).

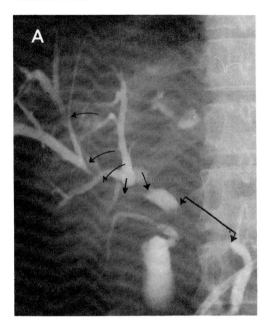

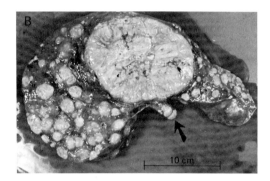

Figure 13   Case 10. *(a)* Percutaneous transhepatic cholaniogram disclosing a curvilinear compression on the right hepatic duct (at arrows) and a filling defect in the common duct (stretch marked) in this 31-year-old male with right upper abdominal colics and jaundice. *(b)* Solitary massive HCC with many intrahepatic mesastases. Tumor was seen growing in the common duct (at arrow).

CASE 10.   M. H., a 31-year-old man, was admitted on March 11, 1972 because of right upper abdominal pain and jaundice. In January he started having dull pain in the right abdomen which turned to colic attacks with jaundice in March. A firm liver was palpated one fingerbreadth below the right costal margin. SGOT was 290 u (K.), AL-P 80 u (K.A.), bilirubin 3.1 mg/100 ml, and AFP positive. Liver scan disclosed a large defect in the central area. Percutaneous transhepatic cholangiography revealed a curvilinear compression over the right major bile duct and a filling defect (Fig. 13a). Exploratory laparotomy was carried out on May 17, but the tumor was not resectable. After the operation, bilirubin started rising and he succumbed to hepatic failure five weeks later. Autopsy disclosed a large mass in the middle portion (the "solitary massive type" by our classification) which was compressing the major bile ducts, and an intraductal growth extending into the common duct (Fig. 13b).

The author has so far experienced four cases including these two. Probably the first detailed description of obstructive jaundice as a presenting symptom of HCC was that of Mallory, which was reported in 1949 (38). In his case, the tumor invaded the cystic duct and a subsequent clot formation in the common duct was the direct cause of obstruction. Fisher (39) operatively removed a cast of tumor with blood clot that had grown from the right hepatic duct into the choledochus. According to Kuroyanagi et al (40), there have been about 20 similar documented cases including 18 HCC, 1 cholangiocarcinoma, and 1 hepatocholangioma. Operation was carried out in 16— choledochotomy in 7, choledochoduodenostomy in 4, hepatectomy in 2, and papillotomy in 1. Except for 2 cases of Rudström (41) and Kuroyanagi (40), all died within 16 days of operation. The content removed from the bile duct by operation was described as "blood clots," "clots with tissue fragments," "greenish friable tissue," "bil-

Table 4   Clinical Forms of Hepatocellular Carcinoma

Classification	Number of Cases	Percentage
Frank type	82	61.6
Cirrhotic type	28	21.1
Occult type	4	3.0
Febrile type	4	3.0
Metastatic type	4	3.0
Hepatitis type	4	3.0
Acute abdominal type	3	2.2
Cholestatic type	1	0.7
Others (not classified)	4	3.0
Total	134	100

iary mud," and "chicken fat." Even though it looks like a blood clot, it usually contains necrotic fragments mixed with viable tissue. Unlike the growth in the portal or hepatic vein, the tumor growing in the bile duct lacks oxygen supply from bathing blood and neovascularization does not occur as readily as in the vein. It necrotizes before forming a long tumor thrombus, is detached, and sometimes occludes the ampulla of Vater (42).

The relative frequency of these eight clinical types is given in Table 4. Of the 130 cases with sufficient data to discern the type, only 20 were atypical not belonging to the frank or the cirrhotic type. A large majority of the patients without clinical evidence of cirrhosis were of the frank type, whereas 1 out of 3 with associated cirrhosis showed the features of the cirrhotic type. Although there were several who had paraneoplastic biochemical syndrome, they were classified by other clinical findings into one of these eight types.

LABORATORY FINDINGS

Urine

Urinalysis is usually unremarkable except for positive urobilinogen and, if there is jaundice, positive bilirubin. Urine volume decreases in patients with ascites and edema as in cirrhosis.

Hematology

The erythrocyte count may decrease with increasing tumor size, but the decrease is much milder in general compared with patients having a carcinoma in the alimentary canal, who often exhibit marked anemias. Anemia in patients with HCC is mostly normochromic normocytic, and sometimes mildly macrocytic. It is impressive to see a patient with a huge liver extending toward the pelvis and who displays no visible anemia. Plethora with increased erythropoietin production has been reported (22), but is very rare. There were several cases in our series who had erythrocyte counts above normal (Fig. 14), but measurements of erythropoietin failed to demonstrate its increase. The leukocyte count was elevated in about one fourth of the patients; it may be elevated in cases with a biliary tract complication or high fever. Leukopenia was mostly associated with splenomegaly.

Blood Chemistry

Biochemical changes in HCC are not much different from those in hepatic cirrhosis or chronic hepatitis except for a few characteristic findings of diagnostic significance. Total serum protein remains within nor-

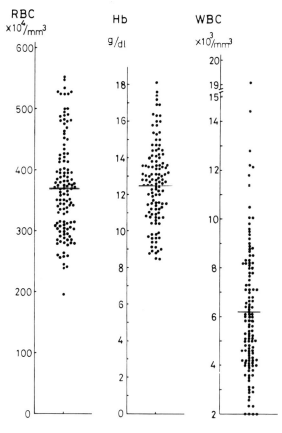

Figure 14 Peripheral blood counts and hemoglobin on admission.

mal limits unless cirrhosis is advanced and ascites removed frequently, or there is the Chiari syndrome. Increase of γ-globulin is more marked in patients with cirrhosis than without (Table 5). It is reflected in abnormal colloid tests such as thymol turbidity and zinc turbidity tests. Polyclonal hyperglobulinemia with plasmacytosis has been reported (43).

Jaundice was seen in about one-third of the patients on admission. The average total serum bilirubin was about 3 mg/100 ml, with the increased conjugated form. An excised liver containing a small HCC, taken from an anicteric patient may have scattered lobules exhibiting distinct cholestatic findings such as bile thrombi. As long as the regurgitated bilirubin is handled by functioning lobules, there will be no overt jaundice. Therefore, increasing serum bilirubin, such as one sees in the cirrhotic patient with HCC, is an ominous sign for prognosis, suggesting a decreasing capacity of the liver parenchyma to metabolize this pigment and other organic anions. In isolated cases, elevated serum bilirubin is due to biliary obstruction as just described.

The mean total cholesterol in serum was normal in our series, and the difference from the report of Alpert et al (44) in African patients is of interest. One of the possible explanations may be the difference in the normal values. Normal serum cholesterol levels are obviously lower in the inhabitants of Uganda. Unlike in the ordinary cholestatic disease, the total cholesterol was not elevated in proportion to the alkaline phosphatase level in sera of pa-

Table 5   Blood Chemistry on Admission

Test	HCC s̄ Cirrhosis (39 Cases)	HCC c̄ Cirrhosis (90 Cases)	Total (129 Cases)
Total protein (g/100 ml)	7.2 ± 0.1	7.1 ± 0.1	7.2 ± 0.1
Albumin (g/100 ml)	3.7 ± 0.1	3.5 ± 0.1	3.4 ± 0.1
γ-Globulin (g/100 ml)	1.3 ± 0.1**	2.0 ± 0.1**	1.8 ± 0.1
Thymol turbidity T. (u)	3.7 ± 0.5**	6.5 ± 0.4**	5.7 ± 0.3
Zinc T.T. (u)	11.3 ± 1.0**	18.6 ± 0.8**	16.4 ± 0.7
Total bilirubin (mg/100 ml)	2.7 ± 0.7	3.4 ± 0.5	3.2 ± 0.4
Total cholesterol (mg/100 ml)	208 ± 13	191 ± 7	196 ± 7
BSP (% at 45 minutes)	16.2 ± 2.0**	24.7 ± 1.8**	21.8 ± 1.4
SGOT (Karmen u)	96 ± 12**	152 ± 14**	135 ± 11
SGPT (Karmen u)	42 ± 5	54 ± 5	50 ± 4
AL-P (K.A. u)	28 ± 3	24 ± 2	25 ± 1
SLDH (Wroblewski u)	421 ± 52*	614 ± 80*	569 ± 29
LAP (u)[a]	360 ± 42	380 ± 36	376 ± 29
γ-GTP (mu/ml)[b]	116 ± 43	175 ± 28	166 ± 25

Figures: Mean ± S.E.
*$p < 0.05$, **$p < 0.01$
[a] Leucine aminopeptidase.
[b] γ-Glutamyl. transpeptidase.

tients with HCC. Choline esterase activities in serum were decreased in all patients, to a greater extent in those with cirrhosis, and decreased protein synthesis or parenchymatous damage was suggested. The bromsulfalein test showed varying degrees of dye retention that were poorly correlated with serum bilirubin in the absence of overt jaundice. This dissociation of BSP from bilirubin was less significant in the diagnosis compared with that between alkaline phosphatase and bilirubin.

Serum levels of transaminases usually remain mildly elevated during the quiescent stage; they rise with the progress of the disease. Elevation of SGOT levels is almost always greater than that of SGPT (Fig. 15), a finding that has long been noted even more so in HCC (45, 46) than in chronic active hepatitis, but little emphasized. If the transaminase levels fluctuate, elevation may be due to liver cell damage by tumor invasion as well as tissue anoxia resulting from neoplastic thrombosis of portal tributaries. When hepatitis exacerbates acutely with a sharp rise in transaminase activities, SGPT level may temporarily be higher than that of SGOT. As the disease advances, the SGOT level increases out of proportion to SGPT level and, toward the terminal phase, the difference between SGOT and SGPT becomes greater, the former being more than threefold the latter (Fig. 16). Thus an increasing difference between SGOT and SGPT activities, greater than a factor of 3, indicates the end stage or approach of the terminus.

In order to explain these characteristic changes of SGOT and SGPT and their relationship, we measured these enzyme concentrations in hepatoma tissue in comparison with the nontumorous portion in the same livers. It was found that on a wet gram basis, tumor tissue contained less transaminase activities compared with liver parenchyma, and that SGOT was always

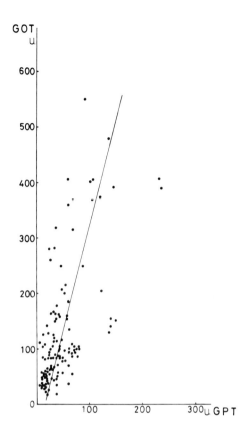

Figure 15 Correlation between SGOT and SGPT on admission. SGOT was almost always greater than SGPT ($r = 0.6877$) with a regession of $23x - 6y - 380 = 0$.

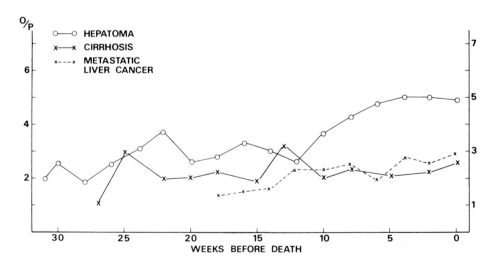

Figure 16 The average ratios of SGOT/SGPT (Karmen units) along the course of HCC (83 cases), cirrhosis (32 cases), and metastatic liver carcinoma (26 cases). Note that this ratio is greater than unity in fully developed cirrhosis and liver cancers, and that it is elevated above 3 several months before death in HCC.

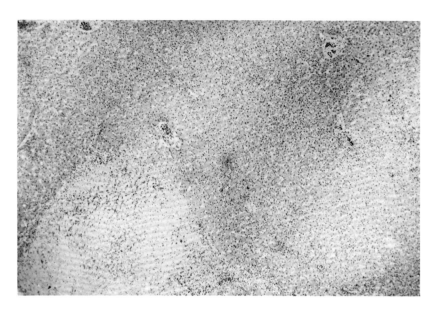

Figure 17 Circumscribed necrosis seen in the noncancerous portion of the resected liver quite apart from the tumor (Case 2). SGOT was 265 u and SGPT 80 u at the time of operation.

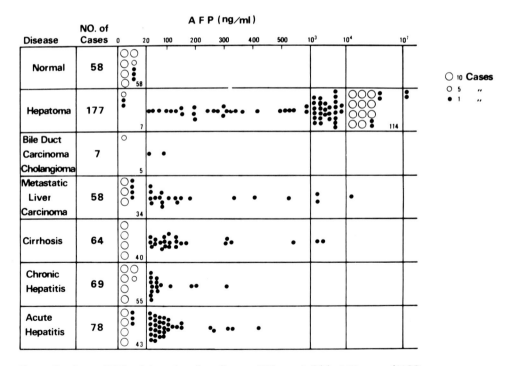

Figure 18 Serum AFP levels in various liver diseases (511 cases). Of the 177 cases of HCC, AFP was above 400 ng/ml in 149 cases (84.2%) and above 1000 ng/ml in 142 cases (80.3%); 7 cases (4%) were below 20 ng/ml and negative. The AFP levels in 58 normal control patients were less than 12 ng/ml.

greater in activity that SGPT. Thus elevated SGOT may be derived from necrosis of carcinoma, growing tumor cells and liver cell damage such as patchy anoxemic necroses constantly occurring in liver parenchyma. The author was surprised to find small necrotic foci in the parenchyma of the liver with a small HCC, excised in an early stage of the disease (Fig. 17). In some patients both SGOT and SGPT are sharply elevated maintaining their ratio shortly before death. This event detailed later is an exaggerated state of widespread anoxemic necroses.

Before the advent of the AFP test, more diagnostic significance was given to the so-called dissociation between alkaline phosphatase and bilirubin than any other biochemical changes (47, 48). In a large proportion of patients, alkaline phosphatase activity becomes elevated in the absence of jaundice or out of proportion to serum bilirubin levels (49). Alkaline phosphatasemia may be caused by cholestasis occurring at the lobular level as is the case with bilirubin. Dissociation between these two tests may be explained by the ability and inability of hepatocytes to dispose of bilirubin and alkaline phosphatase, respectively. Like transaminases, this enzyme activity is also progressively elevated.

Alpha Fetoprotein

We have so far determined AFP in serum using the radioimmunoassay in 511 cases of various liver diseases including 177 of HCC (Fig. 18). The positivity rate varies with the setting of the upper normal limit which depends on the individual investigator. Of the 177 cases of HCC, AFP was above 1000 ng/ml in 142 cases (80.3%), and above 400 ng/ml in 149 (84.2%). The negative values have been calculated from 58 cases of controls to be below 12 ng/ml. Dynamic changes rather than single determination are of diagnostic importance in the low level range (50). We prefer setting

an arbitrary line at 400 ng/ml, based on our observations that in most HCC patients with values below this level at the time the diagnosis of liver tumor has become unmistakable, AFP levels remain low throughout. Values above this level were obtained in 4 of 58 patients with metastatic liver carcinoma, in 3 of 64 cirrhosis patients, and in 1 case of subacute hepatitis. Serum AFP levels lower than 400 ng/ml but above the upper normal limit are frequently encountered in various stages of hepatitis and cirrhosis. It rises after an interval of a few weeks subsequent to acute liver cell damage as indicated by elevated serum transaminase, but comes down quickly. It is very seldom that serum AFP levels remain elevated for more than three months under such circumstances; increased AFP is probably a reflection of very active regenerative processes. Continued study of patients with low but abnormal serum AFP values are most important in the detection of early HCC.

The total activity of serum lactic dehydrogenase (LDH) is elevated in varying degrees (Table 5) and levels continue to rise as the disease progresses, but its correlation with tumor size is not apparent, probably because of the multiple origins on the lactic dehydrogenase group of enzymes. However, the LDH zymogram may be of value in the differentiation from metastatic liver carcinoma—LDH_5 is usually higher than LDH_4 in HCC and a reversed relationship holds for metastatic liver carcinomas (Fig. 19).

Other serum enzyme levels and their changes are also given in Table 5. Gamma-glutamyl transpeptidase (γ-GTP) was elevated considerably in our patients, particularly in those with cirrhosis. This enzyme is contained in high concentrations in Morris hepatoma tissue (51), and the isozyme pattern is similar to that of the fetus. The diagnostic value of this enzyme remains to be assessed since it is increased in other liver diseases. Leucine aminopeptidase (LAP) levels were increased in various de-

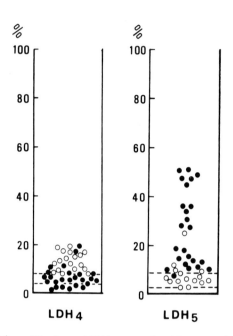

Figure 19 Serum LDH isozymes 4 and 5 expressed as a percentage. LDH5 is more often higher than LDH4 in HCC and vice versa in metastatic liver carcinoma, with some exceptions.

grees but had little diagnostic value because of the lack of specificity.

RADIOLOGY

Changes of the Diaphragm

Elevation of the right diaphragm, general or localized, is frequently seen with limitation of its movement. There may be horizontal streaks of atelectasis in the lung immediately above an extremely elevated diaphragm. Even though the diaphragm looks normal in the posteroanterior projection, the lateral view may reveal an abnor-

mal curvature or elevation of its posterior slope. Introduction of a small quantity of air in the abdominal cavity may demonstrate an irregular surface of the liver (Fig. 20).

Hepatomegaly

Enlargement of the liver may be discerned on a plain abdominal film from the liver density that is bordered by the diaphragm superiorly and by the gas in the ascending colon and duodenal cap inferomedially. The displacement of the stomach and/or compression on the lesser curvature is readily seen in the barium swallow examination. In rare instances, the tumor in the left lobe exerts pressure on the corpus of the stomach posteriorly (Fig. 5).

Other Direct and Indirect Signs

Calcification in the liver may be seen in HCC. It is more frequently seen in hepatoblastoma because of the mesenchymal elements in the tumor. When it occurs in adults, it is usually associated with necrosis of the tumor—calcification occurs subsequent to necrosis within a relatively short period of time (Fig. 21).

Lung metastases may be found on a routine chest film before the tumor is found in the liver. They are usually coin-shaped, but the author has seen two cases that resembled miliary tuberculosis (Fig. 22). Bone metastases can be an early clinical sign and lytic bone lesions may be demonstrated.

Selective Angiography

Selective arteriography using a guide wire through the femoral artery and a pre-shaped synthetic catheter (52, 53), is probably an indispensable procedure for diagnosis. More precise information is obtained if the catheter tip were advanced superselectively to the hepatic artery proper or even further into the first branch (Fig. 23).

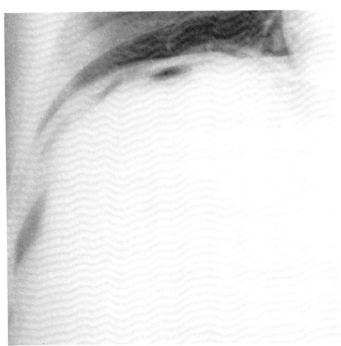

Figure 20 Irregular surface of the liver revealed after introduction of a small amount of air into the abdominal cavity.

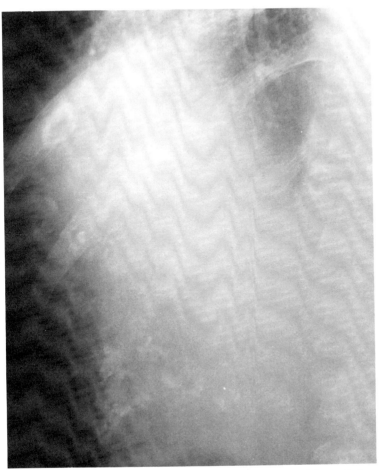

417

Figure 21 Calcification of HCC that occurred after four intraarterial doses of Mitomycin C. This 63-year-old male had had hepatomegaly for several years, and was subsequently found to have a huge encapsulated HCC occupying the entire right lobe.

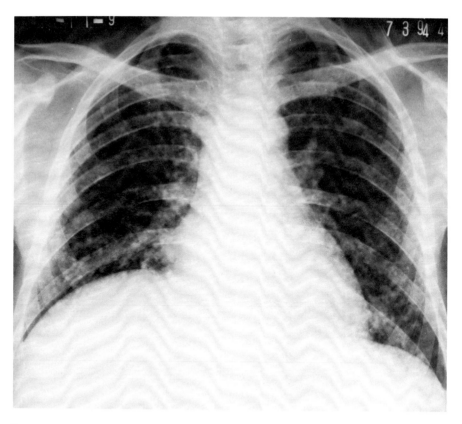

Figure 22 Lung metastases of HCC mimicking miliary tuberculosis. Note the heavier dissemination in the lower lung fields in contrast to hematogenous tuberculosis which produces denser spread in the apex and upper lungs.

The major abnormalities seen in HCC are as follows: (54–67): dilatation of the hepatic artery, displacement or stretching of intrahepatic arteries, increased vascularity, tumor vessels, tumor stain or pooling of the contrast material, arteriovenous shunts in and around the tumor, visualization of portal branches outside the tumor, and retrograde opacification of the portal vein (58). Of these, the last three are pathognomonic for HCC and important in distinguishing from metastatic carconomas.

Although the degree of neovascularization or formation of tumor vessels varies with the gross anatomical types, it is generally more marked compared with metastatic carcinomas. The arterial tumor vessels

in the tumor as described by Yü (54), to be characteristic of HCC, represent not only large vasculature in the stroma between nodules within a massive tumor, but in the encapsulated type they correspond to large irregular vessels in the pseudocapsule— they are filled by arterial blood and drain slowly, acting like venous channels (Fig. 24). During the arterial phase, portal branches of various calibers are opacified as a result of transit of contrast medium into a relatively large branch and, the contrast medium is sent therefrom toward the periphery (Fig. 25). As discussed in the chapter by Dr. Nakashima, portal branches come to act as the efferent vasa for tumor nodules. Should this phenomenon become

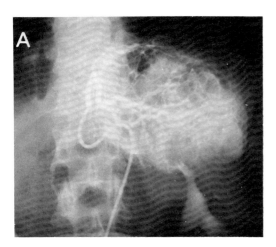

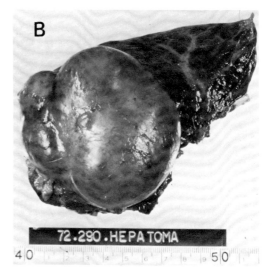

Figure 23 *(a)* Superselective arteriography of the left hepatic artery, demonstrating an oval-shaped area of neovasculature and hypervascularity. *(b)* Resected left lobe containing a 7.5 x 6 x 4 cm HCC. It was the solitary (massive) type by our nomenclature, and the liver parenchyma was mildly cirrhotic (thin septal multilobular type). This 46-year-old man lived 22 months after the operation.

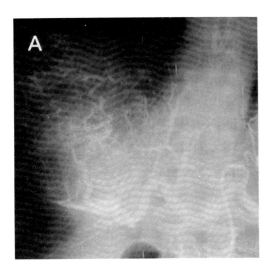

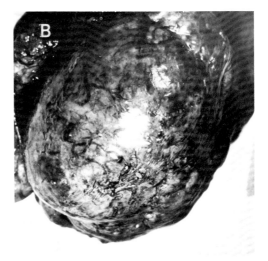

Figure 24 *(a)* Celiac angiogram demonstrating a large mass with typical tumor vessels and displacement of large arteries. Displacement of large vessels is seen only in livers with a large spherical tumor, either the encapsulted or the solitary massive type by our nomenclature (Case 11). *(b)* The encapsulated type of hepatocellular carcinoma. Note the large irregular vessels in the capsule that correspond to some of the tumor vessels in the previous angiogram.

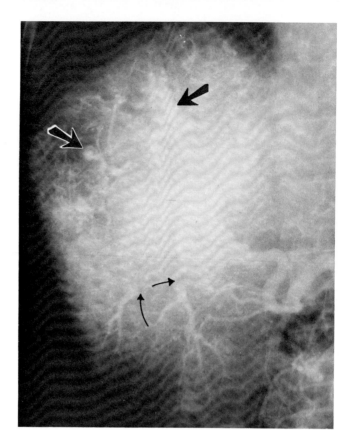

Figure 25 Typical arteriogram of HCC. During the arterial phase, large irregular and tortuous vessels are visualized (tumor vessels) which remain opacified through the capillary phase with transition of contrast medium to similarly large irregular venous channels (upper arrows). Two distinct portal branches are seen in the inferior noncancerous portion (lower arrows), representing typical A-V (A-portal) shunts.

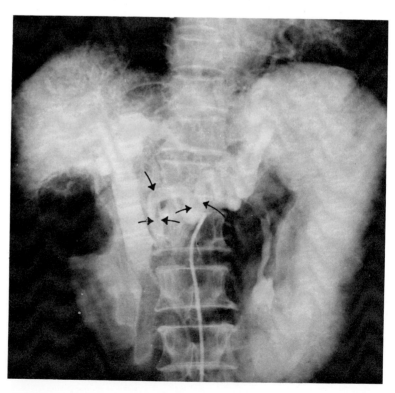

420

Figure 26 Retrograde flow of contrast medium in the portal vein. Note small filling defects in the collateral veins which represent tumor thrombi (arrows) (Okuda, K. et al: *Am. J. Roentgen. Rad. Ther. Nucl. Med.* **119**:419, 1973).

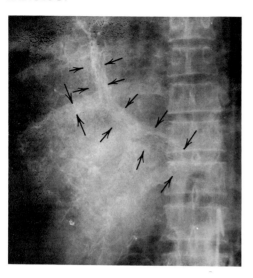

Figure 27 Angiographic demonstration of tumor thrombus growing as a continuous cast or mold in the portal vein. Contrast medium regurgitates in the portal vein with an appearance of a "bundle of thread" (Okuda, K. et al: *Radiology* **117**:303, 1975).

exaggerated, the amount of blood entering the portal vein increases, its pressure surpasses that of portal blood and causes a retrograde flow in the portal trunk. The contrast medium injected intraarterially sometimes opacifies even the collateral veins (Fig. 26). In such cases, tumor thrombi may be seen at autopsy as far as the esophageal varices. The presence of tumor cast is presumed from the "bundle of thread" appearance of the portal vein (Fig. 27). In more than 60 cases we have studied the celiac angiograms in comparison with the changes postmortem or in excised livers in order to correlate angiographic alterations with gross pathology, and we believe that the gross anatomical types can be anticipated from the angiogram with certain accuracy. The anatomical classification that has generally been used is that of Eggel proposed in 1901 (59), which is too simple for clinical purposes. Nakashima and the author have recently described a new gross anatomical classification (19), and the corresponding angiographic characteristics are as follows: the diffuse (type I) and fine no-

dular diffuse (type II)—no displacement of major arteries, little change in the arterial phase, and small irregular poolings in the venous phase (Fig. 28). In multinodular type (III), displacement and stretching of the third and fourth order arterial branches, hypervascularity, and fairly well-demarcated stains in the venous phase are the rule. The cirrhotic oligondular type (IV) features the same vascular alterations that are found in cirrhosis, such as coiling and cork-screw appearance of arteries of the second and third order, sometimes of the first order, shrunk right liver, and tumor stain hardly discernible in the venous phase. Displacement of the fourth or fifth order arteries may be found on careful examination (Fig. 6). The encapsulated type (V) has a round area of hypervascularity containing abnormal tumor vessels in the arterial phase with curvilinear displacement of large vessels that surround the round mass (Fig. 24), and a thin rim of translucency in the venous phase (Fig. 29). The nodular massive type (VI) shows displacement and stretching of the third and fourth order arterial branches with marked hypervascularity, frequent arteriovenous shunts and retrograde portal flow, and strong tumor stains in the venous phase. The solitary massive type (VII), typically a fast growing tumor, is very hypervascular with a round arrangement of large vessels, containing abnormal tumor vessels (Figs. 3*c* and 23*a*); round pooling of contrast medium is seen in the venous phase without a translucent rim. The confluent massive type (VIII), in which small nodules coalesce, has large arteries buried with some encasement in the mass rather than displaced; vascularity is moderate but not marked and the tumor is not linearly demarcated from normal tissue (Fig. 30).

The angiographic findings obtained in 92 cases of HCC are summarized in Table 6. It is to be noted that displacement of large vessels are seen only in cases with a large mass and that diffuse types are infre-

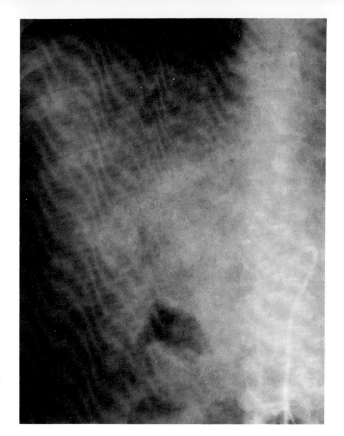

Figure 28 The diffuse type of HCC. Multiple small poolings are seen throughout the liver in the venous phase. The arterial phase is unremarkable.

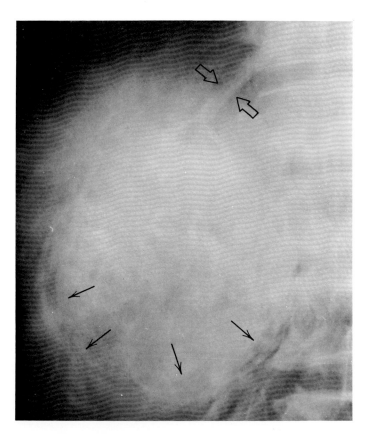

Figure 29 The venous phase of the celiac angiogram exhibiting a thin radiolucent circumferential rim (at arrows), which corresponds to the capsule. Note also the opacified hepatic vein (thick arrows).

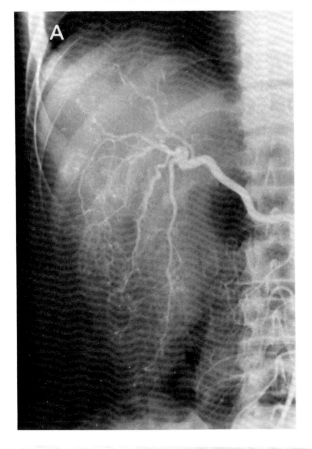

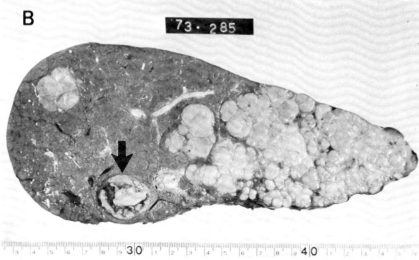

Figure 30 Comparison of celiac arteriogram and resected liver containing the confluent massive type of HCC. Note the irregular encasements of the arterial branches in the right liver inferiorly without displacement of large vessels *(a)*. The encapsulated tumor (at arrow) presumably is the original nodule from which the rest of the tumor had metastasized. Because of the slow growth the original nodule becomes encapsulated.

Table 6 Angiographic Characteristis of HCC and Gross Anatomical Types by Nakashima-Okuda's Classification (92 Cases)[a]

Type	Number of Cases	Hypervascularity (%)	Abnormally Large Arteries (%)	Large Vessel Displacement (%)	Encasement (%)	Arteriovenous Shunt (%)	Portal Regurgitation (%)	Circumferential Lucency (%)
I and II. Diffuse and finenodular diffuse	3	33	0	0	0	0	0	0
III. Multinodular	13	77	38	0	0	77	8	0
IV. Cirrhotic oligonodular	4	50	0	0	0	0	25	0
V. Encapsulated	15	100	73	87	0	73	7	87
VI. Nodular massive	24	92	25	42	17	75	17	0
VII. Solitary massive	18	100	78	89	56	94	11	0
VIII. Confluent massive	15	93	27	7	60	100	7	0
Total	92	87	44	44	25	81	11	14

[a] Types were confirmed by autopsy or resection in half, and presumed from scan and laparoscopy in the rest.

quent and difficult to diagnose. Regurgitation of contrast medium was seen in 13 cases, with little relation to anatomical types.

Scintigraphy

The value of scanning in the early diagnosis of HCC is still limited. Celiac angiography may excel in detecting small lesions (see Case 3), since the scan is incapable of demonstrating with certainty tumors smaller than 3 cm. The two procedures done on the same individual will prove more diagnostic than one method alone. In ^{198}Au colloid scans, clearly demarcated, multiple lesions are more suggestive of metastatic carcinoma (57). It is due to the discrete boundary between the tumor and well-functioning parenchyma. In HCC the surrounding liver tissue is cirrhotic in many instances and takes up colloid poorly. Although the count rate is low with ^{198}Au compared with ^{99m}Tc, it serves in the assessment of blood flow in the liver parenchyma, and hence in the diagnosis of cirrhosis. Should HCC develop in a non-cirrhotic liver, it is usually massive and the defect is single—intrahepatic metastases in this type seldom produce large discrete cold areas. The analysis of scans of 104 cases revealed that the lesion of HCC is either single and large, is poorly demarcated in a mottled liver, or is occupying the right lateral area having a poorly demarcated and advancing boundary with the intact liver. Bieler et al (60) described a type of multiple defect with uneven uptake and rapidly downhill course. It may correspond to our second type. Our statistics on the scans made with ^{198}Au colloid showed that the major defect or lesion was in the right lobe in 62 (73%) out of a total of 85 cases; the lesion was located in the middle area in 10 (11.8%) and in the left lobe in 13 (15.3%). The changes typical of cirrhosis were the predominant findings masking the tumor in 7 cases.

Certain types, but not every type, of HCC concentrates ^{67}Ga-citrate or ^{75}Se-methionine (cf. Case 4). It has not yet been determined whether the degree of incorporation of these radionuclides is related to the degree of differentiation of the tumor cell or the speed of growth. Liver cell adenoma (61) and even well-differentiated HCC take up rose-bengal (62). Use of several radionuclides or sequential imaging with a gamma camera has been recommended to assess vascularity of the mass (63, 64).

DIAGNOSIS

Diagnosis of liver malignancy is not difficult if the liver is enlarged and has increased consistency and surface irregularity. With awareness of the close association of HCC and cirrhosis, and with the aid of the various diagnostic techniques such as laparoscopy, biopsy, and radiology described previously, HCC is seldom missed antemortem in well-equipped large hospitals. Difficulty is encountered, however, in patients who are rushed in for acute abdominal signs and expire before any examination is made, or in those who present with symptoms of advanced cirrhosis (the occult type). In countries where primary liver carcinoma is a rarity, the disease is more often mistaken for metastatic liver carcinoma. According to Moseley (65), a correct diagnosis was made in only 37% of the cases in Boston, whereas in a Chicago series (66), 22 out of 80 cases were correctly diagnosed. In 149 cases of HCC autopsied at Kurume University Hospital, correct diagnosis had been made in 99 cases (66.4%), and the diagnosis of cirrhosis alone in 27 cases (18.1%).

Differential diagnosis of HCC and intrahepatic cholangiocarcinoma is extremely difficult (67). Cholangiocarcinomas arising off the porta hepatis in particular poses a real diagnostic problem because of the absence of jaundice. Other than angiographic hypovascularity and negative AFP, there

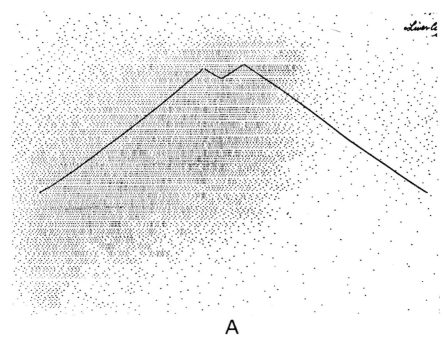

A

are no distinguishing features clinically. In our 22 autopsy cases of cholangiocarcinoma, including those located at the hilum, diagnosis of HCC was made in 7 who had had no jaundice, and in 3 the diagnosis was "either hepatoma or bile duct carcinoma." Only 2 had cirrhosis and this incidence was about the same as reported elsewhere (5, 33, 68). Diagnosis of HCC was made in one case of adenoma (hamartoma) in our series. Scintigraphic demonstration of cellular functions may be helpful in such cases (61).

CLINICAL COURSE

The clinical course is just as variable as the disease itself. Death may intervene within a few days of the onset of symptoms in the abdominal type, or on the other hand, the patient may live for years after the tumor is detected. Some of the typical clinical types have already been described. In the literature, case reports have appeared sporadically about long-term survival (69, 70). They probably represented cases of the encapsulated form of HCC, a specific type that deserves brief discussion. Grossly, the carcinoma is encapsulated or surrounded by a thick "pseudocapsule" formed by accumulation of connective tissue and fibers subsequent to disappearance of liver cells by compression and collagenization of reticulin fibers, and by encompassing remaining portal tracts. Formation of the capsule is indicative of the lack of invasiveness and slowness of the growth of the tumor. Theoretically, surgical resection is best indicated in this type of HCC if detected early; because of the lack of symptoms, the tumor is already large when diagnosis is made in most instances.

CASE 11. C. N., a 71-year-old alcoholic druggist, was first told that he had acute hepatitis in March 1968 when he had grippelike symptoms. He was hospitalized briefly for hepatomegaly and high transaminase levels and treated ambulatorily thereafter. The first liver scan (Fig. 31a), made a year later, already showed a distinct defect, but he refused any surgical

C.N.　71 Yr.　M.

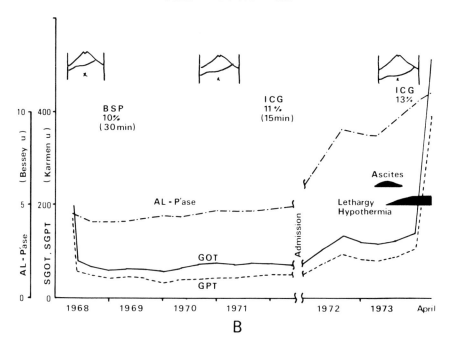

B

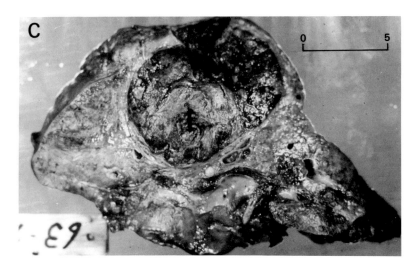

Figure 31 Case 11. (a) Liver scan made four years prior to death already showed a large defect in the right superolateral area. (b) Clinical course that started with an episode mimicking acute hepatitis. Serum enzymes were continuously abnormal with SGOT greater than SGPT, and AFP remained negative throughout. (c) A large hepatocellular carcinoma surrounded by a thick fibrous capsule. The tumor was dark greenish-browh (green hepatoma). There was mild fibrosis in the noncancerous portion.

intervention because of the lack of symptoms. SGOT, SGPT, and AL-P levels were all mildly elevated, and AFP remained less than 3 ng/ml throughout. He was finally admitted in October 1972 because of abdominal distension. Celiac angiography disclosed a typical pattern of the encapsulated HCC (see Fig. 24a). The subsequent course was extremely slow. Ascites was noted only for a short period several months before death. He occasionally ran an unexplained fever. The scintigraphic defect grew somewhat larger but not much during the four years of follow-up from the first scan. Anemia never became severe, serum albumin was within normal limits throughout, γ-globulin was slightly increased, and serum bilirubin increased only terminally and mildly. In the end stage, he was lethargic and hypothermic for almost a month (Fig. 31b). It is to be noted that SGOT levels remained definitely higher than SGPT throughout, and that both were elevated sharply toward the end as discussed below. He succumbed in April 1973, five years after the onset of clinical signs.

Autopsy disclosed one large tumor in the superio-posterior area, surrounded by a thick pseudocapsule, and small intrahepatic metastases (Fig. 31c). Histologically, the carcinoma cells were well-differentiated and producing bilirubin in places. The nontumorous portion was not cirrhotic and compatible with chronic hepatitis with minimal inflammatory activities.

TERMINAL RISE OF SERUM TRANSAMINASES AND LACTIC DEHYDROGENASE

Esophageal varices may rupture toward the terminus, and the patient will lapse into coma from hepatic failure and die soon. Blood withdrawn shortly before death sometimes reveals a phenomenal rise in the serum levels of transaminases and lactic dehydrogenase. The author has experienced at least six cases of such terminal rise, five with HCC and one with extensive metastatic liver cancer. In four, there was an obvious episode of a large blood loss. Autopsy invariably revealed extensive necrosis of liver parenchyma, mostly outside the tumorous tissue. The following case illustrates this terminal event.

CASE 12. I. I., a 54-year-old male, was found to have enlargement of the liver, abnormal blood chemistry, and spider angiomata in December 1967. In April 1971, when AFP was found positive (5400 ng/ml), he was hospitalized for evaluation. There was positive fluid wave with moderately dilated veins

of the abdominal wall. Blood chemistry consisted of the following: SGOT 58 u (K.), SGPT 40 u (K.), AL-P 22 u (K.A.), SLDH 465 u, albumin 3.3 g, γ-globulin 2.3 g, and total bilirubin 1.1 mg/100 ml. Liver scan disclosed a large area of reduced activity in the right lobe, where neovasculature and displacement of large vessels were seen by celiac angiography.

He had massive hematemesis on May 25, and the blood pressure dropped to a level barely measurable. He regained consciousness after vigorous blood transfusions, but succumbed two days later. Blood taken shortly before death showed a remarkable change in chemistry: SGOT and SGPT both above 3000 u, SLDH 4150 u, AL-P 59.8 u (K.A.), and total bilirubin 5.7 mg/100 ml.

Autopsy disclosed an encapsulated HCC in the right lobe of the liver. Although parenchymal necrosis of the liver was suggested from the gross appearance of the cut surface, patchy necroses became evident after formalin fixation (Fig. 32a). Multilobular size necroses were seen mainly in the left lobe where there was no tumor, clearly demarcated by narrow hemorrhagic rims (Fig. 32b). Tumor tissues were spared from necrosis.

We assume that this type of necrosis is caused by hypoxia as a result of sudden drop in blood pressure. The areas that were receiving barely sufficient oxygen for self-sustenance because of portal thrombosis or portal stenosis can no longer live as the blood supply has dropped below the critical level. An irregular multilobular distribution of necroses speaks for the theory that some lobules were receiving less oxygen than others and only the former lose viability at a marginal deficiency of oxygen. That the reduced portal flow is more responsible than reduction in the arterial supply may be evident from the fact that the tumor nodules remain unaffected. If the patient lives for a few more days, bleeding occurs in the periphery of necrotic lesions where blood circulation has recurred after the rise of blood pressure.

COMPLICATIONS

Extrahepatic metastases are found at the

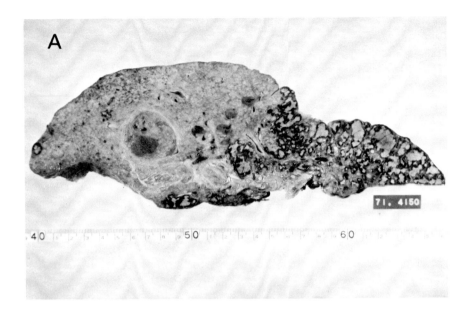

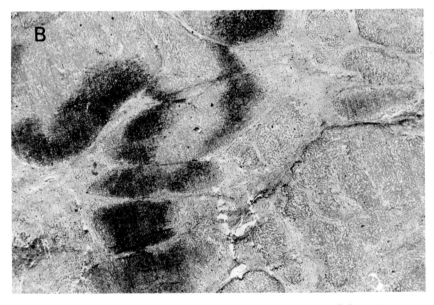

Figure 32 *(a)* Hepatic necrosis occurring as a terminal event in hepatocellular carcinoma. Necroses of varying sizes are seen in the nontumorous left lobe clearly demarcated by hemorrhagic rims. *(b)* Photomicrograph of an area of necrosis. Note the bleeding in the periphery of necrosis that may suggest a regain of blood pressure (10X).

Table 7   Extrahepatic Metastases in 153 Autopsied Cases

Organ	Percentage	Lymph Node	Percentage
Lung	42.7	Lung hilum	11.2
Pancreas	5.6	Periaortic	4.9
Adrenal	5.6	Peribronchial	3.5
Diaphragm	5.6	Perigastric	3.5
Douglas' pouch	4.9	Peripancreatic	3.5
Peritoneum	3.5	Liver hilum	2.8
Rectum	2.1	Retroperitoneal	2.1
Liver hilum	2.1	Mesenteric	2.1
Gallbladder	2.1	Virchow	1.4
Along common duct	2.1		
Bone	1.4		
Omentum	1.4		

time of autopsy in 50 to 86% and lymphatic spread in 30 to 67% (31, 71–73). The organs and lymphnodes with metastases in our autopsied cases are given in Table 7. Clinically, however, symptoms attributable to metastases are much less frequent and seldom the direct cause of death. Lung metastases, which are by far the most common because of the tendency to intravenous growth, were found in 42.7% at autopsy (diagnosed antemortem in only 27.1%). Bone metastases were found in only 1.4% at the time of autopsy. Although small metastatic lesions were sometimes found in the peritoneum or Douglas' pouch during autopsy, none exhibited clinically the signs of peritonitis carcinomatosa, which is characterized by ascites with high protein concentrations, a hard abdominal wall, and palpable mesenteric masses. The author has seen two cases of Virchow's metastasis.

Perihepatic invasion of HCC is rare unless the tumor is anaplastic and highly malignant as in Case 4. There were two cases in which the tumor invaded into the thorax continuously from the liver; in one of them we were able to diagnose it by celiac angiography (Fig. 33). Carcinomatous pleuritis consequent on penetrating invasion has also been reported (71).

Bleeding from the tumor on the liver surface is the most dangerous complication

as already discussed. Tumor growth into the inferior vena cava is not an infrequent occurrence, causing the Budd-Chiari syndrome. The diagnosis may be achieved by cavography (Fig. 34). The tumor grows sometimes into the right atrium as a continuous intravascular cast, and may even reach the lung through the right ventricle (Fig. 35).

It is known that patients with massive ascites develop spontaneous hydrothorax, and the same phenomenon occurs in HCC. In our 134 clinical cases, moderate to massive pleural effusion developed in 10 cases, in the right side in 6 and in the left in 4. Other related complications include rupture of varices and bile duct obstruction (the cholestatic form).

Portal thrombosis by the tumor in the liver is quite common (57, 74), and it was recognized grossly in 71.5% of our autopsy material. Clinically, however, it is seldom diagnosed. Rapid appearance of the signs of portal hypertension is suggestive of the condition, but definite diagnosis is only feasible with celiac angiography (see Figs. 26 and 27).

TREATMENT AND PROGNOSIS

Surgical removal of the tumor before metastasis occurs is the only radical treatment,

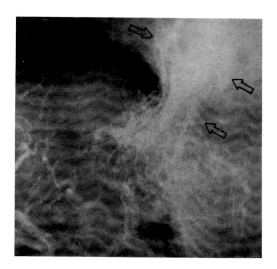

Figure 33 Celiac angiogram demonstrating marked neovasculature in the middle portion of the liver superiorly, entering into the mediastinum.

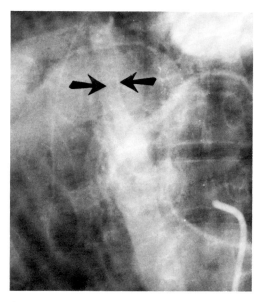

Figure 34 Cavogram obtained in the venous phase of superior mesenteric angiography. Note the abrupt halt of the flow of medium at the level of the diaphragm (at thin arrow), and compression in the hepatic portion caused by tumor (thick arrows).

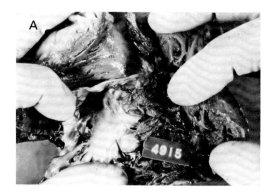

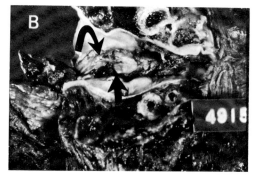

Figure 35 *(a)* Tumor cast growing through the tricuspid values. This 73-year-old man had cirrhosis for 7 years, developed ascites and leg edema 2.5 months previously, and died from rupture of varices. *(b)* Tumor cast growing in the pulmonary artery continuous from the right ventricle.

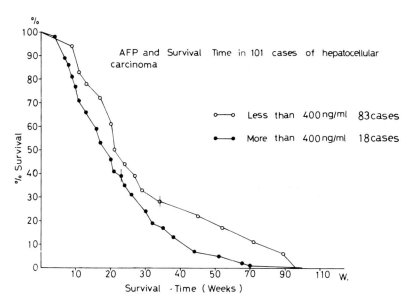

Figure 36 Survival curves for 101 cases of hepatocellular carcinoma. The 50% survival from the onset was about 20 weeks, the longest survival 100 weeks. The average survival was 23 weeks for the group with AFP above 400 ng/ml and 34 weeks for the group less than 400 ng/ml.

Table 8 Cause of Death (128 Cases)

Cause	Number of Patients	Percentage
Hepatic failure	29	22.6
GI bleeding	27	21.1
Cachexia	22	17.2
Intraabdominal bleeding	15	11.7
Postoperative	2	1.6
Sepsis	1	0.8
Intracranial vascular accident	1	0.8
Undetermined between hepatic failure and cachexia	31	24.2

as discussed by Dr. Lin in Chapter 19. After reviewing the livers operated by him through his courtesy and the livers of our own good cases with successful resection, we have concluded that good indication for radical operation is limited to the encapsulated and the solitary and confluent massive types in their early stage, preferably before reaching the size of 5 cm. The majority of Dr. Lin's cases of success had a solitary (massive) type tumor by Nakashima-Okuda's classification (19), and so did ours. Theoretically, an early encapsulated tumor is the best candidate for resection, but in reality, there were more solitary massive type HCC that were resected. It is probably due to the fact that the encapsulated type is clinically insidious and does not develop symptoms before reaching a considerable size. Complicating cirrhosis is infrequent in the massive types. The selection of operable cases should be made carefully, and it is probably best done with celiac angiography (75). Judging from the records of Lin's patients who lived or are living for more than 10 years after resection, the parenchyma of a noncirrhotic liver with a solitary HCC is not necessarily in a precancerous state. It is very unlikely that carcinoma has evolved multicentrically in this type. Patients with overt cirrhosis and HCC are hardly the object of positive chemotherapy, which may adversely affect the remaining liver function so that it is hardly adequate to support life.

There have recently been many papers reporting the results of resection (76–78), surgical ligation of the hepatic artery (79) or portal vein (80), radiation (81), intraarterial radioisotope injection (82), and chemotherapy (83, 84), with varying assessments of the therapeutic effects in prolonging the expected life span. Unless a permanent cure has been brought about, it is difficult to evaluate the effect of any type of treatment using a small number of cases. A patient with an encapsulated type of HCC may live for a comparatively long time and in such cases it is doubtful whether treatment of any kind is capable of extending has allotted life span after diagnosis. It is necessary, therefore, to assess the effect of treatment in comparison with average survival time of untreated patients in each type of this carcinoma.

The mean survival time from the onset or initial symptoms in our series of 134 cases, regardless of treatment, was 6.5 months, with the longest survival time of 24 months. There was little difference between the groups with and without associated cirrhosis, but our statistics suggest a slightly better prognosis in patients with low AFP values (Fig. 36). The reported figures of average survival time have been not much different from ours (73, 85, 86). The direct cause of death in our series was hepatic failure in 22.6% of the cases, gastrointestinal bleeding in 21.2%, cachexia in 17.2%, intraabdominal bleeding in 11.7%, and undetermined in 24.2% (Table 8). Bleeding as a cause of death was more common in patients with cirrhosis, and cachexia or debilitation was more frequent in those without cirrhosis.

REFERENCES

1. Patton TB, Horn RC: Primary liver carcinoma. Autopsy study of 60 cases. *Cancer* **17**:767–764, 1964.

2. Cruickshank AH: The pathology of 111 cases of primary hepatic malignancy collected in the Liverpool region. *J Clin Pathol* **14**:120–131, 1961.

3. Mori W: Cirrhosis and primary cancer of the liver. Comparative study in Tokyo and Cincinnati. *Cancer* **20**:627–631, 1967.

4. Miyaji T: Association of hepatocellular carcinoma with cirrhosis among autopsy cases in Japan (1958–1967). In *Alpha-fetoprotein and Hepatoma*. Hirai H, Miyaji T (Eds). University of Tokyo Press, 1973, pp 179–183.

5. Anthony PP: Primary carcinoma of the liver: A study of 282 cases in Ugandan Africans. *J Pathol Bact* **110**:37–49, 1973.

6. Sherlock S, Fox RA, Niazi SP, et al: Chronic liver disease and primary liver-cell cancer with

hepatitis-associated (Australia) antigen in serum. *Lancet* **1**:1243–1247, 1970.

7. Tong MJ, Sun S-C, Schaffer BT, et al: Hepatitis-associated antigen and hepatocellular carcinoma in Taiwan. *Ann Intern Med* **75**:687–691, 1971.

8. Kubo Y, Sawa Y, Hashimoto H, et al: Hepatitis B antigen and alpha-fetoprotein in primary liver cell carcinoma. *Hepatitis Scientific Memoranda,* H-578, November 1973.

9. Iuchi M, Uchiyama Y, Ishii M, et al: Studies on primary carcinoma of liver associated with schistosomiasis japonica (in Japanese). *Naika* **27**:761–766, 1971.

10. Nakashima T, Okuda K, Kojiro M, et al: Coincidence of hepatocellular carcinoma and chronic schistosomiasis japonica of the liver. A study of 24 necropsies. *Cancer,* **36**:1483–1489, 1975.

11. Hou PC: The relationship between primary carcinoma of the liver and infestation with *Clonorchis sinensis. J Pathol Bact* **72**:239–246, 1956.

12. Gustafson EG: An analysis of 62 cases of primary carcinoma of the liver based on 24,400 necropsies at Bellevue Hospital. *Ann Intern Med* **11**:889–900, 1937.

13. Wells RF, Lundberg GD: Hepatoma: review of 43 cases with comments on syphilis as an etiologic factor. *Gastroenterology* **44**:598–601, 1963.

14. Smoron GL, Battifora HA: Thorotrast-induced hepatoma. *Cancer* **30**:1252–1259, 1972.

15. Berk JE, Lieber MM: Primary carcinoma of the liver in hemochromatosis. *Am J Med Sci* **202**:708–714, 1941.

16. Johnson EL, Feagler JR, Lerner KG, et al: Association of androgenic-anabolic steroid therapy with development of hepatocellular carcinoma. *Lancet* **2**:1273–1276, 1972.

17. Nakamura T, Nakamura S, Aikawa T, et al: Obstruction of the inferior vena cava in the hepatic position and hepatic veins. Report of eight cases and review of the Japanese literature. *Angiology* **19**:479–498, 1968.

18. Berman C: *Primary Carcinoma of the Liver. A Study in Incidence, Clinical Manifestations, Pathology and Aetiology.* Lewis, London, 1951.

19. Nakashima T, Kojiro M, Sakamoto K, et al: Studies of primary liver carcinoma. I. Proposal of new gross anatomical classification of primary liver cell carcinoma. *Acta Hepatol Jap* **15**:279–291, 1974.

20. Kew MC, Dos Antos Ha, Sherlock S: Diagnosis of primary cancer of the liver. *Brit Med J* **4**:408–411, 1971.

21. McFadzean AJS, Todd D, Tsang KC: Polycythemia in primary carcinoma of the liver. *Blood* **13**:427–435, 1958.

22. Nakao K, Kimura K, Miura Y, et al: Erythrocytosis associated with carcinoma of the liver (with erythropoietin assay of tumor extracts). *Am J Med Sci* **251**:161–165, 1966.

23. Landau BR, Wills N, Craig JW, et al: The mechanism of hepatoma induced hypoglycemia. *Cancer* **15**:1188–1196, 1962.

24. Knill-Jones RP, Buckle RM, Parson V, et al: Hypercalcemia and increased parathyroid-hormone activity in a primary hepatoma. Studies before and after hepatic transplantation. *New Engl J Med* **282**:704–708, 1970.

25. Von Felton A, Straub PW, Frick PG: Dysfibrinogenemia in a patient with primary hepatoma. *New Engl J Med* **280**:405–409, 1967.

26. Bell W, Bahr R, Waldmann TA: Cryofibrinogenemia, multiple dysproteinemia, and hypervolemia in a patient with a primary hepatoma. *Ann Intern Med* **64**:658–664, 1966.

27. Santer MA, Waldmann TA, Fallon HJ: Erythrocytosis and hyperlipemia as manifestatin of hepatic carcinoma. *Arch Intern Med* **120**:735–739, 1967.

28. Primack A, Wilson J, O'Conner GT, et al: Hepatocellular carcinoma with the carcinoid syndrome. *Cancer* **27**:1182–1189, 1971.

29. Morgan AG, Walker WC, Mason MK, et al: A new syndrome associated with hepatocellular carcinoma. *Gastroenterology* **63**:340–345, 1972.

30. Ewing J: *Neoplastic Diseases: A Treatise on Tumors,* 4th ed. Saunders, Philadelphia, 1940, pp 738–753.

31. MacDonald RA: Primary carcinoma of liver—Clinicopathologic study of 108 cases. *Arch Intern Med* **99**:532–554, 1957.

32. Okuda K, Shimokawa Y, Yakushiji F: Liver scintillation scanning in the diagnosis of chronic schistosomiasis japonica. *Digestion* **3**:269–278, 1970.

33. Edmondson HA, Steiner PE: Primary carcinoma of the liver. A study of 100 cases among 48,900 necropsies. *Cancer* **7**:462–503, 1954.

34. Ong GB, Taw JL: Spontaneous rupture of hepatocellular carcinoma. *Brit Med J* **4**:146–149, 1972.

35. Talerman A, Magyar E: Hepatocellular carcinoma presenting with pathologic fracture due to bone metastases. *Cancer* **32**:1477–1481, 1973.

36. Ohlsson EGH, Norden JG: Primary carcinoma of the liver. A study of 121 cases. *Acta Pathol Microbiol Scand* **64**:430–440, 1965.

37. Okuda K, Tanikawa K, Emura T, et al: Nonsurgical, percutaneous transhepatic cholangiography—diagnostic significance in medical

CHAPTER 18 DIAGNOSTIC METHODS FOR HEPATOCELLULAR CARCINOMA

TELFER B. REYNOLDS, M.D.

When hepatocellular carcinoma (HCC) is suspected there are a number of tests and procedures that can be used to establish the diagnosis, to evaluate the extent of the tumor, and to assess the presence and severity of any underlying liver disease.

The finding of an abnormal level of alpha fetoprotein in the serum strongly suggests HCC, as discussed in Chapters 16 and 17. If both hepatitis B antigen and excess fetoprotein are present and if acute or subacute hepatitis can be excluded on clinical grounds, then the diagnosis is virtually assured.

Other important diagnostic tests include liver biopsy, celiac angiography, isotope scanning, and laparoscopy. Less useful are portal venography, ultrasonic scanning, and ascitic fluid cytology. The standard "liver function tests" are important in evaluating any underlying liver disease but there is no pattern of abnormality that is consistently helpful in the diagnosis of HCC. Though infrequently present, such extrahepatic abnormalities as hypercalce-

mia, hypoglycemia, erythrocytosis, hypercholesterolemia, or extremely high serum vitamin B_{12} levels are strong clues to the presence of HCC in the right clinical setting.

LIVER BIOPSY

It is difficult to be absolutely certain of a diagnosis of HCC without microscopic examination, since a few cases of metastatic carcinoma of the liver with positive tests for alpha fetoprotein have been reported (1). Liver biopsy is desirable, therefore, in all cases where HCC is suspected. There are two possible reasons for not attempting biopsy. First, needle biopsy in patients with HCC is more hazardous than usual because of an increased risk of bleeding. The frequency with which hepatoma nodules rupture to cause intraperitoneal bleeding is indicative of their tendency toward marked vascularity. There have been two fatalities from hemorrhage after biopsy during the

Table 1   Diagnostic Tests in Hepatocellular Carcinoma [a]

Test	Number	(%)	Test	Number	(%)
Serology			*Peritoneoscopy*		
HbsAg positive [b]	12 of 25	48	Not performed	13	
Alpha fetoprotein positive [c]	16 of 25	64	Cirrhosis plus carcinoma	8 of 12	67
Both tests positive	10 of 25	40	Cirrhosis alone	3 of 12	25
			No abnormality	1 of 12	8
Hepatic Scan [d]			*Liver Biopsy*		
Not performed	1	4			
Pattern of chronic					
liver disease [e]	19 of 24	80	Not performed	5	
Definite filling defect	12 of 24	50	"Blind" biopsy positive	10 of 12	83
Indefinite filling defect	11 of 24	46	Peritoneoscopic biopsy		
			positive	5 of 5	100
No filling defect	1 of 24	4	Surgical biopsy positive	3 of 3	100
"Flow scan" [f] positive	6 of 9	67			
Gallium-67 scan positive	2 of 4	50	*Diagnosis First*		
			Established By		
			"Blind" biopsy	10 of 25	40
Celiac Angiography			Peritoneoscopy	7 of 25	28
Not performed	14		Angiography	3 of 25	12
Vascular tumor	9 of 11	82	Surgery	2 of 25	8
Nonvascular filling					
defect	1 of 11	9	Serology [g]	1 of 25	4
Not abnormal	1 of 11	9	Autopsy	2 of 25	8

[a] Results in 25 consecutive cases with biopsy or autopsy confirmation of the diagnosis seen at LAC–USCMC, 1970–1974.
[b] CEP and RIA.
[c] Immunodiffusion with preliminary concentration of the serum.
[d] ^{99m}Tc sulfur colloid.
[e] Mottling and reduced intensity of the hepatic image with increased uptake in bone marrow and spleen.
[f] Sequential imaging during the first 30 seconds after administration of ^{99m}Tc sulfur colloid.
[g] Both HbsAg and alpha fetoprotein positive.

last six years in our Liver Unit. Second, if hepatic lobectomy for HCC appears feasible, it is probably best to delay biopsy until the time of surgery in order to avoid intraperitoneal spread of tumor.

Technique of Biopsy

Since HCC involvement is often widespread in the liver, a "blind" intercostal, right lobe aspiration biopsy frequently will disclose neoplastic tissue. Analysis of our own case material shows that right lobe needle biopsy obtained neoplastic tissue in approximately 80% of cases in which it was

attempted (Table 1). If liver scan indicates a discrete lesion then the biopsy increases the likelihood of a positive result and for lesions in the left lobe we believe it to be safer than "blind" biopsy. Much of the superior, lateral, and posterior surface of the right lobe cannot be seen at laparoscopy, however.

Soderstrom has described a technique for aspiration biopsy using a fine needle of only 0.7 mm in diameter (2). A small amount of tissue is obtained which is studied by cytological techniques. Rasmussen et al used this method with ultrasonic guidance and claimed it improved the yield of positive biopsies in metastatic cancer (3). Because of the small amount of tissue obtained, there is sometimes a problem in differentiating hepatocellular from metastatic carcinoma (4). Fine needle biopsy may be particularly applicable to the diagnosis of primary HCC because of the claimed lower incidence of postbiopsy bleeding (4). We have had no experience with it in our Liver Unit.

LIVER SCANNING

Liver scanning with isotopes taken up by the reticuloendothelial system [gold or technetium-99 sulfur colloid (Tc-99m)] is potentially useful in the diagnosis of HCC, since there is usually a lack of Kupffer cells in the tumor. However, scanning is considerably less helpful in HCC than in other focal liver defects because of the frequent association with liver cirrhosis. Hepatic uptake of isotopes often is diminished and lacks hemogeneity in patients with cirrhosis, causing the appearance of pseudotumors (5–7). As an example, an unusually discrete pseudotumor in a patient with alcoholic liver disease is shown in Fig. 1. In our patients with HCC at Los Angeles County–USC Medical Center, underlying cirrhosis is the rule, and almost all patients have the scan pattern characteristic of chronic liver disease, with varying degrees of redistribution of isotope from liver to bone marrow and spleen. In spite of this handicap, liver scan shows rather discrete filling defects strongly suggestive of tumor (Fig. 2) in about 50% of our patients (Table 1). The remaining 50% have less discrete (Fig. 3) or no filling defects. In patients who do not have underlying cirrhosis, primary HCC is easily demonstrated on liver scan if the tumor mass is greater than 2 cm in diameter.

Scanning with Gallium-67 has been advocated as a means of distinguishing pseudotumors from tumors (8, 9). Appearance of ^{67}Ga in the "cold spot" indicates metabolism of gallium by the tumor cells (Fig. 4). This technique has been disappointing in our experience, as we have seen examples of apparent gallium uptake in pseudotumors and failure of gallium uptake in filling defects caused by hepatoma. Gallium also may be taken up by liver abscess (9) and is often poorly taken up by metastatic foci of adenocarcinoma (9).

With suitable equipment, a "flow" scan can be recorded during the first 15 to 30 seconds after administration of the colloid. A "hot spot" is an indication of high blood content and, if it coincides with the filling defect seen later in the scanning process, it indicates a vascular tumor (Fig. 4). The "flow scan" suggested a vascular filling defect in six of nine patients with HCC reviewed in Table 1.

CELIAC ANGIOGRAPHY

The profuse hepatic arterial vascular supply of hepatic cell carcinoma often results in a characteristic angiographic appearance of dilated hepatic arteries supplying a rich network of "tumor vessels," with puddling and "tumor staining" during the capillary phase (Fig. 5). There may be evidence of arteriovenous shunting or displacement or stretching of vessels around the tumor. Metastatic tumor nodules are less likely to show as much vascularity except for those from choriocarcinoma and, occasionally, those from hypernephroma, carcinoid, leiomyosarcoma, thyroid, or islet-cell tumor. Some hepatic cell carcinomas contain avascular areas that are necrotic on microscopic examination, so that absence of hypervascularity on arteriography does not exclude this diagnosis.

Abnormal arteriograms are found in the majority of patients with HCC (10, 11). In our own experience approximately 80% of patients have had a "positive" arteriogram (Table 1). The arteriogram alone, how-

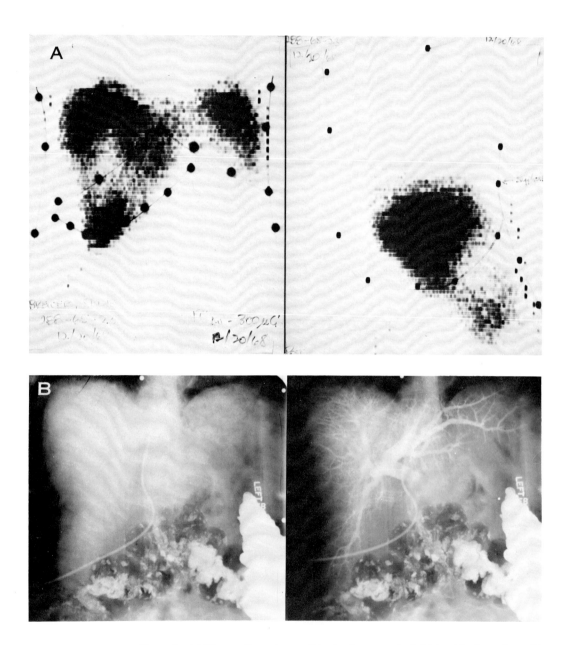

Figure 1 *(a)* Discrete "pseudotumor" in the liver scan (colloidal gold) of a patient with alcoholic cirrhosis. *(b)* Umbilical portogram in the same patient showing normal portal ramifications (right) and relatively homogeneous hepatogram phase (left).

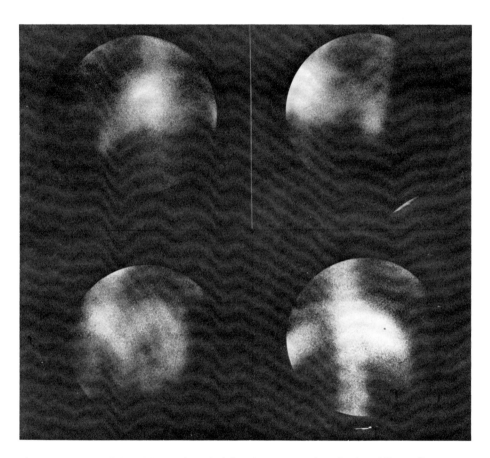

Figure 2 Discrete filling defect in the right lobe of a patient with cirrhosis and liver cell carcinoma (liver scan with ^{99m}Tc sulfur colloid). There is increased isotope uptake in ribs, sternum, and vertebral bone marrow, as well as in the spleen. Upper left: anterior view of right lobe. Upper right: anterior view of left lobe and spleen. Lower left: right lateral view. Lower right: posterior view.

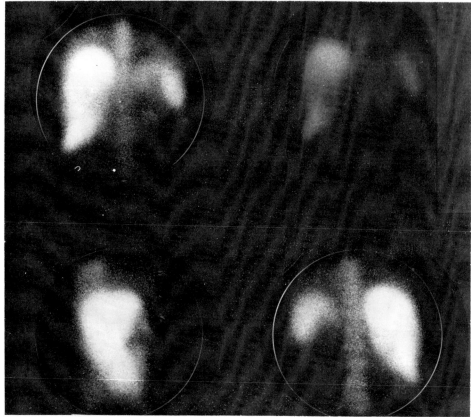

Figure 3 Indefinite filling defect along the medial edge of the right lobe in a patient with cirrhosis and hepatocellular carcinoma (liver scan with ^{99m}Tc sulfur colloid). Upper left: anterior view. Upper right: anterior view with decreased intensity. Lower left: right lateral view. Lower right: posterior view.

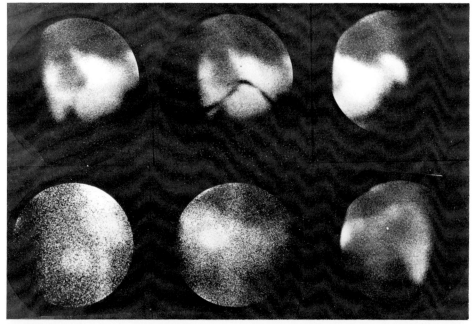

Figure 4 Discrete filling defect in a patient with cirrhosis and liver cell carcinoma (liver scan with ^{99m}Tc sulfur colloid). Upper left: anterior view of right lobe. Upper center: same view with rib markers. Upper right: anterior view of left lobe and spleen. Lower right: posterior view of right lobe. Lower center: Gallium-67 scan, anterior view, showing increased accumulation of isotope in the filling defect. Lower left: "flow scan," anterior view, recorded 10 sec after intravenous administration of ^{99m}Tc sulfur colloid showing increased concentration of isotope in the filling defect and indicating it is a vascular area.

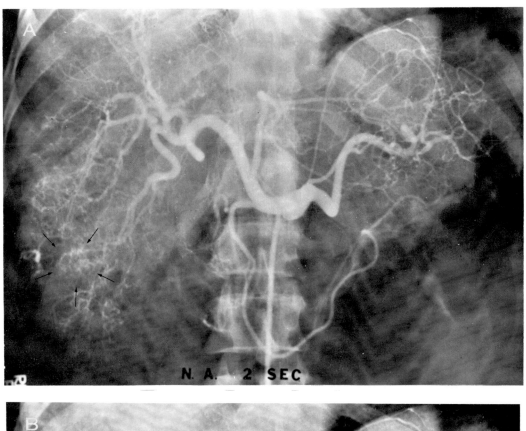

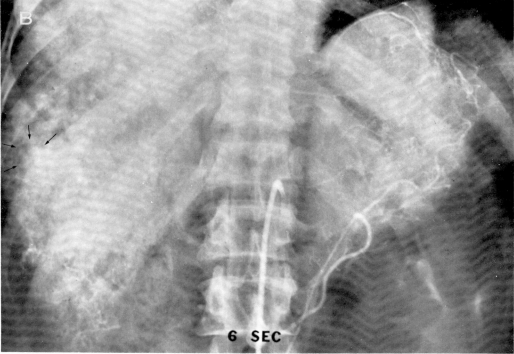

Figure 5 Celiac angiography with 50 ml of contrast media in a patient with cirrhosis and diffuse right lobe hepatocellular carcinoma. *(a)* Shows a large hepatic artery at 2 sec with many areas of tumor neovascularity (arrows) in the right lobe. *(b)* Shows diffuse tumor-staining (arrows) throughout the right lobe at 6 sec.

ever, can not make a definite differentiation between primary and metastatic HCC. Watson and Baltaxe were able to distinguish between the two lesions on the basis of angiographic vascularity with an accuracy of approximately 80% in a group of 78 cases (12).

In addition to providing assistance in the diagnosis of HCC, angiography yields important additional information relative to the portal circulation. Often there is evidence of portal collateral flow due to concomitant cirrhosis. Absence of visualization of the portal vein suggests portal occlusion with tumor, a frequent complication of HCC (13). Angiography may also be useful in assessing the extent of hepatoma in consideration of hepatic lobectomy. Gammill et al correctly predicted whether cancer was present in one or both hepatic lobes in 13 of 14 patients (14). If surgical hepatic artery ligation is used for treatment of HCC, arteriography is helpful preoperatively in delineating the anatomy of the artery.

PORTAL VENOGRAPHY

Portal venography by splenic injection is not much used for diagnosis of HCC. Because of accompanying cirrhosis and portal hypertension, some of the injected contrast often bypasses the liver through portal collateral veins. Therefore, the concentration of contrast media in the sinusoidal phase of the portogram is often insufficient to clearly demonstrate the tumor nodules which appear as filling defects because of their predominantly hepatic arterial blood supply. If the diagnosis of HCC is established and lobectomy is under consideration, then splenoportography may be useful in excluding portal vein occlusion by tumor since this would make curative surgery impossible. Spread of tumor into the portal vein is a relatively frequent complication of HCC, as noted above.

Portal venography by the umbilical route results in "hepatograms" of greater density since a large volume of contrast media can be injected rapidly into the main portal vein near the liver (15). Using this technique, tumors as small as 1 cm in diameter can be seen as filling defects. An example of how relatively small filling defects can be easily seen in the "hepatogram" phase of umbilical portal venography is shown in Fig. 6, which shows distortion and compression of portal veins by a large hepatocellular carcinoma whose blood supply was largely arterial is illustrated in Fig. 7.

LAPAROSCOPY

We have found laparoscopy to be a useful procedure in diagnosis of HCC and in the assessment of its extent, the nature of any underlying liver disease, and the feasibility of hepatic lobectomy.

To diagnose hepatic carcinoma, lesions must be present within the field of view of the laparoscopist which usually includes most of the anterior surface of the left lobe and the lower one-half of the anterior surface of the right lobe. Lesions on the dome of the right lobe or its posterolateral aspect cannot be seen. The operator must have experience in gross liver pathology since it is sometimes difficult to distinguish the nodules of hepatic carcinoma from those of a macronodular cirrhosis. Some of the varying appearances of HCC are shown in Chapter 8.

At the time of laparoscopy a guided biopsy can be made of suspected tumor nodules, either directly through the instrument or by separate insertion of a long Menghini-type needle. If a lesion suspected of being HCC is seen and there is little or no accompanying liver disease, then the possibility of hepatic lobectomy should be considered. It may be best not to perform biopsy in such a patient so as

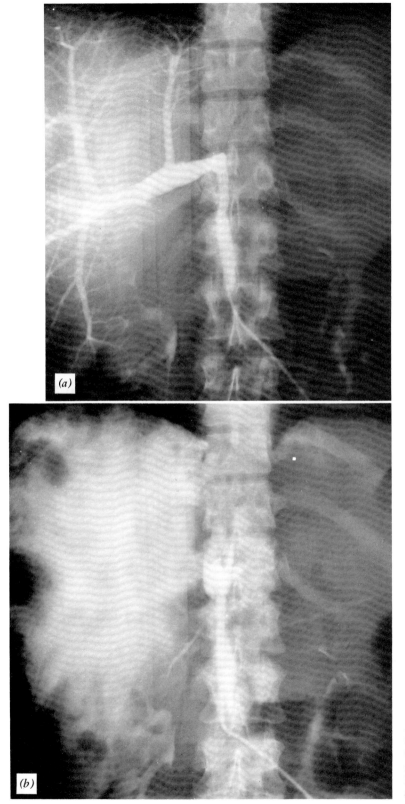

Figure 6 Umbilical portogram in a patient with cirrhosis and several foci of hepatocellular carcinoma in the right lobe. No definite abnormality is seen in the early films (A) but discrete filling defects are evident in the later "hepatogram" (B).

445

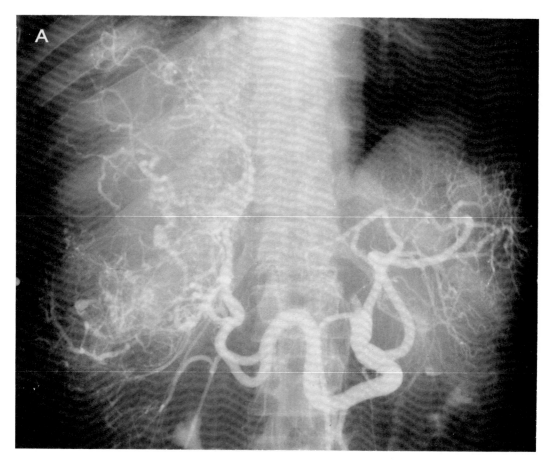

Figure 7   Celiac angiogram and umbilical portogram in a patient with a huge hepatocellular carcinoma occupying most of the right lobe. Characteristic tumor vessels are evident in the arteriogram *(a)* while the portal venogram shows compression and displacement to the left of the portal vessels *(b)*.

to avoid possible seeding of the peritoneum with tumor cells. Every effort should be made to visualize as much as possible of the other hepatic lobe to help establish resectability.

The experience of our own Liver Unit shows that HCC can be diagnosed at laparoscopy in approximately 65% of cases (Table 1). A positive biopsy result was obtained in all instances where neoplasm was suspected from the gross appearance.

ULTRASONIC SCAN

Detection of hepatocellular carcinoma by ultrasound appears to be difficult because

of the similarity in abnormal echoes caused by liver cirrhosis and by carcinoma (16–18). Our own experience with ultrasound has not shown it to be of value in diagnosing HCC but technique and instrumentation are still evolving and it may yet prove to be useful.

SIMPLE TESTS

None of the standard liver function tests are distinctive in patients with HCC. While marked increase in serum alkaline phosphatase (SAP) is a frequent finding in metastatic liver carcinoma, this is often not present with primary liver carcinoma.

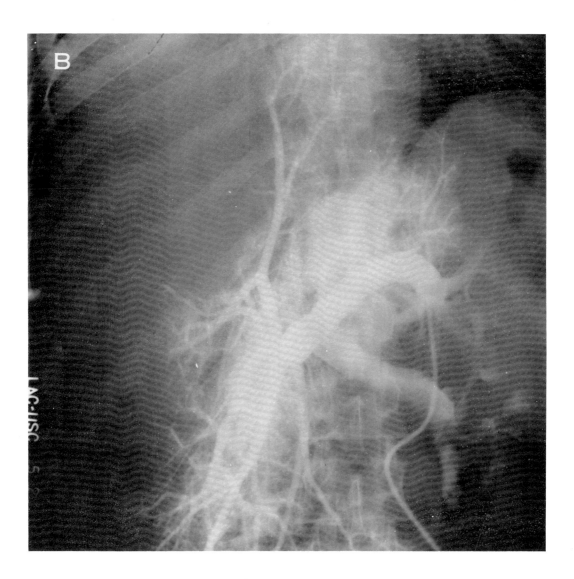

There is invariably some increase in SAP in the latter condition, but it is rarely impressively different than the elevation seen in liver cirrhosis. For example, in 25 recent cases of HCC seen in our Liver Unit, SAP levels at the time of diagnosis ranged from 2.5 to 26 u/liter with a mean of 9.3 Bessey-Lowry μ/liter (normal 1 to 3 μ/liter). Only 15% were higher than 15 units/liter. For comparison SAP levels ranged from 1.4 to 25 with a mean of 7.6 μ/liter in 25 cases of cirrhosis without carcinoma chosen randomly from our files.

When ascites is present with HCC, it is not likely to have an unusually high protein content or malignant cells demonstrable on cytologic exam. Among the 25 cases summarized in Table 1, there was only one report of malignant cells among eight fluids sent for cytologic examination. Protein content was measured in the ascitic fluid of 12 patients with a range of 1.1 to 3.9 and a mean value of 1.8 gm/100 ml. Only one fluid had a protein content greater than 2.5 gm/100 ml and this patient had a concomitant Budd-Chiari syndrome caused by the carcinoma.

REFERENCES

1. Alpert E, Pinn V, Isselbacher K: Alpha-fetoprotein in a patient with gastric carcinoma metastatic to the liver. *New Engl J Med* **285**:1058–1059, 1971.

2. Soderstrom N: *Fine Needle Aspiration Biopsy.* Grune & Stratton, New York, 1966.

3. Rasmussen SN, Holm HH, Kristensen JK, et al: Ultrasonically guided liver biopsy. *Brit Med J* 1:500–502, 1972.

4. Lundquist A: Fine-needle aspiration biopsy for cytodiagnosis of malignant tumor in the liver. *Acta Med Scand* 188:465–470, 1970

5. Johnson RM, Sweeny WA: The false-positive hepatic scan. *J. Nucl Med* 8:451–460, 1967.

6. Klion FM, Dudavsky AZ: False positive liver scans in patients with alcoholic liver disease. *Ann Intern Med* 60:283–291, 1968.

7. Cohen MB: Cirrhosis and the hepatic photoscan. *Radiology* 93:1139–1144, 1969.

8. Suzuki T, Honjo I, Hamamoto K, et al: Positive scintophotography of cancer of the liver with Ga[67] citrate *Am J Roentgenol Radium Ther Nucl Med* 113:92–103, 1971.

9. Lomas F, Dibos PE, Wagner HN: Increased specificity of liver scanning with the use of 67-Gallium citrate. *New Engl J Med* 286:1323–1339, 1972.

10. Yu C: Primary carcinoma of the liver (hepatoma): its diagnosis by selective celiac arteriography. *Am J Roentgenol Radium Ther Nucl Med* 99:142–149, 1967.

11. Boijsen E, Abrams HL: Roentenologic diagnosis of primary carcinoma of the liver. *Acta Radiologica* 3:257–277, 1965.

12. Watson RC, Baltaxe HA: The angiographic appearance of primary and secondary tumors of the liver. *Radiology* 101:539–548, 1971.

13. Albacete RA, Matthews MJ, Saini N: Portal vein thrombosis in malignant hepatoma. *Ann Intern Med* 67:337–348, 1967.

14. Gammill SL, Takahashi M, Kawanami M, et al: Hepatic angiography in the selection of patients with hepatomas for hepatic lobectomy. *Radiology* 101:549–554, 1971.

15. Piccone VA, LeVeen HH, White JJ, et al: Transumbilical hepatography, a significant adjunct in the investigation of liver disease. *Surgery* 61:333–346, 1967.

16. McCarthey CF, Davies ER, Wells PNT, et al: A comparison of ultrasonic and isotope scanning in the diagnosis of liver disease. *Brit J Radiol* 43:100–109, 1970.

17. Holm HH: Ultrasonic scanning in the diagnosis of space-occupying lesions of the upper abdomen. *Brit J Radiol* 44:24–36, 1971.

18. Leyton B, Halpern S, Leopold G, et al: Correlation of ultrasound and colloidal scintiscan studies of the normal and diseased liver. *J Nucl Med* 14:27–33, 1973.

CHAPTER 19 SURGICAL TREATMENT OF PRIMARY LIVER CELL CARCINOMA

TIEN-YU LIN, M.D.

At present, the definitive treatment of hepatocullular carcinoma (HCC) is surgical excision of the tumor. Ligation of the main hepatic artery or portal vein branches or even total extirpation of the liver followed by allograft may be considered when the lesion is so extensive to defy hepatic resection.

HEPATIC RESECTION

This is the most effective measure presently available in treating HCC. History of hepatic resection can be traced back to the last century. The first successful resection of a primary malignant tumor of the liver was performed by Lueke (1) in 1891. The first successful left hepatic lobectomy was done for cancer of the liver by Keen (2) in 1899, and the first right hepatic lobectomy for metastatic carcinoma of the stomach by Wangensteen (3) in 1949. Nevertheless, during the succeeding six to seven decades since the first hepatic resection, surgical treatments of the liver tumor have remained largely within the scope of wedge or partial resections. The lag in hepatic surgery among all abdominal operations might be attributed to the following:

1. The surgical inaccessibility of the liver.
2. The vital functions of the liver precluded large excision for fear of lethal consequences.
3. The liver per se constitutes a huge valcular sponge which is friable with a great capacity for bleeding, not easily controlled by conventional clamping or ligating techniques.

After the clarification of the bilaterality and vascular arrangement of the liver by Cantlie (4) and McIndoe et al (5), and the evolution of the so called "Controlled Method" of hepatic resection by Lortat-Jacob and Robert (6) in 1952, hepatic lobectomy for malignant liver tumor with this technique has been successively reported by Quattlebaum (7), Pack (8), and Clatworthy et al (9). Hepatic surgery has since gradually aroused wide attention of surgeons and emerged to become an important part of general surgery. Based on the modern anatomic terminology, five types of hepatic resection are available at present.

1. Right hepatic lobectomy; namely resection of the anterior and the posterior segments of the right lobe.

2. Extended right hepatic lobectomy; right lobectomy plus median segmentectomy, namely resection of all liver tissue to the right of the falciform ligament.

3. Middle hepatic lobectomy or median segmentectomy; resection of median segment of the left lobe, namely removal of the liver between the main lobar fissure and the left segmental fissure.

4. Left lateral segmentectomy; removal of all liver tissue to the left of the falciform ligament.

5. Left hepatic lobectomy; removal of all tissue to the left of the main lobar fissure, namely resection of the median and the lateral segments of the left lobe.

SURGICAL ANATOMY

The liver is the largest parenchymatous organ of vital importance in the human body. Aside from the hepatic artery and veins, the liver receives ingress of portal blood that drains the splanchnic area and is interlaced with the hepatic biliary system that conveys bile to the intestinal tract. The complicated network of vascular and ductal structures within the liver makes it a fragile, highly vascularized organ that at one time was termed *anoli me tangerel* (do not touch me).

Anatomically, the liver is situated immediately beneath the diaphragm, mostly on the right side, and is enclosed anteriorly and laterally behind the costochondral cage.

There are ligamentous attachments anchoring the liver to the diaphragm. The triangular ligaments, one each at the right and left extremity of the liver, are connected by a coronary ligament on the upper posterior surface of the liver. The falciform ligament runs forward at a right angle to the coronary ligament anchoring the liver where the right and left diaphragmatic leaves meet.

As these ligamentous attachments are the major immobilizing structures of the liver, detachment of these ligaments is all that is required to mobilize and free the liver for hepatic resection.

Externally the liver appears as a single organ. However, it can be divided into right and left lobes based on its internal vascular and ductal structures. The smaller caudate lobe proper and caudate process are relatively unimportant from the surgical point of view. Conventionally, the falciform ligament has been used as the boundary of the right and the left lobe. However, based on the study of the anatomical distribution of hepatic vascular and ductal structures by Cantlie (4), McIndoe and Counseller (5), and others, division between true right and left lobes can be identified by the lobar fissures, a line connecting the gallbladder fossa anterio-inferiorly with the fossa of the inferior vena cava postero-superiorly. The left lobe, which is located sinistrally to the lobar fissure, is further subdivided into the lateral portion, which is to the left of the falciform and the medial segment that is bounded by the lobar fissure on one side and the falciform ligament on the other. The true right lobe is only that portion of the liver dextral to the lobar fissure. The lobar fissure acts as the "surgical plane" for the right and left hepatic lobes. This is the most important surgical boundary of the two main lobes, since the vascular and ductal structures diverge here into each lobe (Fig. 1). The anatomical relationship of hepatic artery, portal vein branches, and bile ducts varies considerably from one individual to another. Although no less than 11 variations have been proclaimed, the majority give rise to their right and left branches of the hepatic

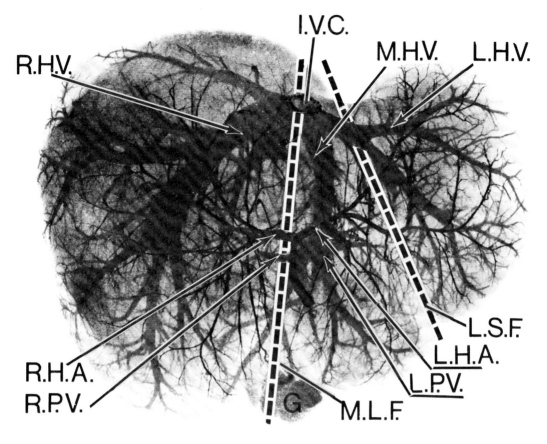

Figure 1 Surgical planes of the liver in relation to the intrahepatic distribution of the hepatic artery, portal vein, and hepatic vein. MLF: main lobar fissure. LSF: lateral segmental fissure. IVC: inferior vena cava. RHV: right hepatic vein. LHV: left hepatic vein. MHV: middle hepatic vein. RHA: right hepatic artery. RPV: right hepatic vein. LHA: left hepatic artery. LPV: left portal vein. G: gallbladder.

artery, portal vein, and hepatic duct regularly at the so-called porta hepatis at the upper end of hepatoduodenal ligament. Furthermore, these branches of the hepatic artery, portal vein, hepatic duct, and even the hepatic veins further branch out within each hepatic lobe and supply or drain particular parts of the lobe. Accordingly, the right lobe can be divided into anterior and posterior segments and the left lobe, medial and lateral segments. Some authors even divide each segment into subsegments by the vascular and ductal distribution, but

it seems to be futile from the surgical point of view.

The hepatic veins, which are usually paired, drain separately the venous blood of the right and left hepatic lobes into the inferior vena cava beneath the diaphragm. The extrahepatic portions of the hepatic veins are extremely short and are predisposed to difficulty in exposure, particularly when the intrahepatic space-taking lesion is large enough to compress against the diaphragm or adhere to the vena cava. There is a subbranch of the left hepatic vein, the middle hepatic vein, that drains the blood of the median segment of the left lobe directly or through the left hepatic vein into the vena cava. It might need be ligated and divided in case of extended right hepatic lobectomy or middle hepatic lobectomy for tumors in the middle part of the liver. The inferior vena cava is of paramount importance during hepatic resection as it runs in close contact with the middle posterior surface of the liver and is so thin-walled as to be overlooked as a mere hepatic capsule, especially when there are adhesions between the two. Hence it is apt to be torn at separation and cause massive hemorrhage and air embolism. Moreover, exposing the vena cava by delivering the huge right hepatic lobe out of abdominal cavity at hepatic resection may result in traction or kinking of the vena cava and cause impeded venous return and cardiac arrest, especially in small infants whose vena cava is of a smaller calibre.

PATHOPHYSIOLOGY OF HEPATIC RESECTION

Resection of more than 70% of normal liver tissue will cause a drop in serum levels of protein, albumin, and total cholesterol and its ester, and a rise in SGOT, SGPT, and bromsulfalein retention from the first to the seventh postoperative days (10, 11). This is invariably noted at the time of right hepatic lobectomy which removes a major part of the liver. These blood chemical changes, however, are gradually restored back toward normal in the second postoperative week and become normal by the third or fourth postoperative week. In a cirrhotic liver, left hepatic lobectomy will result in a similar pattern of blood chemical changes as that produced by resection of normal liver and gradually function will be restored to preoperative (cirrhotic) levels. However, right hepatic lobectomy will cause even more drastic hepatic dysfunc-

tion which further deteriorates as hepatic failure develops in 60% of the patients in one week to three or four months after the resection (10, 12).

The metabolic changes following hepatic resection is accompanied by morphological changes in the residual noncirrhotic liver in animals. Namely, regeneration takes place rapidly and significantly in the residual liver in proportion to the amount resected and in reverse proportion to the size of the animal. In humans, regeneration of the residual liver is apparent on radioisotope scanning by the third postoperative week (10, 13–15). Regeneration of cirrhotic human liver remains equivocal. Lin et al (10) failed to detect any significant change in the size of the residual cirrhotic liver after resection, although some (16) maintain that regeneration does occur.

Based on the pathophysiological observation on liver resection, 80 to 85% resection (that is, extended right hepatic lobectomy) seems to be the upper limit for a noncirrhotic liver, and in the presence of moderately severe cirrhosis (with coarse nodular surface) right hepatic lobectomy is deemed as detrimental or even life-threatening.

OPERATIVE METHOD

Partial Resection of the Liver

Partial resection is indicated when the hepatic tumor is small in size or is located at the periphery of a hepatic lobe. Conventionally, it is done by applying several interrupted mattress sutures on the healthy part of the liver around the tumor and then having the tumor removed (Fig. 2). Blunt needle suture has been advocated in order to minimize injury to the vascular and ductal structure. Lin (12, 17) has secured the treatment of these vascular and ductal structures with clamps as shown in Fig. 3. A hepatic clamp is first applied on the healthy part of the liver near the le-

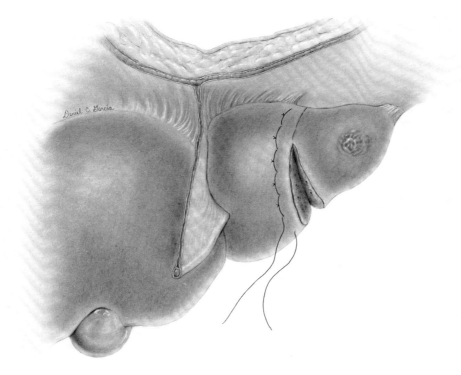

Figure 2   Partial resection of the liver with a series of interlocking mattress sutures.

sion. An incision is made on the Glisson's capsule about 1 cm apart from the hepatic clamp, and then a crush clamp is applied on this incision line so as to crush away the liver substance while remaining vascular and ductal structures in the crush bed are bridging the affected and the healthy part of the liver. These vascular and ductal structures are ligated and divided to complete hepatic resection.

Hepatic Lobectomy

Controlled Method

This was first proposed by Lortat-Jacob and Robert (6) in 1952 and has since gained wide acceptance by most hepatic surgeons. By the "controlled method," the vascular and ductal structures that drain into or out of the hepatic lobes are extrahepatically ligated and divided before starting actual resection of the hepatic lobes, either right or left, in order to control hemorrhage. In principle it is a technique essentially the same as that of pulmonary lobectomy. A large longitudinal incision is used by some surgeons, but upper transverse incision with thoracotomy in case of necessity has been most commonly employed to explore the lesion. On entering the abdominal cavity the triangular and coronary ligaments on the side of attempted lobectomy are divided to free the hepatic lobe from the diaphragm. The teres ligament is divided and held with a clamp on its hepatic end to keep the liver in a suitable position for resection. In attempted right hepatic lobectomy, the cystic

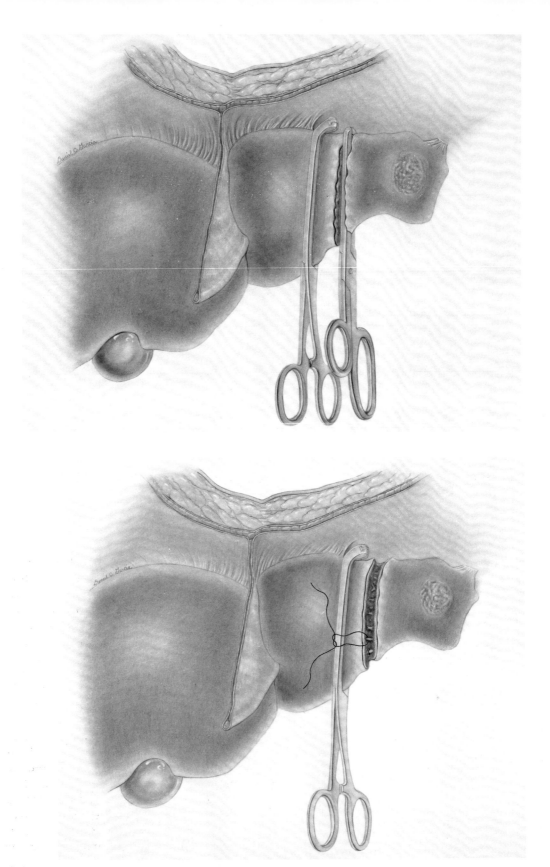

Figure 3 Partial resection with a hepatic clamp and crush clamp. *(a)* The hepatic clamp is shown in place, and the liver parenchyma is crushed with crush clamp through the incision on the superior surface of the Glisson's capsule. *(b)* On release of the crush clamp, the vascular and ductal structures remain as whitish cords bridging the two parts of the liver.

artery and cystic duct are ligated and divided, leaving the gallbladder attached to the right lobe.

After mobilizing the hepatic lobe, the hepatoduodenal ligament at the porta hepatis is dissected to isolate the branches of hepatic artery, portal vein, and hepatic duct of the affected lobe. They are individually ligated and divided. The affected lobe is then rotated clockwise out of the abdominal cavity to expose the inferior vena cava and hepatic veins. The hepatic vein of the affected lobe is then isolated, ligated, and divided. (Fig. 4a).

With the main vascular and ductal structures under control, the liver substance is resected along the surgical plane (main lobar fissure) between the two lobes (Fig. 4b). This is effected by cauterization by some, while others dissect bluntly with fingers or a scalpel. The shortcoming of the controlled method has been that the maneuver of isolating individual vascular or ductal trunk is not only tedious but also is prone to tear the short hepatic vein or even the vena cava during isolation of the hepatic vein with resultant massive bleeding or air embolization. For this potential complication, some advocate applying tape on the vena cava just above and below the liver or using hypothermia to minimize bleeding.

After hepatic transection, the cut surface is covered with an omental (free) graft or gelform sponge to prevent blood oozing. A Penrose drain is placed near the cut surface. Routine use of a T-tube in the common duct has been stressed by some authors, but it seems to be unnecessary in our experience.

Finger Fracture Technique

In 1954 Lin et al (18) devised the finger frature technique in order to overcome the complicated and potentially dangerous maneuvers during isolation of vascular and ductal structures in the controlled method.

By finger fracture technique the lobe in question is prepared for resection by detaching the triangular, coronary, and falciform ligaments, and if it is the right lobe, by dividing the cystic artery and cystic duct. A section line is then made on the Glisson's capsule about 2 to 3 cm apart from the anatomical boundary of the two lobes for insertion of the fingers. With the tumor-bearing lobe supported in one hand, the thumb and index finger of the other hand are inserted directly into the liver substance through the serosal incision and fractures and smashes the liver tissue to pieces with the fingers. Any resistant vessels or ducts that are encountered are clamped, severed, and ligated individually. Usually the maneuver is started first from the hilar region so as to isolate intrahepatically the main branches of the hepatic artery, portal vein, and bile duct of the affected lobe. The hepatic vein is also isolated intrahepatically in the same way at the later part of the transection. (Fig. 5.) This procedure is a departure from the conventional method in that while the lobar ductal and vascular trunks are separated and isolated extrahepatically before transection of the interlobar septum in the controlled method, they are rather isolated and ligated intrahepatically during the transection in the finger fracture technique.

Lin (19) has since performed 82 consecutive hepatic lobectomies by this technique for primary carcinoma of the liver. The simplicity and safety of this method is reflected in its low surgical mortality of 12.1% and requirement of less blood transfusion during operation.

Finger Fracture Technique with Hepatic Clamp

Nevertheless, the finger fracture technique is by no means perfect in controlling bleeding. During the period of finger insertion or fracturing of liver tissue, there still is considerable amount of untoward bleeding that may require rapid transfusion to compensate for blood loss, and a sense of inse-

A

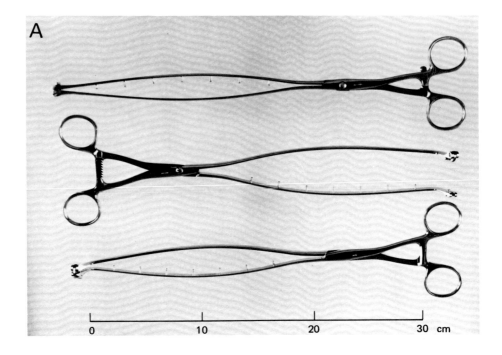

B

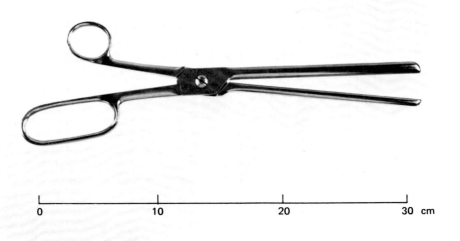

Figure 6   T. Y. Lin's hepatic clamps *(a)* and crush clamp *(b)*.

curity plagues the surgeon. To overcome this handicap, Lin (12) improved the original finger fracture technique by adding a hepatic clamp prior to finger fracture dissection.

The hepatic lobe is exposed and freed as usual. As shown in Fig. 6, a hepatic clamp devised by Lin is then placed on the liver at the anatomical boundary of both lobes. A section line is made about 2 to 3 cm distant from the clamp and Glisson's capsule is incised for insertion of fingers. The remaining procedures such as the fracturing and smashing of liver tissue and isolation and division of the hepatic artery, portal vein branches, hepatic duct, and hepatic veins within the liver are essentially the same as those of the original finger fracture technique (Fig. 7). After completion of the transection, the hepatic clamp is slightly loosened to check bleeding, if any. The hepatic clamp is totally released after securing all bleeding points by ligature. The remaining cut surface is treated in the same way as described.

Lin (12) has applied this method since 1970 in 12 cases of HCC and reported its superiority over original finger fracture technique in that hepatic lobectomy is performed with more safety and almost without blood transfusion.

Crush Method

In 1973 Lin (17) further devised the crush method. Basically, this is similar to the finger fracture technique in principle. The only difference is that instead of fracturing the liver tissue and isolating the unyielding vascular and ductal structures with fingers as in the finger fracture technique, a heavy crush clamp is used to crush the liver tissue exposing these vascular and ductal structures to direct vision (Fig. 8). Lin has used this method in nine hepatic lobectomies for hepatoma and proved it to be the most simplified and excellent method of hepatic lobectomy. By this method, the inexperience in, and the inherent fear of, inserting

the fingers into a vascular sponge organ like the liver and searching for the vascular and ductal components are thus avoided.

The only shortcoming of the crush method is that when the tumor extensively involves a whole hepatic lobe or more, there may be no room available for either a hepatic clamp or crush clamp. In such instances, the controlled method or original finger fracture technique may be resorted to for the hepatic resection.

Middle Hepatic Lobectomy

This is occasionally performed for a tumor of limited extent, confined to the median segment of the left lobe.

The lesion is exposed in the same way as for right hepatic lobectomy by upper transverse incision with right thoracic extension. Prior to incision on the main lobar tissue, a series of interlocking deep sutures of chromicized catgut are placed along tissue from the region to the right of the fossa of the gallbladder inferiorly to the fossa of the inferior vena cava superiorly. After ligating these interlocking sutures the Glisson's capsule is incised, the liver parenchyma is dissected with fingers or a scalpel, and the vessels and hepatic ducts that are encountered are clamped and ligated. When this dissection plane has been completed down to the inferior vena cava, the medial segment is is reflected to the left exposing the middle hepatic vein, which is ligated and transected (Fig. 9a). In a similar manner, interlocking sutures are applied to the left of the left segmental fissue, and the left median segment is dissected bluntly away from the left lateral segment to complete the middle hepatic lobectomy. The bleeders are carefully checked, and transverse large mattress sutures are placed perpendicular to the previously inserted interlocking mattress sutures to permit approximation of the right hepatic lobe with the lateral segment of the left lobe (Fig. 9b). However, Bengmark (20) leaves the section surfaces of the two liver halves

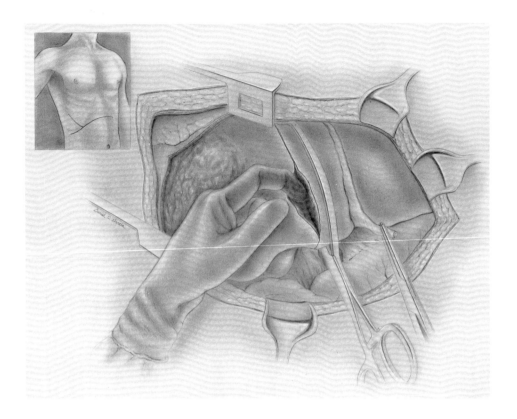

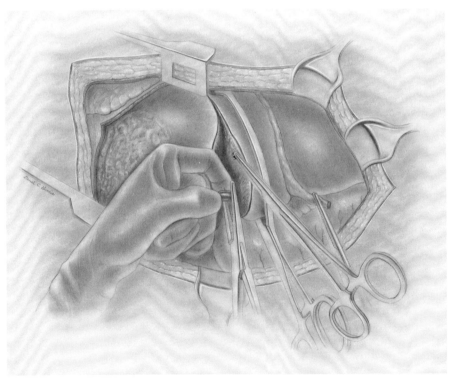

Figure 7 Finger fracture technique with hepatic clamp (Lin, TY: *Ann Surg* **177**:413, 1973). *(a)* With hepatic clamp placed at the anatomical boundary of both lobes, the fingers are

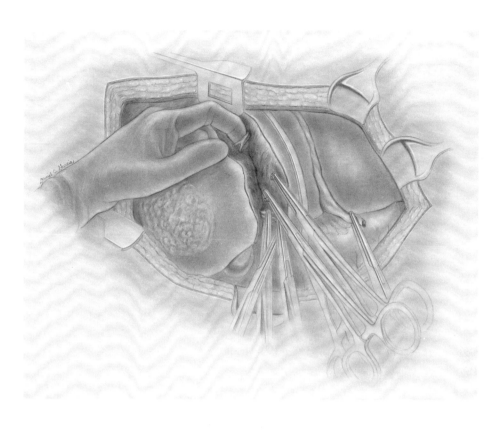

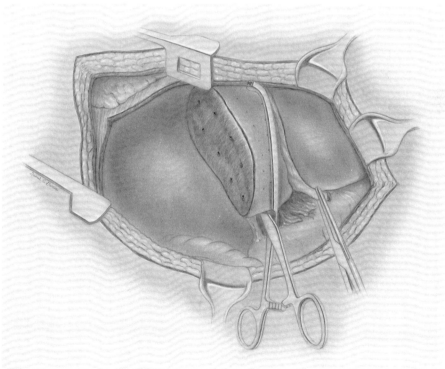

inserted directly into the liver tissue. *(b)* The right branch of the hepatic artery, the portal vein, and the right hepatic vein are exposed to view.

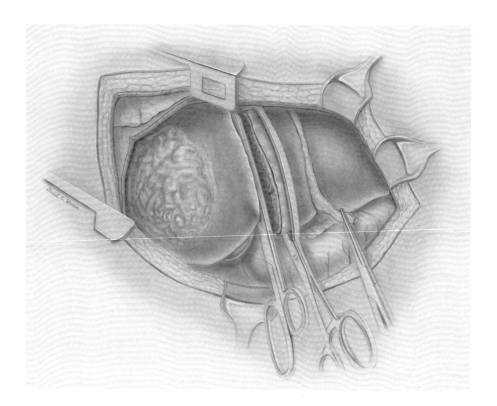

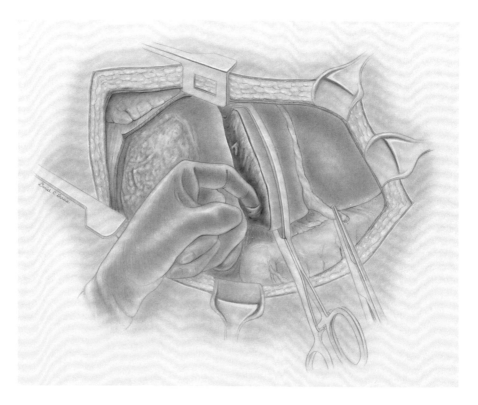

Figure 8   (a) Crush clamp is applied on the incision line and tightened to crush away the friable parenchymatous tissue. (b) On release of the crush clamp, the unyielding vascular and ductal structures appear as bridges between the two compartments of the liver. The right branch of the hepatic artery, the portal vein, and the right hepatic vein are exposed to view.

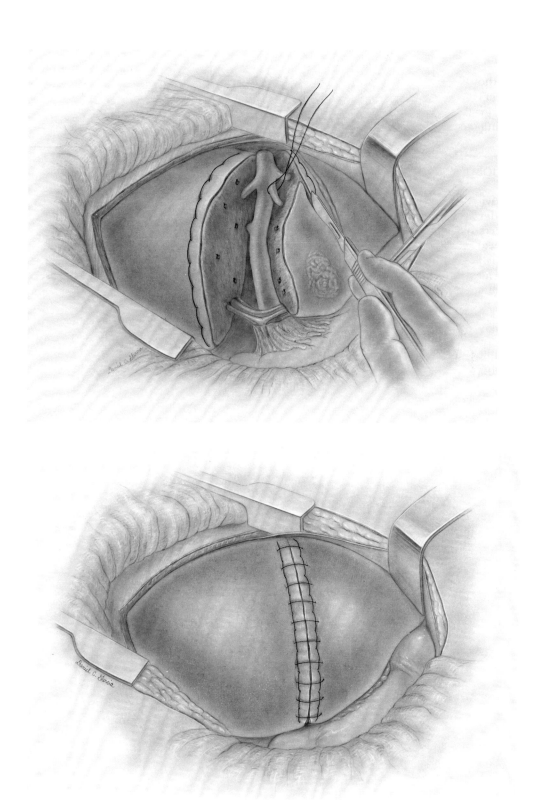

Figure 9 *(a)* Medial segment of the left lobe is removed under interlocking mattress sutures placed on the main lobar fissure and the left segmental fissure. *(b)* Approximation of remaining liver tissue.

open without approximation. The author also covers each section surface with an omental graft after the resection without attempting to approximate them.

INDICATION AND CONTRAINDICATION

Patients with HCC are considered as operable under the following conditions: the general condition of the patient is sufficient to warrant the operation; no definite metastasis is present in the lung, bone, or other organs; palpable hepatic mass or masses, if any, are apparently limited to one lobe of the liver regardless of its size; the other lobe of the liver is not cirrhotic or nodular on palpation; no remarkable jaundice or ascites is present; and laboratory examination reveals no severe impairment in hepatic function.

At the time of operation, massive or nodular types of hepatic carcinoma confined to one hepatic lobe and no metastatic nodule or severe cirrhosis in the other lobe are sufficient and necessary indications for lobectomy.

In the presence of coexisting liver cirrhosis, the advisability of hepatic lobectomy for primary hepatic carcinoma varies with the degree of cirrhosis. Hepatic lobectomy is indicated for either the right or left lobe if the cancer-free lobe is macroscopically normal or only very mildly cirrhotic. In the presence of moderately advanced cirrhosis (with a coarse nodular surface of the liver), lobectomy of the left but not of the right lobe can be undertaken without much danger. When cirrhotic change of the liver is severe, hepatic lobectomy, be it right or left, is contraindicated.

OPERABILITY AND RESECTABILITY

Owing to its high malignancy, early intrahepatic spread, and frequently associated liver cirrhosis, HCC has long been deemed as one of the malignancies of least operability and resectability. Accordingly, it has been treated only occasionally by hepatic lobectomy and is still largely considered to be a hopeless disease.

Nevertheless, Lin (19) reported 72.6% operability and 41.6% resectability among the operable cases based on the aforementioned criteria for indication in 271 cases of HCC experienced between 1954 and 1970. Naturally, early diagnosis is the sole important factor to give higher operability and resectability, and in areas where the disease is common, general survey of the population for alpha fetoprotein may greatly help early detection of this cancer. Furthermore, a more active attitude toward laparotomy along the guidelines provided in the foregoing section, rather than disposing cases as inoperable simply because of a report of liver cirrhosis on needle biopsy, may also increase the number of operable and resectable cases. In view of the brevity of the period between the onset of symptoms and death in this cancer, it is important that surgery be carried out early.

OPERATIVE RISK

The commonly reported operative risks incurred during hepatic lobectomy are bleeding, cardiac arrest, air embolism, and fibrinolysis.

Massive bleeding may occur as a result of a tear of the hepatic vein or vena cava when the short hepatic veins are isolated extrahepatically before hepatic transection and frequently costs large amounts of blood transfusions, up to 10,000 ml or even the patient's life during the operation. It is of utmost importance to pump in blood through the arm vein rather than the saphenous vein for the blood loss in such instances. Air embolism or cardiac arrest may result aside from massive bleeding from the torn vena cava. In order to prevent these lethal complications, some apply a tape around the vena cava above and below the liver before hepatic lobectomy to shut out blood flow in case of vena cava injury. This is, however, unlikely to happen with the finger fracture technique or the crush method.

Cardiac arrest may develop in infants or small children during hepatic lobectomy in the absence of excessive bleeding such as from a torn vena cava. Simple torsion of the small calibered vena cava in children during operative manipulation will cause impeded venous return and cardiac arrest. Because of this hazard in pediatric patients, the heart rate should be carefully monitored through a visioscope during operation, and cardiac resuscitation should be immediately instituted along with rapid removal of the affected hepatic lobe once the heart is arrested.

The other operative risk in hepatic lobectomy is fibrinolysis. Any kind of trauma to the liver including liver resection may activate the fibrinolytic system, deplete fibrinogen, and cause bleeding. In fact, fibrinolysis occurs sometime during or immediately following hepatic resection despite an apparently normal coagulation mechanism before operation. Therefore, it is mandatory to examine the clotting mechanism routinely at the end of operation to eliminate the possibility of fibrinolysis in order that this complication may be prevented and treated in due time.

COMPLICATION, MORTALITY, AND POSTOPERATIVE CARE

Aside from the immediate intraoperative complications listed above, the postoperative complications in hepatic lobectomy are relatively insignificant. They include pleural effusion, wound infection, pneumonia, and, rarely, bile leakage. Occasionally fever of unknown origin is noted, but is readily controlled by administration of

prednisolone. Those cirrhotic patients who are subjected to right hepatic lobectomy in particular are frequently seen to have ankle edema, ascites, and hypoalbuminemia postoperatively and respond well to albumin administration.

Otherwise the postoperative care is essentially the same as that following major operation. Bile leakage will heal spontaneously by conservative treatment unless there is injury to the major hepatic duct.

Immediate postoperative injection of Mitomycin C or 5-FU via the hepatic artery has been tried to kill the unnoticed malignant cells left in the residual lobe of the liver. By the same token, postoperative chemotherapy with these agents given intravenously shortly after the operation may improve the prognosis by killing the circulating hepatoma cells, and hence should be recommended.

Surgical mortality (death within 30 postoperative days) of hepatic lobectomy has steadily been reduced along with the progress in surgical technique. Schweizer et al (21) reported a 35.8% mortality rate in 53 cases and Brunshwig (22), a 29% rate in 24 cases, whereas Lin (19) reported 12.1% mortality in 82 cases treated before 1970 and no mortality in the recent 21 cases treated either with the hepatic clamp and finger fracture technique or with the crush method (12, 17).

RESULTS AND PROGNOSIS

The results of treatment and the prognosis for HCC following hepatic lobectomy depend naturally on the extent of the malignancy, the presence or absence of occult intrahepatic or extrahepatic metastasis, as well as of associated liver cirrhosis. In general, the results of treatment are hardly satisfactory. Of 80 cases of primary carcinoma of the liver who survived hepatic lobectomy in Lin's series (12), two-thirds (53 cases) died within a year after operation

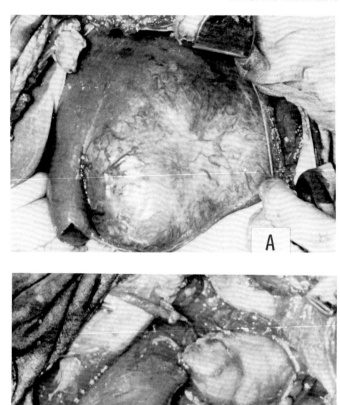

Figure 10   *(a)* A huge hepatoma on the left lobe is shown *(b)* After resection of the left lobe.

either because of local recurrence (26%) or lung metastasis (18.7%) or hepatic failure (11.9%). Nevertheless, hepatic lobectomy for primary carcinoma of the liver in the same series has yielded survival for 1 to 2 years in ten cases, 2 to 3 years in five cases, 3 to 4 years in three cases and more than 5 years in nine cases, of which seven patients are still well for 5 to 13 years (Figs. 10 and 11).

Even though Wang (23) et al reported pessimistically that only two patients survived more than 5 years in a series of 130 hepatic lobectomies for HCC collected from 10 teaching hospitals in China over a period of 20 years, El-Domeiri et al (24) from Sloan-Kettering Hospital reported 15.6% rate of 5-year survival among 32 hepatic lobectomies for primary malignant hepatic tumor over a 20-year period. In Lin's series (12) the 5-year survival rate of hepatic lobectomy in 92 cases of malignant hepatic tumor was 19.1%.

OTHER SURGICAL TREATMENTS

When HCC is so widely spread as to in-

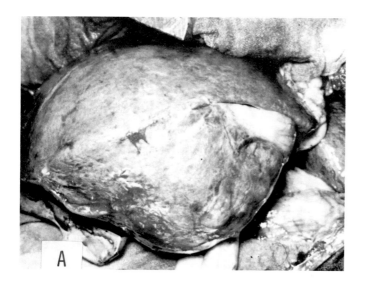

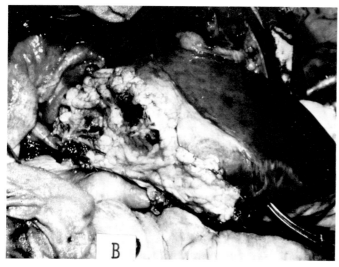

Figure 11 *(a)* A huge massive type hepatoma occupying the right lobe. *(b)* The remaining left lobe after right hepatic lobectomy.

volve the whole liver, or when associated liver cirrhosis is so advanced as to defy hepatic lobectomy, the hepatic artery may be ligated instead. This procedure is based on the concept that a hepatic tumor receives its blood supply exclusively from the hepatic artery, and the interruption of the hepatic artery causes necrosis of the tumor tissue with minimal damage to the surrounding normal liver tissue. Nilsson (25), Plengvanit et al (26), and Almersjo et al (27) have performed hepatic artery ligation in a number of malignant hepatomas but the result has been discouraging. Honjio

(28) reported ligation of the portal vein branch instead of the hepatic artery in 15 cases, with survival of 11.3 months as an average.

In 1968 Starzl (29) did total hepatectomy and whole liver transplantation in 2 cases of hepatoma, who survived 4 months and one year, respectively. Despite its technical feasibility, total hepatectomy for extensive cancer followed by allograft seems to be futile when local spread and remote metastasis remain to be the main stake in hepatoma. However, as soon as the problems regarding rejection and immunosup-

timetabolite, was given in a dosage schedule of 15 mg/kg/day for 3 to 5 days and then 7.5 mg/kg every 2 or 3 days (6, 7). More recently, a weekly intravenous or oral administration of 5-FU, 15 to 20 mg/kg/week to a point of mild toxicity, has been recommended (8). By this modification, the toxic reactions have been lowered without reduction in response rate (9, 10).

In our hospital, antimetabolites are administered daily as a rule, until signs of mild toxicity develop. Schedules are based on experimental studies using tissue culture cells (11). The following are our dosage schedules for various anticancer agents.

1. Oral administration
   a. N_1-(2'-furanidyl)-5-fluorouracil (FT-207), 16 to 24 mg/kg/day, 3 or 4 times daily to mild toxicity (12)
   b. 5-fluorouracil (5-FU), 4 to 8 mg/kg/day, 2 to 4 times daily to mild toxicity.
   c. Cyclophosphamide, 1 to 2 mg/kg/day once a day to mild toxicity.
2. Intravenous administration
   a. Combination chemotherapy, FAMT, 5-FU 10 mg/kg, cyclophosphamide 4 mg/kg, Mitomycin C 0.04 mg/kg, Chromomycin A_3 0.01 mg/kg, twice a week to mild toxicity (13).
   b. Mitomycin C, 0.12 to 0.2 mg/kg, twice a week to mild toxicity, commonly with 3,000 mg dextran sulfate and 2,000 units of urokinase (14).
   c. Cyclophosphamide, 8 mg/kg, twice a week to mild toxicity.
3. Combination chemotherapy, oral antimetabolites with intravenous Mitomycin C.
   Dosage schedules for oral 5-FU and FT-207 are the same as above, and, in addition, Mitomycin C is given in a dose of 0.12 to 0.2 mg/kg, once a week.

RESULTS

The reported response rate varies with investigators. Ramirez et al described a case of unusually long survival following systemic chemotherapy. A patient with disseminated primary liver cancer died of a myocardial infarct after 10 years of therapy with 5-FU, and no viable cancer cells were observed at the time of autopsy (1). Jacob et al reported 2 out of 12 patients with HCC who responded to weekly intravenous 5-FU (9). In the series of Al-Sarraf et al there was no favorable response in any of 18 patients with HCC treated with systemic 5-FU or 5-FU plus vinblastin and other drugs (4).

Table 1 shows our results obtained by systemic chemotherapy using various anticancer agents to primary and metastatic liver carcinomas. Out of 42 patients with primary HCC who entered this study, 26 were evaluable for response, and the remainder not evaluable because of early death (12 cases), toxic reaction (1 case), and change of drugs (3 cases). Of these 26 cases, regression of hepatic tumor was observed in 3 (11.5%). In one additional case, regression of metastases in the lung was observed, but the primary tumor in the liver did not regress in size, and the levels of serum alpha feroprotein (AFP) became higher. This last case was excluded from responders. There were 110 evaluable cases and 22 responders in metastatic to liver cancer (20.0%, 22/110). The response rate was high in patients with liver metastases from the cervix uteri, the stomach, and the lung.

As shown in Table 2, there were responders in the groups of hepatocellular carcinoma treated with FAMT or FT-207, but not in the group treated with Mitomycin C. Treatment by oral FT-207 was also effective for metastatic liver adenocarcinomas (42.9%, 6/14). In metastatic liver car-

Table 1 Results of Systemic Chemotherapy for Primary and Metastatic Carcinomas[a]

Primary site	Total Number of Cases	Number of Evaluable Cases	Number of Responders
Liver	42	26	3
Head and neck	2	2	
Esophagus	2	2	1
Stomach	61	48	11
Colon and rectum	31	29	3
Gallbladder	7	5	
Pancreas	3	3	
Lung	16	7	2
Breast	6	4	1
Uterus	8	7	3
Prostate	1	1	1
Kidney	1	1	
Adrenal	1	0	
Thymus	1	1	
Total	182	136	25

[a] Responders: regression of palpable liver tumor by ≥ 30%.

cinomas of the squamous cell or anaplastic cell type, intravenous Mitocymin C was the most effective with response rate of 30.0% (3/10) and 40.0% (2/5), respectively.

In the responders, regression of hepatic tumor was observed within three weeks, irrespective of anticancer agents employed and of the primary site. With regresion of tumor size, the patients became free from subjective complaints, blood biochemical data improved, and AFP, when positive before treatment, was simultaneously decreased. The regression of hepatic tumor was confirmed by scintigraphy. Prolongation of survival occurred in the patients in whom tumor clearly regressed.

CASE REPORTS

CASE 1. A 55-year-old Chinese man was admitted on November 11, 1967 because of epigastric pain. There was a tumor in the epigastrium, presumably of the liver. Peritoneoscopy on December 5, 1967 disclosed a solitary liver tumor on the surface of the left lobe (Fig. 1). Intravenous drip infusion of combined anticancer agents (FAMT) was performed twice a week from December 7, 1967 to January 17, 1968 for a

total of eight doses. The liver regressed in size and became impalpable at the end of the therapy. On February 2, 1968 a second peritoneoscopic examination was carried out (Fig. 2). The liver tumor was no longer observed, and the surface of the liver portion that had been occupied by the tumor on the first examination was depressed. Left hepatectomy was carried out three months after the last dose of FAMT. The removed specimen revealed hepatocellular carcinoma showing chemotherapeutic effects, but viable cell nests were still demonstrated. The patient is still alive without a sign of recurrence five years after operation. The details will be published elsewhere.

CASE 2. A 58-year-old Japanese man had had frequent colic pain in the right upper abdomen, and laparotomy was performed on December 17, 1973 at another hospital for suspected cholelithiasis. The liver was enlarged with disseminated tumors in both lobes. He was referred to us on January 17, 1974 with a histological diagnosis of HCC. Since the hepatic tumor was already large, oral administration of FT-207 was started with a daily dose of 800 mg/day. By the time of admission on January 31, 1974 the liver had been reduced in size and blood biochemistry markedly improved. The regression of liver continued thereafter with concomitant decrease in serum AFP. On February 4, 1974 the liver became no longer palpable, and he was discharged without complaints on February 14, 1974. His clinical course is summarized in Fig. 3. He

Table 2 Effects of Anticancer Agents on Different Histological Types of Primary and Metastatic Carcinomas[a]

Histological types	Drugs										
	Mitomycin C (i.v)	Cyclophosphamide (i.v)	Cyclophosphamide (p.o)	Adriamycin (i.v)	Bleomycin (i.v)	5-FU (p.o)	FT-207 (p.o)	FT-207 (p.o) with Mitomycin C (i.v)	FAMT (i.v)	Others	Total
Hepatocellular carcinoma	0/7	0/2	0/1	0/1	0/1	0/4	1/4	0/2	2/6	0/2	3/29
Adenocarcinoma	2/25	0/11	1/2	1/5	0/1	1/2	6/14	2/6	1/32	2/17	16/115
Squamous cell carcinoma	3/10		0/2	0/1	1/1				0/3	0/3	4/20
Anaplastic cell carcinoma	2/5		0/1		0/1				0/3	0/1	2/11
Hypernephroma	0/1										0/1
Total	7/48	0/13	1/6	1/7	1/3	1/6	7/18	2/8	3/44	2/23	25/176

[a] Results were obtained from 176 evaluable chemotherapeutic courses carried out in 136 patients.

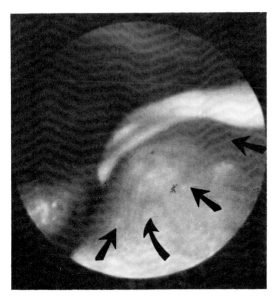

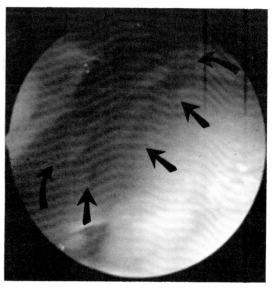

Figure 1 Case 1. The peritoneoscopic picture of the left lobe, before chemotherapy (19). Note the bulge outlined by arrows.

Figure 2 Case 1. The peritoneoscopic picture of the left lobe, after chemotherapy (19). Note the depressed area of the region of the previous tumor (arrows).

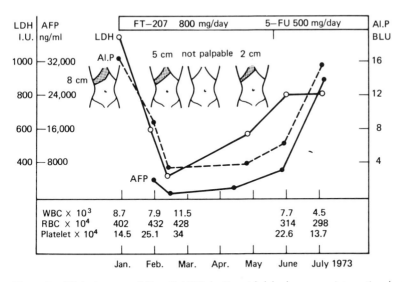

Figure 3 Clinical course of Case 2. LDH: lactic acid dehydrogenase, international units. AFP: alpha fetoproteins, nanograms/milliliters. A1.P: Alkaline phosphatase, Bessey-Lowry units. FT-207: N1-(2'-furanidyl)-5-fluorouracil. 5 FU: 5-fluorouracil.

worked actively until May 11, 1974, when liver tumor again became palpable.

Comments

Recent advances in chemotherapy for cancer has made feasible the selection of various anticancer agents according to the histological type. Most patients with primary HCC have in the past been treated with 5-FU. Our experiences described here also suggest that antimetabolites and their combinations can be employed for the systemic chemotherapy as effective and less toxic (12, 15). The effects of oral FT-207 were remarkable in metastatic adenocarcinomas of the liver. For squamous and anaplastic cell carcinomas, the most favorable results were obtained with Mitomycin C. Likewise, primary HCC seems much less sensitive to hepatic artery infusion chemotherapy (16) than metastatic HCC.

Complete remission cannot be expected by chemotherapy alone at present, although a few exceptional cases are in the literature (1, 2). In 1970 Hermann and Lonsdale reported an infant with hepatoblastoma that became operable after systemic vincristin followed by ^{60}Co teletherapy and systemic cyclophosphamide. Although the resected specimen was composed almost entirely of dense fibrous tissues, active viable cells were still seen in the central portion (17). A similar experience by hepatic artery infusion was made by Hasegawa et al in our hospital (18). In the case described (Case 1), viable cells were also present in the resected specimen, in spite of a striking regression of tumor size following chemotherapy. Therefore, when hepatic tumor has regressed by means of chemotherapy, reconsideration of complete removal of tumor may be made depending on the patient's condition.

CONCLUSION

Primary liver cancer is less sensitive to the currently available chemotherapeutic agents given systemically compared with metastatic liver carcinomas. In our series, whereas 22 out of 110 cases of metastatic carcinoma to liver responded to systemic chemotherapy (20.0%), there were only 3 of 26 patients with HCC (11.5%), who showed a favorable response. Occasionally, however, primary liver carcinoma regresses remarkably following chemotherapy, enabling resection of the tumor.

Among the various anticancer agents, oral FT-207 and intravenous 5-FU in combination were more effective for primary HCC. Of metastatic liver carcinomas, adenocarcinomas responded more favorably to oral FT-207, and squamous and anaplastic cell carcinomas to intravenous Mitomycin C.

REFERENCES

1. Ramirez G, Ansfield FJ, Curreri AR: Hepatoma; Long-term survival with disseminated tumor treated with 5-fluorouracil. *Am J Surg* **120**:400–403, 1970.

2. McSweeney, Dove KE, McAdams AJ: Spontaneous regression of a putative childhood hepatoma. *Am J Dis Child* **125**:596–598, 1973.

3. El-Domeiri AA, Huvas AG, Goldsmith HS, et al: Primary malignant tumors of the liver. *Cancer* **27**:7–11, 1971.

4. Al-Sarraf M, Go TS, Kithier K, et al: Primary liver cancer, a review of the clinical features, blood groups, serum enzymes, therapy and survival of 65 cases. *Cancer* **33**:574–582, 1974.

5. Ariel IM, Pack GT: Treatment of inoperable cancer of the liver by intra-arterial radioactive isotopes and chemotherapy. In *Tumors of the Liver.* Pack GT, Islami AH (Eds). Springer, Berlin, 1970, p 285.

6. Curreri AR, Ansfield FJ, McIver F, et al: The synthesis of 5-fluorouracil. *Cancer Res* **18**:478–484, 1858.

7. Ansfield FJ, Schroeder JM, Curreri AR: Five

years clinical experience with 5-fluorouracil. *JAMA* **181**:295–299, 1962.

8. Brule G, Eckhardt SJ, Hall TC, Winkler A: *Drug Therapy of Cancer.* World Health Organization, 1973, p 47.

9. Jacobs EM, Reeves WJ, Wood DA, et al: Treatment of cancer with weekly intravenous 5-fluorouracil. *Cancer* **27**:1302–1305, 1971.

10. Bateman JR, Pugh RP, Cassidy FR, et al: 5-Fluorouracil given once weekly, comparison of intravenous and oral administration. *Cancer* **28**:907–913, 1971.

11. Shimoyama M, Kimura K: Quantitative study on cytocidal action of anticancer agents. *Saishin-Igaku* **28**:1024–1040, 1973.

12. Konda C, Niitani H, Sakauch N, et al: Chemotherapy of cancer with oral administration of N_1-(2'-furanidyl)-5-fluorouracil. *Jap J Cancer Clin* **19**:495–499, 1973.

13. Kimura K: Combination chemotherapy. *Jap J Cancer Clin* **14**:184–190, 1968.

14. Niitani H: Combined chemotherapy with lyso-some labilizer and Mitomycin C: *Saishin-Igaku* **28**:912–919, 1973.

15. Okazaki N, Hattori N, Ono T, et al: Treatment of liver cancer with oral administration of N_1-(2'-furanidyl)-5-fluorouracil. *Jap J Gastroenterol* **71**:597–601, 1974.

16. Brule G, Eckhardt SJ, Hall YC, Winkle A. *Drug Therapy of Cancer.* World Health Organization, 1973, p 47.

17. Hermann RE, Lonsdale D: Chemotherapy, radiotherapy, and hepatic lobectomy for hepatoblastoma in an infant, report of a survival. *Surgery* **68**:383–388, 1970.

18. Hasegawa H, Mukojima T, Hattori H, et al: Embryonal carcinoma and alpha-fetoprotein, with special reference to hepatoblastoma. In *Alfa-Fetoprotein and Hepatoma,* Hirai H, Miyaji T (Eds). University of Tokyo Press, Tokyo, 1972, p 133.

19. Okazaki N, Hattori N, Arima M, et al: Peritonescopic observation of chemotherapeutic effects in a patient with hepatocellular carcinoma. *Jap J Clin Oncol* **6**:77–78, 1974.

CHAPTER 21 ARTERIAL INJECTION CHEMOTHERAPY

YASUHIKO KUBO, M.D.
YUTAKA SHIMOKAWA, M.D.

Patients with primary liver cancer are usually in an inoperable stage of the disease when the diagnosis is made. The underlying cirrhosis with deteriorated hepatic function drastically reduces the resectability rate even if the tumor is discovered to be small. Inoperable patients are left at the mercy of distressing progress of the tumor, and palliative measures are of no avail. Systemic chemotherapy of primary liver cancer employing various cytotoxic and antimetabolic agents has been attempted, but the results have so far been less satisfactory compared with metastatic liver carcinomas.

Administration of chemotherapeutic agents into an artery was first described by Bierman et al (1) and Klopp et al (2). Their idea was soon applied to the chemotherapy of liver malignancies by utilizing the technique of hepatic artery catheterization by way of the brachial (3) and the femoral arteries (4). The recently developed selective angiography can now be combined with the delivery of a large dose of anticancer agents in one shot into the hepatic artery. Direct transabdominal catheterization was also

carried out by Miller and Griman (5), and has since been used for the same purpose.

Ariel and Pack (6) and Simon and his associates (7) reported administration of radioisotopes such as ^{90}Yttrium microspheres by way of the brachial or femoral artery into the hepatic artery in the treatment of metastatic carcinomas and carcinoid tumor of the liver.

Concurrent with the improvement of techniques for administration, the list of chemotherapeutic agents is rapidly expanding with discovery and synthesis of new compounds. The once bleak outlook of chemotherapy for liver cancer may no longer be the same. The authors have so far treated a total of 64 patients, 40 with chemotherapeutic agents given intraarterially and 24 by supportive measure, and they feel now that with proper selection of patients, intraarterial administration of the agents will bring about a beneficial, if not drastic, response. The available data are still insufficient to enable accurate prediction of the effect at the time of patient selection, and which constitutes a major goal of our current investigation.

METHOD AND RATIONALE OF ARTERIAL INJECTION CHEMOTHERAPY

One of the major difficulties with systemic administration of an anticancer drug is inability to deliver it in sufficient concentrations to the tumor, without causing severe systemic reactions. The rationale for arterial administration is that hepatocellular carcinoma (HCC) is mainly supplied by the hepatic artery rather than the portal vein (8, 9) and that the liver parenchyma can tolerate large doses of chemotherapeutic agents. Furthermore, it is known that extrahepatic metastases are rather uncommon in this carcinoma, except for the lung, since the tumor is confined to the liver for a considerable length of time.

Intraarterial delivery of agents in one injection, which we call "one shot" method, is carried out by the same arteriographic technique originally devised by Seldinger (10) or the procedure now commonly used for celiac angiography. A siliconized teflon catheter, such as the KIFA (Sweden) and Beckton-Dickinson (USA) types currently available, is inserted into the celiac artery from the femoral artery with the aid of a guidewire under fluoroscopic control or, if possible, is threaded further into the hepatic artery superselectively. After arteriography, which determines the position of the catheter tip, a chemotherapeutic agent is delivered through the catheter.

For arterial infusion therapy, placement of the catheter is carried out by two ways. In the first method, or the transabdominal procedure as described by Miller and Griman (5) which has been employed in our study, the catheter is placed in the gastroduodenal or gastroepiploic artery. After laparotomy, the artery is separated from the adjacent tissue, ligated distally, and then a siliconized polyethylene catheter is introduced into the hepatic artery by ar-

teriotomy. The catheter is tied and brought out on the abdominal wall to be attached to the infusion pump. Watkins' chronofuser (USA), Sharp's pump (Japan), or any other type of portable constant infusion pump may be used. They are equipped with a 25 to 50 ml plastic reservoir capable of delivering 5 to 10 ml of fluid per 24 hours. Starting in the operating room, the catheter and reservoir are continuously flushed and filled with sterile saline until the postoperative condition is stabilized. The chemotherapeutic agent is then added to the reservoir to initiate the therapy.

The second method is a closed procedure. Catheterization is carried out through the left brachial or femoral artery (3, 11, 4). Seldinger's guidewire method (10) is more convenient for this transfemoral approach. The closed methods have the benefit of not requiring surgical intervention and general anesthesia. On the other hand, the catheter may not be placed as intended some times, and extrahepatic regions are infused causing toxicity.

In the present study, arterial administration of the agent was carried out by the following two methods: (a) the so-called one shot method via the hepatic artery, in which a large single dose is injected during celiac or hepatic angiography, and (b) long-term continuous infusion via a catheter placed in the right gastroepiploic or gastroduodenal artery.

CHEMOTHERAPEUTIC AGENTS AND DOSAGE

Regardless of the catheterization technique, it is important that the agent flow directly to all areas of involvement and in adequate concentrations. Theoretically, the dosage must be one that is sufficiently large to cause regression of the tumor. Unfortunately, however, patients with hepatocellular carcinoma do not always withstand such a dose because of frequent

Table 1 Mean Survival of Patients with Hepatocellular Carcinoma

	Chemotherapy			Supportive Therapy	Total
	Long Survival [a]	Short Survival [b]	Total		
Number of patients	26	14	40	24	64
Survival after initial signs (months)	10.4	3.6	8.0	4.2	6.6
Survival after start of chemotherapy (months)	5.7	1.6	4.2		

[a] Long survival: longer than 6 months after onset.
[b] Short survival: less than 6 months after onset.

association of liver cirrhosis (12). In such instances, dosage has to be reduced only to palliate subjective symptoms.

The chemotherapeutic agents used for the one shot method were Mitomycin C (MMC), Cyclophosphamide (Endoxan, EX), Cytosine arabinoside (CA), Methotrexate (MTX), Adriamycin, and 5-flurouracil (5-FU). They were given singly or in combinations of two or three. The dose schedules for one shot therapy in our study have been as follows: (1) MMC alone, 0.2 to 0.5 mg/kg of body weight; (2) MMC, 0.2 to 0.4 mg/kg, EX 500 mg and 5FU 500 mg; (3) MMC, 0.2 to 0.4 mg/kg and MTX, 0.5 to 1 mg/kg; (4) MMC (0.2 to 0.5 mg/kg) and CA (1 to 2 mg/kg); and (5) Adriamycin, 1 to 2 mg/kg. Methotrexate was given with its antidote, Leukovorin, as described by Sullivan et al (13). These dosages are lower compared with those generally employed for Caucasians, because Japanese are less tolerant to these agents. One shot delivery was repeated, whenever feasible, with intervals of three to five weeks. The effect is evident when there is relief of pain, the tumor size diminishes, and serum levels of alpha-fetoprotein (AFP), alkaline phosphatase, and lactic dehydrogenase isozyme 5 are decreased. At times, anorexia, leukopenia, thrombocytopenia, and anemia are noted as a reaction. After recovery from these side effects and when

these biochemical indicators are elevated again, a second shot may be considered.

Antimetabolites such as 5-FU and its derivatives are the choice for continuous infusion. The dose schedules in our clinic have been 3 to 5 mg/kg of 5-FU per day. The bag (reservoir) is filled with 25 ml of a saline solution of the agent, and a spring-driven rolling pump delivers 5 ml per 24 hours, impelling the fluid into the catheter and then into the liver. The patient receives the regimen for a period as long as 6 months, or even longer. As most antimetabolites produce antitumor effects by interfering with *de novo* synthesis of nucleic acids, it is mandatory that the duration of administration surpass the tumor doubling time.

CLINICAL MATERIAL AND METHOD OF ANALYSIS

The clinical material for our study was made up of 64 patients, 56 males and 8 females, with unequivocal diagnosis of HCC. Of the 64, 40 were given anticancer chemotherapy either by the one shot method (35 cases) or by continuous infusion (5 cases), and the remainder treated palliatively (Table 1). Diagnosis of HCC was made from the findings of laparoscopy, scintigraphy, biopsy, celiac angiography, and blood tests, particularly AFP, beside physical findings of hepatomegaly and related abnormalities. Subsequent autopsy confirmed the diagnosis in the majority. Intrahepatic cholangiocarcinoma, the incidence of which is very small, could not entirely be excluded, but it was assumed that the vast majority of the patients had HCC.

The overall mean survival time of the total of 64 cases was 6.6 ± 0.6 (SE) months after the initial signs or symptoms, with a range of 2 to 28 months. The patients given chemotherapy lived an average of 8.0 months after the onset of clinical signs and 4.2 months after the start of chemotherapy, as contrasted by a mean survival time of 4.2 months after onset in patients treated with a supportive measure.

In order to facilitate assessment of the effect of chemotherapy, patients were divided into the following three groups: (1) those who had chemotherapy and lived longer than 6 months after onset—long survival group; (2) those who had the same and lived less than 6 months—short survival group; and (3) those who were treated palliatively. Comparison was made among these groups with respect to alleviation of pain, diminution of tumor size, change in AFP level, and in other liver tests.

One of the most important factors that determine prognosis is the associated cirrhosis and its severity. The diagnosis of cirrhosis was made by the same procedures and examinations used for carcinoma, with additional consideration of signs of portal hypertension, ascites, and liver size. Frequency of associated cirrhosis was 80.0% in the long survival group, 71.4% in the short survival group, and 87.5% in the supportive therapy group (Table 2). Although these figures did not indicate associated cirrhosis is deleterious in chemotherapy, neither did it mean that severe cirrhosis is a contraindication, as we discuss below.

RESULTS

Table 3 represents the effect of

chemotherapy on pain, one of the most common and distressing complaints of patients in this disease. It was alleviated in 10 (38.5%) out of 26 cases, and was aggravated in 2 (7.6%). No difference was noted between the long and short survival groups, indicating that relief of pain may be expected even in patients in whom no prolongation of life occurs. In other words, temporary relief of pain is unrelated to the effect on the length of survival time.

The change of the tumor size induced by therapy is summarized in Table 4. No reduction in tumor size was noted in patients in the short survival group as estimated from angiograms, scintiscans, and by palpation, while in the long survival group, considerable reduction in tumor size occured in 14 cases, or in 56% of the patients. The tumor increased in size in 3 patients (23.1%) in the short survival group, but in only 1 (4%) in the long survival group. Thus, there was a definite difference in the response of tumor size between the two groups receiving chemotherapy.

Change of AFP in relation to tumor regression was analyzed by dividing patients treated with chemotherapy into (a) those who exhibited regression and (b) those in whom tumor remained unchanged or increased in size. As the results in Table 5 indicate, in 9 of 12 cases demonstrating tumor regression, AFP was decreased by 26 to 93% of the pretreatment level, with an average of 70%. In the group in which no tumor regression occurred, AFP was decreased in 4 cases, unchanged in 3, and increased in 8, the increase ranging from 19 to 582% (average 203%).

Figure 1 represents the alteration in AFP level during the clinical course in time and in relation to one shot injections (small arrows), making reference to the pretreatment level set at 100%. It is evident from the chart that the patients in whom AFP rose sharply lived for a short time, and those with unchanged or decreased AFP levels lived longer.

Table 2   Relationship between Associated Cirrhosis and Response to Chemotherapy

	Chemotherapy		Supportive Therapy
	Long Survival	Short Survival	
Number of patients	25	14	24
With liver cirrhosis	20	10	21
Percentage	80.0%	71.4%	87.5%

Table 3   Effect of Chemotherapy on Pain

	Total	Long Survival	Short Survival
Number of Patients	26	17	9
Alleviated (%)	10 (38.5)	7 (41.2)	3 (33.3)
No improvement (%)	14 (53.8)	9 (52.9)	5 (55.6)
Aggravated (%)	2 (7.6)	1 (5.9)	1 (11.1)

Table 4   Change in Tumor Size[a] after Chemotherapy

	Long Survival	Short Survival	Total
Number of Patients	25	13	38
Definite regression (%)	14 (56.0)	0	14 (36.8)
No improvement (%)	10 (40.0)	10 (76.9)	20 (52.6)
Increase in size (%)	1 (4.0)	3 (23.1)	4 (10.5)

[a]Tumor size was estimated in angiogram, scintigram, and by palpation.

Table 5   Response of Serum AFP and Tumor Size to Chemotherapy

	Number of Cases	Range of Serum AFP	Response of Serum AFP[a]		
			Decreased	Unchanged	Increased
Regression in tumor size	12	20 to 34 × 10⁴ ng/ml	9 26 to 93% mean 70%	3 ± 5%	0 cases
No regression or enlargment	15	20 to 160 × 10⁴	4 14 to 48% mean 32%	3 ± 5%	8 19 to 582% mean 203%

[a] Maximum change in serum AFP is given in percentage of the pretreatment level.

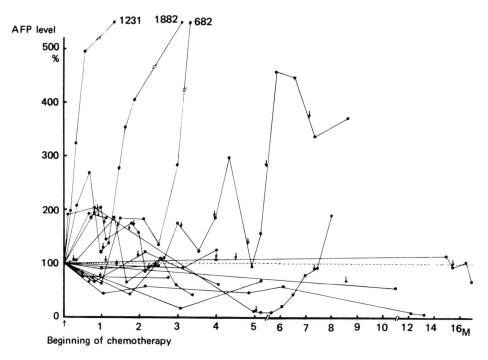

Figure 1 Serum AFP levels during arterial chemotherapy, by one shot method, making reference to the pretreatment level set at 100%. Small arrows indicate each injection.

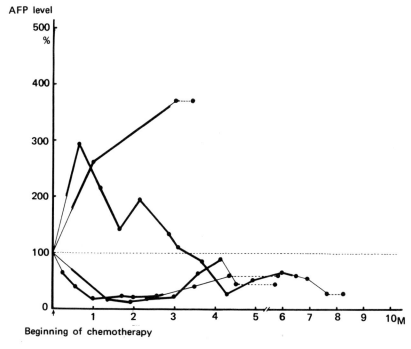

Figure 2 Serum AFP levels during chemotherapy given by hepatic arterial infusion. Thick lines indicate continuous infusion.

The effects of continuous infusion of 5-FU through an indwelling catheter are shown in Fig. 2. Alpha fetoprotein decreased in all three cases in whom tumor regressed, while it increased in another who failed to respond.

In general, there was a close correlation between the changes in serum AFP level and response in terms of tumor size. In some instances, however, serum AFP showed a paradoxical behavior after a prolonged period of chemotherapy; it increased despite tumor regression, or vice versa. The reason is unclear, but it may be that sensitivity of the tumor cells to the drug is altered during long-term therapy in such a way that AFP-producing cells remain sensitive whereas nonproducing cells become resistant or less sensitive. Patients with a low AFP-producing capacity or with serum levels below 400 ng/ml persistently showed low levels regardless of whether treated chemotherapeutically or palliatively.

Changes in blood chemistry or liver function tests were inconsistent and unpredictable. Mild elevation of serum bilirubin, by less than 2 mg/100ml, was noted shortly after chemotherapy in 2 patients (8.0%) out of 25 in the long survival group in whom no overt jaundice had been seen before treatment, and in 6 cases (42.9%) out of 14 in the short survival group. Aggravation of icterus occurred after treatment in 2 patients who had already had jaundice. Serum alkaline phosphatase activity was decreased in 20 (54.1%) of 37 cases with elevated activities before treatment, and in 13 (59.1%) of the 22 in whom tumor regressed. Response of SGOT varied considerably from case to case, displaying little correlation to the chemotherapeutic effect; it fell to normal in some, but it remained around the pretreatment level or was elevated significantly in others. In HCC, SGOT activity is almost invariably higher than SGPT (12, 14) and we have indirect evidence that SGOT is related to tumor growth as well as the state of non-

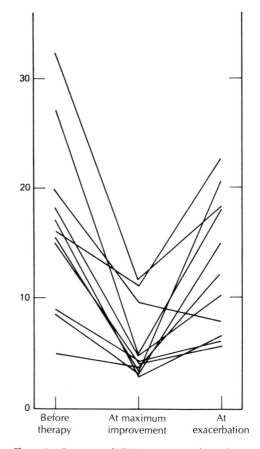

Figure 3   Response of LDH isozyme 5 to chemotherapy.

tumorous portion of the liver (15).

Serum lactic dehydrogenase levels were decreased in 11 (34.3%) of the 32 cases who had exhibited elevated activities at the start of therapy. Fig. 3 shows the response of isozyme 5 of this enzyme, which is usually higher than isozyme 4 in HCC; isozyme 4 is often higher than isozyme 5 in metastatic liver carcinoma as discussed in Chapter 17 by Okuda. There was a close correlation between chemotherapeutic effects and decrease in this isozyme level. Marked decrease was usually accompanied by noticeable clinical response, while reelevation occurring in three to five weeks heralded exacerbation.

Untoward Reactions

The toxic reactions to arterial chemotherapy were minimal in our series. Anorexia was the most common side effect of the one shot therapy, developing in 18 instances out of 56 shots given to 37 patients. Other reactions included nausea, general malaise, abdominal pain, stomatitis, glossitis, and low-grade fever which occurred in several cases. Toxicity was milder during the arterial infusion therapy.

Leukopenia is a common but temporary side effect of practically all anticancer agents. In our study the white cell count dropped below 2000/mm³ on nine occasions with 56 injections, and in one of the five cases given continuous infusion. As a consequence, two of these cases died from infections, one from pneumonia and another, septicemia.

The following two cases illustrate a typical response of the patient to chemotherapy.

CASE 1. R. T., a 68-year-old male, was first noted to have impairment of liver function when he had a gastrectomy in 1965 for a polyp. He was reoperated on in 1972 for recurrence, and liver function test results were again abnormal. He first noted epigastric discomfort in January 1973 and was hospitalized on April 16 because of upper abdominal pain and hepatomegaly. The liver was palpated four fingerbreadths below the right costal margin in the midclavicular line. Laboratory study included: alkaline phosphatase 65 u (K.A.), SGOT 83 u (Karmen), LDH 340 u (Isozyme 1, 40.6%; 2, 39.5%; 3, 12.3%; 4, 1.9%; 5, 5.8%), total bilirubin 1.75 mg/100 ml, total protein 7.0 g/100 ml, BSP test 10% at 45 minutes, and AFP 23,200 ng/ml. Diagnosis of HCC associated with cirrhosis was made from liver scan, laparoscopy, biopsy, and angiography. He had the one shot therapy eight times, the first dose being MCC alone, and a cocktail of 10 mg MMC, 500 mg Ex, and 500 mg 5-FU was given thereafter. Following the first several shots, severe pain subsided, the tumor regressed markedly with a concomitant decrease in serum alkaline phosphatase and AFP levels (Fig. 4). It is to be noted that AFP levels rose despite progressive reduction in tumor size after the fourth injection. Combination of agents was changed to 10 mg MMC, 500 mg EX, and 10 mg CA or MMC, CA, and MTX (100 mg) after the fourth shot, considering possible alterations in sensitivity of AFP-

producing and nonproducing cells. Unfortunately, pancytopenia developed after the eighth shot and he died of pneumonia. He lived 11.5 months. The therapeutic effect obtained in this patient is apparent from the celiac angiograms before and after treatment (Figs. 5 and 6).

CASE 2. H. N., a 53-year-old male, was first found to have a hepatomegaly in May 1972. On admission the liver edge was palpable two fingerbreadths below the right costal margin in the midclavicular line. Serum alkaline phosphatase activity was 28.3 u (K.A.), SGOT level 79 u (Karmen) SGPT 54 u (Karmen), LDH 395 u, total serum bilirubin level was 0.9 mg/100 ml, total serum protein 6.7 g/100 ml, BSP test showed 15.5% retention at 45 minutes, and AFP was 880 ng/ml.

A polyethylene catheter was placed in the right gastroepiploic artery and fixed on the abdominal wall at the time of laparotomy. Infusion chemotherapy was started with 200 mg of 5-FU per day. Alpha fetoprotein, which had been rising sharply, continued to rise at the start and reached a level of 12,500 ng/ml, but it soon dropped precipitously to 850 ng/ml with concomitant shrinkage of the liver (Fig. 7). During the course, three single doses of MMC were given additionally through the catheter. Leukocyte count was decreased to 2500/mm³ after 5 months of continuous infusion. Infection occurred at the site of catheterization, and he finally succumbed to septicemia. Autopsy revealed a large HCC in the middle portion of the liver with softening and necrotization of the interior, indicative of chemotherapeutic effect (Fig. 8). He had lived 12 months after diagnosis of HCC.

SELECTION OF PATIENTS

It is evident from the aforegoing discussion that selection of patients is critical in chemotherapy of primary liver cancer. If properly selected, not only alleviation of patients' complaints but also prolongation of life may be achieved. Chemotherapy can also aggravate the condition and shorten the life of patients. Separation of patients with anticipation of two opposite results may be possible by assessment of the severity of cirrhosis and of remaining liver function. Nakashima, Okuda, and their associates (16) have recently proposed a gross anatomical classification based on 112 necropsies with clinicopathological considerations. A highly atrophic liver containing

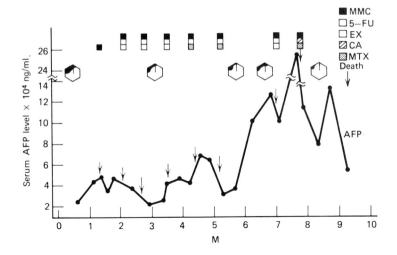

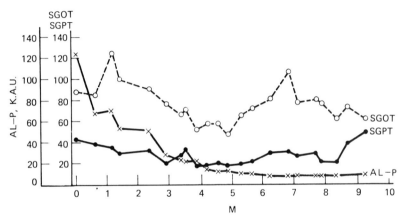

Figure 4 The course of Case 1, HCC with cirrhosis. Arrows in upper diagram indicate one shot injections into the hepatic artery.

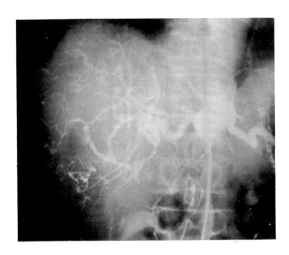

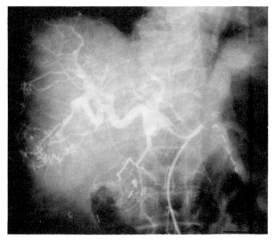

Figure 5 Celiac angiogram of Case 1, made at the first shot.

Figure 6 Celiac angiogram of Case 1, made at the fifth shot. Marked regression of the tumor is seen as compared with Fig. 5.

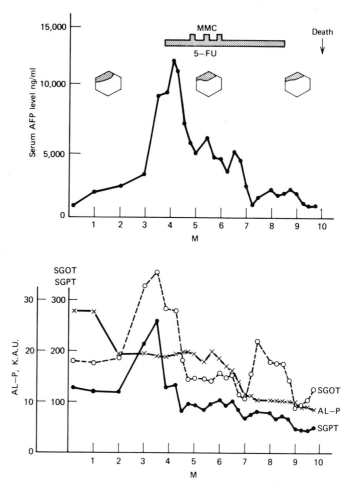

Figure 7 The course of Case 2, HCC with cirrhosis. Shaded bar shows continuous infusion of 5-FU combined with three single doses of MMC.

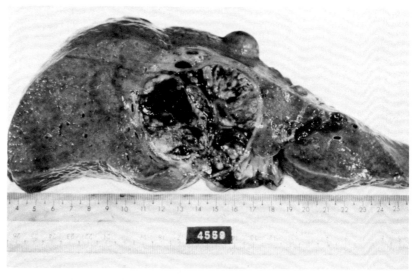

Figure 8 Cut surface of the liver of Case 2. A large tumor surrounded by a thick capsule is seen with softening and necrotization, indicative of chemotherapeutic effect.

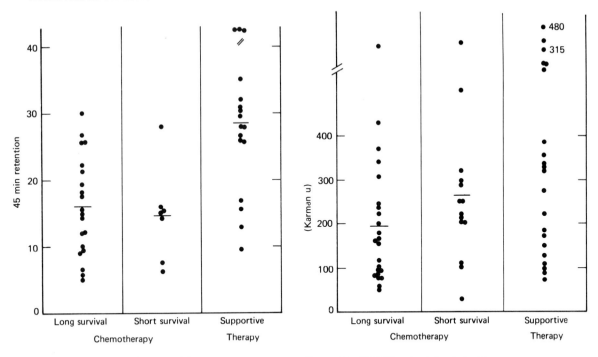

Figure 9 BSP test at the start of therapy.

Figure 10 SGOT levels at the start of therapy.

one or several small hepatoma nodules, which corresponds to Berman's "occult cancer" form (17) and to the "cirrhotic oligonodular" type by Nakashima-Okuda's classification (16), is hardly the object of chemotherapy. Such patients are indistinguishable from noncompensated cirrhosis in clinical manifestations and course, and will eventually succumb to hepatic failure rather than to tumor growth. Chemotherapy is indicated in patients who have a large tumor, a tumor growing rapidly in size, or a relatively small mass with a potential of rapid growth as suggested by rapidly increasing AFP levels. Association of mild cirrhosis does not restrict the use of chemotherapeutic agents as our statistics have indicated. Although Rochlin and Smart (18) set a line at 20% BSP retention and 100 u SGOT, above which no therapeutic effect could be expected, our results have suggested a less strict separat-

ing line; patients with BSP retention below 30% (Fig. 9) and SGOT below 200 Karmen u (Fig. 10) seem to have chances for good response. Total serum protein is seldom reduced in this disease and does not serve as an indicator for selection.

In our patients, serum AFP values at the time of diagnosis were scattered diversely in a range of 10 ng/ml to 1.8×10^6 ng/ml, and showed no correlation with the degree of involvement. Although it increased with tumor growth, the increment of AFP increase per arbitrary unit growth of tumor also varied from case to case. Therefore, the absolute value of AFP in a single determination is of little assistance in determining indication for chemotherapy.

Ascites, if controllable, does not necessarily contraindicate chemotherapy, because the liver is still in a compensated state. It depends more on the capacity of remaining liver function. Rochin et al advocated chemotherapy in patients with obstructive jaundice in the absence of parenchymal damage, since, in their experience, it had alleviated jaundice. According to Ariel et al (6), it is contraindicated in obstructive bile duct diseases when parenchymatous disfunction is apparent. Our experience has been in accord with theirs. Patients with overt jaundice usually have accompanying severe liver damage and a tendency to bleed.

Ariel et al (6) recommend scanning with ^{198}Au colloid and ^{131}I-rose bengal, the former serving to delineate the space occupying lesion and the latter to assess the function of liver parenchyma. They selected for chemotherapy the patients with good ^{131}I-rose bengal pick-up by the liver. When the effects of chemotherapy were analyzed in our series with respect to the locality of the tumor on ^{198}Au colloid scintigrams, it was found that the patients with the tumor in the right lobe and with high activities in the spleen, lived longer than those who had a mass in the middle or the left portion. Clinically, tumors occupying the right lobe cause less symptoms in general, and have ample arterial supply as studied angiographically; chemotherapy proves more effective in such patients.

Summarily stated, our current policy in the selection of patients for arterial chemotherapy are (1) patients with compensated liver function—BSP retention below 30% (at 45 minutes) and SGOT below 200 Karmen u—are candidates. Those with controllable ascites can be considered, if other conditions favor chemotherapy; (2) patients with advanced liver cirrhosis and/or with overt jaundice should not be considered for chemotherapy; (3) chemotherapy is not indicated in patients with widespread extrahepatic metastases.

Unfortunately, no information is as yet available as to what histological type of HCC is amenable to chemotherapy and what type is not. Neither do we know the exact prognosis in term of life span of individual gross anatomical type of this carcinoma.

ASSESSMENT OF THERAPEUTIC EFFECTS

Alleviation of subjective symptoms such as pain and sensation of abdominal fullness not only serves in assessing the effect but is also an aim of the treatment. Other indicators for the response include diminution of the size of the liver and of the tumor as estimated from the scan. Inasmuch as scanning and angiography can not so often be carried out, blood chemistry provides supplementary information—the levels of alkaline phosphatase, LDH, its isozyme 5, SGOT and AFP decline with effective therapy, and rerise with exacerbation. Of these, alkaline phosphatase, LDH isozyme 5, and AFP are the most reliable indications of exacerbation, and serve in deciding whether and when to give the next shot. It is to be remembered that, at times, alkaline phosphatase does not reflect regrowth of tumor once it has declined by therapy. According to Purves et al (19), the clinical improvement obtained by arterial chemotherapy was closely matched by a fall in serum AFP level; the majority of their treatment schedule, however, did not appear to affect the AFP level. Endo et al (20), Kuroyanagi (21), and Hasegawa et al (22) reported correlation between decline of AFP and the effects of arterial chemotherapy. Our results have showed likewise, and furthermore, that at times AFP levels no longer parallel the change of tumor size after prolonged chemotherapy. Beside reduction of AFP, chemotherapy brought about improvement of symptoms, diminution of tumor size, and lowering of alkaline phosphatase and LDH activities in the majority of the long surviving patients. It is a reasonable assumption that chemotherapy was in fact effective in prolonging life, although no definite conclusion is feasible in this regard when analyzed in individual cases.

Trials of systemic chemotherapy are rather few in the literature. Ramirez et al (23) reported on a patient who had lived 10 years with 5-FU treatment, and autopsy after death from heart failure disclosed no remaining tumor. Most other reports interpreted the results as negative in prolonging life. Since the first report by Sullivan et al (13) on intraarterial infusion chemotherapy in 1959, and subsequent similar studies by Byron et al (3) and Clarkson et al (24), this approach has met with some enthusiasm, although interpretation of the results is not entirely unequivocal. Rochlin and his associates (18) obtained regression of tumor by as much as 50% in size in 36% of 51 cases with liver carcinoma, mostly metastatic. They noted objectively some reponse in 2 or 4 patients with hepatoma. In the series of Provan et al (25), which consisted of 200 cases of liver carcinoma, there were 9 cases of HCC and improvement was noted in 6. According to El-Domeiri et al (26), who compared results obtained with systemic chemotherapy in 13 hepatoma patients and with hepatic artery infusion in 6, all of the former died in 12 months while two of the latter lived 2 and 3 years, respectively. Watkins et al (27) reported on significant prolongation of survival obtained in 5 cases with hepatoma after successful infusion treatment. In their series, the median survival was 22 months and the longest survival 32 months from onset of symptoms. Al-Sarraf et al (28), who strongly advocated infusion chemotherapy in hepatoma, observed that 18 cases of hepatoma lived only 11.1 weeks with systemic chemotherapy inducing tumor regression in none, and that tumor diminished in size in 56% of 16 cases with hepatoma by infusion therapy; the average survival time was 62.2 weeks in patients in whom tumor diminution was attained, and it was 5.5 weeks in whom no regression occurred. Based on these results, they considered hepatic artery infusion chemotherapy the treatment of choice when the tumor was unresectable. In our series, the patients classified in the long survival group lived an average of 10.4 months, 4 months longer than the overall survival time and 7 months longer compared with the short survival group. There were 4 cases that lived more than 1 year with the longest survival of 2 years and 4 months.

These results are of significance in view of the fact that the average survival of patients with HCC was only 4 months in Berman's series (29). Since the number of patients treated with hepatic artery infusion chemotherapy was small in our series, comparison of effect between the one shot and the infusion therapy is not feasible, but a statement may be warranted that arterial administration of anticancer agents is indicated in properly selected patients with hepatocellular carcinoma for alleviation of subjective symptoms, tumor regression, and prolongation of life.

REFERENCES

1. Bierman HR, Byron RL, Miller ER, et al: Effects of intraarterial administration of nitrogen mustard. *Am J Med* **8**:535, 1950.

2. Klopp JB, Berry N, Alford C, et al: Fractionated regional cancer chemotherapy. *Cancer Res* **10**:229, 1950.

3. Byron RL, Perez FM, Yonemoto RH, et al: Left brachial arterial catheterization for chemotherapy in advanced intra-abdominal malignant neoplasms. *Surg Gynec Obstet* **112**:689–696, 1961.

4. Wirtanen GW, Bernhardt LC, Mackman S, et al: Hepatic artery and celiac axis infusion for the treatment of upper abdominal malignant lesions. *Ann Surg* **168**:137–141, 1968.

5. Miller TR, Griman OR: Hepatic artery catheterization for liver perfusion. *Arch Surg* **82**:423–425, 1961.

6. Ariel IM, Pack GT: Intra-arterial chemotherapy for cancer metastatic to liver. *Arch Surg* **91**:851–862, 1965.

7. Simon N, Warner RRP, Baron MG, et al: Intra-arterial irradiation of carcinoid tumor of the liver. *Am J Roentgen* **102**:552–561, 1968.

8. Bierman HR, Byron RL, Kelley KH, et al: Studies on blood supply of tumors in man. III. vascular patterns of liver by hepatic arteriography in vivo. *J Natl Cancer Inst* **12**:107–131, 1951.

9. Nakashima T: Vascular changes and hemodynamics in hepatocellular carcinoma. In *Hepatocellular Carcinoma,* Okuda K, Peters RL (Eds). John Wiley, New York, 1976, pp. 169–203.

10. Seldinger SI: Catheter replacement of the needle in percutaneous arteriorgraphy. *Acta Radiol* **39**:368–376, 1964.

11. Brennan MJ, Talley RW, Drake EH, et al: 5-Fluorouracil treatment of liver metastases by continuous hepatic artery infusion via Cournand catheter. *Ann Surg* 158:405–419, 1963.

12. Okuda K: Clinical aspects of hepatocellular carcinoma. In *Hepatocellular Carcinoma,* Okuda K, Peters RL (Eds). John Wiley, New York, 1976, pp. 410–413.

13. Sullivan RD, Miller, E, Spikes RL: Antimetabolite-metabolite combination cancer chemotherapy. *Cancer* **12**:1248–1262, 1959.

14. Kay CJ: Primary hepatic cancer. *Arch Int Med* **113**:96–103, 1964.

15. Kubo Y, Okuda K: to be published.

16. Nakashima T, Kojiro M, Sakamoto K, et al: Studies of primary liver carcinoma. I Proposal of new gross anatomical classification of primary liver cell carcinoma. *Acta Hep Jap* **15**:279–291, 1974.

17. Berman C: *Primary Carcinoma of the Liver.* Lewis & Co., London, 1951, pp 31.

18. Rochlin DB, Smart CR: An evaluation of 51 patients with hepatic artery infusion. *Surg Gynecol Obstet* **123**:535–538, 1966.

19. Purves LR, Bersohn I, Geddes EW: Serum alpha- feto-protein and primary cancer of the liver in man. *Cancer* **25**:1261–1270, 1970.

20. Endo Y, Kanai K, Iino S, et al: Clinical significance of alpha-fetoprotein. In *Alpha-fetoportein and Hepatoma.* Hirai H, Miyaji T (Eds). University of Tokyo Press, Tokyo, 1973, pp 67–78.

21. Kuroyanagi Y: Results in the treatment of hepatocellular carcinoma. In *Alpha-fetoprotein and Hepatoma.* Hirai H, Miyaji T (Eds). University of Tokyo Press, Tokyo, 1973, pp 107–115.

22. Hasegawa H, Mukojima T, Hattori N, et al: Embryonal carcinoma and alpha-fetoprotein. In *Alpha-fetoprotein and Hepatoma.* Hirai H, Miyaji T (Eds). University of Tokyo Press, Tokyo, 1973, pp 129–139.

23. Ramirez G, Ansfield FJ, Curreri AR: Hepatoma: long term survival with disseminated tumor treated with 5-fluorouracil. *Am J Surg* **120**:400–403, 1970.

24. Clarkson B, Young C, Dierick W, et al: Effects of continuous hepatic artery infusion of antimetabolites on primary and metastatic cancer of the liver. *Cancer* **15**:472–488, 1962.

25. Provan JL, Stokes JF, Edward D: Hepatic artery infusion chemotherapy in hepatoma. *Brit Med J* **3**:346–349, 1968.

26. El-Domeiri AA, Huvos AG, Goldsmith HS, et al: Primary malignant tumors of the liver. *Cancer* **27**:7–11, 1971.

27. Watkins E Jr, Khazei AM, Nahra KS: Surgical basis for arterial infusion chemotherapy of disseminated carcinoma of the liver. *Surg Gynecol Obstet* **130**:581–605, 1970.

28. Al-Sarraf M, Go TS, Kithier K, et al: Primary liver cancer, a review of the clinical features, blood groups, serum enzymes, therapy and survival of 65 cases. *Cancer* **33**:574–582, 1974.

29. Berman C: *Primary Carcinoma of the Liver.* Lewis & Co., London, 1951, pp 46–48.

INDEX